Illustrated
Dental Embryology,
Histology, and Anatomy

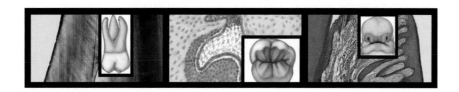

Illustrated
Dental Embryology, Histology, and Anatomy

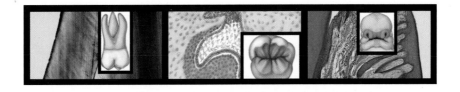

Third Edition

MARY BATH-BALOGH, BA, BS, MS

Instructor, Anatomy and Physiology, Department of Biology
Pierce College, Fort Steilacom
Lakewood, Washington

MARGARET J. FEHRENBACH, RDH, MS

Oral Biologist and Dental Hygienist
Adjunct Instructor, BASDH Degree Program, St. Petersburg College, St. Petersburg, FL
Educational Consultant and Dental Technical Writer, Seattle, Washington

ELSEVIER
SAUNDERS

3251 Riverport Lane
St. Louis, Missouri 63043

ILLUSTRATED DENTAL EMBRYOLOGY, HISTOLOGY, AND ANATOMY   ISBN: 978-1-4377-1730-3
Copyright © 2011, 2006, 1997 by Saunders, an imprint of Elsevier Inc.

Library of Congress Cataloging-in-Publication Data

Bath-Balogh, Mary.
    Illustrated dental embryology, histology, and anatomy / Mary
Bath-Balogh, Margaret J. Fehrenbach ; illustrated by Pat Thomas. -- 3rd ed.
        p. ; cm.
    Includes bibliographical references and index.
    ISBN 978-1-4377-1730-3 (pbk. : alk. paper)
    1. Mouth--Histology. 2. Teeth--Histology. 3. Mouth--Anatomy.
        4. Teeth--Anatomy. I. Fehrenbach, Margaret J. II. Title.
    [DNLM: 1. Tooth--anatomy & histology. 2. Tooth--embryology. 3.
Mouth--anatomy & histology. 4. Mouth--embryology. WC 585]
RK280.B27 2011
611'.31--dc22
                                                                        2010041710

Executive Editor: John Dolan
Managing Editor: Kristin Hebberd
Associate Developmental Editor: Joslyn Dumas
Publishing Services Manager: Julie Eddy
Senior Project Manager: Celeste Clingan
Design Direction: Kim Denando

Printed in the United States of America

Last digit is the print number: 9 8 7 6 5 4 3 2

PREFACE

OVERVIEW

This textbook provides an extensive background for dental professionals in the area of oral biology, as well as graduates of dental professional programs that need to take competency examinations or update their background knowledge in this area. It is divided into four units: Review of Dental Structures, Dental Embryology, Dental Histology, and Dental Anatomy. The textbook was organized into units to accommodate differing curriculum; thus, the units do not have to be presented in any specific order. However, the first chapter, Review of Dental Structures, serves as an outstanding review for the student before further study in oral biology presented in this textbook.

FEATURES

Each of the four units of this textbook consists of several chapters, with each chapter building on the preceding ones. Each chapter begins with an outline, objectives, and new key terms (with pronunciation guide); the terms listed are highlighted for the first time in that chapter. Terms used in other chapters are also bolded for increased emphasis of important concepts. The chapters contain both microscopic and clinical photographs as well as useful tables.

Within each chapter are discussions of clinical and developmental considerations in separate text boxes with identifying icons, which allow for an increased integration of the material into everyday practice for the dental professional. Within each chapter, there are cross-references to other figures or chapters so that the reader can review or investigate interrelated subjects. The content of this edition incorporates additional input from students and educators as well as the latest information from scientific studies and experts.

The textbook concludes with a bibliography, complete glossary of terms using short easy to remember phrases (with pronunciation guide), and appendices that contain a review of anatomical nomenclature, units of measurement, permanent tooth measurements, and developmental information.

The *Workbook for Illustrated Dental Embryology, Histology, and Anatomy* is available for student use. The workbook features activities such as structure identification exercises (both clinical and written), glossary exercises, tooth drawing exercises, infection control for extracted teeth, initial occlusal evaluation, and case studies as well as permanent dentition flash cards.

An Evolve site is also available for both students' and instructors' use. It features discussion questions, supplemental considerations, content updates, as well as PowerPoint programs related to the Workbook activities.

New this time is TEACH, an exciting coordinated effort between a Lesson Plan Manual for all topics covered and the textbook. It features online PowerPoint programs with enrichment exercises and other related materials. The Elsevier sales representative will be able to help introduce this new digital format.

This textbook is coordinated with the *Illustrated Anatomy of the Head and Neck* by Margaret J. Fehrenbach and Susan W. Herring, and as such can be considered a companion textbook to complete the curriculum in oral biology. Many of the figures are also presented in the *Dental Anatomy Coloring Book*, edited by Margaret J. Fehrenbach.

Mary Bath-Balogh
Margaret J. Fehrenbach

ACKNOWLEDGMENTS

We would like to thank Editors John Dolan, Kristin Hebberd, and Joslyn Dumas; Senior Project Manager Celeste Clingan; and the rest of the staff at Elsevier for making this textbook possible. In addition, we would like to thank Heidi Schlei, RDH, BS, Instructor, Waukesha County Technical College of Milwaukee, WI, for reviewing the textbook; Susan Herring, PhD, Professor of Orthodontics, School of Dentistry, University of Washington, of Seattle, WA, for reviewing the embryology unit; Patricia L. Toma, RDH, BS, of Houston, TX, for her clinical expertise.

Also used in the compilation of this text was material on orthodontic therapy from Dona M. Seely, DDS, MSD, Orthodontic Associates of Bellevue, WA. Kimberly K. Benkert, RDH, BSDH, MPH, COM, Midwest Orofacial Myology; MYO USA, Inc., of Countryside, IL, provided material on orofacial myology. Many of the elegant microscopic sections are from the Dr. Bernhard Gottlieb Collection, courtesy of James E. McIntosh, PhD, Professor Emeritus, Department of Biomedical Sciences, Baylor College of Dentistry, of Dallas, TX. Thanks to Pat Thomas, CMI for her contributions to the first edition art program. Her work has been truly beneficial to this text. Finally, we would like to thank our families, colleagues, and students.

Mary Bath-Balogh
Margaret J. Fehrenbach

CONTENTS

CHAPTER 1

Face and Neck Regions

●●● CHAPTER OUTLINE

Study of the face and neck
Regions of the face
   Frontal, orbital, and nasal regions
   Infraorbital and zygomatic regions
   Buccal region

Oral region
Mental region
Regions of the neck

●●● LEARNING OBJECTIVES

- Define and pronounce the key terms in this chapter.
- Locate and identify the regions and associated surface landmarks of the face and neck on a diagram and on a patient.

- Integrate the knowledge of surface anatomy of the face and neck into the clinical practice of patient examination and the understanding of the developmental and histological aspects of these regions.

●●● NEW KEY TERMS

Ala (**ah**-lah) (plural, alae [ah-**lay**])
Angle of the mandible (**man**-di-bl)
Articulating surface of the
   condyle (ar-**tik**-you-**late**-ing **kon**-dyl)
Coronoid (**kor**-ah-noid) **notch, process**
Golden Proportions
Hyoid bone (**hi**-oid)
Labial commissure (**lay**-be-al
   kom-i-shoor)
Larynx (**lare**-inks)
Lymph nodes (limf)
Mandible (**man**-di-bl)
Mandibular condyle (man-**dib**-you-lar
   kon-dyl), **notch, symphysis** (**sim**-fi-sis)

Muscle: masseter (**mass**-et-er),
   sternocleidomastoid (**stir**-no-klii-do-
   mass-toid)
Naris (**nay**-ris) (plural, nares [**nay**-rees])
Nasal (**nay**-zil) **region, septum** (**sep**-tum)
Nose: apex of the, external, root of the
Orbit (**or**-bit)
Parathyroid glands (par-ah-**thy**-roid)
Philtrum (**fil**-trum)
Ramus (**ray**-mus) (plural, **rami** [**rame**-
   eye])
Regions of the face, neck
Region: buccal (**buk**-al), **frontal** (**frun**-tal),
   infraorbital (in-frah-**or**-bit-al), **mental**
   (**men**-tal), **oral, orbital** (**or**-bit-al)

Salivary gland (**sal**-i-ver-ee):
   parotid (pah-**rot**-id), **sublingual**
   (sub-**ling**-gwal), **submandibular**
   (sub-man-**dib**-you-lar)
Temporomandibular joint (tem-poh-
   ro-man-**dib**-you-lar)
Thyroid cartilage (**thy**-roid **kar**-ti-lij),
   gland
Tubercle of the upper lip (**too**-ber-kl)
Vermilion border, zone (ver-**mil**-yon)
Vertical dimension of the face
Zygomatic arch (zy-go-**mat**-ik), **region**

STUDY OF THE FACE AND NECK

Dental professionals must be comfortably familiar with the surface anatomy of the face and neck as discussed in this introduction to Unit I. The superficial features of the face and neck provide essential landmarks for many of the deeper anatomical structures. Dental professionals need to review these underlying structures before continuing further in the study of dental embryology and histology as well as dental anatomy.

Examination of these accessible features, both by visualization and palpation, can give information about the health of deeper tissue.

Some degree of variation in surface features can be considered within a normal range. However, a change in a surface feature in a given person may signal a condition of clinical significance and must be noted in the patient record, as well as correctly followed up by the examining dental professional. Thus, it is not the variations among individuals that should be noted but the changes in a particular individual.

Some of these surface changes in the features of the face and neck may be due to underlying developmental disturbances. Knowledge of the surface features of the face and neck additionally helps dental professionals to understand the associated developmental pattern. Unit II describes the development of the face and neck and associated

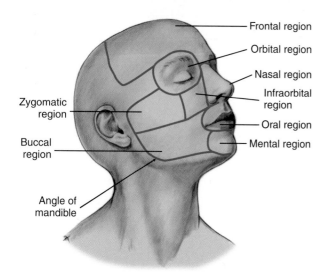

FIGURE 1-1 Regions of the face: frontal, orbital, infraorbital, nasal, zygomatic, buccal, oral, and mental. *(Adapted from Fehrenbach MJ, Herring SW: Illustrated Anatomy of the Head and Neck, ed 3, WB Saunders, Philadelphia, 2007.)*

developmental disturbances. However, other surface changes may be due to underlying associated histological tissue changes as noted in Unit III. This unit describes the histology of the face and neck, discussing what gives them many of their characteristic surface features.

REGIONS OF THE FACE

The study of the face and neck begins with the division of the surface into regions. Within each region are certain surface landmarks. It is important to practice finding these landmarks in each region using a mirror and this textbook, as well as the Workbook for Illustrated Dental Embryology, Histology, and Anatomy, for review in order to improve skills of examination. Later, locate them on peers and then on patients in a clinical setting.

The regions of the face include the frontal, orbital, nasal, infraorbital, zygomatic, buccal, oral, and mental (Figure 1-1). Lymph nodes are located in certain areas of the face and head and, when palpable, should be noted in the patient record (Figure 1-2, A and B, also see Figure 11-15).

In this textbook, the illustrations of the head and neck, as well as any structures associated with them, are oriented to show the patient's head in anatomical position, unless otherwise noted (see Appendix A). This is the same as if the patient is viewed straight on while sitting upright in the dental chair.

FRONTAL, ORBITAL, AND NASAL REGIONS

The frontal region of the face includes the forehead and the area above the eyes (Figure 1-3). In the orbital region of the face, the eyeball and all its supporting structures are contained in the bony socket or orbit.

The main feature of the nasal region of the face is the external nose (Figure 1-4). The root of the nose is located between the eyes, and the tip is the apex of the nose. Inferior to the apex on each side of the nose is a nostril, or naris (plural, nares). The nares are separated by the midline nasal septum. The nares are also bounded laterally by winglike cartilaginous structures, each ala (plural, alae) of the nose.

INFRAORBITAL AND ZYGOMATIC REGIONS

The infraorbital region of the face is located inferior to the orbital region and lateral to the nasal region (see Figure 1-3). Farther laterally is the zygomatic region, which overlies the bony support for the cheek, the zygomatic arch. The zygomatic arch extends from just below the lateral margin of the eye toward the middle part of the ear.

Inferior to the zygomatic arch and just anterior to the external ear is the temporomandibular joint (TMJ). This is where the upper skull forms a joint with the lower jaw (see Figure 19-1). The movements of the joint occur when a person opens and closes the mouth or moves the lower jaw to the right or left. One way to feel the lower jaw moving at the TMJ is to place a finger into the external ear canal.

BUCCAL REGION

The buccal region of the face is composed of the soft tissue of the cheek (see Figure 1-3). The cheek forms the side of the face and is a broad area of the face between the nose, mouth, and ear. Most of the upper cheek is fleshy, mainly formed by a mass of fat and muscles. One of these muscles forming the cheek is the strong masseter muscle, which is felt when a patient clenches the teeth together (see Figure 19-8, A). The sharp angle of the lower jaw inferior to the earlobe is termed the angle of the mandible.

The parotid salivary gland has a small part that can be palpated in the buccal region as well as in the zygomatic region (Figure 1-5, see Figure 11-7). Thus, the parotid is located irregularly from the zygomatic arch down to the posterior border of the lower jaw.

ORAL REGION

The oral region of the face has many structures within it, such as the lips and oral cavity (Figure 1-6, see Figures 2-4 and 2-5). The lips are fleshy folds that mark the gateway of the oral cavity proper. Each lip's vermilion zone has a darker appearance than the surrounding skin. The lips are outlined from the surrounding skin by a transition zone, the vermilion border.

On the midline of the upper lip, extending downward from the nasal septum, is a vertical groove, the philtrum. The philtrum terminates in a thicker area of the midline of the upper lip, the tubercle of the upper lip. The upper and lower lips meet at each corner of the mouth, or the labial commissure.

Clinical Considerations with the Lips

Any loss of the **vermilion border** is very important to note in the patient record. With this loss, it is hard to determine the border between the lips and the surrounding skin (Figure 1-7). This loss may be due to scar tissue from past traumatic incidents, developmental disturbances, or cellular changes in the tissue such as occur with solar damage. These changes may also represent a serious condition associated with cancer; however, this can be verified only with tissue biopsy. If loss is only due to solar damage, protection of the lips (especially the lower lip) with sunscreen is important because sun exposure increases the risk of cancerous changes (as with excessive alcohol consumption and smoking).

Loss of the vermilion border caused by a traumatic incident is important to note given that the rest of the oral cavity may be affected. If loss of the vermilion border is part of a history of a **cleft lip**; this also needs to be noted in the patient record because of its impact on dental treatment (see Figure 4-9).

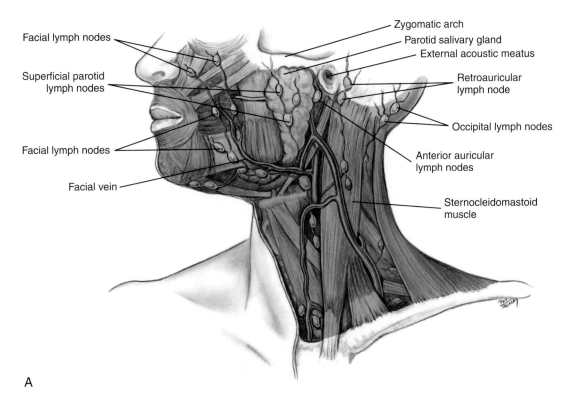

A

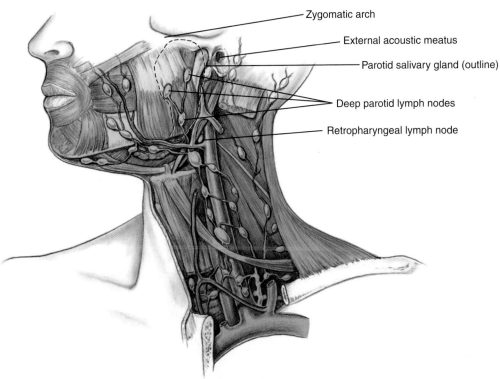

B

FIGURE 1-2 Lymph nodes of the head. **A:** Superficial nodes. **B:** Deep nodes. *(From Fehrenbach MJ, Herring SW: Illustrated Anatomy of the Head and Neck, ed 3, WB Saunders, Philadelphia, 2007.)*

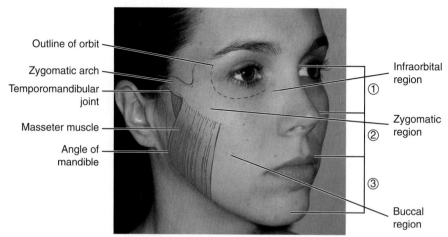

Outline of orbit
Zygomatic arch
Temporomandibular joint
Masseter muscle
Angle of mandible

Infraorbital region
①
Zygomatic region
②
③
Buccal region

FIGURE 1-3 Landmarks of the frontal, orbital, infraorbital, zygomatic, buccal, and mental regions noted. Also illustrated are the three divisions of the vertical dimension of the face. *(From Fehrenbach MJ, Herring SW: Illustrated Anatomy of the Head and Neck, ed 3, WB Saunders, Philadelphia, 2007.)*

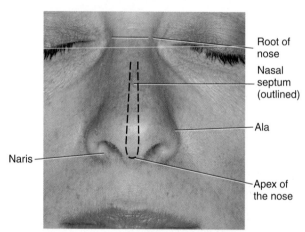

Root of nose
Nasal septum (outlined)
Ala
Naris
Apex of the nose

FIGURE 1-4 Landmarks of the nasal region noted, with the nasal septum highlighted (*dashed lines*). *(From Fehrenbach MJ, Herring SW: Illustrated Anatomy of the Head and Neck, ed 3, WB Saunders, Philadelphia, 2007.)*

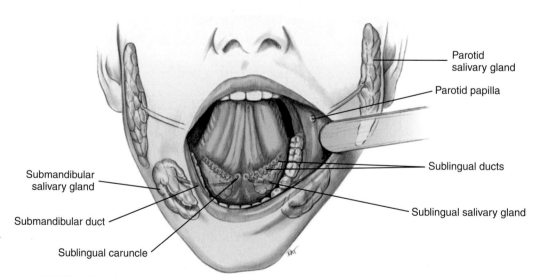

Parotid salivary gland
Parotid papilla
Sublingual ducts
Sublingual salivary gland
Submandibular salivary gland
Submandibular duct
Sublingual caruncle

FIGURE 1-5 Major salivary glands. *(From Fehrenbach MJ, Herring SW: Illustrated Anatomy of the Head and Neck, ed 3, WB Saunders, Philadelphia, 2007.)*

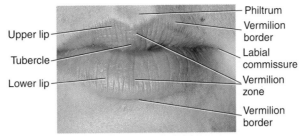

FIGURE 1-6 Lips with vermilion border. *(From Fehrenbach MJ, Herring SW:* Illustrated Anatomy of the Head and Neck, *ed 3, WB Saunders, Philadelphia, 2007.)*

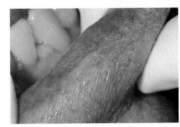

FIGURE 1-7 Loss of vermilion border on the lower lip due to solar damage.

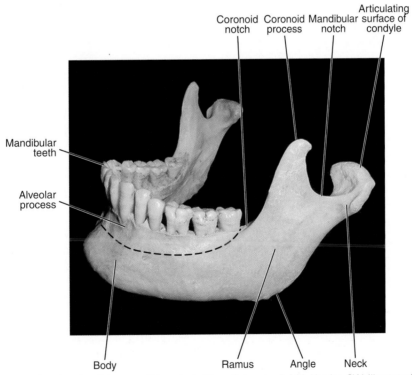

FIGURE 1-8 Landmarks of the mandible noted. *(From Fehrenbach MJ, Herring SW:* Illustrated Anatomy of the Head and Neck, *ed 3, WB Saunders, Philadelphia, 2007.)*

MENTAL REGION

The chin is the major feature of the **mental region** of the face. The bone underlying the mental region is the **mandible,** or lower jaw. The midline is marked by the **mandibular symphysis** (see Figure 4-5).

On the lateral aspect of the mandible, the stout, flat plate of the **ramus** (plural, **rami**) extends upward and backward from the body of the mandible on each side (Figures 1-8 and 1-9). At the anterior border of the ramus is a thin, sharp margin that terminates in the **coronoid process.** The main part of the anterior border of the ramus forms a concave forward curve, the **coronoid notch.**

The posterior border of the ramus is thickened and extends from the angle of the mandible to a projection, the **mandibular condyle**

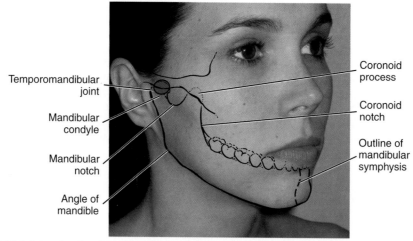

FIGURE 1-9 Landmarks of the mandible integrated with overlying facial features. *(From Fehrenbach MJ, Herring SW:* Illustrated Anatomy of the Head and Neck, *ed 3, WB Saunders, Philadelphia, 2007.)*

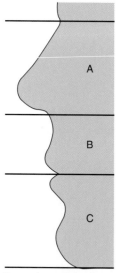

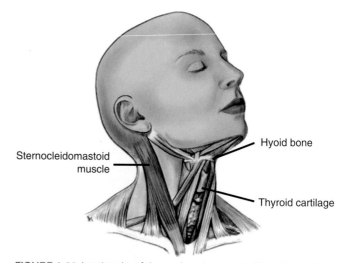

FIGURE 1-10 Golden Proportions of the face with its three divisions illustrating the esthetic considerations of vertical facial dimension: *nasal height* (**A**) is related to *maxillary height* (**B**) as 1.000:0.618; sum of nasal height and maxillary height (**A + B**) are related to *mandibular height* (**C**) as 1.618:1.000; mandibular height (**C**) is related to maxillary height (**B**) as 1.000:0.618; orofacial height (**B + C**) is related to nasal height (**A**) as 1.618:1.000. Note that each ratio is **1.618**, which is integral in these guidelines. These guidelines can also be used when considering the esthetics of a smile.

FIGURE 1-11 Landmarks of the neck region noted. *(From Fehrenbach MJ, Herring SW:* Illustrated Anatomy of the Head and Neck, *ed 3, WB Saunders, Philadelphia, 2007.)*

with its neck. The **articulating surface of the condyle** is an oval head involved in the TMJ (see Figure 19-6). Between the coronoid process and the condyle is a depression, the **mandibular notch**.

REGIONS OF THE NECK

The **regions of the neck** extend from the skull and lower jaw down to the clavicles and sternum (Figure 1-11). Lymph nodes are located in certain areas of the neck and, when palpable, should be recorded (Figure 1-12, *A* and *B*). The regions of the neck can be divided further into different cervical triangles using the large bones and muscles located in the area.

The large strap muscle, the **sternocleidomastoid muscle (SCM)**, is located on each side of the neck (see Figure 1-11) and is used for dividing the neck into further regions. At the anterior midline is the **hyoid bone**, which is suspended in the neck. Many muscles attach to the hyoid bone, which controls the position of the base of the tongue. Also found in the anterior midline, inferior to the hyoid bone, is the **thyroid cartilage**, which is the prominence of the "voice box," or

Clinical Considerations for Facial Dimensions

The face is sometimes thought of as divided into thirds (as are teeth), and this perspective is considered the **vertical dimension of the face** (see Figure 1-3). A discussion of vertical dimension allows a comparison of the three divisions of the face for functional and esthetic purposes using the **Golden Proportions**, a set of guidelines (Figure 1-10). Loss of height in the lower third, which contains the teeth and jaws, can occur in certain circumstances (see Figure 14-22).

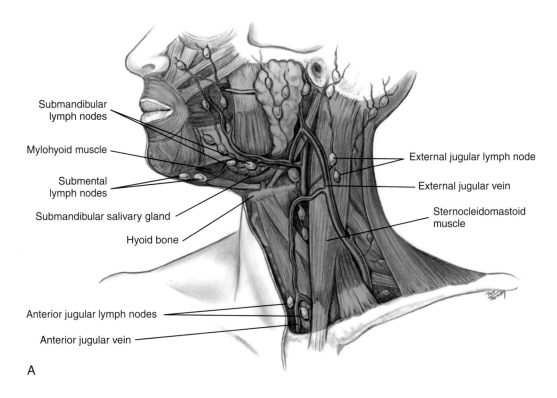

Submandibular lymph nodes

Mylohyoid muscle

Submental lymph nodes

Submandibular salivary gland

Hyoid bone

External jugular lymph node

External jugular vein

Sternocleidomastoid muscle

Anterior jugular lymph nodes

Anterior jugular vein

A

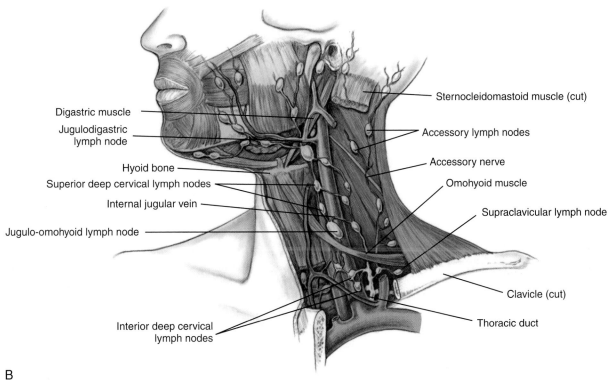

Digastric muscle

Jugulodigastric lymph node

Hyoid bone

Superior deep cervical lymph nodes

Internal jugular vein

Jugulo-omohyoid lymph node

Sternocleidomastoid muscle (cut)

Accessory lymph nodes

Accessory nerve

Omohyoid muscle

Supraclavicular lymph node

Clavicle (cut)

Thoracic duct

Interior deep cervical lymph nodes

B

FIGURE 1-12 Lymph nodes of the neck. **A:** Superficial cervical nodes. **B:** Deep cervical nodes. *(From Fehrenbach MJ, Herring SW: Illustrated Anatomy of the Head and Neck, ed 3. WB Saunders, Philadelphia, 2007.)*

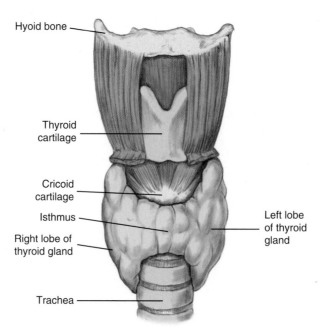

Hyoid bone

Thyroid cartilage

Cricoid cartilage

Isthmus

Left lobe of thyroid gland

Right lobe of thyroid gland

Trachea

FIGURE 1-13 Thyroid gland. *(From Fehrenbach MJ, Herring SW:* Illustrated Anatomy of the Head and Neck, *ed 3, WB Saunders, Philadelphia, 2007.)*

larynx. The vocal cords, or ligaments of the larynx, are attached to the posterior surface of the thyroid cartilage.

The thyroid gland, an endocrine gland, can also be palpated within the midline cervical area (Figure 1-13, see **Chapter 11**). Thus, the thyroid gland is located inferior to the thyroid cartilage, at the junction of the larynx and the trachea. The parathyroid glands are located close to or within the posterior aspect of the thyroid gland and cannot be palpated. The submandibular salivary gland and the sublingual salivary gland can also be palpated in the neck region (see Figures 1-5 and 11-7).

CHAPTER 2

Oral Cavity and Pharynx

●●●CHAPTER OUTLINE

Study of the oral cavity
Divisions of the oral cavity
   Oral vestibules
   Jaws, alveolar processes, and teeth
   Oral cavity proper

Divisions of the pharynx

●●●LEARNING OBJECTIVES

- Define and pronounce the key terms in this chapter.
- Locate and identify the divisions and associated surface landmarks of the oral cavity on a diagram and a patient.
- Outline the divisions of the pharynx.

- Integrate the knowledge of the oral cavity and pharynx into the clinical practice of patient care and later into the understanding of the developmental and histological aspects of this region.

●●●NEW KEY TERMS

Alveolar mucosa (al-**vee**-o-lar mu-**ko**-sah), **processes**
Alveolus (al-**vee**-oh-lus) (plural, **alveoli** [al-**vee**-oh-lie])
Anterior faucial pillar (**faw**-shawl), **teeth**
Arch(es): dental, mandibular (man-**dib**-you-lar), **maxillary** (**mak**-sil-lare-e)
Buccal (**buk**-al), **fat pad**
Canine eminence (**kay**-nine **em**-i-nins)
Canines (**kay**-nines)
Cementum (see-**men**-tum)
Crown
Dentin (**den**-tin)
Duct: parotid (pah-**rot**-id), **sublingual** (sub-**ling**-gwal), **submandibular** (sub-man-**dib**-you-lar)
Enamel (ih-**nam**-l)
Exostoses (eks-ox-**toe**-seez)
Facial (**fay**-shal)
Fauces (**faw**-seez)
Floor of the mouth
Foramen cecum (for-**ay**-men **se**-kum)
Fordyce's spots (for-**die**-seez)
Gingiva (**jin**-ji-vah): **attached, marginal**
Gingival sulcus (**jin**-ji-val **sul**-kus)
Incisors (in-**sigh**-zers)
Labial (**lay**-be-al), **frenum** (**free**-num) (plural, **frena** [**free**-nah])

Laryngopharynx (lah-**ring**-gah-**fare**-inks)
Linea alba (**lin**-ee-ah **al**-bah)
Lingual (**ling**-gwal), **frenum** (**free**-num), **papillae** (pah-**pil**-ay), **tonsil** (**ton**-sil)
Lingual papillae (pah-**pil**-ay): **circumvallate** (serk-um-**val**-ate), **filiform** (**fil**-i-form), **foliate** (**fo**-le-ate), **fungiform** (**fun**-ji-form)
Mandible (**man**-di-bl): **body of the**
Mandibular teeth (man-**dib**-you-lar), **torus** (**tore**-us) (plural, **tori** [**tore**-eye])
Mastication (mass-ti-**kay**-shin)
Maxilla (mak-**sil**-ah): **body of the**
Maxillary (**mak**-si-lare-ee) **sinuses** (**sy**-nuses), **teeth, tuberosity** (too-beh-**ros**-i-tee)
Median lingual sulcus (**lay**-be-al **sul**-kus), **palatine raphe** (**pal**-ah-tine **ra**-fe)
Melanin pigmentation (**mel**-a-nin)
Molars (**mo**-lerz)
Mucobuccal fold (mu-ko-**buk**-al)
Mucogingival junction (mu-ko-**jin**-ji-val)
Mucosa (mu-**ko**-sah): **buccal** (**buk** al), **labial** (**lay**-be-al), **oral**
Nasopharynx (nay-zo-**fare**-inks)
Oral cavity proper
Oropharynx (or-o-**fare**-inks)
Palatal (**pal**-ah-tal), **torus** (**tore**-us)

Palate (**pal**-it): **hard, soft**
Palatine (**pal**-ah-tine) **tonsils** (**ton**-sils), **rugae** (**ru**-ge)
Papilla (pah-**pil**-ah) (plural, **papillae** [pah-**pil**-ay]): **incisive** (in-**sy**-ziv), **interdental** (in-ter-**den**-tal), **parotid** (pah-**rot**-id)
Periodontal ligament (pare-ee-o-**don**-tl)
Plica fimbriata (**pli**-kah fim-bree-**ay**-tah) (plural, **plicae fimbriatae** [**pli**-kay fim-bree-**ay**-tay])
Posterior teeth, faucial pillar (**faw**-shawl)
Premolars (pre-**mo**-lerz)
Pterygomandibular fold (**teh**-ri-go-man-**dib**-yule-lar)
Pulp
Retromolar pad (re-tro-**mo**-ler)
Root(s)
Sublingual fold (sub-**ling**-gwal), **caruncle** (**kar**-unk-kl)
Sulcus terminalis (**sul**-kus **ter**-mi-nal-is)
Taste buds
Teeth permanent, primary
Tongue apex of the, base of the, body of the, dorsal surface of, lateral surface of, ventral surface of
Uvula (**u**-vu-lah)
Vestibular fornix (ves-**tib**-u-lar **fore**-niks)
Vestibules (**ves**-ti-bules)

STUDY OF THE ORAL CAVITY

A dental professional must be totally committed to improving the oral health for every patient. In order to accomplish this, dental professionals must be particularly knowledgeable about their main area of focus, the oral cavity and the adjacent throat or pharynx. To visualize this area of focus successfully, it is important to know the boundaries, terminology, and divisions of the oral cavity and the pharynx as discussed in this second chapter of Unit I. Later, Unit II describes the development of oral tissue and associated developmental disturbances. Following that, Unit III describes the underlying histology of orofacial tissue that gives them many characteristic surface features.

Some degree of variation in the oral cavity and visible divisions of the pharynx can be considered within a normal range. However, a change in any tissue in a given person may signal a condition of clinical significance and must be noted in the patient record, as well as correctly followed-up by the examining dental professional. Thus, it is not the variations among individuals that should be noted but the changes in a particular individual.

DIVISIONS OF THE ORAL CAVITY

The oral cavity is divided into the vestibules, jaws and alveolar processes, teeth, and oral cavity proper. Within each part of the oral cavity are certain surface landmarks. It is important to practice finding these surface landmarks in the oral cavity using a mirror and this textbook, as well as the Workbook for Illustrated Dental Embryology, Histology, and Anatomy, for review in order to improve skills of examination. Later, locate them on peers and then on patients in a clinical setting.

An understanding of the divisions of the oral cavity is aided by knowing its boundaries; many structures of the face and oral cavity mark the boundaries of the oral cavity (Figure 2-1). The lips of the face mark the anterior boundary of the oral cavity, and the pharynx or throat is the posterior boundary. The cheeks of the face mark the lateral boundaries, and the palate marks the superior boundary. The floor of the mouth is the inferior border of the oral cavity.

Many oral structures are identified with orientational terms based on their relationship to other orofacial structures, such as the facial surface, lips, cheek, tongue, and palate (see Figure 2-1). Those structures closest to the facial surface are facial. Those facial structures closest to the lips are labial. Those facial structures close to the inner cheek are buccal. Those structures closest to the tongue are lingual. Those lingual structures closest to the palate are palatal.

ORAL VESTIBULES

The upper and lower horseshoe-shaped spaces in the oral cavity between the lips and cheeks anteriorly and laterally and the teeth and their soft tissue medially and posteriorly are considered the maxillary and mandibular vestibules (Figure 2-2). These oral vestibules are lined by a mucous membrane, or oral mucosa. The inner parts of the lips are lined by a pink labial mucosa. The labial mucosa is continuous with the equally pink buccal mucosa that lines the inner cheek. Both the labial and buccal mucosa may vary in coloration, as do other regions of the oral mucosa, in individuals with pigmented skin (see Figure 9-22).

The buccal mucosa covers a dense pad of underlying fat tissue at the posterior part of each vestibule, the buccal fat pad. The buccal fat pad acts as a protective cushion during mastication, or chewing. On the inner part of the buccal mucosa, just opposite the maxillary second molar, is a small elevation of tissue is the parotid papilla. The parotid

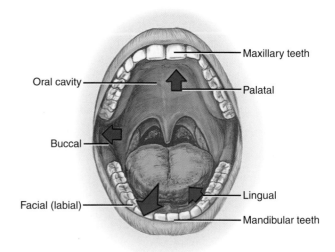

FIGURE 2-1 Oral cavity and the jaws with the designation (*arrows*) of the orientational terms *facial, labial, buccal, palatal,* and *lingual. (From Fehrenbach MJ, Herring SW: Illustrated Anatomy of the Head and Neck, ed 3, WB Saunders, Philadelphia, 2007.)*

papilla protects the opening of the parotid duct (or Stenson's duct) of the **parotid salivary gland** (see Figures 1-5 and 11-7).

Deep within each vestibule is the vestibular fornix, where the pink labial mucosa or buccal mucosa meets the redder alveolar mucosa at the mucobuccal fold. The labial frenum (plural, frena) is a fold of tissue located at the midline between the labial mucosa and the alveolar mucosa on the upper and lower dental arches.

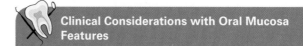

Clinical Considerations with Oral Mucosa Features

Commonly noted on the surface of the labial and buccal mucosa is a normal variation, **Fordyce's spots** (or granules) (Figure 2-3, *A*). These are visible as small, yellowish elevations on the mucosa and are deeper deposits of sebum from trapped or misplaced sebaceous gland tissue, usually associated with hair follicles. Most of the population has these harmless small bumps, however they are more prominent with age due to thinning of the overlying tissue.

Another normal variation noted on the buccal mucosa is the **linea alba** (Figure 2-3, *B*). This is a white ridge of calloused tissue (or hyperkeratinization) that extends horizontally at the level where the maxillary and mandibular teeth come together and occlude; similar ridges of white tissue can sometimes be noted on the tongue perimeter. An additional amount in either surface can be noted with certain oral **parafunctional habits** (see Figure 9-6).

JAWS, ALVEOLAR PROCESSES, AND TEETH

The jaws are deep to the lips and within the oral cavity (Figure 2-4). Underlying the upper lip is the upper jaw, or maxilla. The bone underlying the lower lip is the lower jaw, or mandible.

The maxilla consists of two maxillary bones that are sutured together during development. The maxilla has a nonmovable articulation with many facial and skull bones, and each maxillary bone includes a body and four processes. Each body of the maxilla is superior to the teeth

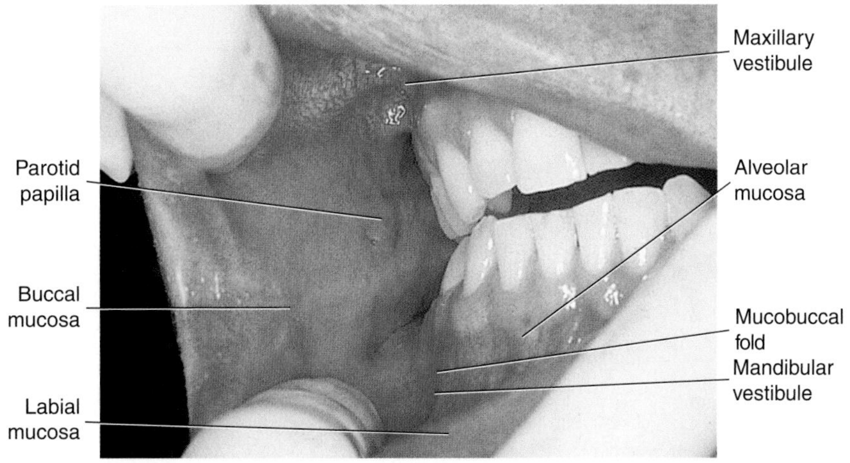

Parotid
papilla

Buccal
mucosa

Labial
mucosa

Maxillary
vestibule

Alveolar
mucosa

Mucobuccal
fold

Mandibular
vestibule

FIGURE 2-2 Vestibules of the oral cavity with landmarks noted. *(From Fehrenbach MJ, Herring SW: Illustrated Anatomy of the Head and Neck, ed 3, WB Saunders, Philadelphia, 2007.)*

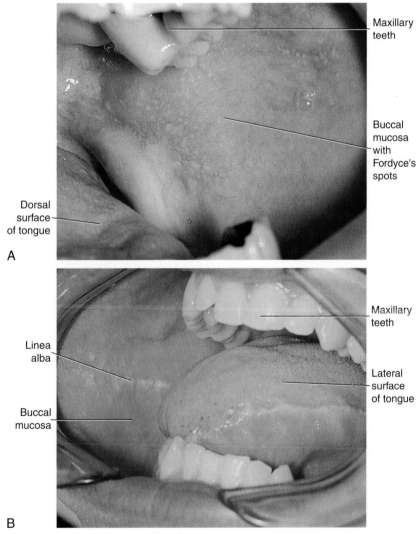

Maxillary
teeth

Buccal
mucosa
with
Fordyce's
spots

Dorsal
surface
of tongue

A

Linea
alba

Buccal
mucosa

Maxillary
teeth

Lateral
surface
of tongue

B

FIGURE 2-3 Buccal and labial mucosa of the oral cavity with normal variations. **A:** Fordyce's visible as small, yellowish elevations. **B:** Linea alba is a white ridge of calloused tissue (or hyperkeratinization) that extends horizontally at the level where the teeth occlude, with a similar white ridge possible on the lateral surface of the tongue.

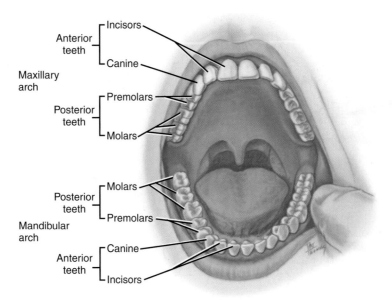

FIGURE 2-4 Diagram of the dental arches and permanent teeth with landmarks noted.

and contains the maxillary sinus. In contrast, the mandible is a single bone with a movable articulation with the temporal bones at each temporomandibular joint. The heavy horizontal part of the lower jaw inferior to the teeth is the body of the mandible.

The alveolar processes, or alveolar bones, are the bony extensions of the maxilla and mandible that contain each tooth socket or alveolus (plural, alveoli) of the teeth (see Figures 2-4 and 2-5). The facial part of the alveolus of the canine, the vertically placed canine eminence, is especially prominent on the maxilla. All the teeth are attached to the bony surface of the alveoli by the fibrous periodontal ligament (PDL), which allows some slight tooth movement within the alveolus while supporting the tooth.

Each of the mature and fully erupted teeth consists of both the crown and the root(s) (see Figures 2-5 and 2-6). The crown of the tooth is composed of the extremely hard outer enamel layer and the moderately hard inner dentin layer overlying the pulp of the tooth. The pulp is the soft innermost layer in the tooth. The moderately hard dentin continues to cover the soft tissue of the pulp of the tooth in the root(s), but the outermost layer of the root(s) is composed of cementum. The bonelike cementum is the part of the tooth that attaches to the periodontal ligament, which then attaches to the alveoli of bone, holding the tooth in its socket.

DENTAL ARCHES

The alveolar processes with the teeth in the alveoli are also called dental arches, the maxillary arch and mandibular arch (see Figure 2-4). The teeth in the maxillary arch are the maxillary teeth, and the teeth in the mandibular arch are the mandibular teeth.

Just distal to the last tooth of the maxillary arch is a tissue-covered elevation of the bone, the maxillary tuberosity. Similarly, on the lower jaw is a dense pad of tissue located just distal to the last tooth of the mandibular arch, the retromolar pad. The tooth types in both arches of the teeth of children, or primary teeth, include incisors, canines, and molars. Adult teeth, or permanent teeth, also include all the same teeth as the primary teeth, as well as premolars. The teeth in the front of the mouth, the incisors and canines, are considered anterior teeth. The teeth located toward the back of the mouth, molars and premolars, if present, are considered posterior teeth. The

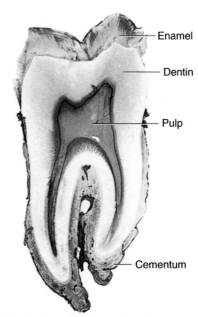

FIGURE 2-5 The distribution of the various tissue types of the tooth. *(From Nanci A: Ten Cate's Oral Histology, ed 7, Mosby, St Louis, 2008.)*

anterior maxillary teeth are supplied by the anterior superior alveolar artery and the maxillary posterior teeth by the posterior superior alveolar artery. The mandibular teeth are supplied by branches of the inferior alveolar artery. The maxillary teeth are drained by the posterior superior alveolar vein and mandibular teeth by the inferior alveolar vein. Later Unit IV discusses the dental anatomy of each tooth of the dentitions, primary and permanent.

GINGIVAL TISSUE

Surrounding the maxillary and mandibular teeth in the alveoli and covering the alveolar processes are the soft tissue gums, or gingiva (or more accurately, but not commonly by the dental community, *gingivae*), composed of a firm pink mucosa (Figure 2-9). The gingival

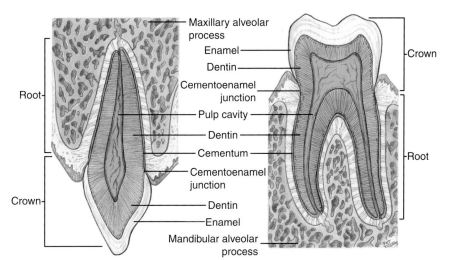

FIGURE 2-6 Diagram of an alveolar process of a single rooted tooth and a multirooted tooth showing the crown and root as well as associated tissue types.

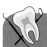

Clinical Considerations with Alveolar Process Features

A normal variation noted usually on the facial surface of the alveolar process of the maxillary arch is **exostoses,** which are localized developmental growths of normal bone with a possible hereditary etiology, and which may be associated with **occlusal trauma** (Figure 2-7, see **Chapter 20**). They may be single, multiple, unilateral, or bilateral raised hard areas, usually in the premolar to molar region and are covered by normal oral tissue, appearing radiographically as radiopaque (light) areas. They may interfere with radiographic analysis, as well as restorative and periodontal therapy, and thus must be noted in the patient record.

Another similar normal variation noted on the lingual aspect of the mandibular arch is the **mandibular torus** (plural, **tori**) (Figure 2-8). Each one is a larger developmental growth of normal bone with a possible hereditary etiology, similar to exostoses, and may also be associated with **bruxism** (grinding). They are usually present bilaterally in the area of the premolars and can present surface clefting, appear lobulated or nodular, or even contact over the midline.

Mandibular tori are covered in normal oral tissue and vary in size. They are slow-growing and asymptomatic and also may be seen on radiographs as radiopaque (light) masses. They may interfere with speech, oral hygiene procedures, radiographic film placement and analysis, as well as prosthesis therapy. The patient may require reassurance, and they must be noted in the patient record.

tissue that tightly adheres to the bone around the roots of the teeth is the **attached gingiva**. The attached gingiva may have areas of **melanin pigmentation** (see Figure 9-22). The line of demarcation between the firmer and pinker attached gingiva and the movable and redder alveolar mucosa is the scallop-shaped **mucogingival junction.**

At the gingival margin of each tooth is the **marginal gingiva** (or free gingiva), which forms a cuff above the neck of the tooth (Figure 2-10). The inner surface of the gingival tissue with each tooth faces a space, the **gingival sulcus**. The gingival tissue between adjacent teeth is an extension of attached gingiva and is considered the *interdental gingiva*, with each extension being an **interdental papilla.**

ORAL CAVITY PROPER

The inside of the mouth is known as the **oral cavity proper** (Figure 2-11). This space is enclosed anteriorly by the maxillary and mandibular arches. Posteriorly, the opening from the oral cavity proper into the pharynx or throat is the **fauces.**

The fauces are formed laterally on each side by the **anterior faucial pillar** and the **posterior faucial pillar**. The **palatine tonsils** are located between these folds of tissue created by underlying muscles and are what patients call their "tonsils," which can become enlarged (see Figure 11-17). Included within the oral cavity proper are the palate, tongue, and floor of the mouth.

PALATE

Within the oral cavity proper is the roof of the mouth or **palate**. The palate separates the oral cavity from the nasal cavity. The palate has two parts: anterior and posterior (Figure 2-12, see Figure 5-6). The firmer anterior part is considered the **hard palate.**

A midline ridge of tissue on the hard palate is the **median palatine raphe,** which overlies the bony fusion of the palate. A small bulge of tissue at the most anterior part of the hard palate, lingual to the anterior teeth, is the **incisive papilla**. Directly posterior to this papilla are **palatine rugae,** which are firm, irregular ridges of tissue radiating from the incisive papilla and raphe.

The looser posterior part of the palate is considered the **soft palate** (see Figure 2-11). A midline muscular structure, the **uvula** of the palate, hangs down from the posterior margin of the soft palate. The **pterygomandibular fold** extends from the junction of hard and soft

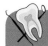

Clinical Considerations with the Palatal Features

A normal variation noted on the midline of the hard palate is the **palatal torus,** similar to the mandibular torus in both etiology and histology (Figure 2-13). It only interferes when prosthesis therapy is considered. However, it needs to be noted in the patient record and patients may need to be reassured. More serious changes in palate such as a history of **cleft palate** need to also be recorded because of its impact on dental treatment (see Figure 5-7).

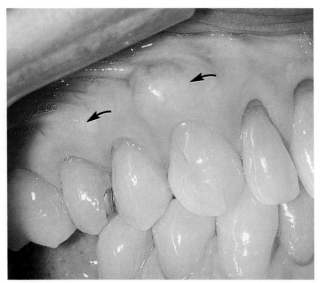

FIGURE 2-7 Normal variation of exostoses (*arrows*) on the facial surface of the maxilla.

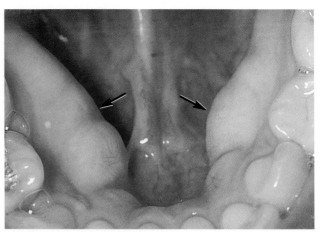

FIGURE 2-8 Normal variation of bilateral mandibular tori (*arrows*) on the lingual surface of the mandible.

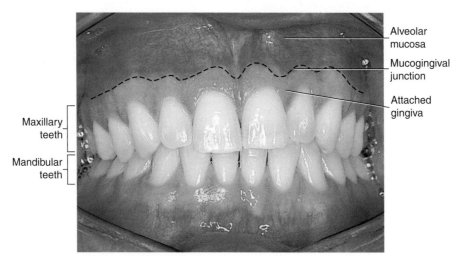

Alveolar mucosa

Mucogingival junction

Attached gingiva

Maxillary teeth

Mandibular teeth

FIGURE 2-9 Gingival tissue with landmarks noted on one arch, with the mucogingival junction highlighted (*dashed line*). (*From Fehrenbach MJ, Herring SW:* Illustrated Anatomy of the Head and Neck, *ed 3, WB Saunders, Philadelphia, 2007.*)

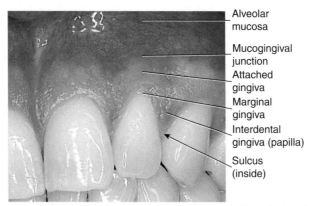

Alveolar mucosa

Mucogingival junction

Attached gingiva

Marginal gingiva

Interdental gingiva (papilla)

Sulcus (inside)

FIGURE 2-10 Close-up of the gingival tissue with landmarks noted. Note the location of the gingival sulcus (*arrow*). (*From Fehrenbach MJ, Herring SW:* Illustrated Anatomy of the Head and Neck, *ed 3, WB Saunders, Philadelphia, 2007.*)

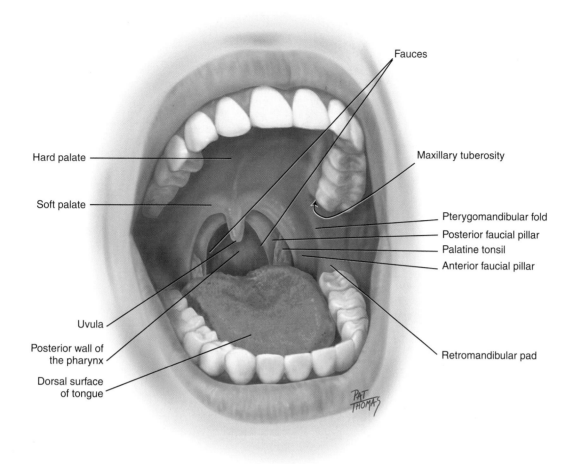

Fauces

Maxillary tuberosity

Pterygomandibular fold

Posterior faucial pillar

Palatine tonsil

Anterior faucial pillar

Retromandibular pad

Hard palate

Soft palate

Uvula

Posterior wall of the pharynx

Dorsal surface of tongue

PAT THOMAS

FIGURE 2-11 Oral cavity proper and the landmarks that form boundaries. *(From Fehrenbach MJ, Herring SW:* Illustrated Anatomy of the Head and Neck, *ed 3, WB Saunders, Philadelphia, 2007.)*

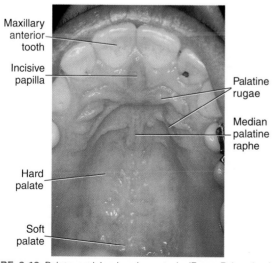

Maxillary anterior tooth

Incisive papilla

Palatine rugae

Median palatine raphe

Hard palate

Soft palate

FIGURE 2-12 Palate and landmarks noted. *(From Fehrenbach MJ, Herring SW:* Illustrated Anatomy of the Head and Neck, *ed 3, WB Saunders, Philadelphia, 2007.)*

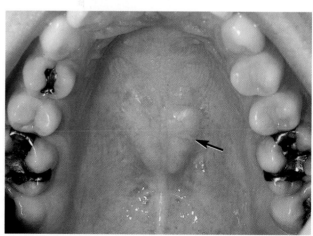

FIGURE 2-13 Normal variation of the palatal torus (*arrow*) on the midline of the hard palate.

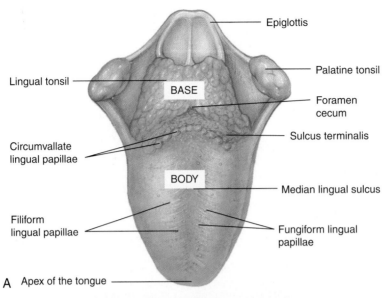

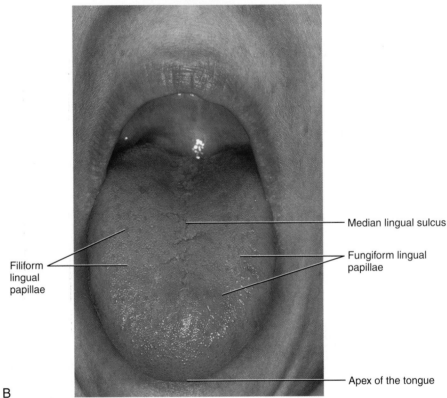

FIGURE 2-14 Dorsal surface of the tongue with landmarks, **A** and **B**. *(From Fehrenbach MJ, Herring SW: Illustrated Anatomy of the Head and Neck, ed 3, WB Saunders, Philadelphia, 2007.)*

palates down to the mandible, just behind the most distal mandibular tooth, and stretches when the mouth is opened wider. This fold covers a deeper fibrous structure and separates the cheek from the throat.

TONGUE

The **tongue** is a prominent feature of the oral cavity proper (Figure 2-14). The posterior one third is the pharyngeal part of the tongue, or **base of the tongue.** The base of the tongue attaches to the floor of the mouth. The base of the tongue does not lie within the oral cavity proper but within the oral part of the throat (discussed later). The anterior

two thirds of the tongue is the **body of the tongue,** which lies within the oral cavity proper. The tip of the tongue is the **apex of the tongue.**

The top, or **dorsal surface of the tongue,** has a midline depression—the **median lingual sulcus**—corresponding to the position of a midline fibrous structure deeper in the tongue and fusion tissue area. Certain surfaces of the tongue have small, elevated structures of **specialized mucosa,** the **lingual papillae,** some of which are associated with **taste buds** (see Figures 9-15 to 9-19). Taste buds are the specialized organs of taste.

The slender, threadlike, whitish lingual papillae are the **filiform lingual papillae,** which give the dorsal surface its velvety texture. The

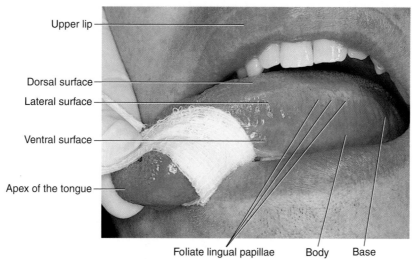

FIGURE 2-15 Lateral surface of the tongue with landmarks noted. *(From Fehrenbach MJ, Herring SW: Illustrated Anatomy of the Head and Neck, ed 3, WB Saunders, Philadelphia, 2007.)*

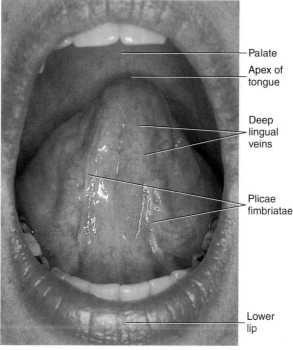

FIGURE 2-16 Ventral surface of the tongue with landmarks noted. *(From Fehrenbach MJ, Herring SW: Illustrated Anatomy of the Head and Neck, ed 3, WB Saunders, Philadelphia, 2007.)*

reddish, smaller mushroom-shaped dots on the dorsal surface are the fungiform lingual papillae. Farther posteriorly on the dorsal surface of the tongue, and more difficult to see clinically, is an inverted V-shaped groove, the sulcus terminalis. The sulcus terminalis separates the base from the body of the tongue, demarcating a line of fusion of tissue during the tongue's development.

The 10 to 14 larger mushroom-shaped lingual papillae, the circumvallate lingual papillae, line up along the anterior side of the sulcus terminalis on the body. Where the sulcus terminalis points backward toward the throat is a small, pitlike depression, the foramen cecum. Even farther posteriorly on the dorsal surface of the base of the tongue is an irregular mass of tissue, the lingual tonsil (see **Chapter 11**).

The side or lateral surface of the tongue has vertical ridges, the foliate lingual papillae (Figure 2-15).

The underside, or ventral surface of the tongue, has large visible blood vessels, the deep lingual veins, which pass close to the surface (Figure 2-16). Lateral to each deep lingual vein is the plica fimbriata (plural, plicae fimbriatae) with fringelike projections.

FLOOR OF THE MOUTH

The floor of the mouth is located in the oral cavity proper, inferior to the ventral surface of the tongue (Figure 2-17). The lingual frenum is a midline fold of tissue between the ventral surface of the tongue and the floor of the mouth.

A ridge of tissue on each side of the floor of the mouth, the sublingual fold, joins in a V-shaped configuration extending from the lingual frenum to the base of the tongue. The sublingual folds contain

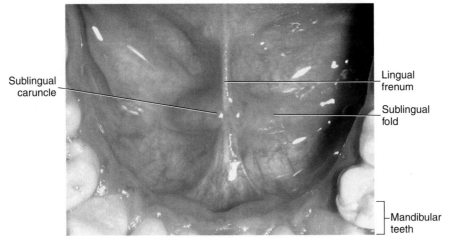

FIGURE 2-17 Floor of the mouth with landmarks noted. *(From Fehrenbach MJ, Herring SW:* Illustrated Anatomy of the Head and Neck, *ed 3, WB Saunders, Philadelphia, 2007.)*

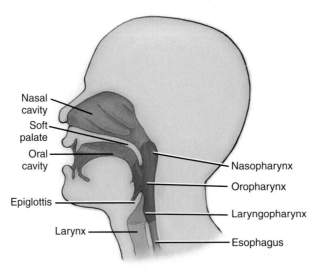

FIGURE 2-18 Midsagittal section of the head with the divisions of the pharynx and associated regions noted. *(From Fehrenbach MJ, Herring SW:* Illustrated Anatomy of the Head and Neck, *ed 3, WB Saunders, Philadelphia, 2007.)*

openings of the sublingual duct from the **sublingual salivary gland** (see Figures 1-5 and 11-7). The small papilla, or sublingual caruncle, at the anterior end of each sublingual fold contains openings of the submandibular duct and sublingual duct (or Wharton's duct and Bartholin's duct, respectively) from both the sublingual as well as the **submandibular salivary gland.**

DIVISIONS OF THE PHARYNX

The oral cavity proper provides the entrance into the throat, or pharynx. The pharynx is a muscular tube that serves both the respiratory and digestive systems. It has three divisions: nasopharynx, oropharynx, and laryngopharynx (Figure 2-18).

The division of the pharynx that is superior to the level of the soft palate is the nasopharynx, which is continuous with the nasal cavity. The division that is between the soft palate and the opening of the larynx is the oropharynx, which is the oral part of the pharynx. The fauces, discussed earlier, marks the boundary between the oropharynx and the oral cavity proper. Only part of the nasopharynx and oropharynx may be visible on an intraoral examination by a dental professional (see Figure 2-11). The laryngopharynx is a more inferior division, close to the laryngeal opening, and thus is not visible on an intraoral examination.

CHAPTER 3

Overview of Prenatal Development

●●●CHAPTER OUTLINE

Prenatal development
  Overview of embryology
Preimplantation period
Embryonic period
  Second week
  Third week
  Fourth week
Fetal period

●●●LEARNING OBJECTIVES

- Define and pronounce the key terms in this chapter.
- Outline the periods of prenatal development, describing the major events that occur during the early weeks.

- Integrate a background on prenatal development into the development of the face, neck, and oral structures and developmental disturbances associated with these structures.

●●●NEW KEY TERMS

Amniocentesis (am-nee-o-sen-**tee**-sis)
Amniotic cavity (am-nee-**ot**-ik)
Bilateral symmetry (**sim**-me-try)
Blastocyst (**blas**-tah-sist)
Cleavage (**kleve**-ij)
Congenital malformations (kon-**jen**-i-til mal-for-**may**-shins)
Cytodifferentiation (site-oh-dif-er-en-she -**ay**-shun)
Differentiation (dif-er-en-she-**ay**-shun)
Down syndrome
Ectoderm (**ek**-toe-derm)
Ectodermal dysplasia (**ek**-toe-derm dis-**play**-ze-ah)
Ectopic pregnancy (ek-**top**-ik)
Embryo (em-bre-oh)
Embryology (em-bre-**ol**-ah-jee)
Embryonic cell layers (em-bre-**on**-ik), **folding, period**
Embryonic disc (em-bre-**on**-ik): **bilaminar** (by-**lam**-i-nar), **trilaminar** (try-**lam**-i-nar)
End: caudal (**kaw**-dal), **cephalic** (se-**fal**-ik)
Endoderm (**en**-doe-derm)
Fertilization (fur-til-uh-**zay**-shun)

Fetal alcohol syndrome (**fete**-il), **period**
Fetus (**fete**-is)
Foregut (**fore**-gut)
Fusion (**fu**-zhin)
Growth: appositional (ap-oh-**zish**-in-al), **interstitial** (in-ter-**stish**-il)
Hindgut (**hind**-gut)
Histodifferentiation (his-toe-dif-er-en-sh e-**ay**-shun)
Implantation (im-plan-**ta**-shin)
Induction (in-**duk**-shin)
Karyotype (**kare**-e-oh-tipe)
Layer: embryoblast (**em**-bre-oh-blast), **epiblast** (**ep**-i-blast), **hypoblast** (**hi**-po-blast), **trophoblast** (**trof**-oh-blast)
Maturation (ma-cher-**ray**-shin)
Meiosis (my-**oh**-sis)
Membrane: cloacal (klo-**ay**-kal), **oropharyngeal** (or-oh-fah-**rin**-je-al)
Mesenchyme (**mes**-eng-kime)
Mesoderm (**mes**-oh-derm)
Midgut (**mid**-gut)
Morphodifferentiation (mor-foe-dif-er-en-she-**ay**-shun)

Morphogenesis (mor-fo-**jen**-is-is)
Morphology (mor-**fol**-ah-je)
Neural crest cells (**noor**-al), **folds, groove, plate, tube**
Neuroectoderm (noor-oh-**ek**-toe-derm)
Ovum (**oh**-vum)
Placenta (pla-**sen**-tuh)
Preimplantation period (pre-im-plan-**ta**-shin)
Prenatal development (pre-**nay**-tal)
Primitive streak
Primordium (pry-**more**-de-um)
Proliferation (pro-lif-er-**ay**-shin)
Rubella (roo-**bell**-ah)
Somites (**so**-mites)
Sperm
Spina bifida (**spi**-nah **bif**-ah-dah)
Syphilis (**sif**-i-lis)
Teratogens (**ter**-ah-to-jens)
Tetracycline stain (tet-rah-**si**-kleen)
Treacher Collins syndrome
Yolk sac
Zygote (**zy**-gote)

PRENATAL DEVELOPMENT

It is important for dental professionals to have an understanding of the major events of prenatal development in order to understand the development of the structures of the face, neck, and oral cavity and the underlying relationships among these structures.

OVERVIEW OF EMBRYOLOGY

Prenatal development begins with the start of pregnancy and continues until the birth of the child; the nine months of gestation is usually divided into three-month time spans or trimesters. Embryology is the study of prenatal development and is introduced in this first chapter of Unit II. Prenatal development consists of three distinct successive periods: preimplantation period, embryonic period, and fetal period (Table 3-1). The preimplantation period and the embryonic period make up the first trimester of the pregnancy, and the fetal period constitutes the last two trimesters.

Each of these structures of the face, neck, and oral cavity has a primordium, the earliest indication of a tissue types or an organ during prenatal development. This information about the embryological background of a structure also helps in the appreciation of any developmental considerations that may occur in these structures, especially if any disturbances occur.

These developmental disturbances can include congenital malformations, or birth defects, which are evident at birth. Most of these occur during both the preimplantation period and the embryonic period and thus involve the first trimester of the pregnancy (discussed later). Such malformations occur in 3 out of 100 cases, and are one of the leading causes of infant death. This does not include anatomical variants, which are common, such as variation in the lesser details of a bone's shape.

Malformations can be due to genetic factors, such as chromosome abnormalities or environmental agents and factors. These environmental agents and factors can include infections, drugs, and radiation and are considered to be teratogens (Table 3-2). Females

TABLE 3-1	Periods of Prenatal Development		
	PREIMPLANTATION PERIOD	**EMBRYONIC PERIOD**	**FETAL PERIOD**
TIME SPAN	**FIRST WEEK**	**SECOND WEEK TO EIGHTH WEEK**	**THIRD TO NINTH MONTH**
Structure(s)*	Zygote / Blastocyst	Blastocyst to disc / Disc to embryo / Embryo	Embryo / Fetus
Structure(s) present	Zygote to blastocyst	Blastocyst to disc to embryo	Embryo to fetus
Description of period	Fertilization and implantation	Induction, proliferation, differentiation, morphogenesis, and maturation to form structures (see Table 3-3)	Maturation of existing structures

*Note that structure size is not accurate or comparative.

of reproductive age should avoid teratogens to protect the developing infant from possible malformations (discussed later).

Malformations in the face, neck, and oral cavity range from a serious cleft in the face or palatal region to small deficiencies of the soft palate or developing cysts underneath an otherwise intact **oral mucosa.** It is important for dental professionals to remember that any orofacial congenital malformations discovered when examining a patient are usually understandable and traceable to a specific time in the embryological development of the individual. Thus, the dental professional must initially understand the development of an individual's orofacial region, including its sequential process to later understand any associated pathology present.

PREIMPLANTATION PERIOD

The first period, the preimplantation period of prenatal development, takes place during the first week after conception. At the beginning of the first week, conception takes place, a female's ovum is penetrated by and united with a male's sperm during fertilization

TABLE 3-2	Known Teratogens Involved in Congenital Malformations
Drugs	Ethanol, tetracycline, phenytoin sodium, lithium, methotrexate, aminopterin, diethylstilbestrol, warfarin, thalidomide, isotretinoin (retinoic acid), androgens, progesterone
Chemicals	Methylmercury, polychlorinated biphenyls
Infections	Rubella virus, syphilis spirochete, herpes simplex virus, human immunodeficiency virus
Radiation	High levels of ionizing type*

*Note that diagnostic levels of radiation such in the dental setting should be avoided when pregnant but have not been directly linked to congenital malformations.

(Figure 3-1). This union of the ovum and sperm subsequently forms a fertilized egg, or zygote.

During fertilization, the final stages of meiosis occur in the ovum. The result of this process is the joining of the ovum's **chromosomes** with those of the sperm. This joining of chromosomes from both biological parents forms a new individual with "shuffled" chromosomes. To allow this formation of a new individual, the sperm and ovum are joined, resulting in the proper number of chromosomes (diploid number of 46). If both these cells, sperm and ovum, instead carried the full complement of chromosomes, fertilization would result in a zygote with *two times* the proper number, resulting in severe congenital malformations and prenatal death.

This situation of excess chromosomes is avoided with meiosis, because, during their development in the gonads, this process enables the ovum and sperm to reduce by one half the normal number of chromosomes (to haploid number of 23). Thus, the zygote has received half its chromosomes from the female and half from the male, with the resultant genetic material a reflection of both biological parents. The photographic analysis of a person's chromosomes is done by orderly arrangement of the pairs in a karyotype, with the sex known by the presence of either having *XX* chromosomes for females or *XY* for males (Figure 3-2).

After fertilization, the zygote then undergoes **mitosis,** or individual cell division with cleavage. After initial cleavage, the solid ball of cells is known as a *morula.* Because of the ongoing process of mitosis and secretion of fluid by the cells within the morula, the zygote becomes a vesicle known as a blastocyst (or blastula) (Figure 3-3). The rest of the first week is characterized by further mitotic cleavage, in which the blastocyst splits into smaller and more numerous cells as it undergoes successive cell divisions by mitosis.

Thus mitosis is a process that takes place during growth or repair and is different from meiosis, which takes place during reproduction (see Table 7-2). Mitosis that occurs during cell division is the self-duplication of the chromosomes of the parent cell and their equal distribution to daughter cells. The result is that the daughter cells have the same chromosome number and hereditary potential as the parent cells. As it grows by cleavage, the blastocyst travels from the site where fertilization took place to the uterus.

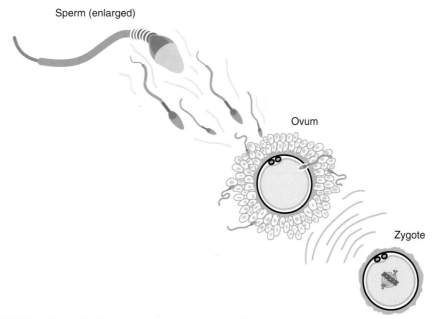

Sperm (enlarged)

Ovum

Zygote

FIGURE 3-1 Sperm fertilizes the ovum and unites with it to form the zygote after the process of meiosis and during the first week of prenatal development. Thus, during this time, both the ovum's and sperm's chromosomes join to form a zygote, a new individual.

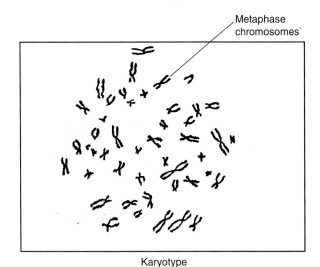

Karyotype

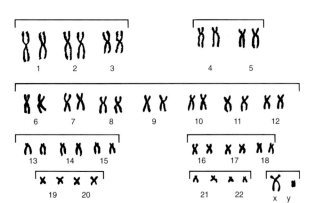

FIGURE 3-2 Example of a karyotype of a male (since it has both *X* and *Y*, with the *Y* determining maleness) showing a photographic analysis of one's chromosomes, which is done by orderly arrangement of the pairs.

By the end of the first week, the blastocyst stops traveling and undergoes implantation and thus becomes embedded in the prepared endometrium, the innermost lining of the uterus on its back wall. After a week of cleavage, the blastocyst consists of a layer of peripheral cells, the trophoblast layer, and a small inner mass of embryonic cells, or embryoblast layer (Figure 3-4). The trophoblast layer later gives rise to important prenatal support tissue. The embryoblast layer later gives rise to the **embryo** during the next prenatal period, the embryonic period.

Developmental Disturbances during Preimplantation Period

If any disturbances occur in meiosis during fertilization, major congenital malformations result from the chromosomal abnormality, which can happen in around 10% of cases. An example of this is **Down syndrome** (or trisomy 21) where an extra chromosome number 21 is present after meiotic division (Figure 3-5). This syndrome presents with flat, broad face with widely spaced eyes, flat-bridged nose, epicanthic folds, oblique eyelid fissures, furrowed lower lip, tongue fissures, lingual papillae hypertropy, and other defects such as various levels of intellectual disability. An arched palate and weak tongue muscles lead to an open mouth position with protrusion of the normal-sized tongue, and articulated speech is often difficult. It may also involve increased levels of periodontal disease and fewer teeth with **microdontia**, presenting challenges to oral hygiene care.

Implantation may also occur outside the uterus, involving the condition of **ectopic pregnancy**, with most occurring in the fallopian tube. This disturbance has several causes but is usually associated with factors that delay or prevent transport of the dividing zygote to the uterus, such as scarred uterine tubes due to pelvic inflammatory disease. In the past, ectopic pregnancies ruptured causing loss of the embryo and threatening the life of the pregnant female but now they are successfully treated with medications.

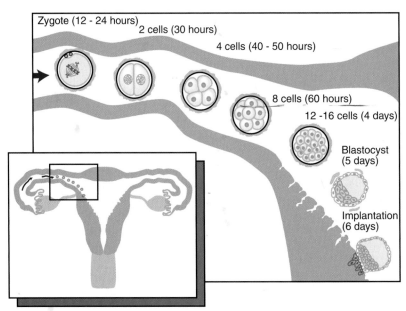

FIGURE 3-3 Zygote undergoing mitotic cleavage to form a blastocyst that travels to become implanted in the endometrium of the uterus.

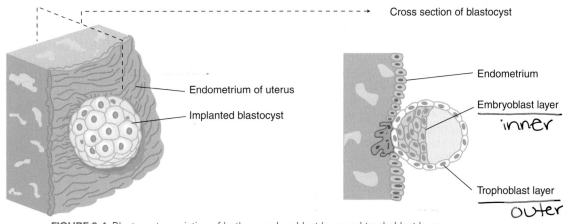

FIGURE 3-4 Blastocyst consisting of both an embryoblast layer and trophoblast layer.

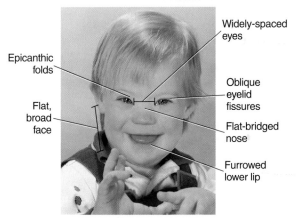

FIGURE 3-5 Down syndrome (or trisomy 21) with an extra chromosome number 21 presents with marked oral and facial features as well as various levels of intellectual disability. *(From Zitelli BJ, Davis HW: Atlas of Pediatric Physical Diagnosis, ed 4, Mosby, St Louis, 2002.)*

TABLE 3-3	Developmental Processes in the Embryo
PROCESS	**DESCRIPTION**
Induction	Action of one group of cells on another that leads to the establishment of the developmental pathway in the responding tissue
Proliferation	Controlled cellular growth and accumulation of byproducts
Differentiation	Change in identical embryonic cells to become distinct structurally and functionally
Morphogenesis	Development of specific tissue structure or differing form due to embryonic cell migration and inductive interactions
Maturation	Attainment of adult function and size due to proliferation, differentiation, and morphogenesis

EMBRYONIC PERIOD

The second period, the **embryonic period** of prenatal development, extends from the beginning of the second week to the end of the eighth week. Certain physiological processes or spatial and temporal events called *patterning* occur during this period, which are considered key to the further development (Table 3-3). These physiological processes include induction, proliferation, differentiation, morphogenesis, and maturation (discussed next). These processes cause the structure of the implanted blastocyst to become, with further development, an **embryo**. These physiological processes also allow the teeth and associated orofacial structures, as well as other organ structures, to develop in the embryo (see Table 6-1).

The first physiological process involved during prenatal development is the process of **induction,** the action of one group of cells on another, which leads to the establishment of the developmental pathway in the responding tissue and which is now considered to be compartmentalized. Over time the populations of embryonic cells vary in the competence of their response to induction. Just what triggers cells to develop into structures from cellular interactions is only beginning to be understood, but many disturbances can result from a failure of induction, leading to a further failure of initiation of certain embryological structures. Induction can also occur in the later stages of development.

Another type of physiological process that follows induction as well as the other processes is the dramatic process of **proliferation,** which is controlled levels of cellular growth present during most of prenatal development. Later migration of these proliferated cells also occurs. Finally, growth also occurs as a result of an accumulation of cellular byproducts.

Growth may be by **interstitial growth,** which occurs from deep within a tissue type or organ. In contrast, growth may be by **appositional growth,** in which a tissue enlarges by the addition of layers on the outside of a structure. Hard tissue growth, such as with mature bone or dental tissue, is usually appositional, whereas soft tissue such skin or gingival tissue increases by interstitial growth. Some tissue types, such as cartilage and immature bone tissue, use both types of growth to attain their final size.

It is important to note that growth is not just an increase in overall size, like a balloon being blown up, but involves differential rates for the different tissue types and organs. An example of this varied rate of growth is tooth eruption in a child, which occurs over many years, allowing for the associated growth of the jaws that will house the teeth.

In the process of **differentiation,** a change occurs in the embryonic cells, which are identical genetically but later become quite distinct structurally and functionally. Thus, cells that perform specialized functions are formed by differentiation during the embryonic period.

Although these functions are minimal at this time, the beginnings of all major tissue types, organs, and organ systems are formed during this period from these specialized cells.

Differentiation occurs at various rates in the embryo. Many parts of the embryo are affected: cells, tissue types, organs, and systems. Various terms describe each one of these types of differentiation, and it is important to note the specific delineation between each of them. **Cytodifferentiation** is the development of different cell types. **Histodifferentiation** is the development of different tissue types within a structure. **Morphodifferentiation** is the development of the differing structure or shape, or **morphology,** for each organ or system.

During the embryonic period, the complexity of the structure and function of these cells increases. This is accomplished by **morphogenesis,** the process of development of specific tissue structure or shape. Morphogenesis occurs due to the migration of embryonic cells, which is followed by the inductive interactions of those cells. As previously mentioned, induction continues to occur throughout the embryonic period as a result of the new varieties of cells interacting with each other, producing an increasingly complex organism.

Finally, the physiological process of **maturation** of the tissue types and organs begins during the embryological period and continues later during the fetal period. It is important to note that the physiological process of maturation of the individual tissue types and organs also involves the processes of proliferation, differentiation, and morphogenesis. Thus, maturation is not the attainment of just the correct adult size but also the correct adult form and function of tissue types and organs.

An **embryo** is easily recognizable at the end of the embryonic period by the eighth week of prenatal development. This chapter discusses only the major events of the second, third, and fourth weeks of the embryonic period. The remaining weeks of prenatal development, as pertinent to dental professionals, are addressed in **Chapters 4** and **5,** which describe the detailed development of the face, neck, and oral cavity.

SECOND WEEK

During the second week of prenatal development, within the embryonic period, the implanted blastocyst grows by increased proliferation of the embryonic cells, with differentiation also occurring resulting in changes in cellular morphogenesis; every ridge, bump, and recess now indicates these increased levels of cellular differentiation. This increased number of embryonic cells creates the **embryonic cell layers** (or germ layers) within the blastocyst. A **bilaminar embryonic disc** is eventually developed from the blastocyst and appears as a flattened, essentially circular plate of bilayered cells (Figure 3-6).

The bilaminar disc (or disk) has both a superior and inferior layer. The superior **epiblast layer** is composed of high columnar cells, and the inferior **hypoblast layer** is composed of small cuboidal cells. After its creation, the bilaminar disc is suspended in the uterus's endometrium between two fluid-filled cavities, the **amniotic cavity,** which faces the epiblast layer, and the **yolk sac,** which faces the hypoblast layer and serves as initial nourishment for the embryonic disc. The bilaminar disc later develops into the **embryo** as prenatal development continues.

Even later, the **placenta,** a prenatal organ that joins the pregnant female and developing embryo, develops from the interactions of the trophoblast layer and endometrial tissue. The formation of the placenta and the developing umbilical circulation permit selective exchange of soluble bloodborne substances between them. This includes oxygen and carbon dioxide as well as nutritional and hormonal substances.

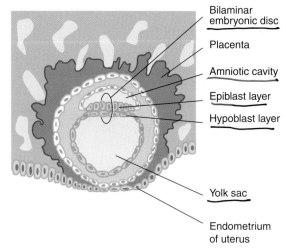

FIGURE 3-6 Blastocyst forming the bilaminar embryonic disc, which consists of the epiblast layer and hypoblast layer surrounded by the amniotic cavity and yolk sac.

THIRD WEEK

During the beginning of the third week of prenatal development, within the embryonic period, the **primitive streak** forms within the bilaminar disc (Figure 3-7). This furrowed, rod-shaped thickening in the middle of the disc results from an increased proliferation of cells in the midline area. The primitive streak causes the disc to have **bilateral symmetry,** with a right half and left half; most of the further development of each half of the embryo mirrors the other half. If looked at from a top view, the embryo would resemble the sole of a shoe with the head end wider than the tail end, and with a slightly narrowed middle.

In addition, during the beginning of the third week, some cells from the epiblast layer move or migrate toward the hypoblast layer only in the area of the primitive streak (Figure 3-8). These migratory cells locate in the middle between the epiblast and hypoblast layers and become **mesenchyme,** an embryonic connective tissue. Mesenchymal cells have the potential to proliferate and differentiate into diverse types of connective tissue, forming cells (such as **fibroblasts, chondroblasts,** and **osteoblasts,** see **Chapter 8**). Some of this tissue begins to create a new embryonic cell layer, the **mesoderm.**

With three layers present, the bilaminar disc has become thickened into a **trilaminar embryonic disc** (Figure 3-9). Thus, the trilaminar disc has three **embryonic cell layers.** With the creation of this new embryonic cell layer of mesoderm, the **epiblast layer** is now considered **ectoderm,** and the **hypoblast layer** is now **endoderm.**

Within the trilaminar disc, each embryonic cell layer is distinct from the others and thus gives rise to specific tissue (Table 3-4, see Table 8-1). The ectoderm gives rise to the skin **epidermis,** the central nervous system, and other structures. The mesoderm gives rise to **connective tissue,** such as skin **dermis, cartilage, bone, blood, muscle,** and other associated tissue. The endoderm gives rise to the **respiratory epithelium** and cells of **glands.**

Mesoderm and associated tissue are found in all areas of the future embryo except at certain embryonic membranes and the pharyngeal pouches (discussed later). In these areas without mesoderm present, both the ectoderm and endoderm fuse together, thereby preventing the migration of mesoderm between them.

Because the trilaminar disc has undergone so much growth during the past three weeks, certain anatomical structures of the disc become apparent. The disc now has a **cephalic end,** or head end. At the cephalic end, the **oropharyngeal membrane** (or buccopharyngeal

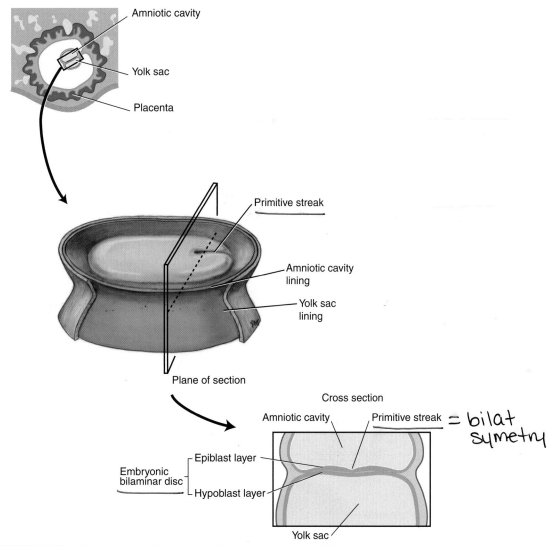

FIGURE 3-7 Bilaminar embryonic disc with primitive streak resulting in bilateral symmetry.

membrane) forms which consists of only ectoderm externally and endoderm internally, without any intermediate mesoderm. This membrane is the location of the future primitive mouth or stomodeum of the embryo and thus the beginning of the digestive tract (see Figure 4-1). The disc also has a caudal end, or tail end (Figure 3-10). At the caudal end, the cloacal membrane forms, which is the location of the future anus, or terminal end of the digestive tract.

During the later part of the third week, the central nervous system (CNS) begins to develop in the embryo. Many steps occur during this week to form the beginnings of the spinal cord and brain (see Table 8-6). First, a specialized group of cells differentiates from the **ectoderm**, and is now considered neuroectoderm. These cells are localized to the neural plate of the embryo, a central band of cells that extends the length of the embryo, from the cephalic end to the caudal end. This plate undergoes further growth and thickening, which cause it to deepen and invaginate inward, forming the neural groove.

Near the end of the third week, the neural groove deepens further and is surrounded by the neural folds. As further growth of the neuroectoderm occurs, the neural tube is formed during the fourth week by the neural folds undergoing fusion at the most superior part. The neural tube forms the future spinal cord as well as other neural tissue (see Table 3-4).

Other areas of the embryo also undergo fusion during the third week and in subsequent weeks, as the embryo develops, but the process occurs differently depending on the structures involved. In the case of the neural tube (and also the palate as discussed in Chapter 5), the process of *fusion*, as the name implies, is the joining of two separate surfaces on the embryo (see Figure 5-1). However, in the case of facial fusion, the process of fusion is mainly the elimination of a groove between two adjacent swellings of tissue or processes on the same surface of the embryo caused by merging of underlying tissue and migration into the groove (see Figure 4-4).

In addition, during the third week, another specialized group of cells, the neural crest cells, develop from **neuroectoderm** (Figure 3-11). These cells migrate from the crests of the neural folds and then disperse within the mesenchyme. These migrated cells are involved in the development of many face and neck structures, such as the branchial arches, because they differentiate to form most of the connective tissue of the head.

On reaching their predetermined destinations, the neural crest cells undergo **differentiation** into diverse cell types that are, in part, specified by local environmental influences. Many embryologists consider the neural crest cells to be a *fourth embryonic cell layer* (see Table 3-4). In the future, these cells become involved in the formation of

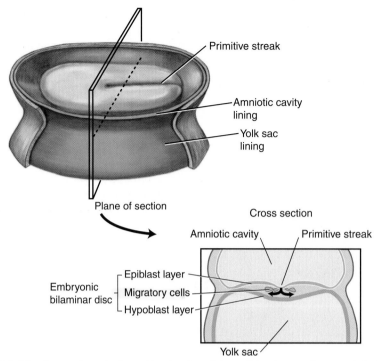

FIGURE 3-8 Bilaminar embryonic disc with migration of the epiblast layer cells toward the hypoblast layer to form the new mesoderm layer.

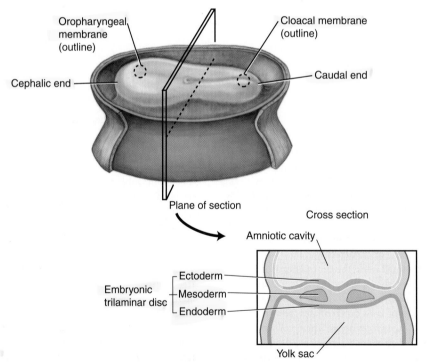

FIGURE 3-9 After the formation of the middle layer of mesoderm, the resulting trilaminar embryonic disc consists of the ectoderm, mesoderm, and endoderm. Note the cephalic and caudal ends on the disc and their associated oropharyngeal and cloacal membranes (*dashed lines*).

TABLE 3-4	Development of Embryonic Cell Layers			
	ECTODERM	**MESODERM**	**ENDODERM**	**NEURAL CREST CELLS***
Origin	Epiblast layer	Migrating cells from epiblast layer	Hypoblast layer	Migrating neuroectoderm
Morphology of the structure	Columnar	Varies	Cuboidal	Varies
Future systemic tissues	Epidermis; sensory epithelium of the eyes, ears, nose, nervous system, and neural crest cells; mammary and cutaneous glands	Dermis, muscle, bone, lymphatics, blood cells and bone marrow, cartilage, reproductive and excretory organs	Respiratory and digestive system linings, liver and pancreatic cells	Components of nervous system pigment cells, connective tissue proper, cartilage, bone, and certain dental tissues

*Note that the **neural crest cells from the neuroectoderm** are included, but they are not present in the embryonic disc until the later part of the third week, and which are considered to be a *fourth embryonic cell layer* by many embryologists.

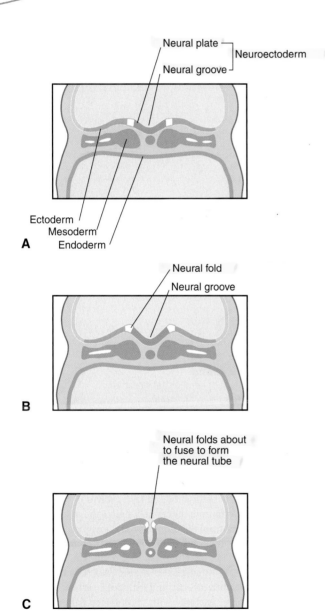

FIGURE 3-10 Embryo's central nervous system beginning to form. **A:** Formation of the neuroectoderm from the ectoderm within the neural plate that thickens to form the neural groove. **B:** Neural groove deepens to become surrounded by the neural folds. **C:** Neural folds meet and fuse, forming the neural tube.

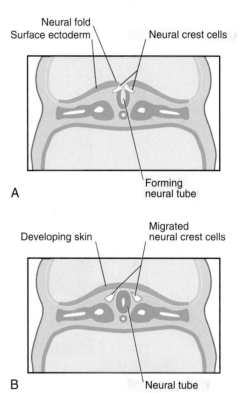

FIGURE 3-11 Neural crest cells from the neural folds **(A)** will migrate and disperse within the mesenchyme **(B)** to affect tissue development.

components of the nervous system, melanocyte pigment cells, connective tissue proper, cartilage, bone, and certain dental tissue (by influencing **ectomesenchyme** as discussed in later chapters), such as the **pulp, dentin, cementum, alveolar bone,** and **periodontal ligament** (see Figure 6-1). Thus, neural crest cells are essential in the development of the face and neck, as well as most oral and dental tissue, except the enamel and certain types of cementum (see Chapters 4, 5, and 6).

By the end of the third week, the mesoderm additionally differentiates and begins to divide on each side of the tube into 38-paired cuboidal segments of mesoderm, forming the **somites** (Figure 3-12). The somites later appear as distinct elevations on the surface of the sides of the embryo and continue to develop in the following weeks of prenatal development, giving rise to most of the skeletal structures of the head, neck, and trunk, as well as the associated muscles and dermis of the skin.

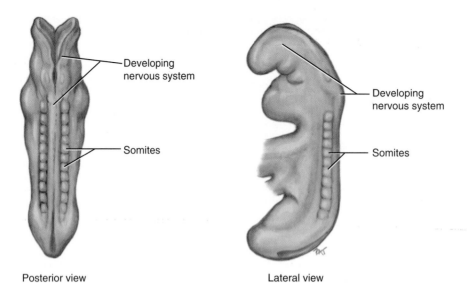

Posterior view   Lateral view

FIGURE 3-12 Differentiated mesoderm gives rise to the somites that are located on both the sides of the developing nervous system.

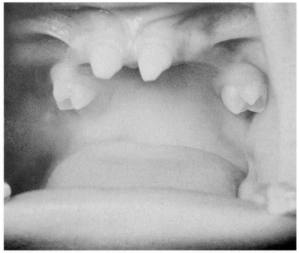

FIGURE 3-13 Ectodermal dysplasia is marked by the abnormal development of ectodermal structures resulting in certain facial features and an absence of teeth, or anodontia (partial in this case).

FOURTH WEEK

During the fourth week of prenatal development, within the embryonic period, the disc undergoes embryonic folding, establishing for the first time the axis, which places forming tissue types into their proper positions for further embryonic development, as well as producing a somewhat tubular embryo (Figure 3-13). This folding results from extensive proliferation of the **ectoderm** and **differentiation** of basic tissue and occurs mainly at the cephalic end, where the brain will form. This tissue grows beyond the **oropharyngeal membrane** to overhang the developing heart.

Folding due to increased growth occurs not only at the cephalic end but also at the caudal end and at the sides of the embryo simultaneously. As a result of this folding, the positions of the embryonic cell layers take on a more recognizable placement for the further development of the embryo.

Thus, after folding of the disc, the endoderm lies inside the ectoderm, with mesoderm filling in the areas between these two layers. This movement of the embryonic cell layers forms one long, hollow tube lined by endoderm from the cephalic end to the caudal end of the embryo—specifically, from the oropharyngeal membrane to the cloacal membrane. This tube is the future digestive tract and is separated into three major regions: foregut, midgut, and hindgut.

The anterior part of this tube is the foregut, which forms the **primitive pharynx**, or primitive throat, and includes a part of the primitive yolk sac as it becomes enclosed with folding (see Figure 4-10). The two more posterior parts, the midgut and hindgut, form the rest of the mature **pharynx**, as well as the remainder of the digestive tract (see Figure 2-18). During development of the digestive tract, four pairs of **pharyngeal pouches** will form from evaginations on the lateral walls lining the pharynx (see Figure 4-11).

Developmental Disturbances during the Embryonic Period

Because the beginnings of all essential external and internal structures are formed during the **embryonic period**, this is considered the most critical period of **prenatal development**. Thus, developmental disturbances occurring during this period may give rise to major **congenital malformations** of the embryo (as discussed earlier).

One syndrome that can occur within this period is ectodermal dysplasia, which involves the abnormal development of one or more structures from **ectoderm** (Figure 3-14). This syndrome has a hereditary etiology and presents with abnormalities of the teeth, skin, hair, nails, eyes, facial structure, and glands, because these are derived from ectoderm or associated tissue. There may be partial or complete **anodontia,** the absence of some or all teeth in each dentition, and the teeth that are present for either dentition have frequent disturbances (see **Chapter 6**). Partial or full dentures are used for both functional and esthetic purposes, but need to be reconstructed periodically as the jaws continue to grow; implants may be considered after growth halts, if enough alveolar bone is present.

If there is failure of migration of the **neural crest cells** to the facial region, **Treacher Collins syndrome** (or mandibulofacial dysostosis) develops in the embryo. This results in failure of full facial development, presenting with downward slanting eyes, micrognathia (small lower jaw), conductive hearing loss, underdeveloped zygomatic bone, drooping in part of the lateral lower eyelids, and malformed or absent ears (Figure 3-15).

In addition, if **teratogens** are present during the active differentiation of an organ or tissue types, after crossing from mother by way of the placenta, this can raise the incidence of congenital malformations. An example of an infective teratogen for the embryo is the virus causing **rubella**, which can result in cataracts, cardiac defects, and deafness. Another infective teratogen is the bacterial spirochete causing **syphilis**, *Treponema pallidum*, because it produces defects in the incisors (**Hutchinson's incisor**) and molars (**mulberry molar**), as well as blindness, deafness, and paralysis (Figure 3-16, see **Chapters 16 and 17**).

An example of the result of a teratogenic drug effect during the embryonic period is **fetal alcohol syndrome**. Ethanol ingested by a pregnant female easily crosses the placenta and can result in prenatal and postnatal growth deficiency, intellectual deficiency, and other anomalies, such as small head circumference, low nasal bridge, short nose, small midface, widely spaced eyes with epicanthic folds and eyelid fissures, indistinct philtrum, and thin upper lip (Figure 3-17). Oral changes, such as crowding of the dentition, mouth breathing, anterior **open bite,** and associated **gingivitis** may occur, possibly because of an increased finger sucking habit.

Direct exposure to high levels of radiation can act as an environmental teratogen during the embryonic period. Radiation may injure embryonic cells, resulting in cell death, **chromosome** injury, and delay of mental and physical growth. The severity of embryonic damage is associated with the absorbed dose, the dose rate, and the state of embryonic or fetal development at the time of exposure.

However, congenital abnormalities have not been directly linked to a diagnostic level of radiation such as that used in the dental setting. Scattered radiation from a radiographic examination of the oral cavity administers a dose of only a few millirads to a pregnant female, which is not known to be teratogenic to an embryo. Nevertheless, even this small dose should be avoided during pregnancy unless an emergency situation requires it; proper protective precautions should be used with all patients at all times and, as always, with the administering dental professionals.

Failure of **fusion** of the **neural tube** results in neural tube defects of the tissue overlying the spinal cord, such as the meninges, vertebral arches, muscles, and skin. One type of neural tube defect is spina bifida, characterized by defects in the vertebral arches and various degrees of disability. Nutritional and environmental factors can also have an important role as teratogens in causing neural tube defects; folic acid supplements are now being recommended during pregnancy to help prevent this defect as well as **cleft lip** and **cleft palate** (see Figures 4-8 and 5-7).

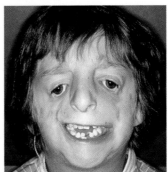

FIGURE 3-14 Treacher Collins syndrome (or mandibulofacial dysostosis) is due to failure of migration of the neural crest cells to the facial region in the embryo. This results in failure of full facial development, presenting with marked features, including a micrognathia (small lower jaw) *(From Kaban LB, Toulis MJ:* Pediatric Oral and Maxillofacial Surgery, *ed 1, Saunders, Philadelphia, 2004.)*

Finally, during the fourth week, the face and neck begin to develop, with the primitive eyes, ears, nose, oral cavity, and jaw areas. The development of the face and neck is discussed in **Chapter 4**, and the development of the associated oral cavity is described in **Chapters 5 and 6**.

FETAL PERIOD

The fetal period of prenatal development follows the embryonic period. It encompasses the beginning of the ninth week, or third month, to the ninth month, with the maturation of existing structures occurring as the embryo enlarges to become a fetus. This process involves not only the physiological process of maturation of the individual tissue types and organs but also further proliferation, differentiation, and morphogenesis, as discussed before with the embryo.

Although developmental changes with the fetus are not as dramatic as those that occur during the embryonic period, they are important because they allow the newly formed tissue types and organs to function. Even though the embryo has been breathing since the third week, by the end of the fourth month, the fetal heartbeat and fetal movements can be noted.

Developmental Disturbances during the Fetal Period

Congenital malformations can also occur during the fetal period of prenatal development. The most common invasive prenatal diagnostic procedure to detect these malformations is **amniocentesis,** where the amniotic fluid is sampled during the fourteenth to sixteenth weeks after the last missed menstrual period. This is usually in older females, when one or both parents have a chromosomal abnormality or neural tube defect, when a previous child was affected, or when the parents are carriers of inborn errors of metabolism or X-linked disorders such as hemophilia.

Systemic tetracycline antibiotic therapy of the pregnant female can act as a teratogenic drug during the fetal period. This therapy can result in **tetracycline stain** within the child's **primary teeth** that are developing at that time. This intrinsic yellow to yellow-brown discoloration of the teeth can occur in slight, moderate, or severe degrees, as the antibiotic becomes chemically bound to the **dentin** for the life of the tooth, and because of the transparency of overlying enamel, this stain is easily visible.

The adult's **permanent teeth** may also be affected, similarly to the primary teeth, if the drug is given during their development (Figure 3-18). If the permanent teeth are involved, treatment may require full-coverage crowns or veneers to improve the appearance of the teeth, although, in some cases, vital tooth whitening may even out the discoloration. Thus, this type of antibiotic therapy should be avoided if possible in pregnant females and children. Studies also show that overuse of amoxicillin in children with ear, nose, and throat infections may be involved in visible changes of the surface smoothness and tooth color in the permanent tooth enamel, resulting in **enamel dysplasia** (see Table 6-3, *H*).

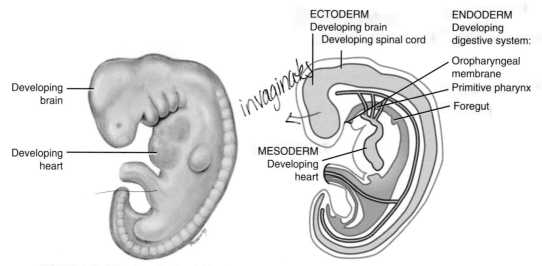

FIGURE 3-15 Trilaminar disc has folded into the embryo as a result of extensive growth of the ectoderm. With folding, the endoderm is now inside the ectoderm, with the mesoderm filling in the areas between the two tissue types, except at the two embryonic membranes as shown on cross section. Note the developing brain with spinal cord, heart, and digestive tract.

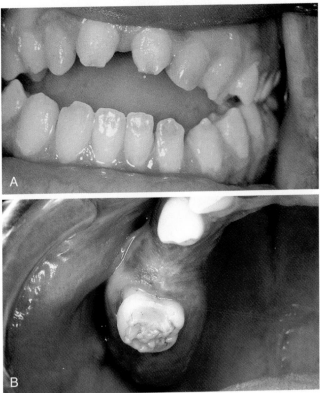

FIGURE 3-16 Dental anomalies from syphilis, an infective teratogen. **A:** Hutchinson's incisors, **B:** Mulberry molar *(From Ibsen OAC, Phelan JA: Oral Pathology for Dental Hygienists, ed 5, WB Saunders, Philadelphia, 2009).*

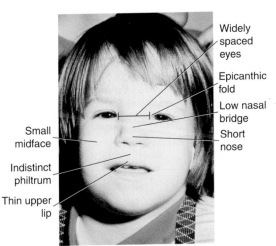

Widely spaced eyes

Epicanthic fold

Low nasal bridge

Short nose

Small midface

Indistinct philtrum

Thin upper lip

FIGURE 3-17 Fetal alcohol syndrome marked by certain facial features and various levels of intellectual disability. This syndrome is caused by the pregnant female's excessive use of ethanol during the embryonic period. *(From Streissguth AP, Landesman-Dwyer S, Martin JC, Smith DW: Teratogenic effects of alcohol in humans and laboratory animals, Science 209:353-361, 1980. Copyright 1980; American Association for the Advancement of Science.)*

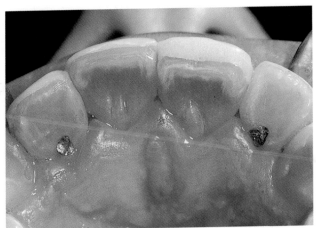

FIGURE 3-18 Lingual view of the permanent maxillary anterior teeth with tetracycline stain that was caused by the ingestion of the drug as a child. This was during the time of development of the permanent dentition. Note the presence of veneer crowns on the facial surface of the affected teeth, which have been placed for esthetic reasons.

CHAPTER 4

Development of the Face and Neck

●●●CHAPTER OUTLINE

●●●LEARNING OBJECTIVES

- Define and pronounce the key terms in this chapter.
- Outline the events that occur during the development of the face and neck, describing each step in their formation.

- Integrate the knowledge of the development of the face and neck into understanding the observed structures and any developmental disturbances of these structures.

●●●NEW KEY TERMS

Branchial apparatus (**brang**-ke-al ap-pah-**ra**-tis), grooves
Branchial arch (**brang**-ke-al): **first, second, third, fourth, fifth, sixth**
Cartilage (**kar**-ti-lij): **Meckel's (mek**-els), **Reichert's (rike**-erts)
Cervical cysts (**ser**-vi-kal)
Cleft lip (kleft)

Hyoid arch (**hi**-oid)
Intermaxillary segment (in-ter-**mak**-si-lare-ee)
Mandibular arch (man-**dib**-you-lar), **processes**
Nasal pits (**nay**-zil)
Oronasal membrane (or-oh-**nay**-zil)
Pharyngeal pouches (fah-**rin**-je-il)

Placodes (**plak**- odz): **lens, nasal (nay**-zil), **otic (o**-tik)
Primitive pharynx (**fare**-inks)
Process(es): frontonasal (frun-to-**nay**-zil), lateral nasal, maxillary (**mak**-si-lare-ee), medial nasal
Stomodeum (sto-mo-**de**-um)

DEVELOPMENT OF THE FACE

Dental professionals must have a clear understanding about the development of the face to further relate the underlying structural relationships to any developmental disturbances that may be present.

OVERVIEW OF FACIAL DEVELOPMENT

The face and its associated tissue begin to form during the fourth week of prenatal development within the **embryonic period** (Box 4-1). During this time, the rapidly growing brain of the embryo bulges over the **oropharyngeal membrane** and developing heart (Figures 4-1 and 4-2). The area of the future face is now squeezed between the developing brain and heart with the formation of the three embryonic layers and resultant **embryonic folding** (see Figure 3-15).

All three embryonic layers are involved in facial development: **ectoderm, mesoderm,** and **endoderm** (Table 4-1). Facial development includes the formation of the primitive mouth, mandibular arch, maxillary process, frontonasal process, and nose. Facial development depends on the five major facial processes (or prominences) that form during the fourth week and surround the embryo's primitive mouth: single frontonasal process and paired maxillary and mandibular processes (Figure 4-3). Thus these facial processes become the centers of growth for the face. If the adult face is divided into thirds—upper, midface, and lower parts—these parts roughly correspond to the centers of facial growth. The upper part of the face is derived from the frontonasal process, the midface from the maxillary processes, and the lower from the mandibular processes.

BOX 4-1 **Facial Development within the Fourth Week of Prenatal Development**

Developmental Events (not in precise order of occurrence)

Disintegration of the oropharyngeal membrane of stomodeum enlarges the primitive mouth, allowing access to the primitive pharynx

Mandibular processes fuse to form mandibular arch, which fuses to form the mandible and lower lip

Frontonasal process forms and gives rise to the nasal placodes, nasal pits, medial and lateral nasal processes, and intermaxillary segment to form the nose and primary palate

Maxillary process forms from mandibular arch

Maxillary process fuses with each medial nasal process to form upper lip and with each mandibular arch to form the labial commissures

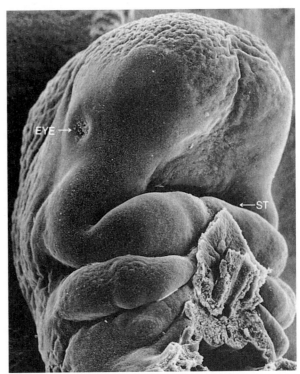

FIGURE 4-2 Scanning electron micrograph of the embryo at the fourth week, showing the developing brain, face, and heart. Note also the stomodeum (*ST*) and lens placode for the eye. (*From Hinrichsen K: The early development of morphology and patterns of the face in the human embryo,* Adv Anat Embryol Cell Biol *98:1-79, 1985.*)

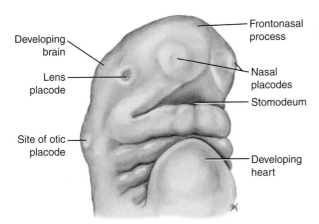

FIGURE 4-1 Embryo at the fourth week of prenatal development showing the developing brain, forming face from the growth of the frontonasal process, and developing heart. Note also the placement of the stomodeum and placodes.

The facial development that starts in the fourth week will be completed later in the twelfth week, within the **fetal period.** The face changes shape considerably as it grows. Thus, overall facial proportions develop during the fetal period. It important to note that the development of the associated oral structures is occurring at the same time and is discussed in Chapters 5 and 6.

Most of the facial structures develop by **fusion** of swellings or tissue on the *same* surface of the embryo (Figure 4-4). A cleft, or furrow, is initially located between these adjacent swellings due to proliferation, differentiation, and morphogenesis (see Table 3-3). However, with facial fusion, these furrows are usually eliminated as the underlying **mesenchyme** migrates into the furrow, making the embryonic facial surface smooth. This migration takes place because adjacent mesenchyme grows and merges beneath the external ectoderm during the maturation of the structure. In some cases, a slight groove or line maybe left on the facial surface, showing where the fusion of the swellings took place. Differing from the fusion that takes place on the facial surface is the type of fusion that occurs during development of the palate (see Figure 5-1). In contrast to facial fusion, palatal fusion involves the fusion of swellings or tissue from *different* surfaces of the embryo, such as that which occurs with the fusion of the neural tube (see Figure 3-10, *C*).

The overall growth of the face is in both an inferior and anterior direction in relationship to the cranial base. The growth of the upper

face is initially the most rapid, in keeping with its association with the developing brain. Subsequently, the forehead ceases to grow significantly after age 12. In contrast, the middle and lower parts of the face grow more slowly over a prolonged period of time and finally cease to grow late in puberty. The eruption of the permanent third molars at approximately 17 to 21 years of age marks the end of the major growth of the lower two thirds of the face. The underlying facial bones, also developing at this time, depend on centers of bone formation by **intramembranous ossification** (see Figure 8-12).

STOMODEUM AND ORAL CAVITY FORMATION

The primitive mouth is now the stomodeum (or stomatodeum), which initially appeared as a shallow depression in the embryonic surface ectoderm at the cephalic end before the fourth week (see Figures 4-1 and 4-2). At this time, the stomodeum is limited in depth by the **oropharyngeal membrane.** This temporary membrane, consisting of external ectoderm overlying endoderm, was formed during the third week of prenatal development. The membrane also separates the stomodeum from the primitive pharynx. The primitive pharynx is the cranial part of the **foregut,** the beginning of the future digestive tract.

The first event in the development of the face, during the fourth week of prenatal development, is disintegration of the oropharyngeal membrane (Figure 4-5). With this disintegration of the membrane, the primitive mouth is increased in depth and enlarges. Access now occurs through the stomodeum from the internal primitive pharynx to the outside fluids of the amniotic cavity that surrounds the embryo. In the future, the stomodeum will give rise to the oral cavity, which will be lined by **oral epithelium,** derived from ectoderm as a result

TABLE 4-1	Embryonic Development of the Face	
EMBRYONIC STRUCTURES	**ORIGIN**	**FUTURE TISSUES**
Stomodeum	Ectodermal depression enlarged by disintegration of oropharyngeal membrane	Oral cavity proper
Mandibular arch (first branchial arch)	Fused mandibular processes and neural crest cells	Lower lip, lower face, mandible with associated tissues (other arch derivatives shown in Table 4-2)
Maxillary process(es)	Superior and anterior swelling(s) from mandibular arch and neural crest cells	Midface, upper lip sides, cheeks, secondary palate, posterior part of maxilla with associated tissues, zygomatic bones, part of temporal bones
Frontonasal process	Ectodermal tissue and neural crest cells	Medial and lateral nasal processes
Nasal pits	Nasal placodes	Nasal cavities
Medial nasal process(es)	Frontonasal process medial to nasal pits	Middle of nose, philtrum region, intermaxillary segment
Intermaxillary segment	Fused medial nasal processes	Anterior part of maxilla with associated tissues, primary palate, nasal septum
Lateral nasal process(es)	Frontonasal process lateral to nasal pits	Nasal alae

of **embryonic folding**. The oral epithelium and underlying tissue will give rise to the teeth and associated tissue types as discussed in Chapter 6 (see Figure 6-1).

MANDIBULAR ARCH AND LOWER FACE FORMATION

After formation of the stomodeum but still during the fourth week, two bulges of tissue appear inferior to the primitive mouth: the two mandibular processes (see Figure 4-5). These processes consist of a core of mesenchyme formed in part by **neural crest cells** that migrate to the facial region, covered externally by ectoderm and internally by endoderm.

These paired mandibular processes then fuse at the midline to form the mandibular arch, the developmental form of the future lower dental arch, the **mandible**. After fusion, the mandibular arch then extends as a band of tissue found inferior to the stomodeum and between the developing brain and heart. In the midline, on the surface of the mature bony mandible, is the **mandibular symphysis**, indicating where the mandible is formed by fusion of right and left mandibular processes (see Figure 1-9). The mandibular arch and its associated tissue are the first parts of the face to form after stomodeum, separating it from the developing cardiac bulge.

The mandibular arch is also considered the *first branchial arch* (discussed later). Thus, this tissue depends on neural crest cells for its formation, as do all the other five branchial arches. During the growth of the mandibular arch, Meckel's cartilage forms within each side of the arch (Table 4-2). Most of this cartilage disappears as the bony mandible forms by **intramembranous ossification** lateral to and in close association with the cartilage; yet, only some small part makes a contribution to it (see Chapter 5). Also, a part of the cartilage participates in the formation of the middle ear bones.

In the future, the mandibular arch directly gives rise to the lower face, including the lower lip. The mandibular arch will also give rise not only to the mandible, but also its **mandibular teeth** and associated tissue. The embryo's mandible initially appears underdeveloped, but it achieves its more characteristic mature form as it develops further during the fetal period (see Figures 4-3 and 4-5).

The mesoderm of the mandibular arch forms the **muscles of mastication** (masseter, temporalis, and pterygoids), as well as some palatal

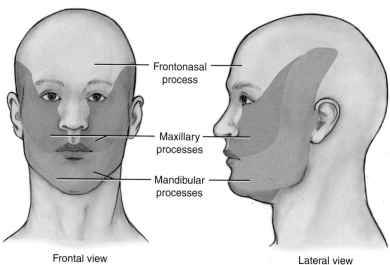

Frontal view   Lateral view

FIGURE 4-3 Adult face with its embryonic derivatives of the five facial processes: single frontonasal process and paired maxillary and mandibular processes.

muscles and suprahyoid muscles (see Figure 19-8). Thus, because these muscles are derived from the mandibular arch they are innervated by the first arch nerve, fifth cranial nerve, and trigeminal nerve (see Table 13-3). The mandibular arch is also involved in the formation of the **tongue** (see Figure 5-11).

During the fifth to sixth week, primitive muscle cells from the mesoderm in the mandibular arch begin to differentiate. These primitive muscle cells become oriented to the site of origin and insertion of the masticatory muscles that they will form. By the seventh week, the mandibular muscle mass has enlarged, and the cells have begun to migrate into the areas where they will begin to differentiate into the four muscles of mastication. Muscle cell migration occurs before bone formation in the facial area.

By the tenth week, the mandibular muscle masses have become well organized bilaterally into the four muscles of mastication. Nerve branches from the trigeminal cranial nerve are incorporated early in these muscle masses. The muscle cells of the masseter and medial pterygoid muscles have formed a vertical sling that inserts into the site that will form the **angle of the mandible.** The temporalis muscle has differentiated in the temporal fossa and is inserting into the

TABLE 4-2	Branchial Arches and Derivative Structures	
ARCHES	**FUTURE NERVES AND MUSCLES**	**FUTURE SKELETAL STRUCTURES AND LIGAMENTS**
First arches (mandibular)	Trigeminal nerve, muscles of mastication, mylohyoid and anterior belly of digastric, tensor tympani, tensor veli palatini muscles	Malleus and incus of middle ear, including anterior ligament of the malleus, sphenomandibular ligament, and parts of sphenoid bone (see also Table 4-1)
Second arches (hyoid)	Facial nerve, stapedius muscle, muscles of facial expression, posterior belly of the digastric muscle, stylohyoid muscle	Stapes and parts of malleus and incus of middle ear, stylohyoid ligament, styloid process of the temporal bone, lesser cornu of hyoid bone, upper portion of body of hyoid bone
Third arches	Glossopharyngeal nerve, stylopharyngeal muscle	Greater cornu of hyoid bone, lower portion of body of hyoid bone
Fourth through sixth arches	Superior laryngeal branch and recurrent laryngeal branch of vagus nerve, levator veli palatini muscles, pharyngeal constrictors, intrinsic muscles of the larynx	Laryngeal cartilages

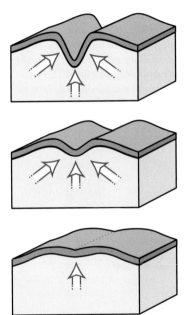

FIGURE 4-4 Facial fusion involves the elimination of a furrow between two adjacent swellings of tissue on the *same* surface of the embryo, unlike palatal fusion, which is the fusion of two separate structures from two *different* surfaces.

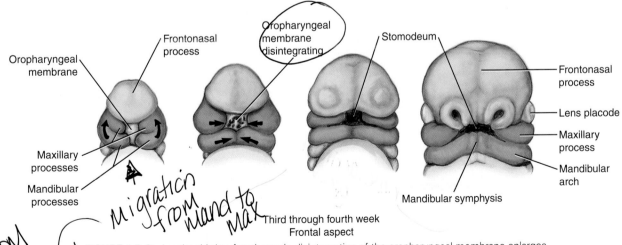

Third through fourth week
Frontal aspect

FIGURE 4-5 During the third to fourth week, disintegration of the oropharyngeal membrane enlarges the stomodeum of the embryo and allows access between the primitive mouth and the primitive pharynx. The frontonasal process also enlarges, helping to form the nasal region. Mandibular processes give rise to the maxillary processes and then fuse together at the mandibular symphysis, forming the mandibular arch inferior to the enlarged stomodeum.

developing **coronoid process.** The lateral pterygoid muscle cells, which arise from the infratemporal fossa, extend horizontally into the **mandibular condyle** and **articular disc.**

FRONTONASAL PROCESS AND UPPER FACE FORMATION

During the fourth week, the frontonasal process (see Figure 4-1) also forms as a bulge of tissue in the upper facial area. This process is at the most **cephalic end** of the embryo and is the cranial boundary of the stomodeum. In the future, the frontonasal process gives rise to the upper face, which includes the forehead, bridge of the nose, primary palate, nasal septum, and all structures associated with the medial nasal processes.

PLACODE DEVELOPMENT

On the outer surface of the embryo are placodes, which are rounded areas of specialized, thickened **ectoderm** found at the location of developing special sense organs. The facial area of the embryo has two lens placodes, which are initially located fishlike on each side of the frontonasal process (see Figures 4-1, 4-2). Later in development, these lens placodes migrate medially from their lateral positions and form the future eyes and associated tissue.

The two otic placodes are even more laterally and posteriorly placed and form pits that create the future internal ear and associated tissue as they appear to rise to their mature position as a result of their relative growth. Parts of the nearby **branchial apparatus** of the embryonic neck later form the external and middle ear (discussed later).

In addition to the lens and otic placodes, the two nasal placodes form in the anterior part of the frontonasal process, just superior to the stomodeum, during the fourth week (see Figure 4-1). These button-like structures form as bilateral ectodermal thickenings that later develop into **olfactory epithelium** for the sensation of smell, located in the mature nose.

NOSE AND PARANASAL SINUS FORMATION

During the fourth week, the tissue around the nasal placodes on the **frontonasal process** undergoes growth, thus starting the development of the **nasal region** and the nose. The placodes then become submerged, forming a depression in the center of each placode, the nasal pits (or olfactory pits) (Figure 4-6). These nasal pits later develop into the **nasal cavity** (see Figure 11-18).

Deepening of the nasal pits produces a nasal sac that grows internally toward the developing brain. At first, the nasal sacs are separated from the stomodeum by the oronasal membrane. This temporary

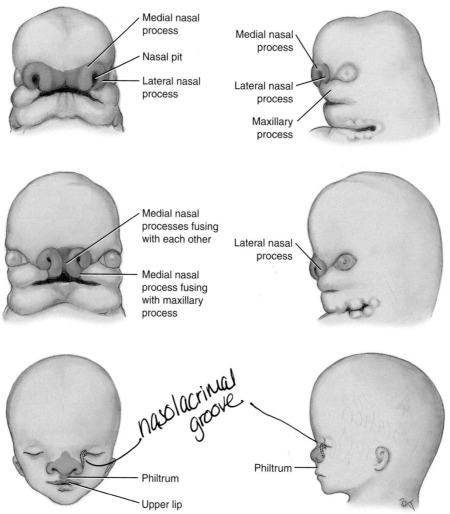

FIGURE 4-6 Development of the nose from the medial and lateral nasal processes; also showing the formation of the upper lip from the medial process fusing with the maxillary process on each side.

membrane disintegrates, bringing the nasal and oral cavities into communication in the area of the primitive choanae, posterior to the developing primary palate. At the same time, the superior, middle, and inferior **nasal conchae** are developing on the lateral walls of the developing nasal cavities.

Some of the **paranasal sinuses** develop later during the fetal period, and others develop after birth. All form as outgrowths of the walls of the nasal cavities and become air-filled extensions of the nasal cavities in the adjacent bones, such as in the maxilla and the frontal bone (see Figure 11-20).

The middle part of the tissue growing around the nasal placodes appears as two crescent-shaped swellings located between the nasal pits. These are the medial nasal processes (see Figure 4-6). In the future, the medial nasal processes will fuse together externally to form the middle part of the nose from the **root of the nose** to the **apex of the nose,** as well as the **tubercle of the upper lip** and **philtrum** (see Figures 1-4 and 1-6).

The paired medial nasal processes also fuse internally and grow inferiorly on the inside of the stomodeum, forming the intermaxillary segment (or premaxillary segment) (Figure 4-7, see Figure 5-2). The intermaxillary segment is involved in the formation of certain **maxillary teeth** (**incisors**) and associated structures, such as the **primary palate** and **nasal septum.**

On the outer part of the nasal pits are two other crescent-shaped swellings, the lateral nasal processes (see Figure 4-6). In the future, the lateral nasal processes form the **alae** of the nose, and the fusion of the lateral nasal, maxillary, and medial nasal processes forms the **nares** (see Figure 1-4). The embryonic nose remains visually flat, however, until the fetal period, when facial development is completed and it has its more mature elevated appearance.

MAXILLARY PROCESS AND MIDFACE FORMATION

During the fourth week of prenatal development, within the embryonic period, an adjacent swelling forms from increased growth of the **mandibular arch** on each side of the **stomodeum,** the maxillary process. Then each maxillary process will grow superiorly and anteriorly around the stomodeum (see Figure 4-5). Because it is formed from the mandibular arch, the maxillary process is also formed from mesenchyme provided by **neural crest cells.**

In the future, the maxillary processes will form the midface. This includes the sides of the upper lip, cheeks, **secondary palate,** and posterior part of the **maxilla** with its **canines,** certain **posterior teeth,** and associated tissue. This tissue also forms the zygomatic bones and parts of the temporal bones.

UPPER AND LOWER LIP FORMATION

During the fourth week, the upper lip is formed when each maxillary process fuses with each medial nasal process on both sides of the stomodeum due to the underlying growth of the mesenchyme (see Figure 4-6). Thus, the maxillary processes contribute to the sides of the upper lip, and the two medial nasal processes contribute to the **philtrum** (see Figure 1-6). Fusion of these processes to form the upper lip is completed during the sixth week of prenatal development, when the grooves between the processes are obliterated. The maxillary

Developmental Disturbances of the Lips and Associated Tissue

Failure of fusion of the maxillary process with the medial nasal process can result in **cleft lip,** with varying degrees of disfigurement and disability (Figures 4-8 and 4-9). This disturbance may be hereditary or associated with environmental factors. It also may be isolated or associated with other developmental abnormalities, such as cleft palate. Cleft lip, with or without **cleft palate,** occurs in about 1 in 1000 cases. The cleft results from a failure of the mesenchyme to grow beneath the ectoderm to obliterate any grooves between these processes, or even a deficiency or absence of mesenchyme in the area.

These clefts of the lip can be located at one side or both sides of the upper lip; it may be unilateral or bilateral and may vary from a notch in the **vermilion border** of the upper lip (incomplete cleft) to more severe cases (complete cleft) that extend into the floor of the naris and through the **alveolar process** of the maxilla.

Cleft lip is more common and more severe in males, more commonly unilateral, and on the left side. It can complicate nursing and feeding of the child as well as speech development and appearance, and it may increase oronasal infection levels. It is treated by oral and plastic surgery, with dental intervention; however, speech and hearing therapy may be needed.

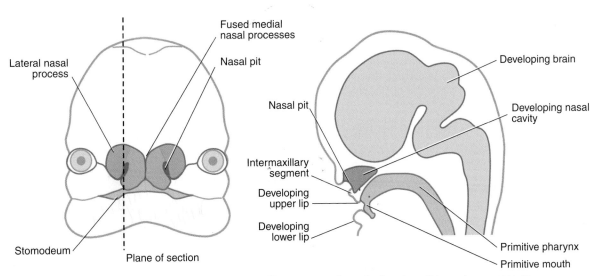

FIGURE 4-7 Development of the intermaxillary segment from the fused medial nasal processes on the inside of the stomodeum, as shown on a cross section of the embryo.

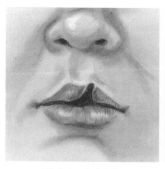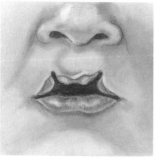

Unilateral cleft lip   Bilateral cleft lip

FIGURE 4-8 Two main types of cleft lip deformities, unilateral and bilateral clefts.

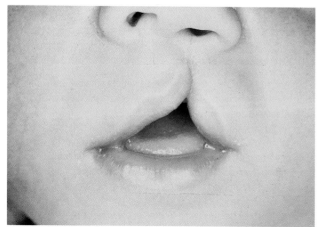

FIGURE 4-9 Unilateral cleft lip that is located at the side of the midline of the oral cavity, where the facial processes failed to fuse.

processes on each side of the developing face partially fuse with the mandibular arch on each side to create each **labial commissure,** because the mandibular arch has already formed the lower lip.

DEVELOPMENT OF THE NECK

The development of the neck parallels the development of the face over time, beginning during the fourth week of prenatal development within the embryonic period, and completed during the fetal period. The neck and its associated tissue develop from the primitive pharynx and the branchial apparatus. Dental professionals must understand the development of the neck to relate its underlying structural relationships to any developmental disturbances that may be present.

PRIMITIVE PHARYNX FORMATION

The beginnings of the embryo's hollow tube are derived from the anterior part of the **foregut** and will form the **primitive pharynx,** the future oral part of the pharynx, or **oropharynx** (Figure 4-10, see Figure 2-18). The foregut is originally derived from the **endoderm** embryonic cell layer (see Figure 3-15). The primitive pharynx widens cranially, where it joins the primitive mouth of the stomodeum and narrows caudally as it joins the esophagus. The endoderm of the pharynx lines the internal parts of the branchial arches and passes into balloon-like areas of the pharyngeal pouches (discussed later). However, this same endoderm, however, does not come to line the oral cavity proper or nasal cavity. Instead, the oral

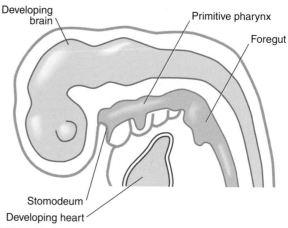

FIGURE 4-10 Foregut gives rise to the primitive pharynx, which will form the oropharynx.

cavity proper and nasal cavities are both lined by ectoderm as a result of embryonic folding.

The caudal part of the primitive pharynx forms the esophagus, which leads to the stomach. A ventral outgrowth forms the **laryngopharynx, larynx,** and trachea and ends in the superior part of the developing lungs. The **thyroid gland** is also an anterior outpocket from the ventral wall of the pharynx (see Figure 11-13).

BRANCHIAL APPARATUS FORMATION

Discussed earlier, the branchial apparatus (or pharyngeal apparatus) consists of the branchial arches, branchial grooves and membranes, and pharyngeal pouches.

BRANCHIAL ARCH FORMATION

During the fourth week of prenatal development, stacked bilateral swellings of tissue appear inferior to the stomodeum and include the mandibular arch. These are the branchial arches (or pharyngeal arches), with the mandibular arch being the first branchial arch and the others numbered in craniocaudal sequence (Figure 4-11). These branchial arches are six pairs of U-shaped bars with a core of mesenchyme formed by neural crest cells that migrate to the neck region (see Chapter 3). The branchial arches are covered externally by ectoderm, lined internally by endoderm, and support the lateral walls of the primitive pharynx.

The branchial arches are located bilaterally, oriented in an anterior-posterior direction on the embryo, bending to surround and support the lateral walls of the developing pharynx. It is important to note that the fifth branchial arch is often so rudimentary that often it is absent in humans or it is included within the fourth branchial arch. The branchial arches will give rise to important structures of the face and neck (see Table 4-2).

Each paired branchial arch has its own developing cartilage, nerve, vascular, and muscular components within each mesodermal core. The first two pairs of arches develop to the greatest extent of all the arches and are also the only ones specifically named. In general, these first pairs of arches form the middle and lower face, and the lower four pairs of arches are involved in the formation of the structures of the neck. The **first branchial arch,** or **mandibular arch,** and its associated tissue were described earlier and include Meckel's cartilage. Forming within the second branchial arch, or hyoid arch, is cartilage

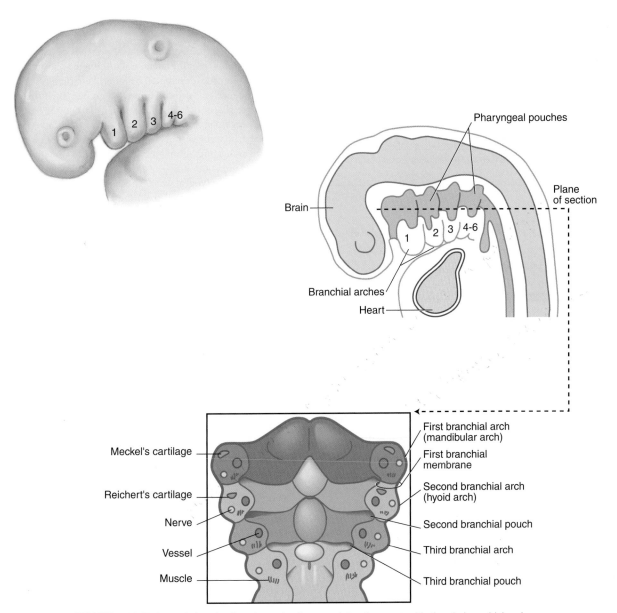

FIGURE 4-11 Embryo during the fourth week of prenatal development with the six branchial arches highlighted, with corresponding pouches on two sections.

similar to that of the mandibular arch, Reichert's cartilage. Most of it disappears during development; however, parts of it are responsible for a middle ear bone, a process of the temporal bone, and parts of the **hyoid bone.**

Additionally, the perichondrium surrounding Reichert's cartilage gives rise to the ligament of the hyoid bone. The mesoderm of the hyoid arches helps form the muscles of facial expression, the middle ear muscles, and a suprahyoid muscle. Because these muscles are derived from the hyoid arches, they are all innervated by the nerve of the second arches, the seventh cranial nerve, and the facial nerve. The hyoid arches, along with the third and fourth branchial arches, are also involved in formation of the tongue (see Figure 5-11).

During the seventh week, the muscle cells from the mesoderm of the hyoid arches have begun to differentiate. These muscle cells then begin to migrate over the mandibular muscle masses. By the tenth week, the muscle cells have migrated superiorly all over the face, forming a thin sheet of muscle masses. Both superficial and deep groups of muscle fibers eventually develop from these muscle masses and become attached to the newly differentiating bones of the facial skeleton as the muscles of facial expression. The nerve from the seventh cranial nerve is incorporated early in these muscle masses.

The third branchial arch has an unnamed cartilage associated with it. This cartilage will be responsible for the formation of parts of the hyoid bone. The only muscle to be derived from the mesoderm of each third arch is a pharyngeal muscle. Each pair of arches is innervated by the ninth cranial nerve, the glossopharyngeal nerve.

Both the fourth branchial arch and the sixth branchial arch also have unnamed cartilage associated with them. These arches fuse and participate in the formation of most of the laryngeal cartilages. The mesoderm of these arches is associated with the muscles of the larynx and pharynx. These structures are innervated by the ninth and tenth cranial nerves, although the nerves of these arches are branches of the tenth cranial nerve or vagus nerve.

TABLE 4-3	Pharyngeal Pouches and Derivative Structures
POUCHES	**FUTURE TISSUES**
First pouches	Tympanic membrane (with first branchial groove), tympanic cavity, mastoid antrum, auditory tube
Second pouches	Crypts and lymphatic nodules of the palatine tonsils
Third and fourth pouches	Parathyroid and thymus glands

BRANCHIAL GROOVE AND MEMBRANE FORMATION

Between neighboring branchial arches, external grooves are noted on each side of the embryo. These are the branchial grooves (or pharyngeal grooves) (see Figure 4-11). Only the first branchial groove, which is located between the first and second branchial arches at approximately the same level as the first pharyngeal pouches, gives rise to a definitive mature structure of the head and neck (discussed later).

The first branchial groove becomes deeper to the extent that the ectoderm of the branchial groove contacts the endoderm of the pharyngeal pouches. At this time, only a thin, double-layered membrane, the first branchial membrane, or pharyngeal membrane, separates the groove from the pouches, although mesenchyme later separates these two layers. This membrane, with its three layers, develops into the tympanic membrane (eardrum). Thus, the first groove forms the external auditory meatus. Other branchial membranes appear in the bottom of each of the four branchial grooves, although, in contrast, they are only temporary structures in the human embryo.

By the end of the seventh week, the last four branchial grooves are obliterated as a result of a sudden spurt of growth experienced by the pair of hyoid arches, which grow in an inferior direction and eventually form the neck. This obliteration of grooves gives the mature neck a smooth surface contour.

PHARYNGEAL POUCH FORMATION

Four well-defined pairs of **pharyngeal pouches** develop as endodermal evaginations from the lateral walls lining the pharynx (see Figure 4-11). The pouches develop as balloon-like structures in a craniocaudal sequence between the **branchial arches**. The fifth pharyngeal pouches are absent or rudimentary. Many structures of the face and neck are developed from the pharyngeal pouches (Table 4-3).

The first pharyngeal pouches form between the first and second branchial arches and become the auditory tubes. The **palatine tonsils** are derived from the lining of the second pharyngeal pouches and also from the pharyngeal walls. The **parathyroid glands** and thymus gland appear to be derived from the lining of the third and fourth pharyngeal pouches. Additionally, a part of the thymus gland may be of ectodermal origin.

The growth and development of the thymus are not complete at birth. The thymus is a relatively large lymphatic organ during the perinatal period and then later starts to diminish in relative size during puberty. By adulthood, the thymus at the top of the breastbone is often scarcely recognizable; however, it still is functioning by secreting thymic hormones and by maturing **T-cell lymphocytes** (see Figure 8-16).

Developmental Disturbances of the Branchial Apparatus

Most congenital malformations in the neck originate during transformation of the **branchial apparatus** into its mature derivatives. Some of these are a result of the persistence of parts of the branchial apparatus that normally disappear during development of the neck and its associated tissue.

The branchial grooves occasionally do not become obliterated, and thus parts remain as cervical cysts (or cervical sinuses). These cysts may drain through sinuses along the neck but may also remain free in the neck tissue just inferior to the angle of the mandible and anywhere along the anterior border of the **sternocleidomastoid muscle**. These cysts do not become apparent until they produce a slowly enlarging, painless swelling.

CHAPTER 5

Development of Orofacial Structures

●●● CHAPTER OUTLINE

●●● LEARNING OBJECTIVES

- Define and pronounce the key terms in this chapter.
- Outline the events that occur during the development of the orofacial structures, describing each step of formation.

- Integrate the knowledge of the development of the orofacial structures into understanding the present structure and any developmental disturbances involved in these structures.

●●● NEW KEY TERMS

Ankyloglossia (ang-ke-lo-gloss-ee-ah)
Cleft palate (kleft pal-it), uvula
Copula (kop-u-lah)

Epiglottic swelling (ep-ee-glot-ik)
Lateral lingual swellings (ling-gwal)
Palatal shelves (pal-ah-tal)

Palate (pal-it): primary, secondary
Tuberculum impar (too-ber-ku-lum im-par)

OROFACIAL DEVELOPMENT

The orofacial structures discussed in this chapter develop during the week to the twelfth week of **prenatal development**, spanning the later **embryonic period** and early **fetal period**. This chapter continues with embryonic development, starting from where the sequence left off with the development of the **stomodeum**, face and neck in Chapter 4 (see Figure 4-1 and Box 4-1). It discusses the development of the associated oral structures: palate, nasal septum, nasal cavity, and tongue, with tooth development discussed in Chapter 6. However, the development of other oral structures, such as the jaws, temporomandibular joint, and salivary glands, is discussed with their associated histology in later chapters.

Dental professionals must have an understanding about the development of the oral structures to relate their underlying structural relationships to any developmental disturbances that may be present.

PALATAL DEVELOPMENT

The formation of the **palate**, initially in the **embryo** and later in the **fetus**, takes place over several weeks of prenatal development (Table 5-1). The formation of the palate starts during the fifth week of prenatal development, within the embryonic period. The palate at this time is formed from two separate embryonic structures: primary palate and secondary palate. The palate is then completed later during the twelfth week, within the fetal period. Thus, the palate is developed in three consecutive stages: formation of the primary palate, formation of the secondary palate, and completion of the final palate.

The completion of the final palate involves the **fusion** of swellings or tissue from *different* surfaces of the embryo to meet and join, similar to that of the fusion of the neural tube (Figure 5-1, see Figure 3-10). In contrast, most of the other structures of the orofacial region develop by facial fusion, the joining of swellings or tissue on the *same* surface of the embryo, which leads to the elimination of furrows between facial tissue (see Figure 4-4).

PRIMARY PALATE FORMATION

During the fifth week of prenatal development, still within the embryonic period, the **intermaxillary segment** forms (Figure 5-2). The intermaxillary segment arises as a result of fusion of the two medial nasal processes within the embryo (see Figure 4-7). The intermaxillary

TABLE 5-1	Development of the Palate
TIME PERIOD	**PALATAL PORTIONS INVOLVED**
Fifth to sixth week	**Primary palate:** intermaxillary segment from fused medial nasal processes
Sixth to twelfth week	**Secondary palate:** fused palatal shelves from maxillary processes
Twelfth week	**Final palate:** fusion of all three processes

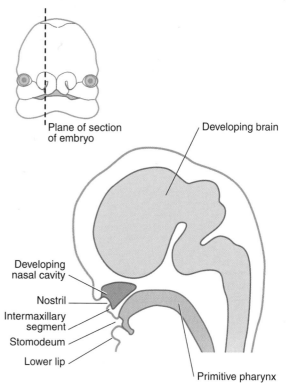

FIGURE 5-2 Intermaxillary segment formation from the fusion of the two medial nasal processes on the inside of the stomodeum of the embryo.

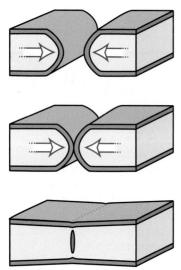

FIGURE 5-1 Process of palatal fusion that involves the joining of swellings or tissue from *different* surfaces of the embryo, unlike facial fusion with the joining of swellings or tissue on the *same* surface of the embryo.

segment is an internal wedge-shaped mass that extends inferiorly and deep to the **nasal pits** on the inside of the stomodeum. It develops into the floor of the **nasal cavity** and the **nasal septum**.

The intermaxillary segment also gives rise to the primary palate (or primitive palate). At this time, the primary palate serves only as a partial separation between the developing oral cavity proper and nasal cavity (Figure 5-3). In the future, the primary palate will form the premaxillary part of the **maxilla**, which is the anterior one third of the final palate. This small part of the **hard palate** is anterior to the **incisive foramen** and will contain certain **maxillary teeth (incisors)** (see Figure 2-12). The formation of the primary palate completes the first stage of palate development.

SECONDARY PALATE FORMATION

During the sixth week of prenatal development, within the embryonic period, the bilateral maxillary processes give rise to two palatal shelves (or lateral palatine processes) (Figures 5-4 and 5-5). These shelves grow inferiorly and deep on the inside of the stomodeum in a vertical direction, along both sides of the developing tongue. The **tongue** is forming on the floor of the **pharynx** at this time, and, as it grows, it initially fills the common nasal and oral cavity (discussed later).

As the developing tongue muscles begin to function, the tongue contracts and moves out of the way of these developing palatal shelves;

thus, the tongue avoids being an obstacle to the future fusion of the shelves by moving both anteriorly and inferiorly. This process is aided by the growth of the lower jaw primordium. The movement of the tongue makes it now confined solely to the oral cavity proper and out of the developing nasal cavity, which is completed around the eighth week of prenatal development.

Because of unknown shelf-elevating forces, the palatal shelves, after growing in a vertical direction, "flip" up in a superior direction within a few hours of the movement of the tongue. Thus, the shelves move into a horizontal position, now superior to the developing tongue. Next, the two palatal shelves elongate and move medially toward each other, meeting and joining, and fusing to form the secondary palate.

The secondary palate will give rise to the posterior two thirds of the hard palate, which contains certain anterior **maxillary teeth (canines)** and **posterior teeth**, posterior to the incisive foramen (Figure 5-6). It also gives rise to the **soft palate** and its **uvula**. The **median palatine raphe** within the mucosa lining and the deeper median palatine suture on the adult bone indicate the line of fusion of the palatal shelves (see Figure 2-12). The formation of the secondary palate completes the second stage of palate development.

COMPLETION OF PALATE

To complete the palate, the posterior part of the primary palate meets the secondary palate, and these structures gradually fuse in an anterior to posterior direction (see Figures 5-4 and 5-5). These three processes completely fuse, forming the final palate, having both hard and soft parts, during the twelfth week of prenatal development. Now the mature oral cavity becomes completely separated from the nasal cavity, which has begun to undergo development of its nasal septum (discussed next).

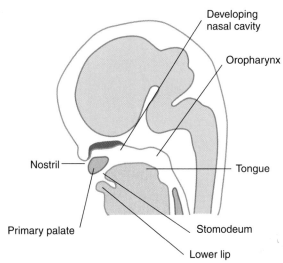

FIGURE 5-3 Primary palate formation from the intermaxillary segment, which serves as a partial separation between the developing nasal and oral cavities.

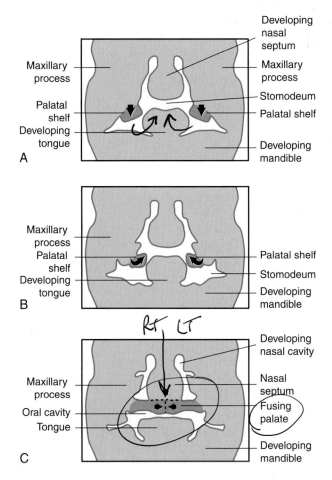

FIGURE 5-4 Developing palate is highlighted. **A:** Palatal shelves formation from the maxillary process deep on the inside of the stomodeum. The growing shelves are vertical (*arrows*) and the position of the developing tongue is between the shelves. **B:** Palatal shelves grow in a horizontal direction toward each other, after "flipping" in a superior direction (*arrows*), to form the secondary palate. **C:** Fusion of the three processes (*arrows*) to complete the final palate in the fetus: primary palate with two palatal shelves to form the secondary palate.

Bone formation (or ossification) has already begun in the anterior hard palate by the time palatal fusion is completed (see Chapter 8). In contrast, in the more posterior soft palate, mesenchyme from the first and second branchial arches migrates into the area to form the palatal muscles that will be involved in swallowing and speech (discussed later).

Small paired nasopalatine canals persist near the median plane of the mature palate at the site of the junction of the primary palate and the secondary palate (see Figure 5-6). These canals are represented in the mature hard palate by the incisive foramen, the common opening for the bilateral incisive canals. An irregular suture extends from the incisive foramen to the alveolar process of the maxilla, between the lateral incisor and canine teeth on each side. It demarcates where the primary and secondary palates fused. This bony fusion is completed within the first year of birth, and the overlying epithelium has already fused by that time.

🔹 **Developmental Disturbances of the Palate and Associated Tissue**

Failure of fusion of the palatal shelves with the primary palate and/or with each other results in cleft palate, with varying degrees of disability (Figure 5-7). This disturbance may be hereditary or associated with environmental factors. **Cleft palate**, with or without **cleft lip** (see Figure 4-8), occurs 1 in 2500 cases. It may also be isolated or associated with other abnormalities, such as cleft lip (Figure 5-8); it may also involve only the soft palate or may extend through to the hard palate. Isolated forms of cleft palate are less common than cleft lip and are more common in females, unlike cleft lip, which is more common in males. **Cleft uvula** is the least complicated example of cleft palate.

Complications can include difficulty with nursing or feeding the child, increased oronasal infections, and problems in speech and appearance. Treatment includes oral and plastic surgery, with dental intervention; however, speech and hearing therapy may also be necessary.

NASAL CAVITY AND SEPTUM DEVELOPMENT

The **nasal cavity** forms in the same time frame as the palate, from the fifth to twelfth week of prenatal development. It will serve as part of the respiratory system (see Figure 11-18). The future **nasal septum** of the nasal cavity is also developing when the palate is forming. The structure of the nasal septum, similar to the primary palate, is a growth from the fused **medial nasal processes** (Figure 5-9). The tissue types that form the nasal septum will grow inferiorly and deep to the medial nasal processes and superior to the **stomodeum**.

The vertical nasal septum then fuses with the horizontally oriented final palate after it forms (Figure 5-10, see Figure 5-5). This fusion begins in the ninth week and is completed by the twelfth week. With the formation of the nasal septum and final palate, the paired nasal cavity and the single oral cavity in the fetus become completely separate. The nasal cavity and oral cavity also undergo development of different types of mucosa, such as **respiratory mucosa** and **oral mucosa**, respectively (see Chapters 9 and 11).

The nasal septum has considerable influence on determining final orofacial form. It transmits septal growth "pull and thrust" to facial bones, such as the maxilla, as it expands its vertical length—a dramatic sevenfold between the tenth week of prenatal development and birth.

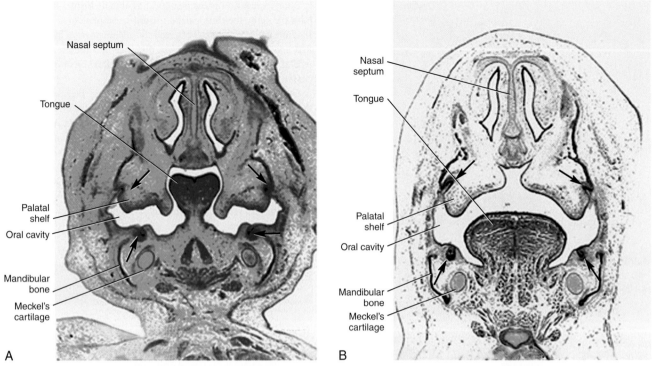

FIGURE 5-5 Photomicrographs of the palatal shelves during the formation of the secondary palate at the seventh week **(A)** and then the ninth week **(B)**. Note that the position of the tongue, oral cavity, and nasal septum (with its nasal cavity), which changes between the two time periods. The teeth in the future dental arches (*arrows*), mandibular bone, and Meckel's cartilage are also developing during this same time period. *(From Nanci A: Ten Cate's Oral Histology,* ed 7, Mosby, St Louis, 2008.)

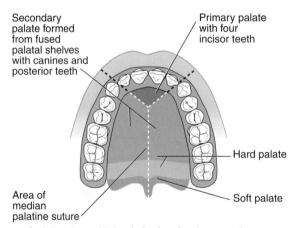

FIGURE 5-6 Diagram of adult palate with its derivative developmental structures. Suture areas highlighted (*dashed lines*) and permanent teeth noted.

TONGUE DEVELOPMENT

The **tongue** develops during the fourth to eighth weeks of prenatal development (Table 5-2). It develops from independent swellings located internally on the floor of the **primitive pharynx**, formed by the first four **branchial arches** (see Table 4-2).

Specifically, the body of the tongue develops from the first branchial arch, and the base of the tongue originates later from the second, third, and fourth branchial arches. The furrows between these swellings are eliminated by fusion similar to that on the external face, with proliferation, migration, and merging of the **mesenchyme** inferior to the **ectoderm** into the furrows.

BODY OF TONGUE FORMATION

During the fourth week of prenatal development, within the embryonic period, the tongue begins its development. The tongue development begins as a triangular median swelling, the tuberculum impar (or median tongue bud) (Figure 5-11, *A* and *B*). The single tuberculum impar is located in the midline, on the floor of the **primitive pharynx**, within the embryo's conjoined nasal and oral cavities (see Figure 4-10).

Later, two oval lateral lingual swellings (or distal tongue buds) develop on each side of the tuberculum impar. It is important to note that these anterior swellings are from the growth of mesenchyme of the **first branchial arch**, or **mandibular arch**. The paired lateral lingual swellings grow in size and merge with each other (see Figure 5-11, *A*).

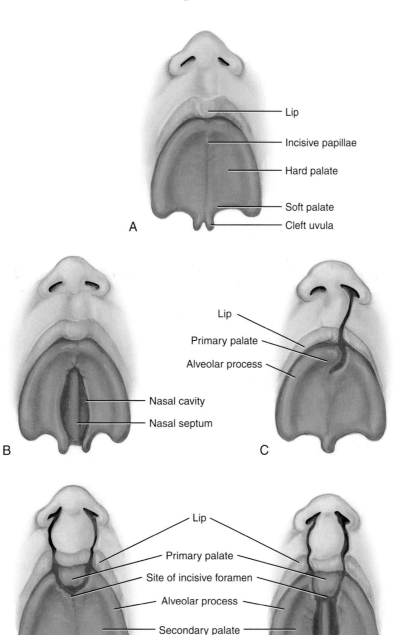

FIGURE 5-7 Various degrees of cleft palate. **A:** Cleft uvula. **B:** Bilateral cleft of the posterior palate. **C:** Complete unilateral cleft of the lip and alveolar process of the maxilla with a unilateral cleft of the primary palate. **D:** Complete bilateral cleft of the lip and alveolar process, with bilateral cleft of the primary palate. **E:** Complete bilateral cleft of the lip and alveolar process, with complete bilateral cleft of both the primary and secondary palates.

Then the two fused swellings overgrow and encompass the disappearing tuberculum impar to form the anterior two thirds, or **body of the tongue,** which lies within the oral cavity proper. The **median lingual sulcus** is a superficial demarcation of the line of fusion of the two lateral lingual swellings, as well as of a deeper fibrous structure (see Figure 2-14). However, the tuberculum impar does not form any recognizable part of the mature tongue. Around the lingual swellings, the cells degenerate, forming a sulcus, which frees the body of the tongue from the floor of the mouth, except for the attachment of the midline **lingual frenum** (see Figure 2-17).

BASE OF TONGUE FORMATION

Immediately posterior to these fused anterior swellings, a pair of swellings, the copula, becomes evident (see Figure 5-11, *B*). The copula is formed from the fusion of mesenchyme of mainly the third and parts of the **fourth branchial arch.** The copula gradually overgrows the **second branchial arch,** or **hyoid arch,** to form the **base of the tongue,** or posterior one third.

Even farther posterior to the copula is the projection of a third median swelling, the epiglottic swelling, which develops from the

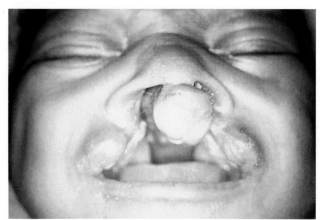

FIGURE 5-8 Complete bilateral cleft of the lip and alveolar process, with complete bilateral cleft of both the primary and secondary palates.

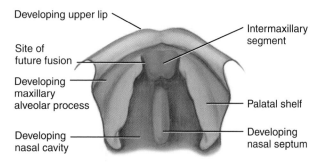

FIGURE 5-9 Growth of the fused medial nasal processes and the early stages in the formation of the nasal septum.

mesenchyme of the posterior parts of the fourth branchial arches (see Figure 5-11, C). This swelling marks the development of the most posterior region of the tongue and of the future epiglottis.

COMPLETION OF TONGUE FORMATION

As the tongue develops still further, the copula of the tongue base, after overgrowing the second branchial arch, merges with the anterior swellings of the first branchial arch of the tongue body during the eighth week of prenatal development (see Figure 5-11, C). This fusion is superficially demarcated by the **sulcus terminalis** in the mature dorsal surface of the tongue, an inverted V-shaped groove marking the border between the base of the tongue and its body (see Figure 2-14).

The sulcus terminalis points backward toward the **oropharynx** at a small pitlike depression, the **foramen cecum,** which is the beginning of the **thyroglossal duct.** This duct is the origin of and pathway showing the migration of the thyroid gland into the neck region. This duct later becomes obliterated (see Figure 11-13). No similar anatomical landmark is found between the base of the tongue and the epiglottic region.

By the end of the eighth week, the tongue has completed the fusion of these swellings. The tongue then contracts and moves anteriorly and inferiorly to avoid becoming an obstacle to the developing palatal shelves. The entire tongue is in the oral cavity proper at birth; its base and epiglottic region descend into the oropharynx by 4 years of age, while the body remains in the oral cavity proper. Thus, the tongue moves out of the pharynx into its proper place in the oral cavity

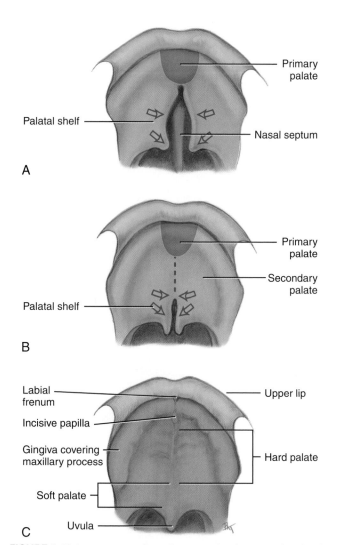

FIGURE 5-10 Later stages of nasal septum development showing its fusion with the final palate (**A** and **B**) in order to separate the nasal and oral cavities completely (**C**).

TABLE 5-2	Development of the Tongue
TIME PERIOD	**TONGUE PORTIONS INVOLVED**
Fourth to eighth week	**Body**: Tuberculum impar and lateral lingual swellings appear
	Base: Copula overgrowing second branchial arches
Eighth week	**Completed Tongue**: Merging of anterior swellings of body and copula of base

proper. The tongue normally doubles in length, breadth, and thickness between birth and puberty, when it reaches its maximum size in most persons.

The intrinsic muscles of the tongue are believed to originate from the mesoderm of the occipital **somites** and not from the branchial arches (see Figure 3-12). Primitive muscle cells from these somites migrate into the developing tongue, taking their motor nerve supply—the twelfth cranial nerve or hypoglossal nerve. Reviewing the discussion in this chapter, explains how the single structure of the

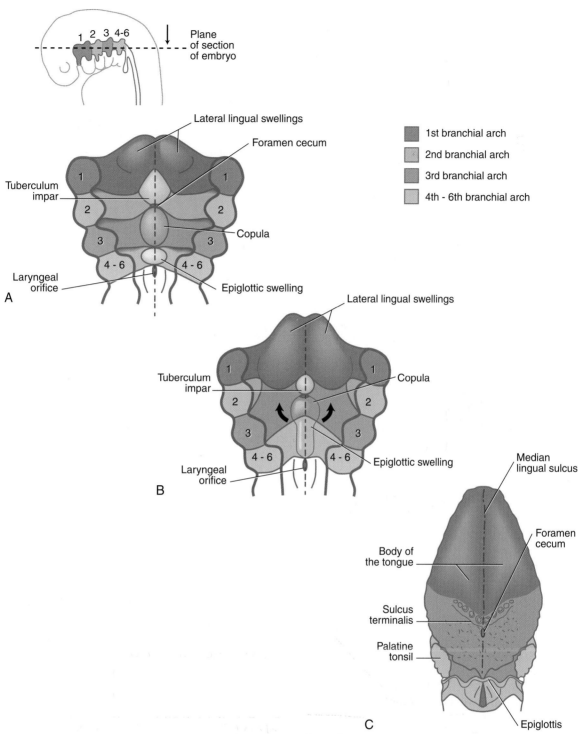

FIGURE 5-11 Diagram of the development of the tongue, with branchial arches highlighted. **A:** Tuberculum impar and lateral lingual swellings forming the body of the tongue. **B:** Copula and its involvement forming the base of the tongue (*arrows*). **C:** Final fusion of the anterior swellings and the posterior swellings to complete the tongue.

Developmental Disturbances of the Tongue

Abnormalities of the tongue are uncommon. However, one type that is more common than others is **ankyloglossia,** described as "tongue-tied," which results from a short attachment of the lingual frenum that extends to the tongue apex (Figure 5-12). This restricts the movement of the tongue to varying degrees and may be associated with other craniofacial abnormalities. However, the lingual frenum usually stretches with time (see Figure 2-17). However, if it has not adjusted over time, and movement is still not functional, **orofacial myofunctional therapy (OMT)** may be attempted before surgery is considered (see **Chapter 20**).

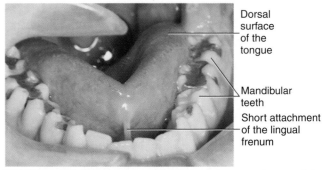

Dorsal surface of the tongue

Mandibular teeth

Short attachment of the lingual frenum

FIGURE 5-12 Ankyloglossia resulting from a short attachment of the lingual frenum that extends to the tongue apex.

tongue is innervated by various cranial nerves: It develops from the first four pairs of branchial arches (each with its own cranial nerve) and the occipital somites.

The **lingual papillae,** small elevated structures of specialized mucosa on the dorsal surface, appear toward the end of the eighth week (see Figures 2-14 and 9-15 to 9-19). The circumvallate and foliate appear first, close to the terminal branches of the glossopharyngeal nerve. The fungiform appear later, near the terminations of the chorda tympani branches of the facial nerve. Finally, the filiform develop during the early fetal period, which comprises the tenth to eleventh weeks.

The **taste buds** that are associated with certain lingual papillae develop during the eleventh to thirteenth weeks by inductive interaction between the epithelial cells of the tongue and invading nerve cells from the chorda tympani of the facial nerve and the glossopharyngeal nerve.

CHAPTER 6

Tooth Development and Eruption

●●● CHAPTER OUTLINE

●●● LEARNING OBJECTIVES

- Define and pronounce the key terms in this chapter.
- Outline the events that occur during the development of the teeth and associated structures and during tooth eruption, describing each step of formation.
- Integrate the knowledge of the development of the teeth and associated structures and tooth eruption into understanding the present anatomy of these structures and any developmental disturbances.

●●● NEW KEY TERMS

Accessory roots
Alveolar bone
Ameloblasts (ah-**mel**-oh-blasts)
Amelogenesis (ah-mel-oh-**jen**-i-sis), imperfecta (im-per-**fek**-tah)
Anodontia (an-ah-**don**-she-ah)
Apposition (ap-oh-**zish**-in)
Cells of the dental papilla (pah-**pil**-ah): central, outer
Cementoblasts (see-**men**-tah-blasts)
Cementocytes (see-**men**-toe-sites)
Cementogenesis (see-men-toe-**jen**-i-sis)
Cementoid (see-**men**-toyd)
Cervical loop (**ser**-vi-kal)
Concrescence (kahn-**kres**-ens)
Dens in dente (denz in **den**-tay)
Dental lamina (**lam**-i-nah), papilla (pah-**pil**-ah), sac
Dentigerous cyst (den-**ti**-jer-os)
Dentin dysplasia (**den**-tin dis-**play**-ze-ah)
Dentinal tubule
Dentinogenesis (den-tin-oh-**jen**-i-sis), imperfecta (im-per-**fek**-tah)

Dentition (den-**tish**-in): permanent, period, primary, mixed
Ectomesenchyme (**ek**-toe-mes-eng-kime)
Enamel epithelium (ep-ee-**thee**-lee-um): inner, outer
Enamel knot, organ, dysplasia (dis-**play**-ze-ah), pearl
Epithelial rests of Malassez (ep-ee-**thee**-lee-al mal-ah-**say**)
Eruption: active, passive
Fusion (fu-**zhin**)
Gemination (jem-i-**nay**-shin)
Hertwig's epithelial root sheath (**hirt**-wigz)
Junction: dentinocemental, dentinoenamel
Macrodontia (mak-roe-**don**-she-ah)
Matrix (**may**-triks): enamel (ih-**nam**-l)
Microdontia (mi-kro-**don**-she-ah)
Nasmyth's membrane (**nas**-miths)
Nonsuccedaneous (non-suk-seh-**dane**-ee-us)
Odontoblasts (oh-**don**-toe-blasts)

Odontoclasts (oh-**don**-toe-klasts)
Odontogenesis (oh-don-to-**jen**-eh-sis)
Oral epithelium (ep-ee-**thee**-lee-um)
Periodontal ligament
Preameloblasts (pre-ah-**mel**-oh-blasts)
Predentin
Process: odontoblastic (oh-**don**-toe-blast-ik), Tomes' (tomes)
Proliferation (pro-lif-er-**ay**-shin)
Reduced enamel epithelium (ih-**nam**-l ep-ee-**thee**-lee-um)
Repolarization (re-po-ler-i-**za**-shun)
Stage: bell, bud, cap, initiation
Stellate reticulum (**stel**-ate reh-**tik**-u-lum)
Stratum intermedium (**stra**-tum in-ter-**mede**-ee-um)
Succedaneous (suk-seh-**dane**-ee-us)
Successional dental lamina (suk-**sesh**-shun-al)
Supernumerary teeth (soo-per-**nu**-mer-air-ee)
Tooth fairy, germ
Tubercles (**tu**-ber-kls)

TOOTH DEVELOPMENT

Dental professionals must have a clear understanding of the stages of odontogenesis or tooth development and their physiological basis. Developmental disturbances can occur within each stage of odontogenesis, affecting the physiological processes taking place. These developmental disturbances can have ramifications that may affect the clinical treatment of a patient.

DEVELOPMENT OF THE DENTITIONS

The term dentition is used to describe the natural teeth in the jaws (see Chapter 15). There are two dentitions: primary dentition and permanent dentition. A child's primary dentition develops during the prenatal period and consists of 20 teeth, which erupt and are later shed or exfoliated (see Chapter 18). As the primary teeth are shed and the jaws grow and mature, the permanent dentition, consisting of as many as 32 teeth, gradually erupts and replaces the primary dentition (see Chapters 16 and 17). An overlapping period between the primary and permanent dentition during the preteen years is referred

to as the *mixed dentition* period, when an individual has some teeth from both dentitions (see Figures 15-4 and 18-17).

This chapter initially focuses on the development of the primary dentition, and then its eruption and shedding. The final discussion centers on the eruption of the permanent dentition. The process of development for both dentitions is similar; only the associated time frame for each is different. The overall general dental anatomy associated with both these dentitions is discussed further in Chapter 15.

Odontogenesis takes place in stages, which occur in a stepwise fashion for both dentitions (Table 6-1). Odontogenesis is a continuous process until completed, and there is no clear-cut beginning or end point between stages. However, these stages are used to help focus on the different events in odontogenesis and are based on the appearance of the developing structures. After initiation of odontogenesis, identifiable stages in tooth development include the bud stage, the cap stage, and the bell stage. Odontogenesis then progresses to the stage of apposition with the formation of the hard dental tissue types, such as enamel, dentin, and cementum, and then finally to the stage of maturation for these structures (Table 6-2).

TABLE 6-1	Stages of Tooth Development		
STAGE/TIME SPAN*	**MICROSCOPIC APPEARANCE**	**MAIN PROCESSES INVOLVED**	**DESCRIPTION**
Initiation stage/sixth to seventh week		Induction	Ectoderm lining stomodeum gives rise to oral epithelium and then to dental lamina; adjacent to deeper ectomesenchyme, which is influenced by the neural crest cells. Both tissue types are separated by a basement membrane
Bud stage/eighth week		Proliferation	Growth of dental lamina into bud shape that penetrates growing ectomesenchyme
Cap stage/ninth to tenth week		Proliferation, differentiation, morphogenesis	Formation of tooth germ as enamel organ forms into cap shape that surrounds inside mass of dental papilla, with an outside mass of dental sac, both from the ectomesenchyme.
Bell stage/eleventh to twelfth week		Proliferation, differentiation, morphogenesis	Differentiation of enamel organ into bell shape with four cell types and dental papilla into two cell types

Handwritten annotations: "successional dental lamina", "primordium of succedaneous tooth", "enamel organ", "dental papilla", "dental sac", "tooth germ"

TABLE 6-1	Stages of Tooth Development—cont'd		
STAGE/TIME SPAN*	MICROSCOPIC APPEARANCE	MAIN PROCESSES INVOLVED	DESCRIPTION
Apposition stage/varies per tooth		Induction, proliferation	Dental tissue types secreted in successive layers as matrix
Maturation stage/varies per tooth		Maturation	Dental tissue types fully mineralize to mature form

*Note that these are approximate prenatal time spans for the development of the primary dentition.

TABLE 6-2	Comparison of Dental Hard Tissue Types			
	ENAMEL	DENTIN	CEMENTUM	ALVEOLAR BONE
Embryological background	Enamel organ	Dental papilla	Dental sac	Mesoderm
Tissue source or type	Epithelium	Connective tissue	Connective tissue	Connective tissue
Formative cells	Ameloblasts	Odontoblasts	Cementoblasts	Osteoblasts
Incremental lines	Lines of Retzius	Imbrication lines of von Ebner	Arrest and reversal lines	Arrest and reversal lines
Mature cells	None, lost in reduced enamel epithelium with eruption	None within, only dentinal tubules with processes, found instead in pulp	Cementocytes	Osteocytes
Resorptive cells	Odontoclasts	Odontoclasts	Odontoclasts	Osteoclasts
Mineral levels (approximate)	96%	70%	65%	60%
Organic and water levels (approximate)	1% organic, 3% water	20% organic, 10% water	23% organic, 12% water	25% organic, 15% water
Formation after eruption	None, only may undergo remineralization	Possible	Possible	Possible
Vascularity	None	None	None	Present
Innervation	None	Possibly present within dentinal tubule, found instead in pulp	None	Present

During these stages of odontogenesis, many physiological processes occur. In many ways, these parallel the processes that occur in the formation of other embryonic structures, such as the face. These physiological processes include **induction, proliferation, differentiation, morphogenesis,** and **maturation** (see Table 3-3). Except for the induction process, many of these processes overlap and are somewhat continuous during odontogenesis. However, one individual process does tend to be predominant and mark each stage of odontogenesis.

In the past, the study of odontogenesis included a discussion of *developmental lobes* that were thought to be growth centers during tooth development. These parts of the crown of the tooth are both microscopically and clinically visible by the presence of associated depressions. Whether there may be any justification for including them in a discussion of tooth formation remains controversial; developmental lobes may simply be evidence of the tooth form only, but information concerning lobes are included in this textbook for completeness.

Not all the teeth in each dentition begin to develop at the same time across each arch of the jaws. The initial teeth for both dentitions develop in the anterior mandibular region, followed later by the anterior maxillary region, and then development progresses posteriorly in both jaws. This posterior progression of odontogenesis allows time for

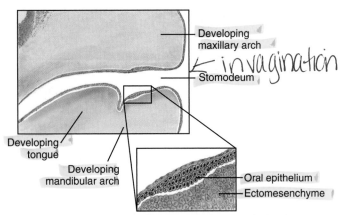

FIGURE 6-1 Initiation stage of odontogenesis, or tooth development, of the primary teeth on cross section, highlighting the developing mandibular arch. The stomodeum is now lined by oral epithelium, with the deeper ectomesenchyme influenced by neural crest cells. A similar situation is occurring in the maxillary arch.

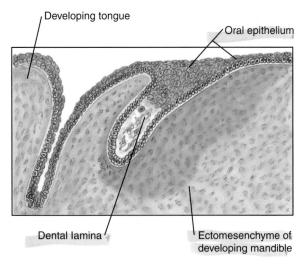

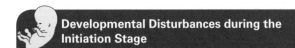

FIGURE 6-2 Development of the dental lamina from the oral epithelium in the mandibular arch, where primary teeth will later form during the initiation stage, surrounded by ectomesenchyme. A similar situation is also occurring in the maxillary arch.

the jaws to grow to accommodate the increased number of primary teeth, the larger primary molars, and then finally the overall larger permanent teeth.

The primary dentition develops during both the **embryonic period** and **fetal period** of **prenatal development**. Most of the permanent dentition is formed during the fetal period. Tooth development continues for years after birth, however, especially considering the formation of the permanent second and third molars; see Unit IV and Appendix D for tooth development timelines. Thus, teeth have the longest developmental period of any set of organs in the body.

INITIATION STAGE

Odontogenesis of the primary dentition begins between the sixth and seventh week of prenatal development, during the embryonic period (Figure 6-1). This first stage of tooth development, known as the initiation stage, involves the physiological process of **induction,** which is an active interaction between the embryological tissue types. Studies show that mesenchymal tissue must influence the ectodermal tissue in order to initiate odontogenesis, but the exact mechanisms are unknown at this time.

At the beginning of the sixth week, the embryo's **stomodeum,** or primitive mouth, is lined by ectoderm (see Chapter 4). The outer part of the ectoderm gives rise to **oral epithelium.** The oral epithelium initially consists of two horseshoe-shaped bands of tissue at the surface of the stomodeum, one for each future arch or jaw. At the same time, deep to the forming oral epithelium, there is a type of mesenchyme originally from the ectoderm, ectomesenchyme, which is influenced by **neural crest cells** that have migrated to the area (see Figure 6-1).

An important acellular structure that separates the oral epithelium and the ectomesenchyme within the stomodeum is the **basement membrane.** This basement membrane is similar to the one separating all epithelium and connective tissue (see Figure 8-4).

During the later part of the seventh week, the oral epithelium grows deeper into the ectomesenchyme and is induced to produce a layer, the dental lamina (Figure 6-2). This growth occurs in the developing jaw areas where the two future curved **dental arches** of the primary dentition will form. The dental lamina then begins to form initially in the midline for both arches and progresses posteriorly.

Developmental Disturbances during the Initiation Stage

Lack of **initiation** within the **dental lamina** results in the absence of a single tooth (partial) or multiple teeth (complete), producing anodontia (Table 6-3, *A*). However, partial anodontia (hypodontia) is more common and most commonly occurs (listed in order of occurrence) with the permanent maxillary lateral incisors, third molars, and mandibular second premolars. Anodontia can be associated with the syndrome of **ectodermal dysplasia,** because many parts of the tooth are indirectly or directly of ectodermal origin (see Figure 3-13.)

Anodontia can also result from endocrine dysfunction, systemic disease, and exposure to excess radiation, such as that in radiation therapy used with cancer treatment, and may cause disruption of occlusion and esthetic problems. Patients may need partial or full dentures, bridges, or implants to replace the missing teeth. If severe, it can result in disruption of the complete development of the jaws.

In contrast, abnormal **initiation** may result in the development of one or more extra teeth, or **supernumerary teeth** (hyperdontia) (see Table 6-3, *B*). These extra teeth are initiated from the **dental lamina** and have a hereditary etiology. Certain areas of both dentitions commonly have supernumerary teeth, such as (listed in order of occurrence) between the maxillary central incisors (**mesiodens**, see Chapter 16), distal to the maxillary third molars (distomolar or "fourth molar"), and in the premolar region (perimolar) of both dental arches. They are smaller than normal, and most are accidentally discovered on radiographic examination. These extra teeth may be either erupted or noneurupted and in both cases may cause dentition displacement, crowding, and delayed eruption to the adjacent teeth, as well as occlusal disruption; thus, removal by surgery is often necessary.

BUD STAGE

The second stage of odontogenesis is considered the bud stage and occurs at the beginning of the eighth week of prenatal development for the primary dentition (Figures 6-3 and 6-4). This stage is named for an extensive **proliferation** of the dental lamina into buds or oval masses that penetrate into the ectomesenchyme. At the end of the

TABLE 6-3	Common Dental Developmental Disturbances and Involved Stage			
DISTURBANCE	**STAGE**	**DESCRIPTION**	**ETIOLOGICAL FACTORS**	**CLINICAL RAMIFICATIONS**
A. Anodontia (missing maxillary lateral incisors) (missing mandibular second premolars)	Initiation stage	Absence of single or multiple teeth	Hereditary, endocrine dysfunction, systemic disease, excess radiation exposure	May cause disruption of occlusion and esthetic problems. May need partial or full dentures, bridges, and/or implants to replace teeth
B. Supernumerary teeth (mesiodens) 	Initiation stage	Development of one or more extra teeth	Hereditary	Commonly found between the maxillary centrals, distal to third molars and premolar region. May cause crowding, failure of normal eruption, and disruption of occlusion

Continued

TABLE 6-3	Common Dental Developmental Disturbances and Involved Stage—cont'd			
DISTURBANCE	**STAGE**	**DESCRIPTION**	**ETIOLOGICAL FACTORS**	**CLINICAL RAMIFICATIONS**
C. Microdontia/ macrodontia 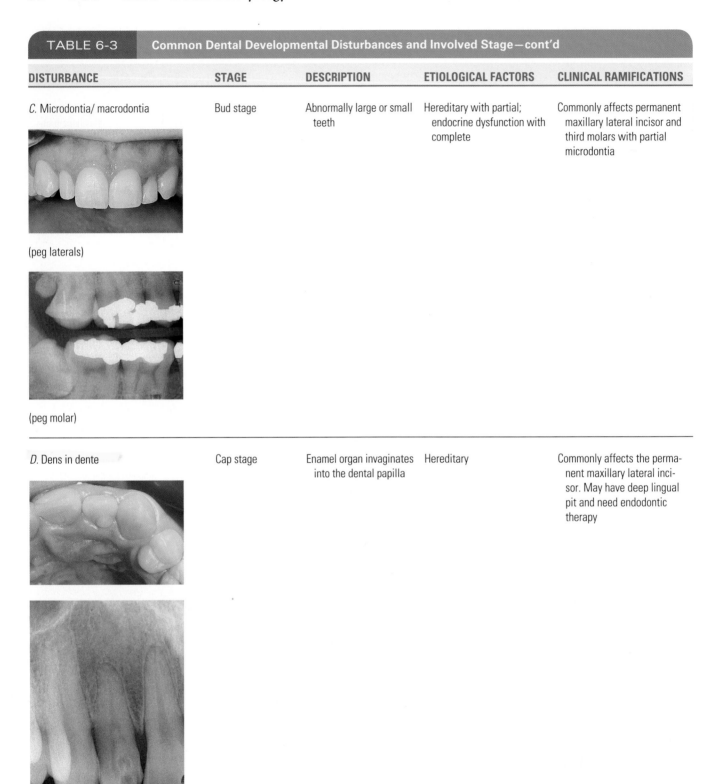 (peg laterals) (peg molar)	Bud stage	Abnormally large or small teeth	Hereditary with partial; endocrine dysfunction with complete	Commonly affects permanent maxillary lateral incisor and third molars with partial microdontia
D. Dens in dente	Cap stage	Enamel organ invaginates into the dental papilla	Hereditary	Commonly affects the permanent maxillary lateral incisor. May have deep lingual pit and need endodontic therapy

TABLE 6-3	Common Dental Developmental Disturbances and Involved Stage—cont'd			
DISTURBANCE	**STAGE**	**DESCRIPTION**	**ETIOLOGICAL FACTORS**	**CLINICAL RAMIFICATIONS**
E. Gemination	Cap stage	Tooth germ tries to divide	Hereditary	Large single-rooted tooth with one pulp cavity, with "twinning" in crown area. Normal number of teeth in dentition. May cause problems in appearance and spacing
F. Fusion	Cap stage	Union of two adjacent tooth germs	Pressure on area	Large tooth with two pulp cavities. One fewer tooth in dentition. May cause problems in appearance and spacing

Continued

TABLE 6-3	Common Dental Developmental Disturbances and Involved Stage—cont'd			
DISTURBANCE	**STAGE**	**DESCRIPTION**	**ETIOLOGICAL FACTORS**	**CLINICAL RAMIFICATIONS**
G. Tubercle	Cap stage	Extra cusp from affect on enamel organ	Trauma, pressure or metabolic disease	Commonly found on permanent molars or cingulum of anterior teeth
H. Enamel dysplasia	Apposition and maturation stages	Faulty development of enamel from interference involving ameloblasts	Local or systemic; hereditary	Pitting and intrinsic color changes in enamel, with changes in thickness of enamel possible. Problems in function and esthetics
I. Concrescence	Apposition and maturation stages	Union of root structure of two or more teeth by cementum	Traumatic injury or crowding of teeth	Commonly affects permanent maxillary molars. Problems with extraction

TABLE 6-3	Common Dental Developmental Disturbances and Involved Stage—cont'd			
DISTURBANCE	**STAGE**	**DESCRIPTION**	**ETIOLOGICAL FACTORS**	**CLINICAL RAMIFICATIONS**
J. Enamel pearl	Apposition and maturation stages	Sphere of enamel on root	Displacement of ameloblasts to root	May be confused as calculus deposit on root

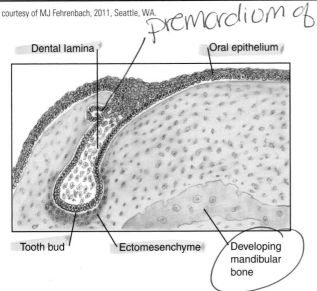

All courtesy of MJ Fehrenbach, 2011, Seattle, WA.

Premordium of succadaneous tooth

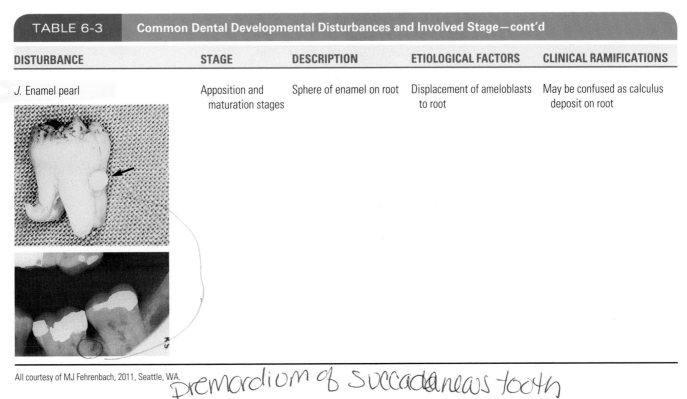

FIGURE 6-3 Bud stage, which involves extensive proliferation of the dental lamina into the ectomesenchyme in the form of buds, the future tooth germs.

proliferation process involving the primary dentition's dental lamina, both the future maxillary arch and the future mandibular arch will each have 10 buds. The underlying **ectomesenchyme** also undergoes adjacent proliferation. However, a **basement membrane** remains between the bud and the surrounding growing ectomesenchyme.

Each of these buds from the dental lamina, together with the surrounding ectomesenchyme, will develop into a **tooth germ** with its associated supporting tissue during the next stage. Thus, all the teeth and their associated tissue types develop from both ectoderm and the mesenchymal tissue, ectomesenchyme, which is influenced by **neural crest cells**.

However, only proliferation of these two tissue types occurs during this stage; no structural change occurs in the cells of either the dental lamina or ectomesenchyme as later occurs with differentiation and morphogenesis of these tissue types. In areas where teeth will not be

Developmental Disturbances during the Bud Stage

Abnormal **proliferation** can cause a single tooth (partial) or the entire dentition (complete) to be larger or smaller than normal. Abnormally large teeth result in **macrodontia**; abnormally small teeth result in **microdontia** (see Table 6-3, *C*). Individual teeth can sometimes appear larger than normal as a result of splitting of the enamel organ or fusion of two adjacent tooth germs, but this is not true case of partial macrodontia (these other disturbances are discussed later), or appear smaller by being in a large set of jaws (relative). Hereditary factors are involved, and teeth commonly affected with true partial microdontia are the permanent maxillary lateral incisor (**peg lateral**, see Chapter 16) and permanent third molars (**peg molars**, see Figure 17-50).

Complete microdontia of either dentition rarely occurs but can occur with hypopituitarism (dwarfism) or **Down syndrome** (see Figure 3-5). In contrast, systemic conditions such as childhood hyperpituitarism (gigantism) can produce complete macrodontia. However, some population groups have overall larger teeth than other groups; one of these is the Inuit people of arctic regions of North America.

developing, the dental lamina only remains thickened; it lines the stomodeum but does not produce buds. Later, this non–tooth-producing part of the dental lamina disintegrates as the developing oral mucosa comes to line the maturing oral cavity.

CAP STAGE

The third stage of odontogenesis is considered the cap stage and occurs for the primary dentition between the ninth and tenth week of prenatal development, during the fetal period (Figures 6-5 and 6-6). The physiological process of **proliferation** continues during this stage, but the tooth bud of the dental lamina does *not* grow into a large sphere surrounded by ectomesenchyme. Instead, there is unequal

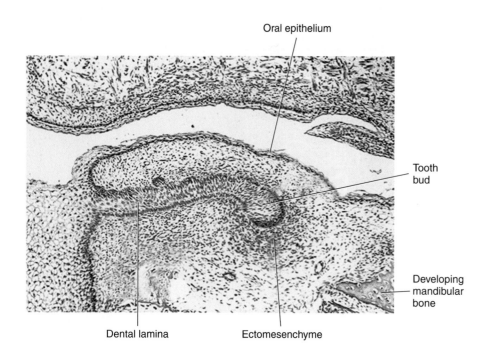

Oral epithelium

Tooth bud

Developing mandibular bone

Dental lamina   Ectomesenchyme

FIGURE 6-4 Photomicrograph of the bud stage, which involves extensive proliferation of the dental lamina into the ectomesenchyme in the form of buds, the future tooth germs. *(From Nanci A:* Ten Cate's Oral Histology, *ed 7, Mosby, St Louis, 2008.)*

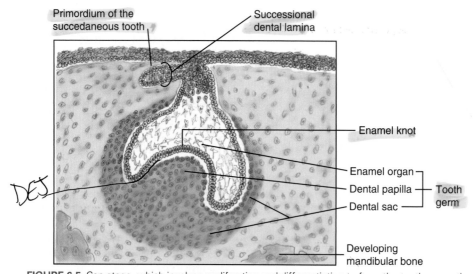

Primordium of the succedaneous tooth

Successional dental lamina

Enamel knot

Enamel organ
Dental papilla — Tooth germ
Dental sac

Developing mandibular bone

FIGURE 6-5 Cap stage, which involves proliferation and differentiation to form the tooth germ, the primordium of a primary tooth. Tooth germ consists of the enamel organ with enamel knot, dental papilla, and dental sac. Note that the primordium of the permanent succedaneous tooth, from the growth of the successional dental lamina (*circle*), is located lingual to the primary tooth germ and is in the bud stage.

growth in different parts of the tooth bud, leading to formation of a cap shape attached to the dental lamina.

Thus, not only does proliferation characterize this stage, but various levels of **differentiation,** including the more specific processes of cytodifferentiation, histodifferentiation, and morphodifferentiation, are also active during the cap stage. Additionally during this stage, a primordium of the tooth (or tooth germ) develops with a specific form. Therefore, the predominant physiological process during the cap stage is one of **morphogenesis.**

From these combined physiological processes, a depression results in the deepest part of each tooth bud of dental lamina, forming the cap, or enamel organ. It is important to note that the enamel organ was originally derived from **ectoderm,** making enamel an ectodermal product. In the future, the enamel organ will produce enamel on the outer surface of the tooth. The innermost margin of the cap shape of the enamel organ orchestrates the tooth's future crown form, such as

cusps; specifically, this may occur through nondividing cells in the enamel knot seen in the developing molars.

A part of the **ectomesenchyme** deep to the buds has condensed into a mass within the concavity of the cap of the enamel organ. This inner mass of ectomesenchyme is now considered the dental papilla. The dental papilla will produce the future dentin and pulp for the inner part of the tooth. Note that the dental papilla is originally derived from ectomesenchyme, which is influenced by **neural crest cells.** Thus, dentin and pulp are of mesenchymal origin. However, a **basement membrane** still exists as before, but now it is between the enamel organ and the dental papilla, being the site of the future **dentinoenamel junction.**

The remaining ectomesenchyme surrounding the outside of the cap or enamel organ condenses into the dental sac, or dental follicle. In the future, the capsule-like dental sac will produce the **periodontium,** the supporting tissue types of the tooth: cementum, periodontal

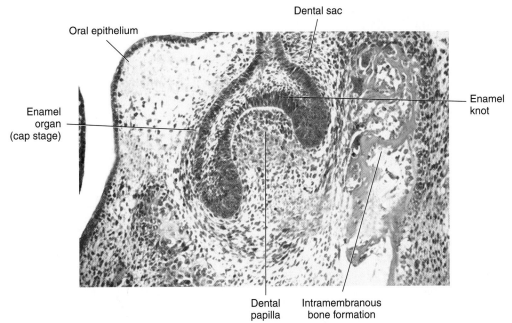

FIGURE 6-6 Photomicrograph of the cap stage showing the enamel organ from the dental lamina, as well as the adjacent dental papilla and dental sac from the ectomesenchyme. Note that oral epithelium is still lining the stomadeum, and intramembranous bone formation is also occurring. *(From Nanci A: Ten Cate's Oral Histology, ed 7, Mosby, St Louis, 2008.)*

TABLE 6-4	Components of Tooth Germ during Cap Stage	
COMPONENT	**DESCRIPTION OF COMPONENT**	**FUTURE DENTAL TISSUE TYPE PRODUCED**
Enamel organ	Formation of tooth bud in a cap shape with deep central depression	Enamel
Dental papilla	Condensed mass of ectomesenchyme within the concavity of the enamel organ	Dentin and pulp
Dental sac	Condensed mass of ectomesenchyme surrounding outside of the enamel organ	Cementum, periodontal ligament, alveolar bone

ligament, and alveolar bone. It is important to note that the dental sac is originally derived from **ectomesenchyme**; thus, this supporting dental tissue is of mesenchymal origin. A similar **basement membrane** also separates the enamel organ and dental sac.

At the end of the cap stage, these three embryological structures—the enamel organ, dental papilla, and dental sac—are now considered together to be the tooth germ, which is the **primordium** of the tooth (Table 6-4). These initial 10 tooth germs housed within each of two developing **dental arches** will develop into the **primary dentition**.

Already at the tenth week of prenatal development, during the cap stage for each primary tooth, initiation is occurring for the anterior teeth of the permanent dentition. Each primordium for these initially formed permanent teeth appears as an extension of the dental lamina into the ectomesenchyme lingual to the developing primary tooth germs. Its site of origin is the successional dental lamina (see Figure 6-26).

Permanent teeth formed with primary predecessors are considered to be succedaneous and include the anterior teeth and premolars, which replace the primary anterior teeth and molars, respectively. The crown of the permanent succedaneous will erupt lingual to the root(s) of its primary predecessor, if the primary tooth has not been fully shed or lost.

In contrast, the permanent molars are nonsuccedaneous and have no primary predecessors. Instead the six permanent molars per dental arch develop from a posterior extension of the **dental lamina** distal to the dental lamina of the primary second molar and its associated ectomesenchyme for each of the four quadrants.

BELL STAGE

The fourth stage of odontogenesis is considered the bell stage (Figures 6-7 and 6-8), which occurs for the primary dentition between the eleventh and twelfth week of prenatal development. It is characterized by continuation of the ongoing processes of proliferation, differentiation, and morphogenesis. However, **differentiation** on all levels occurs to its furthest extent, and as a result, four different types of cells are now found within the enamel organ (Table 6-5). These cell types form layers to include: inner enamel epithelium, outer enamel epithelium, stellate reticulum, and stratum intermedium. Thus, the cap shape of the enamel organ, evident during the last stage, now assumes a bell shape with this stage.

The outer cuboidal cells of the enamel organ are the outer enamel epithelium (OEE). The OEE will serve as a protective barrier for the rest of the **enamel organ** during enamel production. The innermost tall columnar cells of the enamel organ are the inner enamel epithelium (IEE). In the future, the IEE will differentiate into enamel-secreting cells (**ameloblasts**). However, a basement membrane still remains between the IEE and the adjacent dental papilla.

Developmental Disturbances during the Cap Stage

During the cap stage, the **enamel organ** may abnormally invaginate into the **dental papilla**, resulting in **dens in dente** or dens invaginatus (see Table 6-3, *D*). The teeth most commonly affected are the permanent maxillary incisors, especially the lateral incisor, and may be associated with hereditary factors (see **Chapter 16**). The invagination produces an enamel-lined pocket extending from the lingual surface. This usually leaves the tooth with a deep lingual pit in the area where the invagination occurs and may appear as a "tooth within a tooth" on radiographic examination. This lingual pit may lead to pulpal exposure and pathology, and subsequent endodontic therapy; therefore, early detection is important.

Another disturbance that can occur during the cap stage is **gemination** (see Table 6-3, *E*). This disturbance occurs as the single **tooth germ** that tries unsuccessfully to divide into two tooth germs, which results in a large single-rooted tooth with a common pulp cavity. The tooth exhibits "twinning" in the crown area, resulting in a broader, falsely macrodontic tooth, similar to fusion (discussed next). However, when this is verified by radiographic examination, it shows only one pulp cavity, and the number of teeth in either dentition with this disturbance is usually normal. The appearance of splitting can be detected as a cleft with varying depths in the incisal surface, or it may manifest as two crowns. It usually occurs in the anteriors in either dentition, may be due to hereditary factors, and can create problems in appearance, spacing, and thus periodontal health

Another disturbance that can occur during the cap stage is **fusion** (see Table 6-3, *F*). This results from the union of two adjacent **tooth germs**, possibly resulting from pressure in the area, which leads to a broader, falsely macrodontic tooth similar to gemination, but when it is verified by radiographic examination, it shows two distinct **pulp cavities**, with the enamel, dentin, and pulp united. Fusion usually occurs only in the crown area of the tooth, but it can involve both the crown and root, and the arch of the dentition with this disturbance has one less tooth. It occurs more commonly with the anteriors of the primary dentition and can present problems in appearance and spacing.

Teeth may also have **tubercles** or extra **cusps** (see Table 6-3, *G*, **Chapters 16 and 17**) that appear as small, round, enamel extensions. They are noted mainly on the **occlusal surface** of permanent molars, especially the third molars, and may also be present as a lingual extension on the **cingulum** on permanent maxillary anteriors, especially lateral incisors and canines, but can be found on any tooth in both dentitions. This disturbance may be due to trauma, pressure, or metabolic disease that affects the **enamel organ** as it forms the crown area.

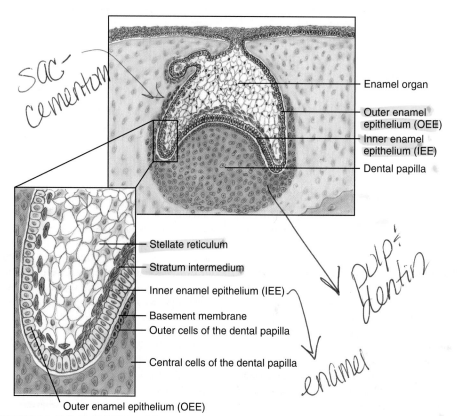

FIGURE 6-7 Bell stage, which exhibits differentiation of the tooth germ to its furthest extent. Both the enamel organ and dental papilla have differentiated into various layers in preparation for the apposition of enamel and dentin.

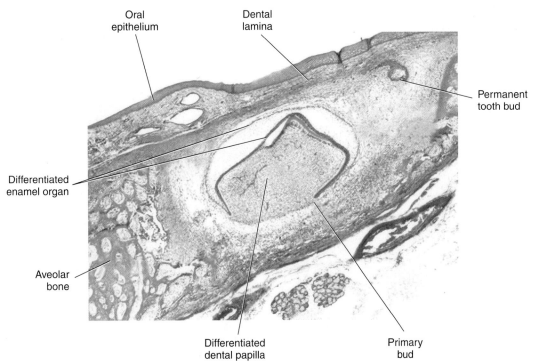

Oral epithelium

Dental lamina

Permanent tooth bud

Differentiated enamel organ

Aveolar bone

Differentiated dental papilla

Primary bud

FIGURE 6-8 Photomicrograph of the bell stage of the primary tooth, which exhibits differentiation of the tooth germ to its furthest extent. Both enamel organ and dental papilla have differentiated into various layers in preparation for the apposition of enamel and dentin. *(From Nanci A:* Ten Cate's Oral Histology, *ed 7, Mosby, St Louis, 2008.)*

TABLE 6-5	Cell Layers of the Tooth during the Bell Stage (from Outer to Inner)	
CELL LAYERS	**DESCRIPTION OF LAYER**	**ROLE IN TOOTH FORMATION**
Dental sac	Increasing amount of collagen fibers forming around the enamel organ	Will differentiate into cementum, periodontal ligament, and alveolar bone
Outer enamel epithelium (OEE)	Outer cuboidal cells of enamel organ	Serves as protective barrier for enamel organ
Stellate reticulum	More outer star-shaped cells in many layers, forming a network within the enamel organ	Supports the production of enamel matrix
Stratum intermedium	More inner compressed layer of flat to cuboidal cells	Supports the production of enamel matrix — nutritive value
Inner enamel epithelium (IEE)	Innermost tall, columnar cells of enamel organ	Will differentiate into ameloblasts that form enamel matrix
Outer cells of dental papilla	Peripheral layer of cells of the dental papilla nearest the inner enamel epithelium of the enamel organ (note the presence of basement membrane between this outer layer and the IEE)	Will differentiate into odontoblasts that form dentin matrix
Central cells of dental papilla	Inner cell mass of the dental papilla	Will differentiate into pulp tissue

Between the outer and inner enamel epithelium are the two innermost layers, the stellate reticulum and stratum intermedium. The outermost stellate reticulum consists of star-shaped cells in many layers, forming a network. The innermost stratum intermedium is made up of a compressed layer of flat to cuboidal cells. Both of these two intermediately placed layers of the enamel organ help support the future production of **enamel**.

At the same time, the **dental papilla** within the concavity of the enamel organ is also undergoing extensive differentiation so that it now consists of two types of tissue in layers: outer cells of the dental papilla and central cells of the dental papilla (see Table 6-5). In the future, the outer cells of the dental papilla (or peripheral cells) will differentiate into dentin-secreting cells (**odontoblasts**), whereas the central cells (or inner cells) become the **primordium** of the **pulp**. The outermost dental sac increases only its amount of collagen fibers at this time and thus undergoes differentiation into its mature dental tissue types of cementum, periodontal ligament, and alveolar bone later than that of both the enamel organ and dental papilla.

STAGES OF APPOSITION AND MATURATION

The final stages of odontogenesis include the stage of apposition or secretory stage, during which the enamel, dentin, and cementum are secreted in successive layers. These hard dental tissue types are initially secreted as a matrix, which is an extracellular substance that is partially mineralized, yet serves as a framework for later mineralization.

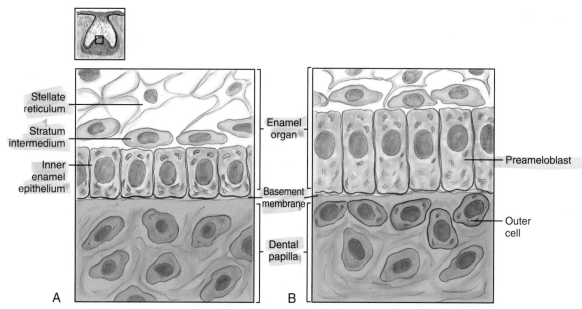

FIGURE 6-9 Close-up of inner enamel epithelium of the enamel organ differentiating into the pream-eloblasts, the future cells that will secrete enamel matrix. **A:** Inner enamel epithelial cells, with their central nuclei, line up along the basement membrane. **B:** Inner enamel epithelial cells that have elongated and repolarized their nuclei to become preameloblasts. Note the outer cells of the dental papilla are lined up on the other side of basement membrane.

The stage of **maturation** is reached when the matrices of the hard dental tissue types subsequently fully mineralize. It is important to note that the period of time for these two final stages varies according to the tooth involved but overall involves the same chronology as the initiation of odontogenesis. The results of the maturation of each hard dental tissue are noted in Table 6-2; this table should be again consulted during the histological study of each dental tissue in Unit III.

During the stage of apposition, many **inductions** occur between the ectodermal tissue of the enamel organ and mesenchymal tissue of the dental papilla and dental sac. Studies show that these interactions are necessary for the production of enamel, dentin, and cementum by the proliferation of cellular byproducts; these are examples of the biological concept known as *reciprocal induction*. Acting not only as a boundary between the two tissue types, the basement membrane conveys communications between the cells of the enamel organ, the dental papilla, and the dental sac, allowing these tissue interactions.

This part of the chapter mainly focuses on the production of enamel and coronal dentin, with the development of the crown of the tooth discussed first (maturation and histology are discussed in Chapters 12 and 13, respectively). This follows the same timeline as tooth development, given that development begins in the crown and then proceeds to the root, which is evident on most periapical or panoramic radiographs of a mixed dentition (see Figure 6-27, *A*). Root development with root dentin and cementum formation is discussed later in this chapter. The events in the production of enamel and coronal dentin include the formation of preameloblasts, odontoblasts and dentin matrix, ameloblasts, dentinoenamel junction, and enamel matrix (see Table 6-5).

FORMATION OF PREAMELOBLASTS

After the formation of the IEE in the bell-shaped enamel organ, these innermost cells grow even more columnar or elongate as they differentiate into preameloblasts (Figure 6-9). During this **differentiation** process, the **nucleus** in each cell moves away from the center of the cell to the position farthest away from the **basement membrane** that

separates the enamel organ from the dental papilla. This movement of all the nuclei in the IEE cells occurs during cellular repolarization, and studies show its importance in the change of the IEE cells into preameloblasts. In the future, the preameloblasts will first induce dental papilla cells to differentiate into dentin-forming cells (odontoblasts), and then will differentiate into cells that secrete enamel (ameloblasts).

FORMATION OF ODONTOBLASTS AND DENTIN MATRIX

After the IEE differentiates into preameloblasts, the **outer cells of the dental papilla** are induced by the preameloblasts to differentiate into odontoblasts (Figures 6-10 and 6-11). These cells also undergo **repolarization**, which results in their **nuclei** moving from the center to a position in the cell farthest from the separating **basement membrane**. These repolarized cells also line up adjacent to the basement membrane but in a mirror-image orientation compared with the preameloblasts. After the differentiation and repolarization, the odontoblasts now begin dentinogenesis, which is the apposition of **dentin matrix**, or predentin, on their side of the basement membrane. Thus, the odontoblasts start their secretory activity some time before enamel matrix production begins. This timing difference in production explains why the dentin layer in any location in a developing tooth is slightly thicker than the corresponding layer of enamel matrix.

FORMATION OF AMELOBLASTS, DENTINOENAMEL JUNCTION, AND ENAMEL MATRIX

After the differentiation of odontoblasts from the outer cells of the dental papilla and their formation of predentin, the **basement membrane** between the preameloblasts and the odontoblasts disintegrates. This disintegration of the basement membrane allows the preameloblasts to contact the newly formed predentin, which induces the **preameloblasts** to differentiate into ameloblasts.

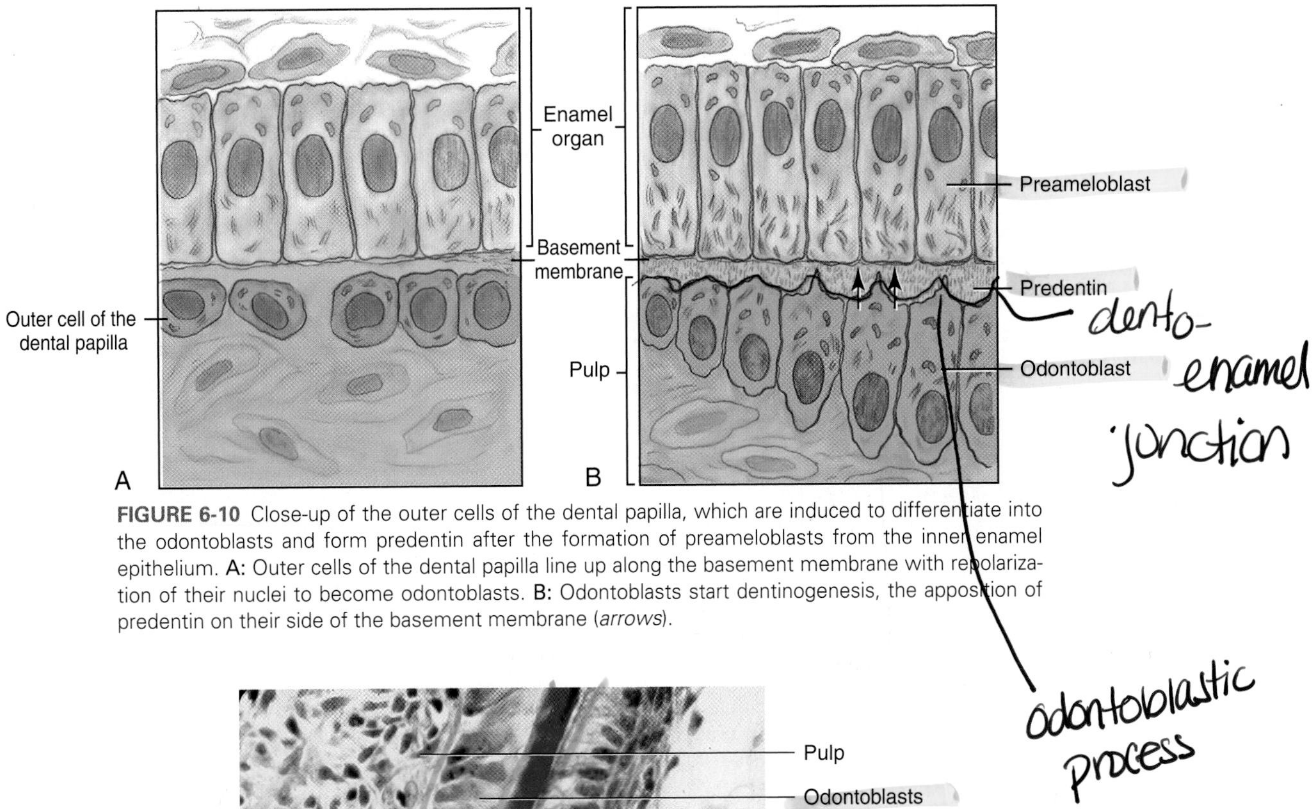

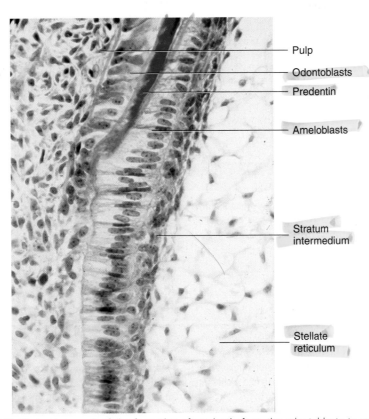

FIGURE 6-10 Close-up of the outer cells of the dental papilla, which are induced to differentiate into the odontoblasts and form predentin after the formation of preameloblasts from the inner enamel epithelium. **A:** Outer cells of the dental papilla line up along the basement membrane with repolarization of their nuclei to become odontoblasts. **B:** Odontoblasts start dentinogenesis, the apposition of predentin on their side of the basement membrane (*arrows*).

FIGURE 6-11 Photomicrograph of the formation of predentin from the odontoblasts to enclose the forming pulp from the dental papilla. The enamel organ has its layers on the other side of the basement membrane that includes the ameloblasts, stratum intermedium, and stellate reticulum. (*From Nanci A: Ten Cate's Oral Histology, ed 7, Mosby, St Louis, 2008.*)

After differentiation, the ameloblasts begin amelogenesis, or the apposition of enamel matrix, laying it down on their side of the now disintegrating basement membrane (Figures 6-12, 6-13, 6-14, and 6-15). The enamel matrix is secreted from Tomes' process, an angled part of each ameloblast that faces the disintegrating basement membrane created as the ameloblasts move away from the dentin interface.

With the newly formed enamel matrix in contact with the predentin, mineralization of the disintegrating basement membrane now occurs, forming the dentinoenamel junction (DEJ), the inner junction between the dentin and enamel tissue. Continued apposition of both types of dental matrix becomes regular and rhythmic, as the cellular bodies of both the odontoblasts and

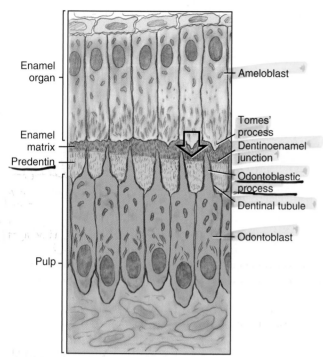

FIGURE 6-12 Preameloblasts being induced to differentiate into ameloblasts and beginning amelogenesis from Tomes' process (*large arrow*), with the apposition of enamel matrix on their side of the basement membrane. Later this membrane will disintegrate and mineralize to form the dentinoenamel junction. Note that the predentin is thicker than the enamel matrix because the odontoblasts differentiate and start matrix production earlier than the ameloblasts. The predentin forms around the dentinal tubules that contain the odontoblastic process attached to the odontoblasts.

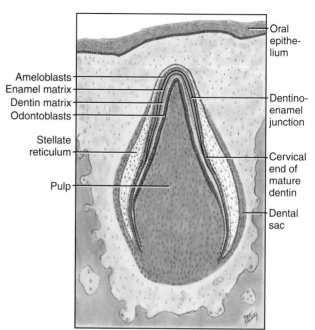

FIGURE 6-13 Stage of apposition showing both enamel and dentin matrix formation.

Developmental Disturbances during Stages of Apposition and Maturation

Certain factors may interfere with the metabolic processes of the **ameloblasts**, resulting in **enamel dysplasia**, which is the faulty development of enamel (see Table 6-3, *H*). Many different types are possible, and have either a local or a systemic etiology. Local enamel dysplasia may result from trauma or infection occurring to a small group of ameloblasts. Systemic enamel dysplasia involves larger numbers of ameloblasts and may result from traumatic birth, systemic infections, nutritional deficiencies, or dental fluorosis (excess systemic fluoride level).

Any tooth in which **amelogenesis** is active during the metabolic interference may be affected, and changes in either focal areas or the entire tooth, or even the complete dentition may be noted. A type of enamel dysplasia, enamel hypoplasia, results from a reduction in the *quantity* of enamel matrix. As a result, the teeth appear with pitting and grooves in the enamel surface.

Enamel hypoplasia can be noted in the presence of **Hutchinson's incisors** and **mulberry molars**, which is caused by the **teratogen of syphilis** (see Figure 3-16, **Chapters 16** and **17**). From the labial view, Hutchinson's incisors have a crown with a screwdriver shape that is wide cervically and narrow incisally, with a notched incisal edge. Mulberry molars have enamel tubercles on the occlusal surface.

Enamel dysplasia may also involve enamel hypocalcification. This disturbance results in reduction in the *quality* of the enamel maturation. The teeth appear more opaque, yellower, or even browner because of an intrinsic staining of enamel. A single affected area or white "sparkle spot" is called *Turner's spot* and if the permanent crown is affected, *Turner's tooth*.

Enamel hypoplasia and hypocalcification may occur together and affect entire dentitions, a common finding in dental fluorosis (see Figure 12-5).

A certain type of enamel dysplasia, **amelogenesis imperfecta**, has a hereditary etiology and can affect all teeth of both dentitions (Figure 6-16). With this disturbance, the teeth have very thin enamel that chips off or have no enamel at all. Thus, the crowns are yellow because they are composed of mainly softer dentin and undergo extreme **attrition**, the mechanical loss of tooth material resulting from **mastication**; full-coverage crowns are needed for esthetic appearance, as well as to prevent further attrition.

In addition, **dentin dysplasia**, or the faulty development of **dentin**, can result from an interference with the metabolic processes of the **odontoblasts** during **dentinogenesis**. This condition is rarer than enamel dysplasias but can also be due to local or systemic factors, similar to enamel dysplasias, and can involve either dentin hypoplasia or hypocalcification or both.

One type of dentin dysplasia is **dentinogenesis imperfecta**, which has a hereditary basis (Figure 6-17). This disturbance results in blue-gray or brown teeth with an opalescent sheen. The enamel is normal but chips off because of a lack of support by the abnormal underlying dentin, leaving crowns of dentin; the dentin has an irregular maturation quality (**interglobular dentin**) (see Figure 13-4). The result is severe **attrition** because the dentin is less mineralized overall; full-coverage crowns are needed for esthetic appearance, as well as to prevent further attrition. Several types of the condition are recognized; most are Type II, while Type I is involved with osteogenesis imperfecta.

ameloblasts retreat away from the DEJ, forming their perspective tissue types.

However, the odontoblasts, unlike the ameloblasts, will leave attached cellular extensions in the length of the predentin, the odontoblastic process as they move away from the DEJ. Each odontoblastic process is contained in a mineralized cylinder, the dentinal tubule. The mineralization or maturation of each type of matrix occurs later and is a different process for both enamel and dentin. However, the cell bodies of odontoblasts will remain within pulp attached by the odontoblastic processes. In contrast, the cell bodies of the ameloblasts will be involved in active eruption and mineralization process but will be lost after eruption (see later discussion).

ROOT DEVELOPMENT

The process of root development takes place long after the crown is completely shaped and the tooth is starting to erupt into the oral cavity (see Figure 6-22 and note the root development over time). Most find it remarkable that the tooth is formed starting with the crown and then moving to the apex of the root, unless they are in dental studies or looked closely at their dental office radiographs (see Figure 6-27, A). The structure responsible for root development is the cervical loop (Figure 6-18, A). The cervical loop is the most cervical part of the **enamel organ**, a bilayer rim that consists of only IEE and OEE.

To form the root region, the cervical loop begins to grow deeper into the surrounding ectomesenchyme of the dental sac, elongating and moving away from the newly completed crown area to enclose more of the dental papilla, forming Hertwig's epithelial root sheath (HERS) (Figures 6-18, B and C). The function of this sheath or membrane is to shape the root(s) by inducing dentin formation in the root area so that it is continuous with coronal dentin. Thus, HERS will determine if the root will be curved or straight, short or long, as well as single or multiple. This chapter first discusses root development in single-rooted teeth and then later in multirooted teeth.

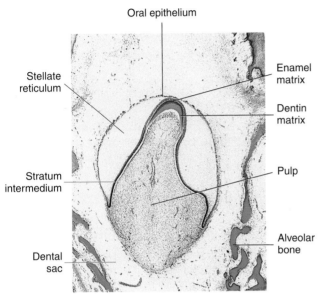

FIGURE 6-14 Photomicrograph during the stage of apposition showing enamel and dentin matrix formation. *(From Nanci A: Ten Cate's Oral Histology, ed 7, Mosby, St Louis, 2008.)*

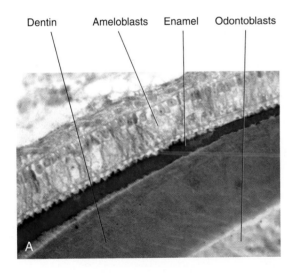

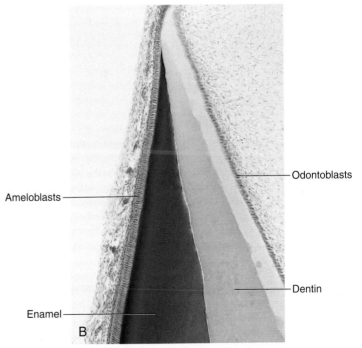

FIGURE 6-15 Photomicrographs of enamel formation from ameloblasts and dentin formation from odontoblasts. Note the stratum intermedium and stellate reticulum covering the ameloblasts. *(A: From Nanci A: Ten Cate's Oral Histology, ed 7, Mosby, St Louis, 2008. B: Courtesy of James McIntosh, PhD, Assistant Professor Emeritus, Department of Biomedical Sciences, Baylor College of Dentistry, Dallas, TX.)*

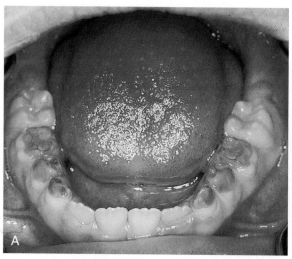
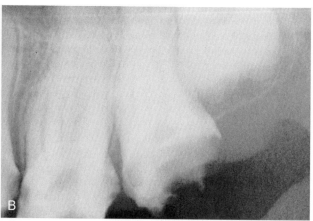

FIGURE 6-16 Amelogenesis imperfecta in the permanent dentition, a hereditary type of enamel dysplasia, where the teeth have either no enamel or very thin enamel that chips off, leaving the yellow crowns of dentin, which undergo extreme attrition. **A:** Clinical view. **B:** Radiograph.

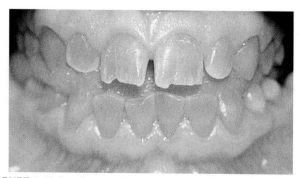

FIGURE 6-17 Dentinogenesis imperfecta in the permanent dentition, a hereditary type of dentin dysplasia that results in blue-gray teeth with an opalescent sheen, chipped enamel, and crowns of dentin with severe attrition.

ROOT DENTIN FORMATION

Root dentin forms when the outer cells of the dental papilla in the root area undergo **induction** and then **differentiation** and become **odontoblasts** (Figure 6-19). This induction occurs similarly to the process that happens in the crown area to produce coronal dentin, under the influence of the IEE of HERS. Lacking the intermediate layers of the stellate reticulum and stratum intermedium, HERS induces odontoblastic differentiation but fails to have IEE differentiate into enamel-forming ameloblasts. This accounts for the usual absence of enamel in the roots.

After the differentiation of odontoblasts in the root area, these cells undergo **dentinogenesis** and begin to secrete **predentin**. As in the crown area, a **basement membrane** is located between the IEE of the sheath and the odontoblasts in the root area.

When root dentin formation is completed, this part of the basement membrane also disintegrates, as does the entire HERS. After this disintegration of the root sheath, its cells may become the *epithelial rests of Malassez*. These groups of cells of **epithelium** become located in the mature **periodontal ligament** but can become cystic, presenting future periodontal infections (see Figure 14-26).

CEMENTUM AND PULP FORMATION

The apposition of **cementum**, or *cementogenesis,* in the root area also occurs when HERS disintegrates (Figure 6-20). This disintegration of the sheath allows the undifferentiated cells of the **dental sac** to contact the newly formed surface of root dentin. This contact of the dental sac cells with the dentin surface induces these cells to become immature *cementoblasts.*

The cementoblasts move to cover the root dentin area and undergo cementogenesis, laying down cementum matrix, or *cementoid.* Unlike ameloblasts and odontoblasts, which leave no cellular bodies in their secreted products, many cementoblasts become entrapped by the cementum they produce and become mature *cementocytes* in the later stages of apposition. As the cementoid surrounding the cementocytes becomes mineralized, or matured, it is then considered *cementum* (see Figure 14-2).

As a result of the apposition of cementum over the dentin, the *dentinocemental junction (DCJ)* is formed in the area where the disintegrating **basement membrane** between the two tissue types was located. Also at this time, the **central cells of the dental papilla** are forming into the **pulp**, which later becomes surrounded by the newly formed dentin (see Figure 13-11).

Developmental Disturbances with Cemental Formation

Excess **cementum** formation can rarely occur with **concrescence** (see Table 6-3, *I*). This is the union of the root structure of two or more teeth through the cementum only, mainly occurring with permanent maxillary molars (see **Chapter 17**). The teeth involved are originally separate but join because of the excessive cementum deposition on one or more teeth after eruption. Traumatic injury or crowding of the teeth in the area during the apposition and maturation stage of tooth development may be the cause. This may present problems during extraction and endodontic treatment, and thus preoperative radiographs are important in the detection of this disturbance.

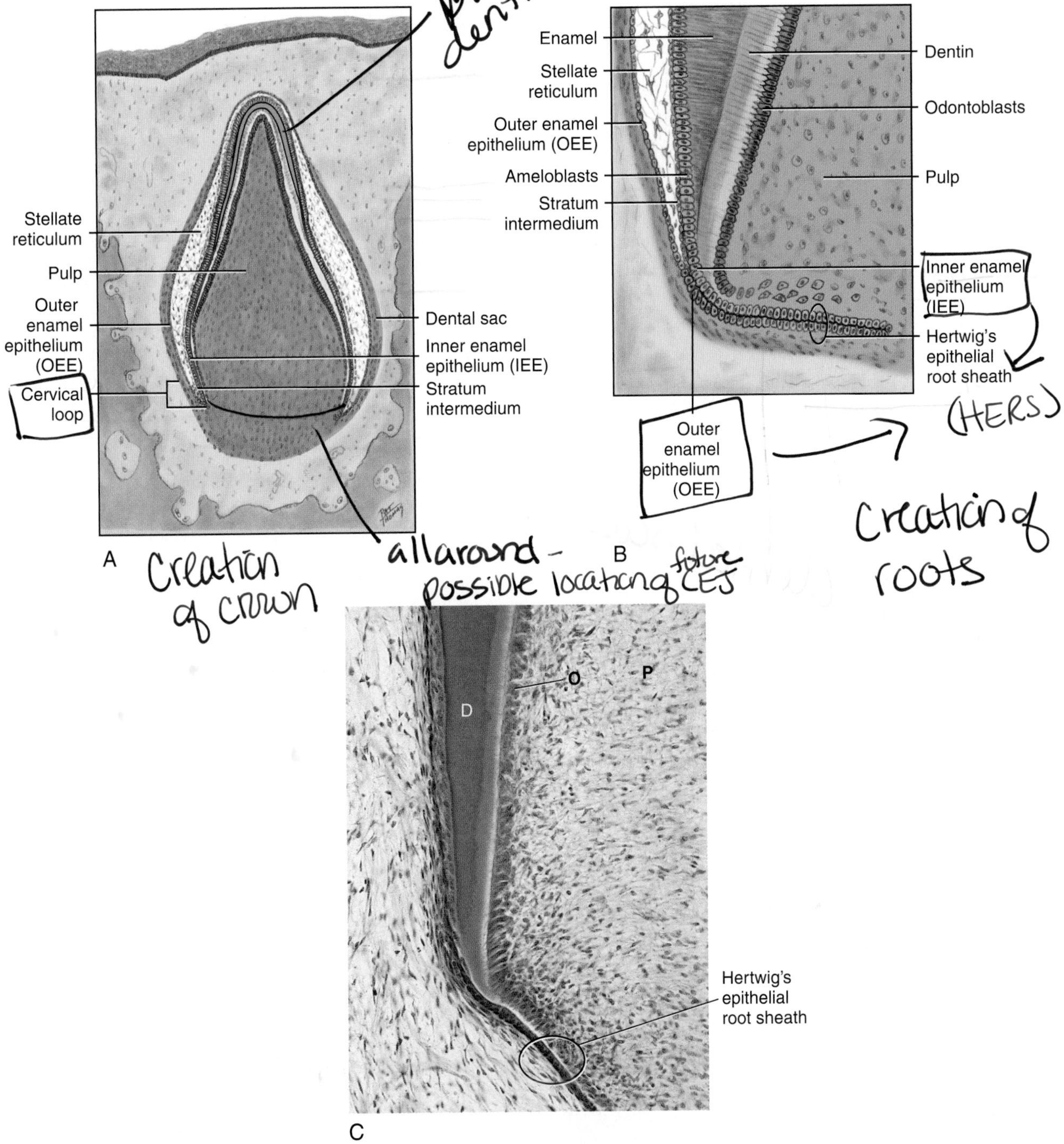

Handwritten annotations:
- *Whitishyellow Prewash dentin* (top)
- *Creation of crown* (below A)
- *all around - possible location of future CEJ*
- *Creation of roots* (right)
- *(HERS)*

Labels in figure A: Stellate reticulum; Pulp; Outer enamel epithelium (OEE); Cervical loop; Dental sac; Inner enamel epithelium (IEE); Stratum intermedium

Labels in figure B: Enamel; Stellate reticulum; Outer enamel epithelium (OEE); Ameloblasts; Stratum intermedium; Dentin; Odontoblasts; Pulp; Inner enamel epithelium (IEE); Hertwig's epithelial root sheath; Outer enamel epithelium (OEE)

Labels in figure C: D; O; P; Hertwig's epithelial root sheath

FIGURE 6-18 Root development. **A:** Cervical loop of a primary tooth, which is composed of the most cervical part of the enamel organ and is responsible for root development. Note that it is composed of only the inner (IEE) and outer enamel epithelium (OEE). **B:** Hertwig's epithelial root sheath is formed from elongation of the cervical loop (*circle*), which is responsible for the shape of the root (or roots) and the induction of root dentin. **C:** Microscopic view of the root sheath (*circle*). Odontoblasts (*O*) are within the pulp tissue (*P*) after forming dentin (*D*). (*Courtesy of James McIntosh, PhD, Assistant Professor Emeritus, Department of Biomedical Sciences, Baylor College of Dentistry, Dallas, TX.*)

DEVELOPMENT OF MULTIROOTED TEETH

Like anterior teeth, **multirooted** premolars and molars originate as a single root on the base of the crown. This part of posterior teeth is considered the **root trunk.** The cervical cross section of the root trunk initially follows the form of the crown. However, the root of a posterior tooth divides from the root trunk into the correct number of root branches for its tooth type (see Figure 17-34). Differential growth of **HERS** causes the root trunk of the multirooted teeth to divide into two or three roots (Figure 6-21). During the formation of the **enamel organ** on a multirooted tooth, elongation of its **cervical loop** occurs, which allows the development of long, tongue-like horizontal epithelial extensions or flaps within it. Two or three such extensions can be present on multirooted teeth, depending on the similar number of roots on the mature tooth.

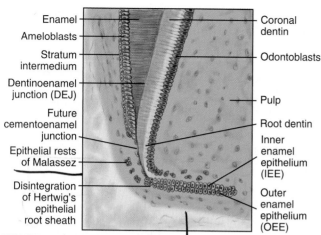

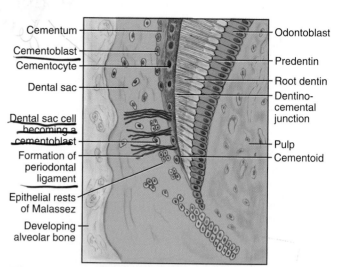

FIGURE 6-19 Apposition of dentin in the root area resulting from the induction of the outer cells of the dental papilla to differentiate into odontoblasts. Note the disintegration of Hertwig's epithelial root sheath to produce the epithelial rests of Malassez.

FIGURE 6-20 Apposition of cementum in the root area after Hertwig's epithelial root sheath disintegration and the induction of dental sac cells to differentiate into cementoblasts. The cementoblasts produce cementoid, and cells become entrapped to become cementocytes. Note both development of the periodontal ligament and alveolar bone.

dental sac

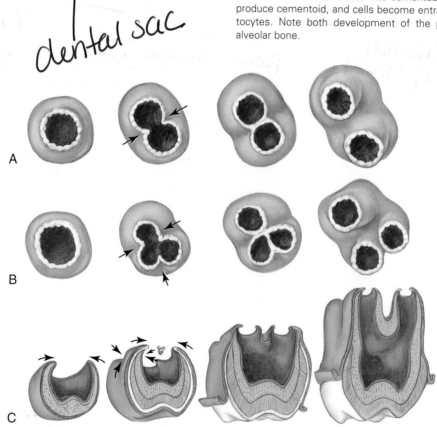

FIGURE 6-21 Apical view of multiroot development from horizontal extensions (*arrows*) of the cervical loop for (**A**) a two-rooted tooth, and (**B**) a three-rooted tooth. Cross section that shows the division that produces three roots (**C**) on a permanent maxillary molar.

The usually single cervical opening of the coronal enamel organ is then divided into two or three openings by these horizontal extensions. On the pulpal surfaces of these holes, dentin formation starts after the induction of the odontoblasts and disintegration of HERS and the associated basement membrane. Cementoblasts are induced to form cementum on the newly formed dentin only at the periphery of each opening. Root development then proceeds in the same way as described for a single-rooted tooth.

PERIODONTAL LIGAMENT AND ALVEOLAR BONE DEVELOPMENT

As the crown and root develop, the surrounding supporting tissue types of the tooth are also developing from the **dental sac** (see Figure 6-20). The **ectomesenchyme,** from the dental sac, begins to form the periodontal ligament (PDL) adjacent to the newly formed cementum. This process involves forming **collagen fibers** that are

Developmental Disturbances during Root Formation

In some cases, misplaced **ameloblasts** can migrate to the root area, causing **enamel** to be abnormally formed over the cemental root surface, which produces an **enamel pearl** (see Table 6-3, *J*). It appears as a small, spherical, enamel projection on the root surface, especially at the **cementoenamel junction (CEJ)**, or in the **furcations** on molars where the roots divide. It may have a tiny dentin and pulp core and appear radiopaque (light) on radiographs. An enamel pearl may be confused with a calculus deposit upon exploration of the root surface but cannot be removed by scaling alone.

Another disturbance that can occur during root development is **dilaceration**, resulting in either distorted root(s) or crown angulation in a formed tooth (see **Chapter 16**, and Figure 17-36). Dilaceration is caused by a distortion of **HERS** due to an injury or pressure; it can occur in any tooth or group of teeth during tooth development. It can cause problems during extraction and endodontic therapy and underlines the importance of preoperative radiographic examination; sometimes the bend is pronounced enough to prevent eruption. This is in contrast to the disturbance of *flexion*, which is a deviation or bend restricted just to the root; usually the bend is less than 90 degrees or a right angle.

Teeth may also have extra or **accessory roots** (or supernumerary roots). This disturbance may be due to trauma, pressure, or metabolic disease that affects **HERS**. Any tooth may be affected, but it occurs mainly with the permanent third molars and is rare in incisors. These accessory roots can present problems in extraction and endodontic therapy; thus, again preoperative radiographic examination is necessary to rule out this disturbance.

immediately organized into the fiber bundles of the PDL (see Figure 14-27). The ends of these fibers insert into the outer layers of the cementum and the surrounding alveolar bone to support the tooth (**Sharpey's fibers**). The ectomesenchyme of the dental sac also begins to mineralize to form the tooth sockets or **alveoli** of the alveolar bone surrounding the PDL (see Figure 14-15).

PRIMARY TOOTH ERUPTION AND SHEDDING

Eruption of the primary dentition takes place in chronological order, as does the permanent dentition (Figure 6-22). This process involves **active eruption**, which is the actual vertical movement of the tooth. This is not the **passive eruption**, which occurs with aging, when the gingival tissue recedes but no actual tooth movement takes place. Passive eruption is usually completed by age 24 ± 6.2 years, and only 12% of patients exhibited any amount of delayed passive eruption. In a fully erupted tooth, the gingival margin becomes located on the enamel 0.5 to 2.0 mm coronal to the CEJ. The timelines for eruption and root completion are useful for the clinician to know while using approximate ages (for primary dentition, see Table 18-1 and Figure 20-5 for sequence; for permanent dentition, see Table 15-2, **Appendix D**, and Figure 20-6, for sequence).

How active eruption occurs is understood, but *why* can only be theorized. No one can certify what forces "push" teeth through the oral soft tissue or can identify the timing mechanism that coincides with these eruptions; each theory for eruption presents a problem in its conception. Root growth, existence of a temporary ligament, vascular pressure, contractile collagen, and hormonal signals to genetic targets all have been used to explain eruption.

Active eruption of a primary tooth has many stages in the movement of the tooth. After enamel apposition ceases in the crown area of each primary or permanent tooth, the **ameloblasts** place an acellular dental cuticle on the newly formed outer enamel surface. In addition, the layers of the **enamel organ** become compressed, forming the reduced enamel epithelium (REE) (Figures 6-23 and 6-24). The REE appears as a few layers of flattened cells overlying the enamel surface. When this formation of the REE occurs for a primary tooth, it can then begin to erupt into the oral cavity.

The external cells of the REE are mostly from the stratum intermedium cells, but possibly cellular remnants of the stellate reticulum and OEE; thus these undifferentiated epithelial cells will divide and multiply and eventually give to the junctional epithelium.

To allow for the eruption process, the REE first has to fuse with the **oral epithelium** lining the oral cavity (Figure 6-25). Second, enzymes from the REE then disintegrate the central part of the fused tissue, leaving an epithelial tunnel for the tooth to erupt through the surrounding **oral epithelium** into the oral cavity. This tissue disintegration causes an inflammatory response known as "teething," which may be accompanied by tenderness and edema of the local tissue. Proper homecare can reduce the amount of inflammation and, thus, the discomfort associated with these oral changes in infants as their first teeth erupt, as well as in young adults when their third molars erupt.

As a primary tooth actively erupts, the coronal part of the fused epithelial tissue peels off the crown, leaving the cervical part still attached to the neck of the tooth like a banana being peeled. This fused tissue that remains near the CEJ after the tooth erupts then serves as the initial **junctional epithelium** of the tooth, creating a seal between the tissue and the tooth surface. This tissue is later replaced by a definitive junctional epithelium as the root becomes completely formed (see Figure 10-1).

The primary tooth is then lost, exfoliated, or shed, as the **succedaneous** permanent tooth develops lingual to it. The process involving shedding of the primary tooth consists of differentiation of multinucleated **osteoclasts** from fused macrophages, which absorb the **alveolar bone** between the two teeth from their *ruffled borders* (see Figure 8-15). In addition, similar cells, **odontoclasts** from undifferentiated **mesenchyme**, are also formed. These cells cause resorption, or removal of parts of the primary's root of **dentin** and **cementum**, as well as small parts of the enamel crown. Special **fibroblasts** (fibroclasts) destroy any remaining **collagen fibers**.

The process of shedding the primary tooth is intermittent ("on again/off again"), because at the same time that osteoclasts differentiate to resorb bone and odontoclasts differentiate to resorb dental tissue, the always-ready odontoblasts and cementoblasts work to replace the resorbed parts of the root. Thus, a loose primary tooth may become tightened just when the supervising adult takes a child to have it checked, because the child playing with it is driving the adult crazy. When the primary tooth is finally lost, the tooth fairy (and helpers) goes into action, with rates of return now approaching very high levels.

PERMANENT TOOTH ERUPTION

The **succedaneous** permanent tooth usually erupts into the oral cavity in a position **lingual** to the roots of the shedding or shed primary tooth, just as it develops that way (Figures 6-26, 6-27, and 6-28). The

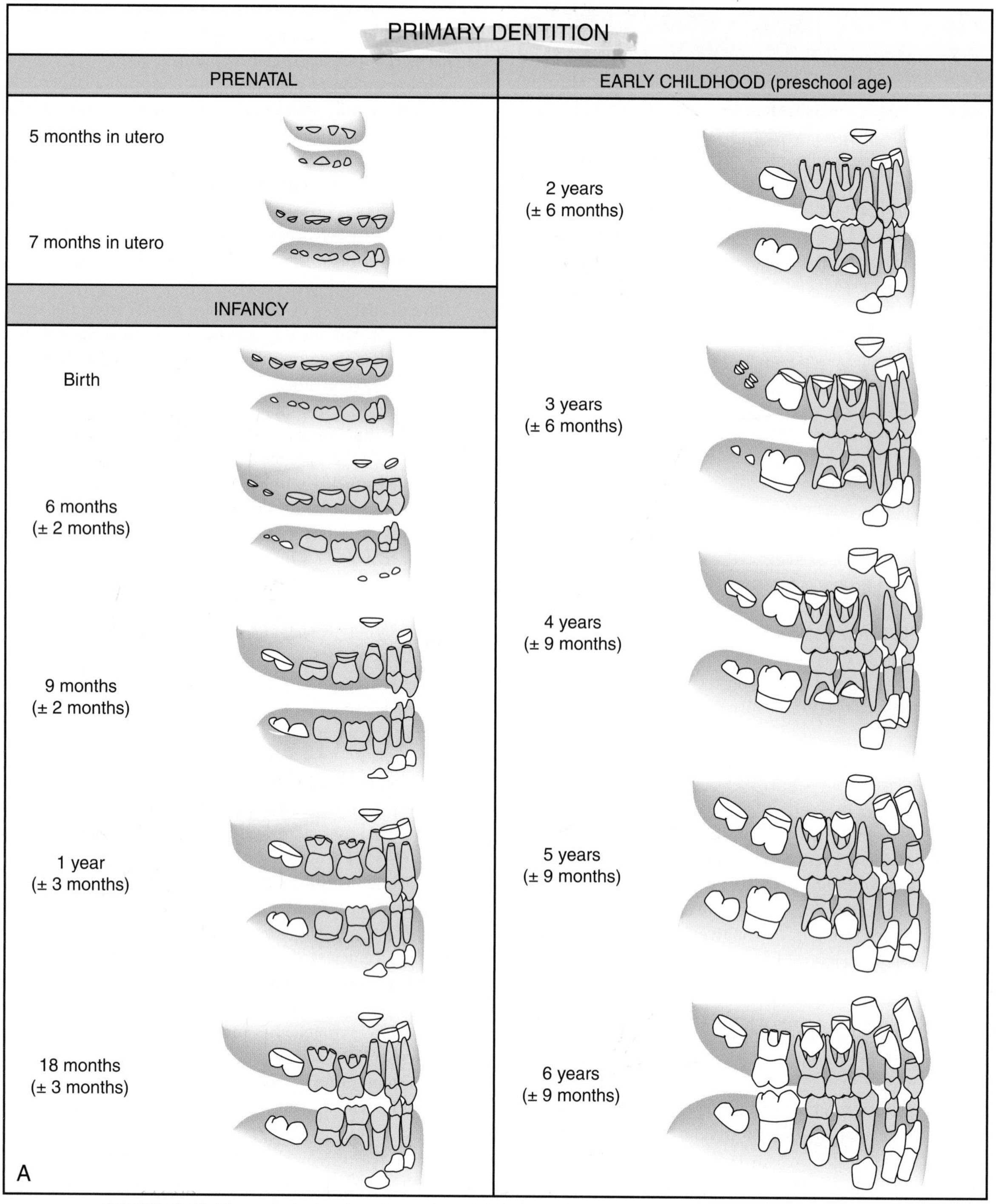

PRIMARY DENTITION	
PRENATAL	**EARLY CHILDHOOD (preschool age)**

FIGURE 6-22 Chronological order of eruption of (**A**) the primary (*blue*) dentition, and (**B**) the permanent (*white*) dentition. *(Adapted with permission from Schour I, Massler M: The development of the human dentition, J Am Dent Assoc 28:1153–1160, 1941.)*

only exception to this is the permanent maxillary incisors, which move to a more facially placed position as they erupt into the oral cavity.

The process of eruption for a succedaneous permanent tooth is the same as for the primary tooth: The REE fuses with the oral epithelium to create a tissue that degenerates, leaving an epithelial-lined eruption tunnel. The process of the nonsuccedaneous permanent tooth's eruption is similar also, but no primary tooth is shed. Both succedaneous and nonsuccedaneous permanent teeth erupt in chronological order (see Figure 6-22).

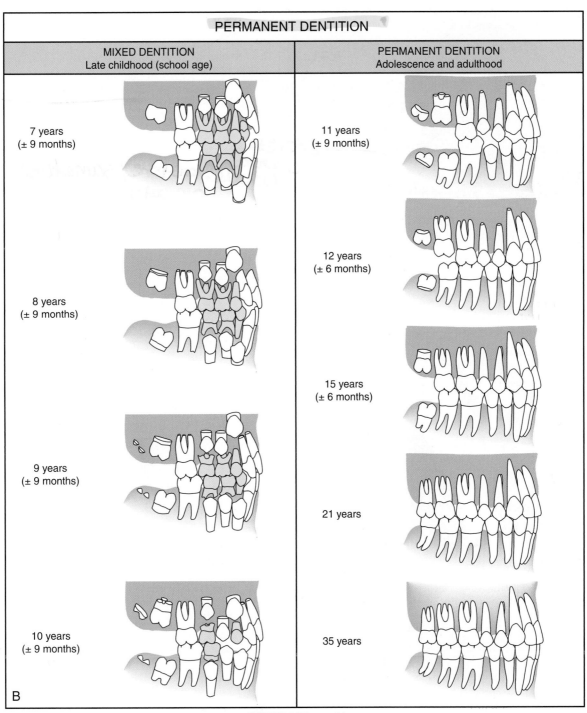

FIGURE 6-22, cont'd

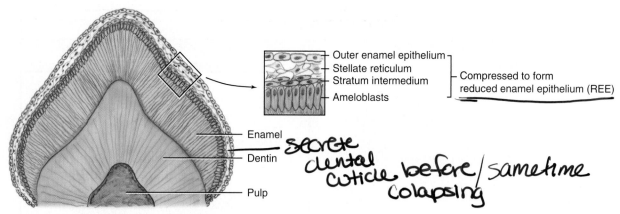

- Outer enamel epithelium
- Stellate reticulum
- Stratum intermedium — Compressed to form reduced enamel epithelium (REE)
- Ameloblasts

Enamel

secrete dental cuticle before/sametime colapsing

Dentin

Pulp

FIGURE 6-23 Reduced enamel epithelium produced after the completion of enamel apposition when the enamel organ undergoes compression of its many layers on the enamel surface.

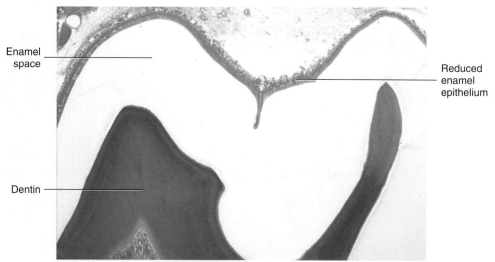

Enamel space

Reduced enamel epithelium

Dentin

FIGURE 6-24 Photomicrograph of reduced enamel epithelium after the completion of enamel apposition when the enamel organ undergoes compression of its many layers on the enamel surface (enamel space). *(From Nanci A: Ten Cate's Oral Histology, ed 7, Mosby, St Louis, 2008.)*

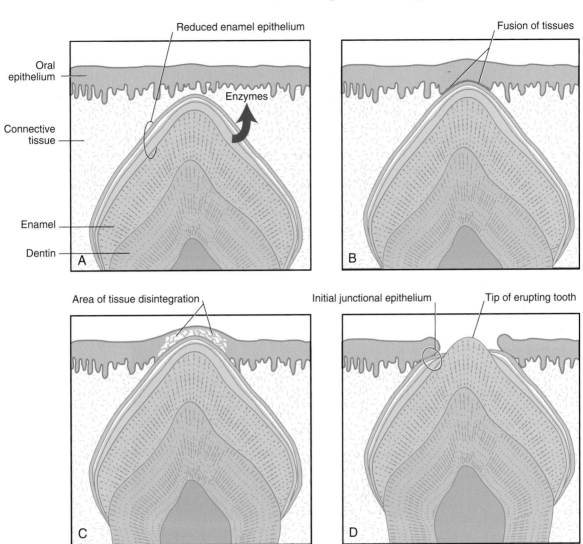

FIGURE 6-25 Process of tooth eruption. **A:** Oral cavity before the eruption process begins with reduced enamel epithelium (*circle*) covering the newly formed enamel; enzymes from the epithelium are present for tissue disintegration (*arrow*). **B:** Fusion of the reduced enamel epithelium with the oral epithelium. **C:** Disintegration of the central fused tissue, leaving a tunnel for tooth movement. **D:** Coronal fused tissue peel back from the crown during eruption, leaving the initial junctional epithelium (*circle*) near the cementoenamel junction.

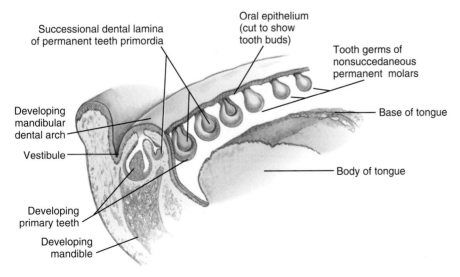

Section through fetal mandible

FIGURE 6-26 Development of the succedaneous permanent teeth in a lingual position to the primary teeth on a section of a fetal mandible.

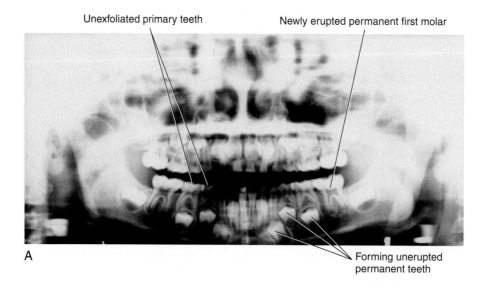

Unexfoliated primary teeth

Newly erupted permanent first molar

Forming unerupted permanent teeth

A

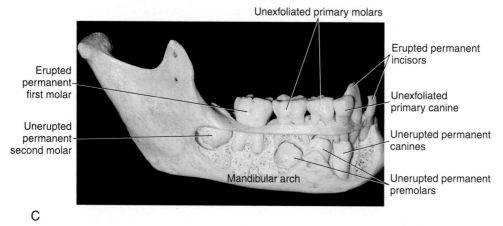

Unerupted permanent canine

Unerupted permanent premolars

Maxillary arch

Unerupted permanent second molar

Erupted permanent incisors

Unexfoliated primary molars

Unexfoliated primary canine

B

Unexfoliated primary molars

Erupted permanent incisors

Erupted permanent first molar

Unexfoliated primary canine

Unerupted permanent second molar

Unerupted permanent canines

Mandibular arch

Unerupted permanent premolars

C

FIGURE 6-27 Mixed dentition with primary teeth being shed and the permanent dentition erupting within the jaws of each arch. **A:** Panoramic radiograph. **B** and **C:** Maxilla and mandible, with a section of facial compact bone removed.

FIGURE 6-28 Photomicrograph of a sagittal section of the mandible showing a mixed dentition of posterior teeth, primary and permanent. Note the root resorption of the primary molars and position of the permanent premolars, as well as the formation of the roots of the nonsuccedaneous permanent first molar. *(From Nanci A:* Ten Cate's Oral Histology, *ed 7, Mosby, St Louis, 2008.)*

Clinical Considerations with the Eruption Process

A permanent tooth often starts to erupt before the primary tooth is fully shed, possibly creating problems in spacing. Interceptive orthodontic therapy can prevent some of these situations. Thus, it is important for children with prolonged retention of any primary teeth to seek early dental consultation. Root fragments from primary molars may be left from the process and create periodontal complications for the permanent dentition; panoramic radiographs of the mixed dentition are important in order to monitor on tooth development (see Figure 6-27, *A*).

A residue may form on newly erupted teeth of both dentitions that may leave the teeth extrinsically stained. This green-gray residue, **Nasmyth's membrane,** consists of the fused tissue of the **REE** and **oral epithelium,** as well as the dental cuticle placed by the **ameloblasts** on the newly formed outer enamel surface (Figure 6-29). Nasmyth's membrane then easily picks up stain from food debris and is hard to remove except by selective polishing. The child's supervising adults may need reassurance that it is only an extrinsic stain on a child's newly erupted teeth.

In addition, because the crown forms before the root, prevention of traumatic injury to the permanent teeth before they are fully anchored into the jaws is very important. Mouth guards, which consist of individually formed plastic coverings for the teeth, are recommended for children active in all types of sports. Any injury to children's dentition, such as **avulsion,** must be seen promptly by their dental professionals to rule out injury to the forming teeth and supporting tissue types.

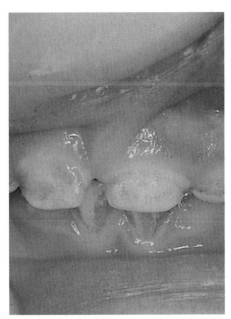

FIGURE 6-29 Staining of Nasmyth's membrane after eruption of the teeth. The entire crown of the primary dentition may be affected, as well as the permanent dentition.

Developmental Disturbances during Eruption

An odontogenic cyst that forms from the **REE** after the crown has completely formed and matured is the **dentigerous cyst,** or follicular cyst (Figure 6-30). This initially asymptomatic cyst forms around the crown of a nonerupted impacted or developing tooth, most commonly the permanent third molars. When this cyst becomes larger within the bone of the jaws, it may cause displaced teeth, jaw fracture, and pain; it must be completely removed surgically, because it may become neoplastic otherwise.

If a dentigerous cyst appears on a partially erupted tooth, it is considered an *eruption cyst* and appears as fluctuant, blue, vesicle-like gingival lesion (Figure 6-31). Unlike the other types of dentigerous cysts, the eruption cyst disintegrates with eruption of the tooth and no further treatment is needed. Because it appears to enlarge as the tooth erupts, supervising adults may need reassurance that this lesion is not serious.

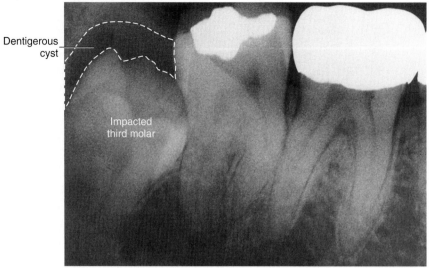

FIGURE 6-30 Radiograph of a dentigerous cyst (*dashed lines*) that is formed around the crown of an unerupted impacted permanent mandibular third molar.

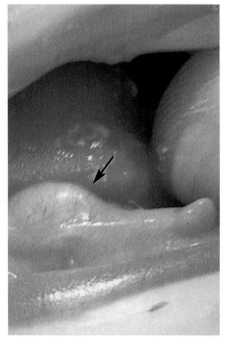

FIGURE 6-31 Eruption cyst (*arrow*) in a child. This less serious type of dentigerous cyst has formed over an erupting primary mandibular incisor.

CHAPTER 7

Overview of the Cell

●●● CHAPTER OUTLINE

The cell
  Anatomy of the cell
  Cell membrane and cytoplasm
  Organelles
  Inclusions

Cell division
Extracellular materials
Intercellular junctions

●●● LEARNING OBJECTIVES

- Define and pronounce the key terms in this chapter.
- Indicate and discuss the components of the cell, including the cell membrane, cytoplasm, organelles, and inclusions.
- Outline cell division and describe the phases of mitosis that are involved.

- Describe the extracellular materials surrounding the cell and its intercellular junctions.
- Integrate the knowledge of a background of the cell into the promotion and understanding of healthy orofacial tissue and any pathology that may occur within them.

●●● NEW KEY TERMS

Anaphase (an-ah-faz)
Cell, membrane
Centrioles (sen-tree-ols)
Centromere (sen-tro-mere)
Centrosome (sen-tro-some)
Chromatids (kro-mah-tids)
Chromatin (kro-mah-tin)
Chromosomes (kro-mah-somes)
Cytoplasm (cy-to-plazm)
Cytoskeleton (site-oh-**skel**-it-on)
Desmosome (des-mo-som)
Endocytosis (en-do-sigh-**toe**-sis)
Endoplasmic reticulum (en-do-**plas**-mik rey-**tik**-u-lum)
Exocytosis (ek-so-sigh-**toe**-sis)

Golgi complex (gol-jee)
Hemidesmosome (hem-eye-**des-**mo-som)
Histology (his-**tol**-oh-jee)
Inclusions (in-**kloo**-zhins)
Intercellular junctions
Intercellular substance
Intermediate filaments (fil-ah-ments)
Interphase (in-ter-faz)
Lysosomes (li-sah-somes)
Metaphase (met-ah-faz)
Mitochondria (mite-ah-**kon**-dree-ah)
Mitosis (my-**toe**-sis)
Microfilaments (my-kroh-**fil**-ah-ments)
Microtubules (my-kroh-**too**-bules)

Nuclear envelope (noo-kle-er), **pores**
Nucleolus (noo-**kle**-oh-lis)
Nucleoplasm (noo-kle-ah-plazm)
Nucleus (noo-kle-is) (plural, **nuclei,** noo-kle-eye)
Organ
Organelles (or-gah-**nels**)
Phagocytosis (fag-oh-sigh-**toe**-sis)
Prophase (pro-faz)
Ribosomes (ry-bo-somes)
System
Telophase (tel-oh- faz)
Tissue, fluid
Tonofilaments (ton-oh-fil-ah-ments)
Vacuoles (vak-you-oles)

THE CELL

As an introduction to Unit III, the organization of the body's histology is discussed in this chapter. Histology is the study of the microscopic structure and function of cells and associated tissue. Another term for histology is *microanatomy* because the dimensions of the anatomical structures studied are on a microscopic scale (see Appendix B). A dental professional must have a clear understanding of the basic unit of the body, the cell and its components, as well as understanding the larger concepts involved in the histology of tissue, such as those found in the oral cavity. This chapter gives an overview of the cell and its various components, and then Chapter 8 presents a review of basic tissue types in the body. A discussion of the histology of each of the tissue types in the oral cavity follows in later chapters of Unit III.

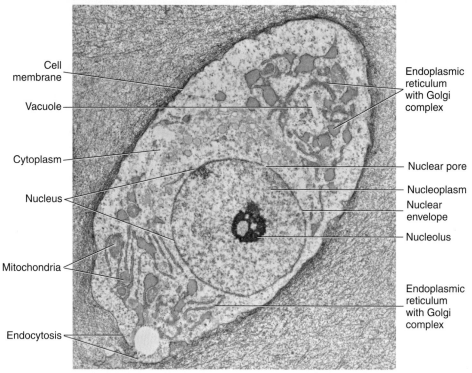

FIGURE 7-1 Electron micrograph of the cell and its most visible contents, such as its cell membrane and nucleus.

ANATOMY OF THE CELL

The smallest living unit of organization in the body is the cell, because each cell is capable of performing any necessary functions without the aid of other cells (Figures 7-1 and 7-2, Table 7-1). Each cell has a cell membrane, cytoplasm, organelles, and inclusions. Thus, every cell is a world unto itself, like a gated small city, surrounded by a boundary, having "factories" and other "industries" that make it almost self-sufficient.

Cells also interact with one another as a city reacts with other cities. Cells with similar characteristics of form and function are grouped together to form a tissue (see Table 7-1), as countries are formed from cities for a common goal. Thus, a tissue is a collection of similarly specialized cells, most often surrounded by extracellular materials. Various tissue types are then bonded together to form an organ, a somewhat independent body part that performs a specific function or functions, similar to organizations formed from countries. Organs can function together as a system.

Cells in a tissue undergo cell division (or mitosis) to reproduce and replace the dead tissue cells. As a result of the division process, two daughter cells that are identical to each other and to the original parent cell are formed. This process consists of different phases, which are discussed later with regard to different components of the cell.

However, cells also interact with the extracellular environment in many ways. Cells can perform exocytosis, which is an active transport of material from a vesicle within the cell out into the extracellular environment. Exocytosis occurs when there is fusion of a vesicle membrane with the cell membrane and subsequent expulsion of the contained material.

The uptake of materials from the extracellular environment into the cell is endocytosis. Endocytosis can take place as an invagination of the cell membrane. Endocytosis can also take the form of phagocytosis, which is the engulfing and then digesting of solid waste and foreign material by the cell through enzymatic breakdown of the material (discussed later).

CELL MEMBRANE AND CYTOPLASM

The cell membrane (or plasma membrane) surrounds the cell (see Figures 7-1 and 7-2). Despite its fragile microscopic appearance, it is a tough and resourceful "gatekeeper" for the cell's interior. The usual cell membrane is an intricate bilayer, consisting predominantly of phospholipids and proteins. The phospholipids serve largely as a diffusion regulator. The proteins of the cell membrane serve as structural reinforcements, as well as receptors for specific hormones, neurotransmitters, and immunoglobulins (antibodies). The cell membrane is associated with many of the mechanisms of intercellular junctions and other functions of the cell.

The cytoplasm includes the semifluid part contained within the cell membrane boundary, as well as the skeletal system of support or cytoskeleton (discussed later). The cytoplasm contains not only a number of structures but also spaces or cavities called vacuoles.

ORGANELLES

The organelles are metabolically active specialized structures within the cell (see Figures 7-1 and 7-2). The organelles allow each cell to function according to its genetic code. Organelles also subdivide the cell into compartments. The major organelles of the cell include the nucleus, mitochondria, ribosomes, endoplasmic reticulum, Golgi complex, lysosomes, and cytoskeleton.

NUCLEUS

The nucleus (plural, nuclei) is the largest, densest, and most conspicuous organelle in the cell when it is viewed microscopically (Figure 7-3, see Figures 7-1 and 7-2). A nucleus is found in all cells of the body except mature red blood cells, and most cells have a single nucleus. However, some cells are multinucleated, such as **osteoclasts** or **skeletal muscles** (see Figures 8-15 and 8-18).

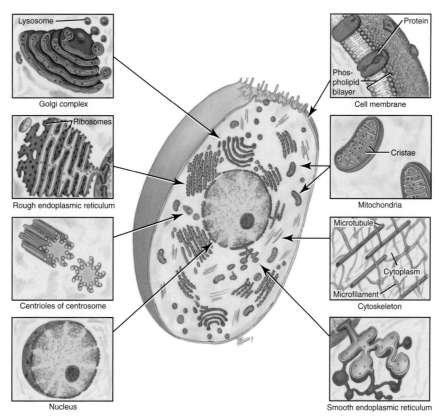

FIGURE 7-2 The cell with its organelles and cell membrane examined.

TABLE 7-1	Components of the Body and Examples
Cell	Smallest living unit of organization: epithelial cell, neuron, myofiber, chondrocyte, osteocyte, fibroblast, erythrocyte, macrophage, sperm
Tissue	Collection of similarly specialized cells: epithelium, nervous tissue, muscle, cartilage, bone, connective tissue, blood
Organ	Independent body part formed from tissue: skin, brain, heart, liver
System	Organs functioning together: central nervous system, respiratory system, immune system, cardiovascular system

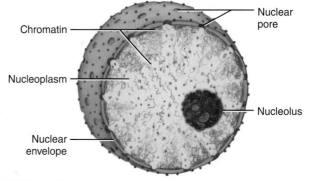

FIGURE 7-3 Nucleus and its various components: chromatin, nucleoplasm, nuclear envelope, nuclear pore, and nucleolus.

When stained with histological dyes, the chief nucleic acid in the nucleoplasm is deoxyribonucleic acid (DNA), in the form of chromatin, which looks like diffuse stippling when the cell is viewed microscopically. In an actively dividing cell, the chromatin condenses into microscopically visible, discrete, rodlike chromosomes. Each chromosome has a centromere, a clear, constricted area near the middle. Chromosomes become two filamentous, or threadlike, chromatids (daughter chromosomes) joined by a centromere during cell division. After cell division, major segments of the chromosomes again become uncoiled and dispersed among the other components of the nucleoplasm.

The nucleus is the cell's "data bank," because it stores the genetic code. From its sequence of nucleotides in the chromatin, the DNA and ribonucleic acid (RNA) give directions for everything the cell is and will become. Thus, they control all functions the cell performs. The nucleus is also the "command center" of the cell, controlling the other organelles in the cell; it is influenced by what occurs inside the cell as well as outside the cell. Only certain genes are "turned on" to participate in the production of specific proteins at any particular time.

The chemical messages that result in genes switching on or off in the nucleus come from the cytoplasm, where, in turn, they are generated as a result of interaction between the surface membrane and the environment. Although genes contain the total range of the cell's possibilities, the cellular environment dictates which of these possibilities for differentiation, growth, development, and specialization will be expressed.

As would be expected, the nucleus is constantly active. Before cell division, new DNA must be synthesized and every single gene must be replicated. These genes, linked into chromosomes, are then separated into duplicate sets during cell division. In the nucleus, three very important types of RNA are produced: messenger RNA (mRNA) molecules, which are complementary copies of distinct segments of DNA;

transfer RNA (tRNA) molecules, which are molecules capable of specifically binding to and transporting amino acid units for protein synthesis; and ribosomal RNA (rRNA), which will be discussed later.

In addition to all the hereditary activity associated with cell division, genes on the DNA selectively direct the synthesis of thousands of enzymes and other integral and cytoplasmic proteins, as well as any secretory products. This process involves transcription of information from various parts of the DNA molecules into new strands of mRNA, which carry the encoded instructions into the cytoplasm for processing through the process of translation, which involves tRNA, rRNA, and amino acids.

The fluid part within the nucleus is the nucleoplasm, which contains important molecules used in the construction of ribosomes, nucleic acids, and other nuclear materials. The nucleus is surrounded by the nuclear envelope, a membrane similar to the cell membrane, except that it is double-layered. The nuclear envelope is associated with many other organelles of the cell. The nuclear envelope may be pierced by nuclear pores, which act as avenues of communication between the inner nucleoplasm and the outer cytoplasm. The number and distribution of these nuclear pores vary with the cell type, with the level of cell activity, and with states of differentiation level of the same cell type.

Contained in the nucleus is the nucleolus, a prominent, rounded nuclear organelle that is centrally placed in the nucleoplasm when the cell is viewed microscopically (see Figure 7-3). The nucleolus mainly produces rRNA and the nucleotides of the two other types of RNA. Without a nucleolus, no protein synthetic activity would occur within the cell; it acts almost like a "city hall." The roles of the nucleolus and ribosomes with rRNA in protein synthesis are discussed later.

MITOCHONDRIA

The mitochondria are the most numerous organelles in the cell. They are associated with energy conversion, and thus are the "power plants" for the cell. They are a major source of adenosine triphosphate (ATP), and therefore are the site of many metabolic reactions (see Figures 7-1 and 7-2). Microscopically, mitochondria resemble small bags with a larger bag fitted inside, because each bag is folded back on itself. These inner folds exist to increase the surface area for more dense packing of the particular proteins and enzyme molecules involved in aerobic cellular respiration. Internal to the folds, mitochondrial DNA, calcium and magnesium granules, enzymes, electrolytes, and water are present in a matrix.

Most of a cell's energy comes from mitochondria, produced by two of the pathways of aerobic cellular respiration. These involve both Krebs cycle, with its multienzyme system, and the hydrogen pathway, which uses the electron transport chain of enzymes. Besides supplying energy, mitochondria help balance the concentration of water, calcium, and other ions in the cytoplasm. Cells with high levels of mitochondria are known for their high levels of activity, such as with young fibroblasts; the reverse is noted with the cellular changes encountered with periodontal disease (see Chapter 8).

RIBOSOMES

The ribosomes are the tiny sphere-shaped organelles in the cell (see Figure 7-2). The ribosomes are made in the nucleolus from rRNA and protein molecules and are assembled in the cytoplasm. They function as roving "protein factories" for the cell; their location changes based on the type of protein being made for the cell. They can be within mitochondria, free in the cytoplasm, or bound to membranes, either

to the outer nuclear membrane or onto the surface of the rough endoplasmic reticulum (discussed next).

Ribosomes can also be found singly or in clusters within the cell. As many as 30 separate ribosomes may be attached sequentially to a single molecule of mRNA, with each ribosome making its own protein copy as it works its way along the length of the mRNA transcript. Within these ribosomes, free amino acids are being joined together according to the particular order specified by the mRNA transcript corresponding to the sequence of the required protein chain.

ENDOPLASMIC RETICULUM

Endoplasmic reticulum (ER) is so called because it is more concentrated in the cell's inner or endoplasmic region as compared to the peripheral or ectoplasmic region (see Figures 7-1 and 7-2). The ER consists of parallel membrane-bound channels. All the membranes of the ER interconnect, forming a system of channels and folds microscopically, and are continuous with the nuclear envelope, a "highway" system for the cell.

The ER can be classified as either smooth or rough, which is determined by the absence or presence of ribosomes, each giving a different microscopic appearance to the structure, as well differing in function. The smooth ER (SER), which is free of ribosomes, appears microscopically smooth in surface texture. Rough ER (RER) is dotted with ribosomes on its outer surface, which makes it appear microscopically rough.

The outer layer of the nuclear envelope connects with all the ER in the cell, both smooth and rough. The ER's primary functions are modification, storage, segregation, and finally transport of proteins that the cell manufactures (on the ribosomes) for use in other sections of the cell or even outside the cell.

GOLGI COMPLEX

Once the ER has modified the new protein, it is then transferred to the Golgi complex for subsequent segregation, packaging, and transport of protein compounds (see Figures 7-1 and 7-2), just like a "packaging plant" for the cell. The Golgi complex is the second largest organelle after the nucleus and is composed of stacks of three to twenty flattened, smooth-membrane vesicular sacs arranged parallel to one another.

Vesicles of protein molecules from the RER fuse with the Golgi complex, transferring protein molecules to be further modified, concentrated, and packaged by the Golgi complex. After this modification and packaging, the Golgi complex wraps up large numbers of these molecules into a single membranous vesicle and then sends it on its way to the cell's surface to be released by the process of exocytosis. These protein molecules, which include hormones, enzymes, and other secretory products, are released into the extracellular space or into capillaries, as these vesicles fuse with the cell membrane. These products that are put together in the Golgi complex can include such substances as mucus secretory product for the salivary glands or insulin for the pancreas.

The modifications by the Golgi complex to the protein molecules include adding carbohydrates, thus forming glycoproteins, as it does in the production of mucus. The Golgi complex also may remove part of a polypeptide chain, as it does in the case of insulin. The Golgi complex not only prepares proteins for export by exocytosis but also produces a separate organelle, lysosomes (discussed next).

LYSOSOMES

The lysosomes are organelles produced by the Golgi complex (see Figure 7-2) and function in both intracellular and extracellular digestion by the cell. This digestive function is due to their ability to lyse, or digest, various waste and foreign materials in or around the cell, which occurs during **phagocytosis** (Figure 7-4)—like a "sewer system" for the cell. Lysosomes break down many kinds of molecules using the powerful hydrolytic and digestive enzymes contained within them (see Figure 8-15). The main hydrolytic enzyme in lysosomes is hyaluronidase. Lysosomes are membrane-bound vesicles that develop as a bud that pinches off the end of one of the Golgi complex's flattened sacs. The enzymes of the lysosomes originally are produced on the RER and then are transported for packaging in the Golgi complex, where the lysosomes originate.

As the substances are broken down into sufficiently small and simple products, the usable material diffuses out of the lysosome into the cell's cytoplasm to be incorporated into new molecules being synthesized, a situation of cellular recycling. Indigestible material remains in the lysosome and becomes a residual body. It either migrates to the cell surface to be released by exocytosis or remains as a remnant in the lysosome and becomes an inclusion (discussed later). Although all cells, except red blood cells, are capable of some digestive activity, other cells, such as certain **white blood cells**, have differentiated to specialize in digestive processes, especially **phagocytosis** (see Figure 8-17). Phagocytosis is very active even at the junction between healthy **gingival tissue** and the tooth surface (see Chapter 10).

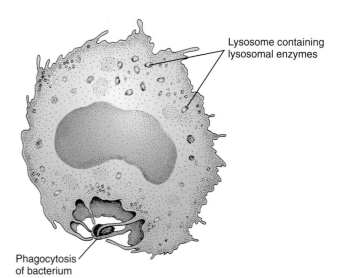

Lysosome containing lysosomal enzymes

Phagocytosis of bacterium

FIGURE 7-4 Phagocytosis, which is the engulfing and digesting of solid waste and foreign material (such as with the bacterium shown here) by a white blood cell (monocyte) through enzymatic breakdown of the matter from its enclosed lysosomes. *(From Fehrenbach MJ: Inflammation and repair. In Ibsen OAC, Phelan JA (eds):* Oral Pathology for Dental Hygienists, *ed 5, WB Saunders, Philadelphia, 2009.)*

CENTROSOME

The centrosome is a dense, somewhat oval-shaped organelle that contains a pair of cylindrical structures, the centrioles. The centrosome is always located near the nucleus, which is important because it plays a significant role in forming the mitotic spindle apparatus during cell division or mitosis. There are two centrioles within the centrosome, and each is composed of triplets of microtubules arranged in a cartwheel pattern. Without this self-replicating centriole-centrosome unit, an animal cell cannot reproduce (discussed later). *90° to each other*

CYTOSKELETON

The interior of the cell is neither liquid nor gel in nature but somewhat between the two. It also has a three-dimensional system of support, the cytoskeleton. The components of the cytoskeleton include microfilaments, intermediate filaments, and microtubules. This design lends basic stability to the cell as a whole, functioning like reinforced girders. It also acts to compartmentalize the cytoplasm, creating preferred "freeways" for the movement of molecules formed by cellular processes.

Both microfilaments and microtubules consist of specialized proteins. Microfilaments are delicate, threadlike microscopic structures. Microtubules are slender, hollow, tubular microscopic structures that may appear individually, doubly, or as triplets. Microtubules assist microfilaments in the maintenance of overall cell shape and in the transport of intracellular materials. Additionally, microtubules form the internal framework of cilia and flagella, centrioles, and the mitotic spindle for cell division (discussed later).

Certain cells exhibit projections that help move substances along the surface of the cell, or are for moving the entire cell in the extracellular environment. If the projections on the cell are shorter and more numerous, they are considered *cilia*; if the projections are fewer and longer, they are considered *flagella*.

Both cilia and flagella are useful in human reproduction. An **ovum** is propelled within the fallopian tube by cilia, and **sperm** are propelled by their own flagella (see Figure 3-1). Structurally, there is no major difference between cilia and flagella except for their relative lengths. Both consist of pairs of multiple microtubules that form a ring around two single microtubules. Cilia are also noted in the **respiratory**

mucosa lining the **nasal cavity** and **paranasal sinuses** as they move the mucous coating of these tissue types.

The intermediate filaments are of various types of thicker, threadlike microscopic structures within the cell. One type of intermediate filament, a tonofilament, has a major role in intercellular junctions (discussed later). Another type of intermediate filament is one that forms **keratin,** which is found in calloused-type of **epithelium,** many of which are located in the oral cavity, such as on the surface of the **tongue** (see Figure 9-1).

INCLUSIONS

The cell also contains inclusions, which are metabolically inert substances that are also transient over time in the cell (see Figure 7-2). These include masses of organic chemicals and often are recognizable microscopically. These inclusions are released from storage by the cell and used as demand dictates. Lipids and glycogen can be decomposed for energy from inclusions in the cell. Melanin is stored as inclusions in certain cells of the skin and **oral mucosa** and is responsible for the **pigmentation** of these tissue types (see Figures 9-22 and 23). Inclusions also include residual bodies: spent lysosomes and their digested material.

CELL DIVISION

Cell division or mitosis is a complex process involving many of the organelles of the cell (Table 7-2). Mitosis functions during tissue growth or replacement, and its activity is dependent on the length of the individual cell's life span. Before cell division, the DNA is replicated during interphase as part of the cell cycle, which is the cell's "living" time. Interphase has three phases: Gap 1, or *G1* (initial resting phase: cell growth and functioning), Synthesis, or *S* (cell DNA synthesis by duplication), and Gap 2, or *G2* (second resting phase: resuming cell growth and functioning).

Following interphase, mitosis occurs with the cell's nuclear material dividing so that the resulting production is of two daughter cells that are identical to the parent cell as well as to each other (see Chapter 3). Then, at the same time, the other cytoplasmic components of the cell also are

TABLE 7-2	Process of Interphase Followed by Phases of Mitosis during Cell Cycle

CELL CYCLE PHASES	MICROSCOPIC APPEARANCE	
INTERPHASE: G1, S, G2 PHASES Cells between divisions engage in growth, metabolism, organelle replacement, and substance production, including chromatin and centrosome replication.	 Chromatin	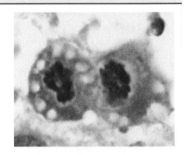
MITOSIS PHASES **Prophase** Chromatin condenses into chromosomes in cell. Replicated centrioles migrate to opposite poles. Nuclear membrane and nucleolus disintegrate.	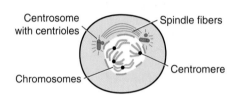 Centrosome with centrioles — Spindle fibers — Centromere — Chromosomes	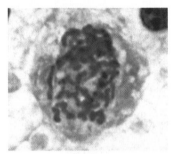
Metaphase Chromosomes move so that their centromeres are aligned in the equatorial plane. Mitotic spindle forms.	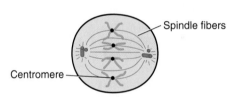 Spindle fibers — Centromere	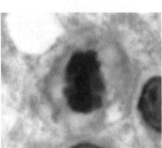
Anaphase Centromeres split, and each chromosome separates into two chromatids. Chromatids migrate to opposite poles by the mitotic spindle.	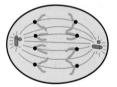	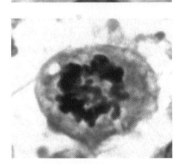
Telophase Division into two daughter cells occurs. Nuclear membrane reappears.	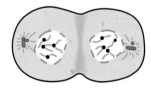	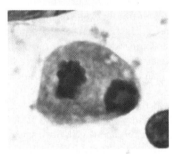

Electron micrographs from Stevens A, Lowe J: *Human Histology*, ed 3, Mosby, St Louis, 2005.

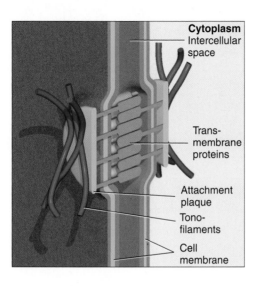

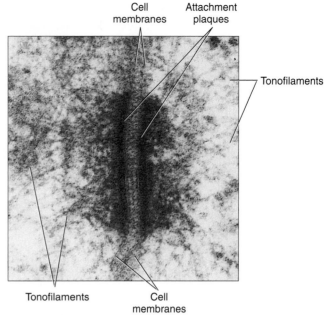

FIGURE 7-5 Intercellular junctions between cells, with its cell adhesion between cell membranes mediated by transmembrane proteins shown in an electron micrograph. Note the attachment plaque, which is the attachment device involving tonofilaments. *(From Stevens A, Lowe J:* Human Histology, *ed 3, Mosby, St Louis, 2005.)*

divided. The cell division that takes place during mitosis consists of four phases: prophase, metaphase, anaphase, and telophase, which is then followed again by interphase so as to continue the cell cycle.

EXTRACELLULAR MATERIALS

The cells in each tissue type are surrounded by extracellular materials, which include both tissue fluid and intercellular substance. Tissue fluid (or interstitial fluid) provides a medium for dissolving, mixing, and transporting substances and for carrying out chemical reactions. Similar to blood **plasma** in its content of ions and diffusible substances, tissue fluid contains a small amount of plasma proteins.

Tissue fluid enters the tissue to surround the cells by diffusing through the capillary walls as a filtrate from the plasma of the blood. Tissue fluid then drains back into the blood as **lymph** through osmosis, via the **lymphatics** (see Chapter 8). The amount of tissue fluid varies from tissue to tissue, with smaller variations occurring over time within any one tissue. An excess amount can accumulate when an injured tissue undergoes an inflammatory response, leading to tissue enlargement or edema (see Figure 10-3).

Intercellular substance (or ground substance) is shapeless, colorless, and transparent. It fills the spaces between cells in a tissue. It serves as a barrier to the penetration of foreign substances into the tissue. It also serves as a medium for the exchange of gases and metabolic substances. The surrounding cells produce the intercellular substance, and one of its most common ingredients is hyaluronic acid.

INTERCELLULAR JUNCTIONS

Some cells in certain tissue are joined by the mechanism of intercellular junctions. These are mechanical attachments formed between cells, and also between cells and nearby noncellular surfaces. With the formation of these intercellular junctions, the cell membranes come close together but do not completely attach. Higher-power microscopes are needed to visualize these attachments, which appear as dense bodies; all intercellular junctions involve some sort of intricate attachment device. The attachment device includes an attachment plaque that is located within the cell as well as adjacent tonofilaments.

An intercellular junction between cells is formed by a desmosome, such as that seen in the upper layers of the skin (Figure 7-5). The desmosome appears to be disc-shaped, and can be likened to a "spot weld" within the structure of a tissue. The desmosomal junctions are also released during tissue turnover and then become reattached in new locations as the cells migrate, such as during repair after an injury to the skin or oral mucosa (see Figure 8-3).

Desmosomes can cause an artifact when cells in the **stratified squamous epithelium** are fixed for prolonged microscopic study, because they tend to cause the regularly plump cells to appear prickled or star-shaped as the desmosomes still maintain their junctional stronghold between the shrinking cells (see Figure 9-8).

Another type of intercellular junction is formed by a hemidesmosome, which involves an attachment of a cell to an adjacent noncellular surface (Figure 7-6). This type of attachment is used for attaching the epithelium to connective tissue, such as with the **basement membrane** in the **oral mucosa** (see Figure 8-4). The attachment device of a hemidesmosome looks like half of a desmosome, because it involves a smaller attachment plaque and tonofilaments from only the cellular side. Thus, it appears as a thinner disc because the noncellular surface cannot produce the other half of the attachment mechanism. Hemidesmosomes are also involved as a mechanism allowing **gingival tissue** to be secured to the tooth surface by the **epithelial attachment** (see Figures 10-8), as well as with the attachment between the nails and nail beds.

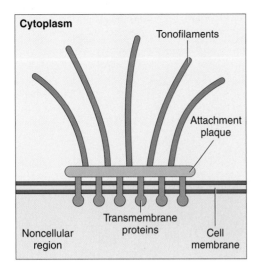

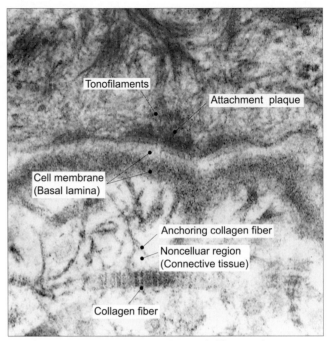

FIGURE 7-6 Hemidesmosomal intercellular junctions shown in an electron micrograph. The attachment of cells is to an adjacent noncellular surface, with the adhesion to the noncellular surface mediated by transmembrane protein. This type occurs at the basement membrane between epithelial and connective tissue (as shown here), as well as at the attachment of gingival tissue to the tooth surface. Note the smaller attachment plaques of the hemidesmosomal junction and tonofilaments on the cellular side. *(From Stevens A, Lowe J:* Human Histology, *ed 3, Mosby, St Louis, 2005.)*

Basic Tissue

●●●CHAPTER OUTLINE

●●●LEARNING OBJECTIVES

- Define and pronounce the key terms in this chapter.
- List and describe each of the basic histological types of tissue.
- Integrate the knowledge of the basic histology into an understanding of the specific histology of the orofacial region and its promotion of health as well as any related pathology that may occur.

●●●NEW KEY TERMS

Basal lamina (bay-sal lam-i-nah)
Basement membrane
Basophil (bay-sah-fil)
Blood
Bone: cancellous (kan-sel-us), compact (kom-pak), immature, marrow (mar-oh), mature, secondary
Calcium hydroxyapatite (hy-drox-see-ap-ah-tite)
Canaliculi (kan-ah-lik-u-lie)
Cartilage (kar-ti-lij): hyaline (hi-ah-line), elastic
Cell: B-, mast, NK-, red blood, T-, white blood
Chondroblasts (kon-dro-blasts)
Chondrocytes (kon-dro-sites)

Connective tissue: adipose (ad-i-pose), dense, elastic (e-las-tik), loose
Connective tissue papillae (pah-pil-ay), proper
Dermis (der-mis)
Endosteum (en-dos-te-um)
Endothelium (en-do-thee-lee-um)
Eosinophil (e-ah-sin-ah-fil)
Epidermis (ep-i-der-mis)
Epithelium (ep-ee-thee-lee-um): pseudostratified columnar (soo-doh-strat-i-fide), simple, stratified (strat-i-fide), stratified squamous (skway-mus)
Fibers: anchoring collagen (kol-ah-jen), collagen, elastic
Fibroblast (fi-bro-blast)

Fibrocartilage (fi-bro-kar-ti-lij)
Granulation tissue (gran-yoo-lay-shin)
Haversian system (hah-ver-zi-an), canal
Immunogen (im-un-ah-jen)
Immunoglobulin (im-u-nah-glob-ul-in)
Lacuna (plural, lacunae) (lah-ku-nah, lah-ku-nay): Howship's (how-ships)
Lamellae (lah-mel-ay)
Layer: papillary (pap-i-lar-ee), dense
Lines: arrest, reversal
Lymphocyte (lim-fo-site)
Macrophage (mak-rah-faje)
Matrix (may-triks)
Monocyte (mon-ah-site)
Muscle: skeletal
Nerve
Neuron (noor-on)

Odontoclast (o-**don**-to-klast)
Ossification (os-i-fi-**kay**-shun):
   endochondral (en-do-**kon**-dril),
   intramembranous (in-trah-**mem**-
   bran-us)
Osteocytes (os-tee-oh-sites)
Osteoid (os-te-oid)
Osteoblasts (os-te-oh-blasts)
Osteoclast (os-te-oh-klast)

Osteons (os-te-onz)
Perichondrium (per-ee-**kon**-dre-um)
Periosteum (per-ee-**os**-te-im)
Plasma (plaz-mah)**, cells**
Platelets (plate-lits)
Polymorphonuclear leukocyte (pol-ee-
   mor-fah-**noo**-klee-er **loo**-ko-site)
Resorption (re-**sorp**-shun): **generalized,**
   localized

Rete ridges (ree-tee)
Reticular connective tissue (re-**tik**-u-ler),
   fibers, lamina (**lam**-i-nah)
Squames (skwaymz)
Synapse (**sin**-aps)
Turnover time
Trabeculae (trah-**bek**-u-lay)
Volkmann's canals (**volk**-manz)

BASIC TISSUE

Dental professionals must have a clear understanding of the histology of these basic tissue types before studying the distinct tissue types present in the oral cavity and associated regions of the face and neck. This information will help dental professionals fully understand the processes involving tissue repair during patient care to promote orofacial health, as well as the underlying pathological processes that can occur in these regions.

ANATOMY OF BASIC TISSUE

Cells with similar characteristics of form and function are grouped together to form a **tissue** as was discussed in Chapter 7. A tissue is a collection of similarly specialized cells that will then form into **organs**. Tissue types are categorized according to four basic histological types. These basic histological tissue types include epithelial, connective, muscle, and nerve tissue (Table 8-1, see Table 7-1). These basic tissue types have subcategories that serve specialized functions. It is during prenatal development that embryonic cell layers differentiate into the various basic embryological tissue types: **ectoderm, mesoderm,** and **endoderm** that will later form the basic histological tissue types of the body (see Table 3-4).

Most tissue of the body can be renewed as the individual cells die and are removed from the tissue. The turnover time is the time it takes for the newly divided cells to be completely replaced throughout the tissue. The turnover time differs for each of the basic tissue types, as well as for specific regions of the oral cavity. A complete understanding of turnover time may be the future basis for how aging and disease processes in the body are fought, including those occurring in the oral cavity.

EPITHELIUM

Epithelium is the tissue type that covers and lines both the external and internal body surfaces, including vessels and small cavities. Epithelium not only serves as a protective covering or lining but is also involved in tissue absorption, secretin, sensory, and other specialized functions. It serves to protect the more complex inner structures from physical, chemical, and pathogenic attack, as well as dehydration and heat loss by the formation of an epithelial barrier.

Depending on their classification, epithelial tissue can be derived from any of the three **embryonic cell layers**. Those of the skin and oral mucosa are of ectodermal origin. Those lining the respiratory and digestive tract are of endodermal origin, and those of the urinary tract are derived from mesoderm.

HISTOLOGY OF EPITHELIUM

Epithelium generally consists of closely grouped polyhedral cells surrounded by very little or no **intercellular substance** or **tissue fluid** (Figure 8-1). This tissue is capable of rapid turnover. In fact,

TABLE 8-1	Classification of Basic Tissue Types
TISSUE	**TYPES**
Epithelium	**Simple:** squamous, cuboidal, columnar, pseudostratified
	Stratified: squamous (keratinized, nonkeratinized), cuboidal, columnar, transitional
Connective tissue	**Solid soft:** connective tissue proper, specialized (adipose, fibrous, elastic, reticular)
	Solid firm: cartilage
	Solid rigid: bone
	Fluid: blood, lymph
Muscle	**Involuntary:** smooth, cardiac
	Voluntary: skeletal
Nerve	**Afferent:** sensory
	Efferent: motor

epithelium is highly regenerative because its deeper germinal cells are capable of reproduction by **mitosis** (see Table 7-2). Epithelial cells usually undergo cellular differentiation as they move from the deeper germinal layers to the surface of the tissue.

Epithelial cells are tightly joined to one another by **intercellular junctions** in the form of **desmosomes,** except in the more superficial layers. The epithelial cells are also tightly joined in some cases to nearby noncellular surfaces by **hemidesmosomes,** such as with the basement membrane (see Figures 7-5 and 7-6).

The **basement membrane** is located between most epithelium and deeper connective tissue, such skin and **oral mucosa**, and is produced by both the epithelium and the adjoining connective tissue.

Epithelium is avascular, having no blood supply of its own. Cellular nutrition consisting of oxygen and metabolites is obtained by diffusion from the adjoining connective tissue, which is usually highly vascularized, providing its own source of nutrition.

CLASSIFICATION OF EPITHELIUM

Epithelium can be classified into two main categories based on their arrangement into layers of cells: simple and stratified. Simple epithelium consists of a single layer of epithelial cells. The further classification of tissue involves different types of epithelial cells according to cellular shape; they can be simple squamous, simple cuboidal, or simple columnar (Table 8-2).

Simple squamous epithelium consists of flattened platelike epithelial cells, or squames, lining blood and lymphatic vessels, heart, and serous cavities, as well as interfaces in the lungs and kidneys (see

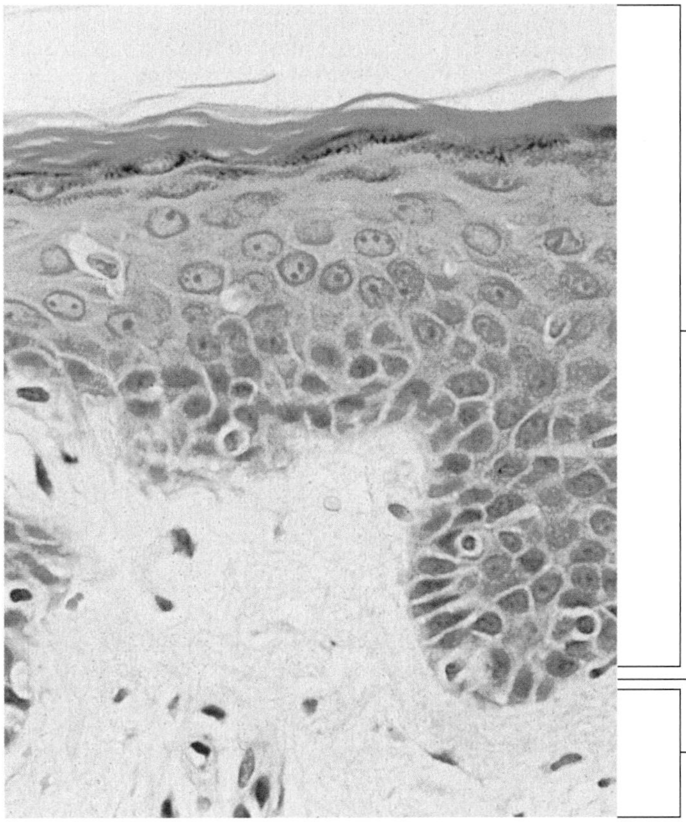

FIGURE 8-1 Microscopic sections of the skin showing epidermis and dermis, epithelium and connective tissue, respectively. A basement membrane is located between these two tissue types. (*A: From Stevens A, Lowe J: Human Histology, ed 3, Mosby, St Louis, 2005; B: Courtesy of James McIntosh, PhD, Assistant Professor Emeritus, Department of Biomedical Sciences, Baylor College of Dentistry, Dallas, TX.)*

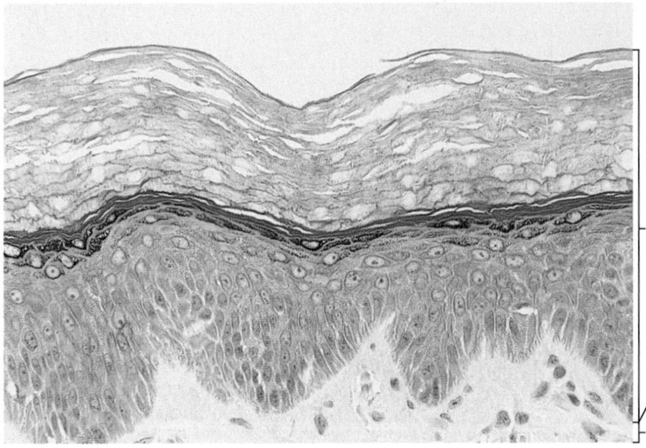

Table 8-2). The special term endothelium is used to refer to the simple squamous epithelium lining of these vessels and serous cavities.

Simple cuboidal epithelium consists of cube-shaped cells that line the **ducts** of various glands, such as certain ducts of the **salivary glands**. Simple columnar epithelium consists of rectangular or tall cells, such as in the lining of other salivary gland ducts, as well as the **inner enamel epithelium**, whose cells become enamel-forming **ameloblasts** (see Figures 6-9 and 11-6).

Epithelium can also be classified as pseudostratified columnar epithelium (Figure 8-2). This epithelium falsely appears as multiple

cell layers when viewed under low-power microscopic magnification, because the cells' nuclei appear at different levels (see Table 8-1). However, in reality, under higher microscopic magnification, cells of different heights are seen. Thus, this is a type of simple epithelium because all the cells line up to contact inner the basement membrane, but not all reach the outer surface of the tissue. Pseudostratified columnar epithelium lines the upper respiratory tract, including the **nasal cavity** and **paranasal sinuses** (see Figure 11-19). This type of epithelium may have cilia or be nonciliated at the tissue surface.

TABLE 8-2	Types of Epithelial Cells

CELLS WITH DESCRIPTION/EXAMPLES	MICROSCOPIC APPEARANCE IN TISSUE*
Squamous cells Flattened cells with cell height much less than cell width i.e., blood vessel lining (endothelium)	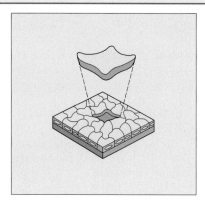 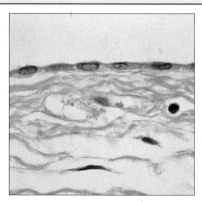
Cuboidal cells Cube-shaped cells with approximately equal cell height and cell width i.e., salivary gland	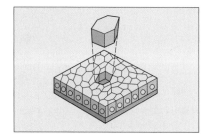 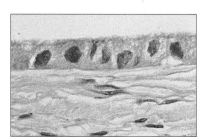
Columnar cells Rectangular or tall cells in which cell height exceeds cell width i.e., salivary gland ducts	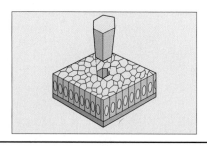 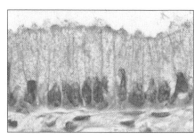

*Note that these epithelial cells are shown within *simple epithelium*. Diagrams from Stevens A, Lowe J: *Human Histology*, ed 3, Mosby, St Louis, 2005.

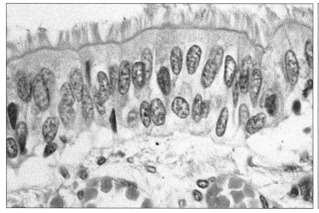 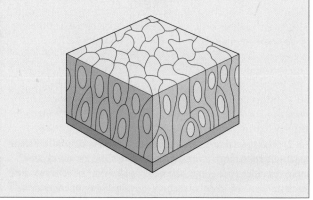

FIGURE 8-2 Microscopic view and diagram of pseudostratified columnar epithelium, such as present lining the respiratory system. It falsely appears as multiple cell layers when viewed under low-power microscopic magnification, because the cells' nuclei appear at different levels. However, in reality, cells of different heights are present, and because all have a direct relationship with the basement membrane, it is simple epithelium. *(From Stevens A, Lowe J:* Human Histology, *ed 3, Mosby, St Louis, 2005.)*

Stratified epithelium consists of two or more layers of cells, with only the deepest layer lining up to contact the basement membrane (see Table 8-1). It is important to note that only the cellular shape of the most superficial or surface layer is used to determine the classification of stratified epithelium. Thus, stratified epithelium can consist of cuboidal, columnar, or squamous epithelial cells, or a combination of types, as seen in a transitional epithelium.

Most epithelium in the body is stratified squamous epithelium, which includes the superficial layer of the skin and oral mucosa (see Figures 8-1 and 8-7 and Chapter 9). Only the most superficial layers of this tissue are flat cells, or **squames**; the deeper cells vary from the deeper cuboidal to the more superficial polyhedral. Interdigitation of the outer epithelium with the deeper connective tissue, having a basement membrane between them, appear on two-dimensional microscopic sections as the rete ridges (or rete pegs).

Stratified squamous epithelium can be keratinized or nonkeratinized. **Keratin** (see Chapter 7) is a tough, fibrous, opaque, waterproof protein that is impervious to pathogenic invasion and resistant to friction. Keratin is produced during the maturation of the *keratinocyte* epithelial cells as they migrate from near the basement membrane to the surface of the keratinized tissue, which occurs in certain regions of the **oral mucosa** found in the oral cavity (see Figure 9-11).

Another example of keratinized stratified squamous epithelium is epidermis, which is the superficial layer of the skin (see Figures 8-1 and 8-7). The epidermis overlies a basement membrane and the adjoining deeper layers of connective tissue (dermis and hypodermis, respectively; discussed later). The skin has varying degrees of keratinization depending on the region of the body; areas such as the palms of the hands and bottom of the feet have thicker layers of keratin, which form calluses. However, the keratin is less densely packed in both the skin and oral cavity, as compared with the densely packed hard keratin of the nails and hair.

EPITHELIUM TURNOVER AND REPAIR

Turnover of epithelium occurs as the newly formed deepest cells migrate superficially from their formation near the basement membrane. Thus, the **turnover time** is the time needed for a cell to divide and pass through the entire thickness of tissue. In order to migrate, the cells release and then regain their desmosomal connections at their **intercellular junctions** in the more superficial location. The turnover time is higher for all types of epithelium, as compared to connective tissue. This higher turnover time is a result of the higher level of **mitosis** in those deepest dividing cells near the basement membrane. Thus, the older, superficial epithelial cells are being shed or lost at the same rate as the deeper germinal cells are dividing into more cells.

These overall higher turnover times vary slightly for the different types of epithelium. However, the epithelium of the **oral mucosa** generally has a higher turnover time than the **epidermis** of the skin (see Table 9-6). More specifically, within the oral cavity, the epithelium that lines the cheek tissue (**buccal mucosa**) has a higher turnover time (14 days) than the epithelium that covers the skin (27 days). This difference becomes apparent when dental professionals sadly note a traumatic superficial injury to the facial skin lasting for weeks, and, at the same time, happily observe the quicker healing in the cheek area after the patient accidentally bites the superficial oral mucosa.

Thus the differences of turnover time are especially noted during repair or healing of the tissue after injury. Immediately after an injury to either the skin or oral mucosa, a clot from blood products forms in the area, and the inflammatory response is triggered by the blood's **white blood cells (WBCs)** as they migrate into the tissue (Figure 8-3). If the source of injury is removed, tissue repair can begin within the next few days. The epithelial cells at the periphery of the injury will lose their desmosomal intercellular junctions and migrate to form a new epithelial surface layer beneath the clot.

Thus, a clot is very important in repair of the epithelium and must be retained in the first days of repair because it acts as a guide to form a new surface. A clot stays moist in the oral cavity but dries out on the skin (called a *scab* when on the skin). Later, after the epithelial surface is repaired, the clot is broken down by enzymes because it is no longer needed. Repair of the epithelium is a process that is also tied to repair in the deeper connective tissue (discussed later).

BASEMENT MEMBRANE

As discussed earlier, the basement membrane is a thin, acellular structure always located between any form of epithelium and its underlying connective tissue, as noted in both the skin and oral mucosa (Figure 8-4, see Figures 7-6 and 8-7). This type of structure is even present embryologically between the two types of tissue of the tooth germ during tooth development (see Figure 6-7).

The details of the basement membrane are not seen when it is viewed by scanning or lower-power microscopic magnification; only its location can be indicated. A higher-power magnification, such as that afforded by an electron microscope, is needed to see the intricacies of the basement membrane. The basement membrane consists of two layers: basal lamina and reticular lamina. The terms *basement membrane* and *basal lamina* are sometimes used interchangeably, but the basal lamina is, in fact, only a part of the basement membrane. The term "basal lamina" is usually used with electron microscopy, while the term "basement membrane" is usually used with lower-power light microscopy.

The superficial layer of the basement membrane is the basal lamina and is produced by the epithelium, and it is about 40 to 50 nm

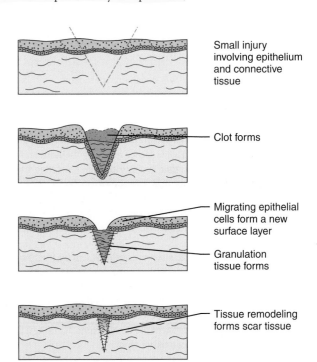

FIGURE 8-3 Repair process of the skin or oral mucosa after an injury. Note the initial formation of the clot and migrating epithelial cells from the surrounding intact tissue, and formation of granulation tissue in the later days of repair. Later, the tissue will remodel and form scar tissue. *(From Fehrenbach MJ: Inflammation and repair. In Ibsen OAC, Phelan JA (eds).* Oral Pathology for Dental Hygienists, *ed 5, WB Saunders, Philadelphia, 2009.)*

Small injury involving epithelium and connective tissue

Clot forms

Migrating epithelial cells form a new surface layer

Granulation tissue forms

Tissue remodeling forms scar tissue

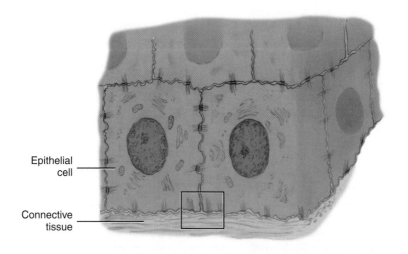

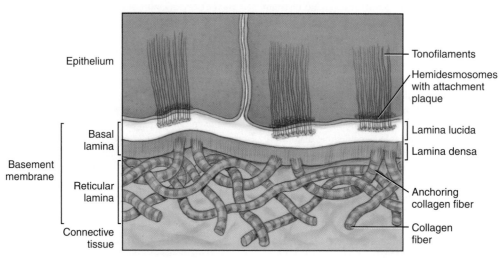

FIGURE 8-4 Basement membrane, with its basal lamina and reticular lamina, as well as the attachment devices from the epithelium (hemidesmosomes and tonofilaments with attachment plaques) and connective tissue (anchoring collagen fibers), respectively.

thick. Microscopically, the basal lamina consists of two sublayers: The *lamina lucida* is a clear layer that is closer to the epithelium, and the *lamina densa* is a dense layer that is closer to the connective tissue. The deeper layer of the basement membrane is usually the reticular lamina (the exception is lung alveoli and kidney, with fusion of basal laminae). The reticular lamina consists of collagen fibers and reticular fibers produced and secreted by the underlying connective tissue (discussed later).

Attachment mechanisms are also part of the basement membrane. These involve **hemidesmosomes** with the attachment plaque, **tonofilaments** from the epithelium and the anchoring collagen fibers from the connective tissue (see Figure 7-6). The tonofilaments loop through the attachment plaque, whereas the collagen fibers of the reticular lamina loop into the lamina densa of the basal lamina, forming a flexible attachment between the two tissue types.

It is important to note that the interface between the epithelium and connective tissue of the skin and oral mucosa where the basement membrane is located is not two-dimensional, as seen in microscopic cross sections of the tissue where there are rete ridges and connective tissue papillae (discussed next). Instead, in reality, the interface consists of three-dimensional *interdigitation* of the two tissue types. This complex arrangement increases the amount of surface area for

the interface, thus increasing the mechanical strength of the interface, as well as the nutrition potential of the avascular epithelium from the vascularized connective tissue.

CONNECTIVE TISSUE

All of the connective tissue of the body, when taken together represents, by weight, the most abundant type of basic tissue in the body—even if it is epithelium that is mainly seen when clinically viewing the body. Connective tissue is derived from the **somites** during prenatal development (see Figure 3-12). The functions of connective tissue are varied; connective tissue is involved in support, attachment, packing, insulation, storage, transport, repair, and defense (see Table 8-1).

HISTOLOGY OF CONNECTIVE TISSUE

Compared with epithelium, connective tissue is usually composed of fewer cells spaced farther apart and containing larger amounts of matrix between the cells (except in adipose connective tissue). This matrix is composed of **intercellular substance** and fibers.

Most connective tissue is renewable because its cells are capable of **mitosis,** and because most of its cells can even produce their own

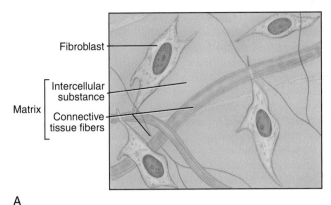

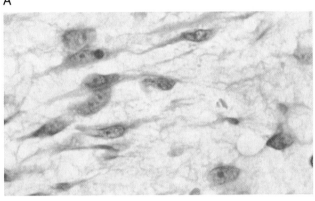

A

B

FIGURE 8-5 Diagram and related microscopic view of fibroblasts within loose connective tissue, showing their spindle or fusiform shape. It forms the fibers of the connective tissue, as well as the intercellular substance between the tissue components. (**B** *from Stevens A, Lowe J: Human Histology, ed 3, Mosby, St Louis, 2005.*)

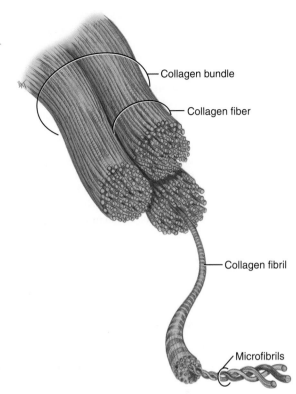

FIGURE 8-6 Collagen bundle that is composed of fibers, and smaller subunits—fibrils and microfibrils.

TABLE 8-3	Types of Collagen
MAIN TYPES OF COLLAGEN	**DESCRIPTION**
Type I	Most common type in skin dermis, lamina propria, bone, teeth, tendons, and virtually all connective tissue
Type II	In hyaline and elastic cartilage
Type III	In granulation tissue, produced quickly by young fibroblasts before tougher Type I synthesized, thus commonly found alongside Type I
	Main component of reticular fibers but also found in artery walls, skin, intestines, and uterus
Type IV	In basal lamina, eye lens, and filtration system of capillaries and kidney's nephron glomeruli

matrix of intercellular substance and fibers. In most cases, connective tissue is vascularized (except cartilage), having own blood supplies.

Differing cells are found within the various types of connective tissue. The most common cell in all types of connective tissue is the **fibroblast** (Figure 8-5). Fibroblasts synthesize certain types of protein fibers and intercellular substances needed to sustain the connective tissue. They are flat, elongated cells with cytoplasmic processes at each end. Subpopulations of fibroblasts may be possible in connective tissue. Fibroblasts are considered fixed cells in connective tissue, because they do not leave the tissue to enter the blood, as compared to cells with mobility, such as WBCs.

Young fibroblasts that are actively engaged in the production of fibers and intercellular substances appear to have large amounts of cytoplasm, mitochondria, and rough endoplasmic reticulum. Fibroblasts can show aging and inactivity, with a reduction in cytoplasm, mitochondria, and rough endoplasmic reticulum, such as seen in the later stages of periodontal inflammation (see **Chapter 10**). If adequately stimulated during repair, however, fibroblasts can revert to a more active state.

Other cells found in connective tissue include migrated **WBCs** from the blood supply, such as monocytes (macrophages), basophils (mast cells), lymphocytes (including plasma cells), and neutrophils (discussed later). Certain other transient cell types are found in specific classifications of connective tissue and are discussed later.

Different types of protein fibers are found in various types of connective tissue. Collagen fibers are the main connective tissue fiber type found in the body (Figure 8-6). Tissue containing a large amount

of collagen fibers is considered a *collagenous connective tissue,* but all connective tissue (except blood) contain some collagen fibers. Collagen fibers are composed of the protein collagen, including distinct types that have been shown by immunological study to have great tensile strength. All collagen fibers are composed of smaller subunits, or *fibrils,* which are composed of *microfibrils*—similar to a strong, intact rope that is composed of smaller entwined strands of roping material.

Over 29 types of collagen have been identified and described; however, over 90% of the collagen in the body or in fetal tissue is composed of only Types I-IV (see Table 8-3). The most common type of collagen protein is Type I, which is found in the skin **dermis**, **lamina propria**, **bone**, **dentitions**, tendons, and virtually all other types of connective tissue. Cells responsible for the synthesis of Type I include **fibroblasts** and **osteoblasts,** which produce bone, as well as **odontoblasts,** which produce dentin (see Figure 6-11).

Elastic fibers are another type of fiber, composed of **microfilaments** embedded in the protein elastin, which results in a very elastic type of tissue. Thus, this tissue has the ability to stretch and then to return to its original shape after contraction or extension. Certain regions in the oral cavity, such as the **soft palate,** contain elastic fibers in the lamina propria to allow this type of tissue movement (see Figure 9-9).

Reticular fibers are found in relationship to an embryonic tissue and thus are found more rarely in the body. Reticular fibers are composed of the protein reticulin and are very fine, hairlike fibers that branch, forming a network in the tissue that contain them. Reticular connective tissue predominates in the **lymph nodes** and spleen.

CLASSIFICATION OF CONNECTIVE TISSUE

One method of classifying connective tissue is according to texture, which can be soft, firm, rigid, or fluid in nature (see Table 8-1). Soft connective tissue includes the tissue found in the deeper layers of the skin and oral mucosa, such as a connective tissue proper. Firm connective tissue consists of different types of cartilage. Rigid connective tissue consists of bone. Fluid connective tissue consists of blood with all its components and lymph.

CONNECTIVE TISSUE PROPER

Soft connective tissue can be classified as loose, dense, or specialized. Both loose and dense types of connective tissue are found together in two layers as connective tissue proper. The connective tissue proper is found deep to the epithelium and basement membrane, in the deeper layers of the skin and oral mucosa.

The connective tissue proper in the skin is the dermis and is found deep to the epidermis (discussed earlier; see Figures 8-1 and Figure 8-7). Even deeper to the dermis is the *hypodermis*, which is composed of loose connective tissue and adipose connective tissue, a specialized connective tissue, as well as glandular tissue, large blood vessels, and nerves. Cartilage, bone, and muscle can be present deep to the hypodermis of the skin, depending on the region of the body. In **oral mucosa,** the connective tissue proper is considered the **lamina propria,** which is discussed in Chapter 9, and the deeper connective tissue is the **submucosa,** similar to the hypodermis (see Figures 9-1 and 9-7).

Loose Connective Tissue The superficial layer of both the dermis of the skin and lamina propria of the oral mucosa is composed of loose connective tissue (see Figure 8-7). In the dermis or lamina propria, this layer of loose connective tissue is also considered the papillary layer. The papillary layer has connective tissue papillae, which are interdigitations of loose connective tissue with the epithelium (see earlier discussion of rete ridges). This papillary layer has no overly prominent connective tissue element; all the components of the papillary layer are present in equal amounts. Thus, equal amounts of cells, intercellular substance, fibers, and tissue fluid are in an irregular and loose arrangement. This loose layer of the connective tissue proper serves as protective padding for the deeper structures of the body.

Dense Connective Tissue Deep to the loose connective tissue is dense connective tissue, such as that found in the deepest layers of the dermis or lamina propria (see Figure 8-7). Similar to loose connective tissue, all the same components of connective tissue are still present. However in contrast to loose connective tissue, dense connective tissue is tightly packed, with a regular arrangement, and it also consists mainly of protein fibers, which give this tissue its strength.

The dense connective tissue in the dermis and lamina propria is also considered the dense layer (or *reticular layer*). Thus, the dense layer is deep to the papillary layer in these types of connective tissue proper. In contrast, tendons, aponeuroses, and ligaments are a type of dense connective tissue that has a regular arrangement of strong, parallel collagen fibers with few fibroblast cells.

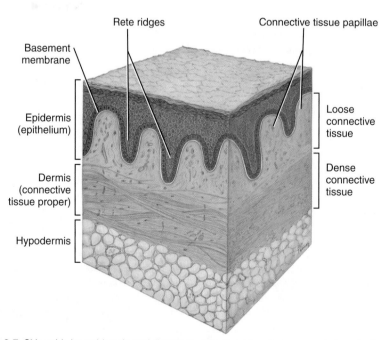

FIGURE 8-7 Skin with its epidermis and dermis layers. Hypodermis is present deep to the dermis. Note the interdigitating rete ridges of the epidermis with the connective tissue papillae.

Connective Tissue Turnover and Repair Turnover of both the connective tissue proper in skin or oral mucosa occurs as a result of the production of fibers and intercellular substance by the fibroblasts. Other types of cells can also undergo mitosis and create additional cells, such as certain WBCs and endothelial cells. The overall turnover time for a connective tissue proper is slower than its adjacent epithelium; it also demonstrates individual variance from region to region.

When injured, the connective tissue proper in the skin or oral mucosa goes through stages of repair that are related to the events in the more superficial epithelium (see Figure 8-3). After a clot forms and an inflammatory response is triggered with WBCs: **Fibroblasts** migrate to produce an immature connective tissue deep to the clot and newly forming epithelial surface.

This immature connective tissue is considered **granulation tissue** and has few fibers and an increased amount of blood vessels. Granulation tissue appears as a redder, soft tissue that bleeds easily. This tissue may become abundant and can interfere with the repair process. Surgical removal of excess granulation tissue may be necessary to allow for optimum repair. This sometimes occurs after the extraction of teeth or with periodontal disease.

Later, during the repair process, this temporary granulation tissue is replaced by paler and firmer scar tissue in the area. Scar tissue contains an increased amount of fibers and fewer blood vessels. The amount of scar tissue varies, depending on the type and size of the injury, amount of granulation tissue, and movement of tissue after injury. Interestingly, the skin shows more scar tissue both clinically and microscopically after repair than does the oral mucosa. This difference may be based on differing developmental origins of the tissue producing differing types of fibroblasts and thus different types of fibers.

AGING AND THE SKIN

At birth, the skin has not developed a sufficient protective layer, or facilitated the synthesis of immune cells. It often looks to be transparent, and therefore is sensitive to damage, and must be protected by extra clothing and kept away from environmental stress. At puberty, glandular and hair development, as well as the immune system, begins to function at an increased rate, giving extra protection for the skin against the coming adult world. During this time, the skin is in a very active state but still vulnerable to sensitization by allergens.

By age 20, however, the skin begins to deteriorate, and by the age of 50 is in a rapid state of degradation. Collagen fibers begin to fall apart; elastic fibers stiffen and thicken, wrinkling the skin. Oil glands in skin cease production, and melanin production decreases, leading to more pallid color and grey hairs. Keratin cells also cease production and so become thin and stiff. Skin begins to heal poorly after injury (see earlier discussion). It also becomes susceptible to disease states that include inflammation (such as with dermatitis), infection (such as with herpes zoster), and cancer (such as with basal cell carcinoma). Exposure to ultraviolet light will accelerate the aging process in skin, as does increased environmental toxicity (excessive alcohol and tobacco use).

SPECIALIZED CONNECTIVE TISSUE

Specialized connective tissue includes adipose, elastic, or reticular. **Adipose connective tissue** is a fatty tissue that is found beneath the skin, around organs and various joints, and in regions of the oral cavity. Unlike most connective tissue, this type of connective tissue has cells packed tightly together with little or no matrix. After fibroblasts, the predominant type of cell found in this tissue is the adipocyte, which stores fat intracellularly.

Elastic connective tissue has a large number of elastic fibers in its matrix, which combine strength with elasticity, such as in the tissue of the vocal cords. **Reticular connective tissue** is a delicate network of interwoven reticular fibers forming a supportive framework for blood vessels and internal organs.

CARTILAGE

Cartilage is a firm, nonmineralized connective tissue that serves as a skeletal tissue in the body (Figure 8-8). Cartilage forms much of the temporary skeleton of the **embryo** and serves as structural support for certain soft tissue after birth. Additionally, cartilage serves as a model or template in which certain bones of the body subsequently develop. Cartilage is also present at articular surfaces of most freely movable joints, such as the **temporomandibular joint (TMJ)** (see Figure 19-3). Further, in regard to the TMJ, cartilage may form abnormally within an aging **articular disc** that is normally composed of dense fibrous connective tissue, possibly causing clinical difficulties.

HISTOLOGY OF CARTILAGE

The connective tissue surrounding most cartilage is the **perichondrium**, a fibrous connective tissue sheath containing blood vessels.

Cartilage is composed of cells and matrix. Its matrix is composed of fibers, mainly collagen, and intercellular substance. Thus, this matrix is similar to soft connective tissue in composition, except that the matrix of cartilage is firmer.

Two types of cells found in cartilage are the immature **chondroblasts**, which lie internal to the perichondrium and produce cartilage matrix, and the **chondrocytes**, which are mature chondroblasts that maintain the cartilage matrix (see Figure 8-8). After the production of cartilage matrix, the chondrocyte becomes surrounded and enclosed by the matrix. Only a small space surrounds the chondrocyte within the cartilage matrix, the **lacuna** (plural, **lacunae**).

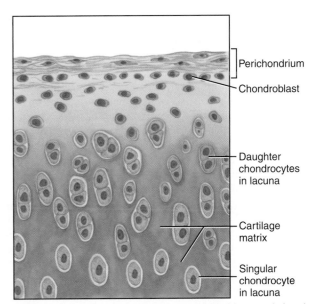

Perichondrium

Chondroblast

Daughter chondrocytes in lacuna

Cartilage matrix

Singular chondrocyte in lacuna

FIGURE 8-8 Cartilage, including its cells, chondroblasts and chondrocytes, as well as the outer layer of perichondrium, a formative connective tissue sheath.

The three types of cartilage—hyaline, elastic, and fibrocartilage—have slightly differing histological features. Histologists believe that this distinction between types of cartilage is not to be stressed, and that most cartilage contains a combination of the different types.

Hyaline cartilage is the most common type found in the body and contains only collagen fibers as part of its matrix. The associated collagen fibers of hyaline cartilage are much finer in substance than those within dense connective tissue. Hyaline cartilage can be found in the embryonic skeleton and in growth centers, such as the **mandibular condyle** (see Figure 19-7). All cartilage starts as hyaline cartilage and are then modified into the other two types of cartilage, according to need.

Elastic cartilage is similar to hyaline, except that it has numerous elastic fibers in its matrix, in addition to its numerous collagen fibers. Elastic cartilage is found in the external ear, auditory tube, epiglottis, and parts of the **larynx**.

Fibrocartilage is never found alone and merges gradually with its neighboring hyaline cartilage, such as in the outer part of the **TMJ** (see Figure 19-3). Unlike elastic cartilage, fibrocartilage is not merely a modification of hyaline. Rather, it is a transitional type of cartilage between hyaline cartilage and dense connective tissue of tendons and ligaments. The cells of the tissue are enclosed in capsules of matrix, giving it great tensile strength. Unlike both elastic and hyaline cartilage, fibrocartilage has no true perichondrium overlying it.

DEVELOPMENT OF CARTILAGE

Cartilage can develop or grow in size in two different ways: **interstitial growth** and **appositional growth** (see Chapter 3). Interstitial growth is growth from deep within the tissue by the **mitosis** of each chondrocyte, thus producing larger numbers of daughter cells within a single lacuna (each of which secretes more matrix), and expanding the tissue (see Figure 8-8). This interstitial growth is important in the development of bone that uses cartilage as a model for its own formation (endochondral ossification is discussed next).

Appositional growth is layered growth on the outside of the tissue from an outer layer of chondroblasts within perichondrium. This layer of chondroblasts is always present on the external surface of cartilage to allow appositional growth of cartilage after an injury or remodeling.

REPAIR AND AGING OF CARTILAGE

Unlike rigid bone, cartilage has some flexibility resulting from its fibers in the matrix; however, it has no inorganic (or mineralized) materials. Cartilage, unlike most connective tissue, is also avascular. Much like epithelium, this tissue depends on its surrounding connective tissue for its cellular nutrition, such as oxygen and metabolites. Since it has no vascularity of its own, cartilage takes longer to repair than does vascularized bone. Cartilage also has no nerve supply within its tissue. Thus, cartilage even when subjected to trauma or surgery does not produce overly painful symptoms.

Thus, during repair of the avascular cartilage, it is dependent on neighboring connective tissue from the perichondrium for nutrition to transform it slowly into cartilage. With this transformation, the newly formed cartilage slowly proliferates and fills in the defect by appositional growth. In contrast, fractured mature cartilage is often united by dense connective tissue, and if vascularization is initiated, then healing cartilage may eventually be replaced by bone.

As cartilage ages, it becomes less cellular, with its chondrocytes dying. It may start to contain firm fibers in parallel groups, or it may even form areas of scattered mineralization. These tend to coalesce over time, with the tissue becoming hard and brittle and losing flexibility.

BONE

Bone is a rigid connective tissue that constitutes most of the mature skeleton (Figure 8-9). Thus, bone serves as protective and structural support for soft tissue and as an attachment mechanism. It also aids in movement, manufactures blood cells through its red bone marrow, and is a storehouse for calcium and other minerals. It also surrounds the teeth with their **alveoli** as the **alveolar bone proper** (see Figure 14-15*B*).

Because bone is vascularized with its own blood supply, it repairs quickly compared with avascular cartilage. Even though bone is rigid, it is important to remember that it does not consist of an inanimate inner rod being moved by the **skeletal muscles**. Instead, it is a living and functioning tissue in the body. Bone has also undergone the most developmental **differentiation** of all the connective tissue.

ANATOMY OF BONE

When bone is examined grossly, the outer part of bone is covered by periosteum (see Figure 8-9). Periosteum is a double-layered, dense connective tissue sheath. The outer layer contains blood vessels and nerves. The inner layer contains a single layer of cells that give rise to bone-forming cells, the osteoblasts.

Deep to the periosteum is a dense layer of compact bone. Deep to the compact bone is a spongy bone, or cancellous bone. Both compact bone and cancellous bone have the same cellular components, but each has a different arrangement of those components (discussed next).

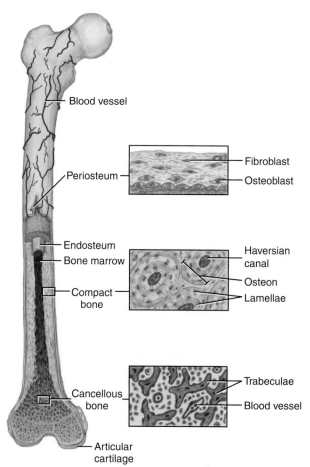

FIGURE 8-9 Anatomy of bone showing close-up views of its periosteum and compact or cancellous bone. Note the endosteum and bone marrow.

It is important to understand that the differences between these two types of bone include the relative amount of solid bone and also the size and number of soft tissue spaces in each; however, no sharp boundary exists between these two types of bone within an individual bone. Each bone type is located where it best serves the needs for either strength or lightness of weight. Compact bone is strong because it has fewer soft tissue spaces, but it is heavy. In contrast, cancellous bone is light because it is formed by pieces of solid bone that join to form a lattice; it is not as strong because it has more soft tissue spaces.

Lining the medullary cavity of bone on the inside of the layers of compact bone and cancellous bone is the endosteum (see Figure 8-9). The endosteum has the same composition as the periosteum but is thinner. On the innermost part of bone in the medullary cavity is the bone marrow. This gelatinous substance is where the stem cells of the **blood** are located, and **lymphocytes** are created and **B-cells** mature (discussed later). These stem cells can continue to produce most of the cells of the blood.

HISTOLOGY OF BONE

Bone consists of cells and a partially mineralized matrix that is 50% inorganic (or mineralized) material (Figure 8-10). It is this inorganic substance in a crystalline formation of mainly calcium hydroxyapatite, having the chemical formula $Ca_{10}(PO_4)_6(OH)_2$, that gives bone its hardness. This same type of inorganic crystal is found in differing percentages in the hard dental tissue, such as enamel, dentin, and cementum (see Table 6-2 for comparison of dental hard tissue types). Smaller amounts of other minerals, such as magnesium, potassium, calcium carbonate, and fluoride, are also present. This inorganic material has matrix packed between its bone cells. The matrix is composed of organic collagen fibers and intercellular substance.

Bone matrix is initially formed as osteoid, which later undergoes mineralization. The osteoid is produced by osteoblasts, cuboidal cells that arise from fibroblasts. Osteoblasts are also involved in the later mineralization of osteoid to form bone. Always present in the periosteum is a layer of osteoblasts at the external surface of the compact bone; it allows remodeling of bone and repair of injured bone.

Within fully mineralized bone are osteocytes, which are entrapped mature osteoblasts. Similar to the chondrocyte, the cell body of the osteocyte is surrounded by bone, except for the space immediately around it, the **lacuna** (plural, **lacunae**). The cytoplasmic processes of the osteocyte radiate outward in all directions in the bone and are located in tubular canals of matrix, or canaliculi. These canals provide for interaction between the osteocytes. However, unlike chondrocytes, osteoblasts never undergo mitosis during tissue formation, and thus only one osteocyte is ever found in a lacuna.

Bone matrix in compact bone is formed into closely apposed sheets, or lamellae. Within and between the lamellae are embedded osteocytes with their cytoplasmic processes in the canals. This highly organized arrangement of concentric lamellae in compact bone is the Haversian system.

In the Haversian system, these lamellae form concentric layers of matrix into cylinders or osteons (Figure 8-11). The osteon is the unit of structure in compact bone and consists of 5 to 20 lamellae. This arrangement in the osteon is similar to the growth rings in a cross section of a tree trunk. However, unlike tree rings that form at a rate of one per year, an entire Haversian system is produced all at the same time, no matter the number of concentric lamellae that may be involved.

The Haversian canal (or osteonic or central canals) is a central vascular canal within the each osteon surrounded by the lamellae. It contains longitudinally running blood vessels, nerves, and a small amount of connective tissue and is lined by endosteum. The Haversian canals communicate not only with each other but also with the osteocytic processes in the canaliculi and also provide cellular nutrition for the surrounding bone. This system of bone is noted within the structure of the **alveolar bone** (see Figure 14-16).

Located on the outer part of the Haversian system in compact bone are Volkmann's canals, or similar nutrient canals that contain the same vascular and nerve components as the Haversian canals, being also lined by **endosteum**. Volkmann's canals pass obliquely or at right angles to the Haversian canals of the osteons and communicate with them, as well as with the larger blood supply external to the bone. These canals are noted with the tooth socket or **alveolus** (plural, **alveoli**) so that it is sometimes referred to as the *cribriform plate* (see Figure 14-15, *B*).

In contrast to the highly organized compact bone, cancellous bone has its bone matrix formed into trabeculae, or joined matrix pieces forming a lattice (see Figure 8-9). Lamellae of the matrix of cancellous bone are not arranged into concentric layers around a central blood vessel as with the compact bone, but rather their concentric rings are

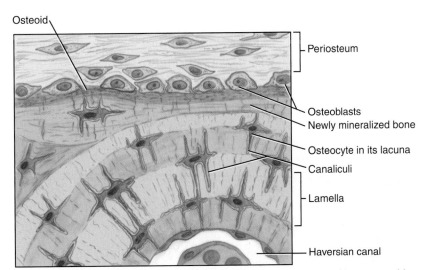

Osteoid
Periosteum
Osteoblasts
Newly mineralized bone
Osteocyte in its lacuna
Canaliculi
Lamella
Haversian canal

FIGURE 8-10 Histology of bone (in this case, compact bone). Note the cells of bone, osteoblasts, and osteocytes, as well as the periosteum, the outer formative sheath of connective tissue. The initial bone matrix or osteoid will mineralize later into mature bone.

formed into cone-shaped spicules. Osteocytes in lacunae with their cytoplasmic processes are located between the lamellae of the trabeculae. Surrounding the trabeculae are soft tissue spaces that consist of vascular canals with blood vessels, nerves, and varying amounts of connective tissue. These spaces also serve as a nutritional source for the lattice structure of bone.

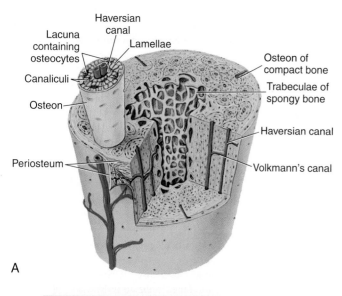

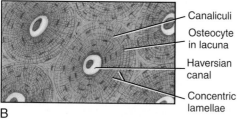

FIGURE 8-11 Haversian system in compact bone. **A:** Lamellae forming osteons. Note Volkmann's canal and its communication with larger blood vessels external to the bone. **B:** Close-up view highlighting osteons with their central Haversian canals, osteocytes, and canaliculi. *(From Applegate EJ: The Anatomy and Physiology Learning System, ed 3, WB Saunders, Philadelphia, 2006.)*

DEVELOPMENT OF BONE

Bone development, or ossification, has two methods of development: intramembranous and endochondral ossification. The bone produced by both these developmental methods is microscopically the same; only the process of formation is different. **Intramembranous ossification** is formation of osteoid between two dense connective tissue sheets, which then eventually replaces the outer connective tissue (Figure 8-12). During intramembranous ossification, mesenchymal cells differentiate into osteoblasts to form the osteoid.

Intramembranous ossification uses a method of appositional growth similar to that of cartilage, with layers of osteoid being produced. The osteoid later becomes mineralized to form bone. Certain bones in the body, such as the flat bones and clavicle, can form this way, enlarging over time as the appositional growth of bone occurs. The **maxilla** and the majority of the **mandible** are formed by intramembranous ossification (see Chapter 14).

Endochondral ossification is the formation of the osteoid within a hyaline cartilage model that subsequently becomes mineralized and dies (Figure 8-13). Osteoblasts penetrate the disintegrating cartilage and form primary ossification centers that continue forming osteoid toward the ends of the bone during prenatal development. Thus, bone matrix eventually replaces the earlier cartilage model. This type of ossification first uses the method of interstitial growth of the initial cartilage tissue to form the model, or pattern, of the future bone's shape. Later, appositional growth of osteoid, with layers laid down on the outer perimeter, occurs to complete the final bone mass within the model.

Most long bones of the body are formed this way, because it allows bone to grow in length from deep within the tissue. Later after birth, secondary ossification centers, which allow further growth of the bones, are also formed. In particular, the head of the **mandibular condyle** is formed by endochondral ossification that has a multidirectional growth capacity (see Chapter 14, Figure 19-4).

Regardless of its method of development, bone also goes through specific stages (Figure 8-14). The first bone to be produced by either method of ossification is considered woven bone, or immature bone. In immature bone, the lamellae are indistinct because of the irregular arrangement of the collagen fibers and lamellae, whether located within the Haversian system or trabeculae.

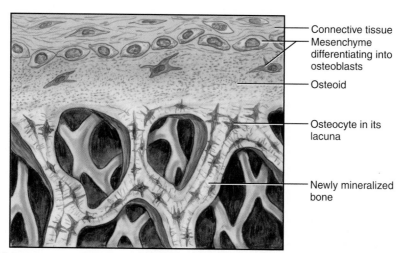

FIGURE 8-12 Intramembranous ossification, which is the formation of osteoid within two dense connective tissue sheets that eventually replace the connective tissue. During intramembranous ossification, mesenchyme differentiates into osteoblasts to form osteoid, which later matures into bone.

Immature bone is a temporary tissue that is replaced by a more mature secondary bone. Depending on the specific needs of the bone in any given area, secondary bone can be compact or cancellous (see Figure 8-11). In contrast to immature bone, secondary bone has a well-organized arrangement of collagen fibers and distinct lamellae.

BONE REPAIR, REMODELING, AND AGING

After bone fracture and during the repair of bone, bone goes through the stages of bone formation, no matter how the bone initially developed. In the area to be repaired, bone forms initially as immature bone, which matures into secondary bone to complete the repair. The repair of bone depends on adequate blood supply, the presence of periosteum with active osteoblasts, and adequate mineral and vitamin levels.

Thus, it becomes apparent that a bone's overall structure is not static and, therefore, never remains the same. Throughout life, bone in the body is constantly being remodeled or replaced. Bone undergoes removal in certain areas and new bone formation in other areas, with the two processes balancing each other within a healthy body. Appositional growth, with layered formation of bone along its periphery, is accomplished by the osteoblasts, which later become entrapped as osteocytes (see Figure 8-10).

Resorption can involve the removal of bone (Figure 8-15). The cell that causes resorption of bone is the osteoclast. The osteoclast is a large multinucleated cell located on the surface of secondary bone in a large, shallow pit created by this resorption, Howship's lacuna. Each osteoclast contains a large number of lysosomes in its cytoplasm, and these are discharged into the surrounding tissue as bone breaks down when the cell attaches by way of its *ruffled border*. It is formed from the fusion of numbers of macrophage blood cells (discussed later).

Localized resorption occurs in a specific area of a bone as a result of infection, altered mechanical stress, or pressure on the bone so that it adapts by remodeling. Resorption can occur in an uncontrolled manner during active periodontal disease, which is in contrast to that occurring in a controlled manner with orthodontic therapy (see Chapters 14 and 20). In contrast, generalized resorption occurs over the entire skeleton in varying amounts because of endocrine activity to increase blood levels of calcium and phosphate needed by the body. Excess generalized bone resorption, as well as excess bone appositional growth, can occur in certain bone disorders when the two processes are no longer balanced.

Microscopically, a cross section of bone demonstrates layers related to its development that look like growth rings in a tree when stained, similar to those noted in cementum (see Figures 8-10, 8-15, 14-9, and 14-13). The arrest lines, or resting lines, appear as smooth lines between the layers of bone because of osteoblasts having rested, formed bone, and then rested again after appositional growth. Thus, arrest lines show the incremental or layered nature of appositional growth. In contrast, reversal lines appear as scalloped lines between the layers of bone. Reversal lines represent areas where bone resorption has first taken place, followed quickly by appositional growth of new bone.

As a person grows from fetal life through childhood, puberty, and finishes growth as a young adult, the bones of the skeleton change in size and shape; these can be noted on radiographs. The "bone age" of a child is the average age at which children reach this stage of bone maturation, and a child's current height and bone age can be used to predict adult height.

Bone mass or density is lost as people age, especially in women after menopause, with the bones losing calcium and other minerals. This can become accelerated with osteoporosis, especially for older women. The spinal column also becomes curved, compressed, and shorter; bone spurs may also form on the vertebrae that have become thinner with mineral and fluid loss; now bones become more brittle and may break more easily.

BLOOD

Blood is a fluid connective tissue that serves as a transport medium for cellular nutrients, such as respiratory gases like oxygen and carbon dioxide, as well as metabolites for the entire body. Blood is carried in endothelium-lined blood vessels, and its medium consists of plasma and cells (Table 8-4).

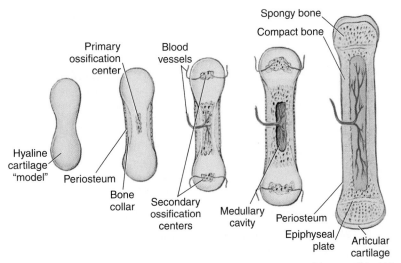

FIGURE 8-13 Endochondral ossification over time, which is the formation of the osteoid within a cartilage model that subsequently becomes mineralized and dies (**A** through **E**). Osteoblasts penetrate the disintegrating cartilage and form a primary ossification center that continues forming osteoid toward the ends of the bone during prenatal development. Later, after birth, secondary ossification centers form, which allows further growth of bones. (*From Applegate EJ:* The Anatomy and Physiology Learning System, *ed 3, WB Saunders, Philadelphia, 2006.*)

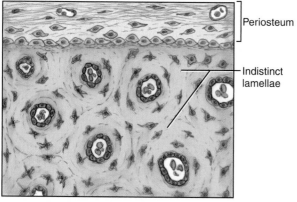

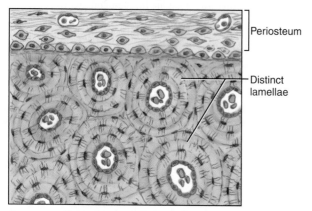

A   Immature bone (compact)

B   Secondary bone (compact)

FIGURE 8-14 Stages of bone development from immature bone (**A**) to secondary bone (**B**), in this case, compact bone. These two stages occur during both methods of ossification, as well as during the repair of bone.

PLASMA

Plasma is the fluid substance in the blood vessels that carries the plasma proteins, blood cells, and metabolites. It is more consistent in composition than **tissue fluid** and **lymph**; yet it contains most of the same materials with the addition of red blood cells (see Chapter 7). Serum, another fluid product, is distinguished from the plasma from which it is derived due to the removal of clotting proteins. If a sample of blood is treated with an agent to prevent clotting and is spun in a centrifuge, the plasma fraction is the least dense and will float as the top layer. Bone repair is being enhanced by the use of platelet-rich plasma (PRP) in alveoli with periodontal surgery of periodontal defects and implant placement.

BLOOD CELLS AND RELATED TISSUE CELLS

Blood cells and associated derivatives are also called the *formed elements* of the blood. Most blood cells come from a common stem cell in the **bone marrow** (Figure 8-16). The formed elements of the blood include the red blood cells. Not only are these cells present in the blood and its vessels, but also certain related components are also present in surrounding connective tissue.

The most common cell in the blood is the red blood cell (RBC), or erythrocyte (see Table 8-4). An RBC is a biconcave disc that contains

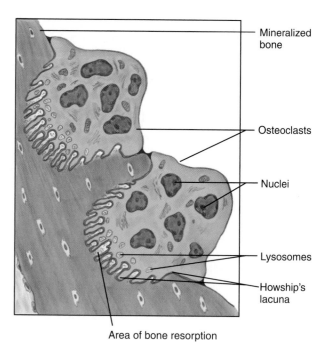

FIGURE 8-15 Osteoclasts within Howship's lacunae resorbing bone from their ruffled borders. Note the multiple nuclei within their cytoplasm, which contain lysosomes, and which, when discharged into the tissue, break down the bone.

hemoglobin, which binds and then transports the oxygen and carbon dioxide. It has no nucleus and does not undergo mitosis because it is formed from the bone marrow's stem cells. There are 5 to 6 million per cubic milliliter of blood, and thus are more common than other blood cells. In centrifuged blood, the RBCs settle to the bottom because they are denser than the rest; this fraction is the *hematocrit*.

The blood also contains platelets (or thrombocytes), which are smaller than RBCs, disc shaped, and also have no nucleus. However, this formed element is not considered a true blood cell, but instead a fragment of another blood cell and is found in lesser numbers at 250,000 to 400,000 per cubic milliliter. Platelets function in the clotting mechanism.

In even smaller numbers in the blood is the white blood cell (WBC) (or leukocyte) (see Tables 8-4 and Table 8-5). Like RBCs, WBCs form from bone marrow stem cells. WBCs later mature in the bone marrow or in various lymphatic organs. They are involved in the defense mechanisms of the body, including the inflammatory and immune responses. Thus, WBCs are also normally found in small numbers in both epithelium and connective tissue after they migrate from the blood by moving through openings between the cell junctions of the endothelial lining of the vessel to participate in defense mechanisms.

WBCs differ from RBCs because they possess a **nucleus**, have more **cytoplasm**, and have the power of active amoeboid movement in order to migrate from the blood to the tissue; thus, unlike RBCs, WBCs perform their functions not only in the blood but also in other tissue. They are also less numerous than RBCs (only 5,000 to 10,000 per cubic milliliter). There are five main types based on their microscopic appearance: neutrophils, lymphocytes, monocytes, eosinophils, and basophils. All are colorless and must be stained so that their differences may be observed. The fraction of centrifuged blood that settles on the surface of the hematocrit consists of the WBCs along with platelets, forming the intermediate *buffy coat*, with the plasma fraction superior to it.

The most common WBC in the blood is the polymorphonuclear leukocyte (PMN) or neutrophil (Figure 8-17). These are the first cells

TABLE 8-4	**Blood Cells and Related Tissue Cells**		
TYPE	**MICROSCOPIC APPEARANCE**	**DESCRIPTION**	**FUNCTION**
Red blood cell (erythrocyte)		Biconcave disc without nucleus	Binds and transports oxygen and carbon dioxide
Platelets (thrombocytes)		Discs without nucleus; cell fragments derived from special line of blood cell	Clotting mechanism
White blood cell (leukocyte)	See Table 8-5	Rounded cells with nucleus, many variations (see Table 8-5)	Inflammatory response and immune response

to appear at an injury site when the inflammatory response is triggered; thus, large numbers of the PMNs can be present in the suppuration, or pus, in certain cases seen locally at the injury site. PMNs constitute 54% to 62% of the total blood WBC count. They have a short life span, contain lysosomal enzymes, are active in **phagocytosis**, and respond to chemotactic factors (see Chapter 7).

The second most common WBC in the blood is the lymphocyte, which makes up 25% to 33% of the count. There are three functional types: B cell, T cell, and NK cell. B cells mature in the bone marrow and gut-associated lymphoid tissue such as lymph nodes (see Figure 11-16), whereas T cells mature in the thymus (see Figure 8-16). NK-cells also mature in the bone marrow. NK-cells (or natural killer cells) are large cells that are involved in the first line of defense against tumor- or virally infected cells by killing them and thus are not considered part of the immune response.

Cytokines are produced by B and T cells and are chemical mediators of the immune response. Thus, both these types of lymphocytes are involved in the immune response (see Table 8-5). In the past, the immune response was broken into two strict divisions: humoral and cell-mediated. However, the distinction between the two divisions is less important because they are strongly related.

One important difference between the two divisions remains: The B-cell lymphocytes divide during the immune response to form plasma cells. Once mature, plasma cells produce an immunoglobulin (Ig or antibody), one of the blood proteins. There are five distinct classes of immunoglobulins: IgA (serum or secretory types), IgE, IgD, IgG, and IgM (Table 8-6). Each plasma cell produces only one specific class of immunoglobulin in response to a specific immunogen (or antigen). Immunogens are mainly proteins that are seen by the body as foreign and are capable of triggering an immune response.

Although immunoglobulin structure overall is very similar, a small region at the tip of the protein (hypervariable region) is extremely variable, allowing generation of an infinite number with slightly different tip structures, or antigen binding sites, to exist. An immunoglobulin, along with its specific immunogen (its variable region is the epitope), often forms an immune complex in an effort to render the immunogen unable to cause disease. Immunoglobulins can be extracted from the blood of recovering patients and used for passive immunization against certain infectious diseases.

The most common WBC in the connective tissue proper is the macrophage, which is considered a monocyte before it migrates from

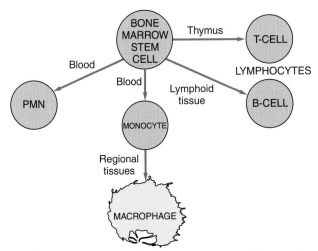

FIGURE 8-16 Flowchart showing that most blood cells come from a common stem cell type in the bone marrow. B-cell lymphocytes stay and mature in the bone marrow, and T-cell lymphocytes travel to mature in other glands or tissue in the body, such as the thymus. Later, both types of lymphocytes will engage in immune responses throughout the body. Note also the polymorphonuclear leukocyte (PMN) (or neutrophil) and monocyte (or macrophage). *(From Fehrenbach MJ: Immunity. In Ibsen OAC, Phelan JA (eds): Oral Pathology for Dental Hygienists, ed 5, WB Saunders, Philadelphia, 2009.)*

the blood into the tissue. They have a longer lifespan than PMNs but constitute only 2% to 10% of the WBC count. After migration, macrophages arrive at the site of injury later and in fewer numbers than PMNs when the inflammatory response is triggered. Macrophages contain lysosomal enzymes, are involved in **phagocytosis** (as are PMNs), are actively mobile, and have the ability to respond to chemotactic factors and cytokines (see Figure 7-4). Macrophages also assist in the immune response to facilitate immunoglobulin production. In certain disease states, numbers of macrophages may fuse together, forming giant cells with multiple nuclei. In bone connective tissue, these are then considered **osteoclasts** that will resorb bone (discussed earlier).

The eosinophil is normally only 6% of the WBC count, but its percentage is increased during a hypersensitivity response (allergy) and in parasitic diseases because its primary function seems to be the phagocytosis of immune complexes.

TABLE 8-5	Blood Cells and Related Tissue Cells		
Cells	**MICROSCOPIC APPEARANCE**	**DESCRIPTION**	**FUNCTIONS**
Polymorphonuclear leukocyte (PMN) (neutrophil)		Multilobed nucleus with granules	Inflammatory response: phagocytosis
Lymphocyte		Eccentric round nucleus without granules: B, T, and NK cells	B and T cell: immune response: humoral and cell-mediated NK; defense against tumor- and virally infected cells
Plasma cell		Round cartwheel nucleus derived from B-cell lymphocytes	Humoral immune response: produces immunoglobulins (antibodies)
Monocyte (blood)/ **macrophage** (tissue)		Bean-shaped nucleus with poorly staining granules	Inflammatory and immune response: phagocytosis, as well as process and present immunogens (antigens)
Eosinophil		Bilobed nucleus with granules	Hypersensitivity response
Basophil		Irregularly shaped bilobed/trilobed nucleus with granules	Hypersensitivity response
Mast cell (tissue)		Irregularly shaped bilobed nucleus with granules	Hypersensitivity response

The **basophil** is normally found in less than 1% of the WBC count and is also involved in the hypersensitivity response. Other WBCs located in the connective tissue include the **mast cell,** which is similar in appearance to the basophil. As with basophils, mast cells are also involved in the hypersensitivity response. However, even though both cells are derived from the bone marrow, they probably originate from different stem cells.

MUSCLE

The muscle in the body is part of the muscular system, and similar to connective tissue, most muscles are derived from somites. Each muscle shortens under neural control, causing soft tissue and bony structures of the body to move. The three types of muscle are classified according to structure, function, dend innervation: skeletal, smooth, and cardiac (see Table 8-1).

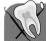

Clinical Considerations for Cells in the Blood and Tissue

Dental professionals must understand certain laboratory procedures that patients may have undergone, when viewing the medical record. These procedures include a complete blood count (CBC), which is an evaluation of both RBC and WBC types to detect infections, anemia, or leukemia. A platelet count can also be performed to determine the platelet number if bleeding problems are a consideration, and a coagulation (bleeding) test can also be performed to test platelet function. These procedures may also be recommended to the patient if there is clinical evidence of unusual periodontal diseases such as an aggressive periodontitis, with its uncontrolled periodontal support loss.

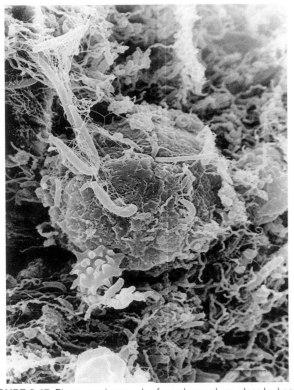

FIGURE 8-17 Electron micrograph of a polymorphonuclear leukocyte (PMN), or neutrophil, which is the most common white blood cell. *(Courtesy of Jan Cope, RDH, MS, Associate Professor, Oregon Institute of Technology, Klamath Falls, OR.)*

TABLE 8-6	Known Immunoglobulins (Antibodies) from Plasma Cells
IgA	Has two subgroups: serous in blood; secretory in saliva, tears, and breast milk; both aid in defense against pathogens in body fluids
IgD	Functions in activation of B-cell lymphocytes as antigen receptor; has been shown to activate basophils and mast cells to produce antimicrobial factors
IgE	Involved in hypersensitivity response; binds to mast cells and basophils, and releases bioactive substances such as histamine
IgG	Has four subgroups; major immunoglobulin in blood serum and can pass placental barrier to form first passive immunity for newborn
IgM	Involved in early immune responses against pathogens because of involvement with IgD in activation of B-cell lymphocytes before sufficient IgG production

CLASSIFICATION OF MUSCLE

Each type of **muscle** has its own type of action, which is the movement accomplished when the muscle cells contract. Smooth muscle and cardiac muscle are considered involuntary muscles because they are under autonomic nervous system control (discussed next). Smooth muscles are located in organs, glands, and the linings of blood vessels. Cardiac muscle is in the wall of the heart (myocardium).

Skeletal muscles are considered voluntary muscles because they are under voluntary control, involving the somatic nervous system (Figure 8-18). All the major muscles of the body's appendages and trunk are skeletal muscles. Thus, skeletal muscles are usually attached to bones of the skeleton. Skeletal muscles also include the muscles of the facial expression, **tongue**, **mastication, pharynx,** and upper esophagus.

HISTOLOGY OF SKELETAL MUSCLE

Skeletal muscles are also called *striated muscles* because the muscle cells appear striped microscopically. Each muscle is composed of numerous muscle bundles, or fascicles, which then are composed of numerous muscle cells or *myofibers*. Each myofiber extends the entire length of the muscle and is composed of smaller *myofibrils* surrounded by the other organelles of the cell. Each myofibril is composed of even smaller *myofilaments*.

NERVE TISSUE

Nerve tissue forms the nervous system in the body, being derived from the neuroectoderm within the embryo (Table 8-7, see Figure 3-10). Nerves function to carry messages or impulses based on electrical potentials. Nerve tissue in the body causes muscles to contract, resulting in facial expressions and joint movements, such as those associated with mastication and speech. The tissue stimulates glands to secrete hormones and regulates many other systems of the body, such as the cardiovascular system. It also allows for the perception of sensations such as pain, touch, taste, and smell.

HISTOLOGY OF NERVE TISSUE

A **neuron** is the functional cellular component of the nervous system and is composed of three parts: one neural cell body with two different types of neural cytoplasmic processes (Figure 8-19). The neural cell body is not involved in the process of impulse transmission but provides the metabolic support for the entire neuron.

One type of process associated with the cell body is an *axon*, a long, thin, singular, cable-like process that conducts impulses away from the cell body. An axon is encased in its own cell membrane, with nerve excitability and conduction due to changes that develop in the nerve membrane; certain axons can be additionally covered by layers of a lipid-rich myelin sheath.

The myelin sheath consists of tightly wrapped layers of phospholipid-rich membrane surrounding the Schwann cell cytoplasm; there is very little cytoplasm sandwiched between them. It is only in the outermost layer of the myelin sheath where the Schwann cell and its nucleus are located. Along a myelinated axon are the nodes of Ranvier, which form a gap between the adjacent Schwann cells. The insulating properties of the myelin sheath and its gaps allow the axon to conduct impulses more quickly. The other type of process associated with the cell body is the *dendrite*, a threadlike process that usually contains multiple branches, which functions to receive and conduct impulses toward the cell body.

A **nerve** is a bundle of neural processes outside the central nervous system and in the peripheral nervous system. A **synapse** is the junction between two neurons or between a neuron and an effector organ, such as a muscle or gland, where neural impulses are transmitted by chemical means (neurotransmitter substance). To function, most tissue or organs have innervation, a supply of nerves. A nerve allows information to be carried to and from the brain, which is the central information center. An aggregation of neuron cell bodies outside the central nervous system is termed a *ganglion* (plural, *ganglia*).

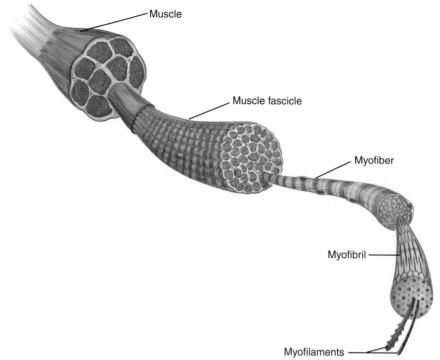

FIGURE 8-18 Skeletal muscle showing its striations composed of smaller muscle bundles, fascicles, myofibers, myofibrils, and myofilaments.

The two functional types of nerves are afferent and efferent nerves. An *afferent nerve*, or sensory nerve, carries information or relays impulses from the periphery of the body to the brain (or spinal cord). Thus, an afferent nerve carries sensory information, such as taste, pain, or proprioception, to the brain. Proprioception is information concerning the movement and position of the body. This sensory information is sent on to the brain to be analyzed, acted upon, associated with other information, and stored as memory.

An *efferent nerve*, or motor nerve, carries information away from the brain to the periphery of the body. Thus, an efferent nerve carries information to the muscles or glands in order to activate them, often in response to information received by the afferent nerve pathway. One motor neuron with its branching fibers may control hundreds of muscle fibers. Autonomic nerves are (by definition) always efferent.

NERVOUS SYSTEM

The nervous system has two main divisions: the central nervous system (CNS) and the peripheral nervous system (PNS) (see Table 8-7). These two systems are not separate but rely on each other and thus constantly interact. The CNS consists of the brain and spinal cord. The PNS consists of the spinal and cranial nerves, and includes both the somatic and the autonomic nervous systems. The spinal nerves extend from the spinal cord to the periphery of the body. The cranial nerves are initially attached to the brain, which then pass through openings in the skull. The somatic nervous system operates with conscious control of the individual to move the skeletal muscles.

The autonomic nervous system (ANS) is a part of the PNS and operates without conscious control as the caretaker of the body. Autonomic nerves are efferent processes, and they are always in two-neuron circuits. The first neuron carries autonomic impulses to a ganglion, where they are transmitted to the body of the second neuron. The ANS itself has two divisions: a sympathetic system and a

TABLE 8-7	Divisions of the Nervous System
DIVISIONS	**COMPONENTS**
Central nervous system (CNS)	Brain and spinal cord
Peripheral nervous system (PNS)	Spinal and cranial nerves of the somatic nervous system and autonomic nervous system (ANS) (includes sympathetic and parasympathetic systems)

parasympathetic system. Most tissue or organ systems are supplied by both divisions of the autonomic nervous system.

The sympathetic nervous system is involved in fight-or-flight responses, such as in the inhibition of **salivary gland** secretion (**hyposalivation**). Such a response by the sympathetic system leads to a dry mouth (**xerostomia**) (see Figure 11-8). Sympathetic neurons arise in the spinal cord and synapse in ganglia arranged in a chain extending nearly the length of the vertebral column on both sides. Therefore, all the sympathetic neurons in the head have already synapsed in a ganglion. Sympathetic fibers reach the cranial tissue that they supply by traveling with the arteries.

The parasympathetic nervous system is involved in rest-or-digest responses, such as the stimulation of salivary gland secretion. Such a response leads to salivary flow to aid in digestion. Parasympathetic fibers associated with glands of the head and neck region are carried in various cranial nerves, and their ganglia are located in the head. Therefore, parasympathetic neurons in this region may be either preganglionic neurons (before synapsing in the ganglion) or postganglionic neurons (after synapsing in the ganglion).

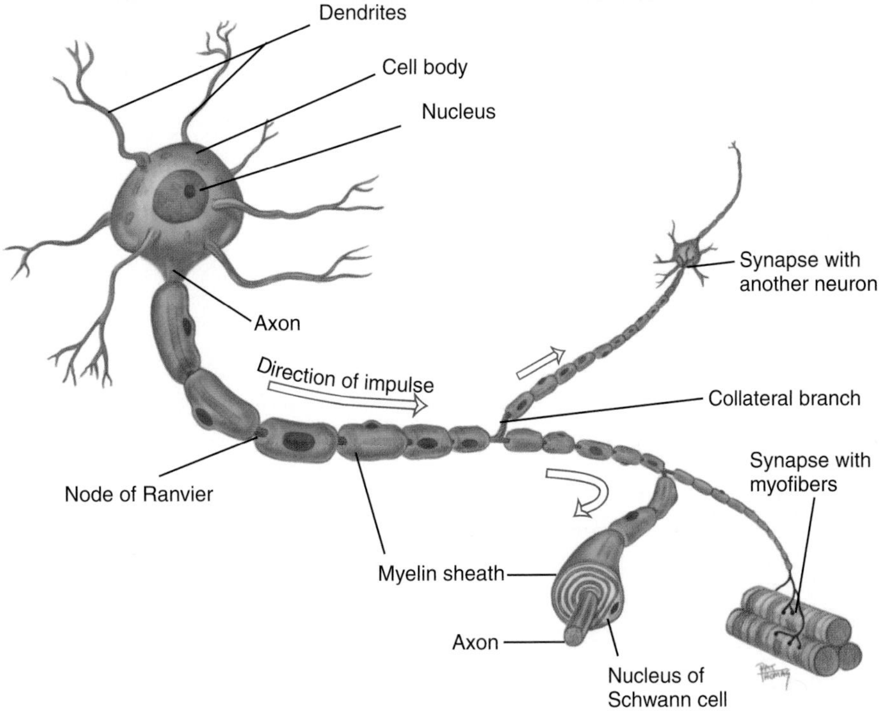

FIGURE 8-19 Neuron with its dendrites, cell body, and axon, showing a synaptic relationship with the muscle, as well as with another neuron.

CHAPTER 9

Oral Mucosa

●●●CHAPTER OUTLINE

●●●LEARNING OBJECTIVES

- Define and pronounce the key terms in this chapter.
- List and describe the types of oral mucosa, characterizing each of the different types of epithelium associated with each region in the oral cavity, including the tongue.
- List and discuss the clinical correlations associated with the regional differences in the oral mucosa.

- Discuss the turnover times for different regions of the oral mucosa and their clinical correlations, as well as repair and aging considerations.
- Integrate the knowledge of the histology with an understanding of the promotion of oral mucosal health and any related pathology that may occur within it.

●●●NEW KEY TERMS

Capillary plexus (**cap**-ih-lary)
Hyperkeratinization (hi-per-ker-ah-tin-**zay**-shun)
Keratin (**ker**-ah-tin)
Keratohyaline granules (ker-ah-toe-**hi**-ah-lin)
Lamina propria (**lam**-i-nah **pro**-pree-ah)
Layer: basal (**bay**-sal), **granular, intermediate, keratin** (**ker**-ah-tin), **prickle, superficial**

Mucoperiosteum (mu-ko-per-ee-**os**-te-um)
Mucosa (mu-**ko**-sah): **lining, masticatory** (mass-ti-**ka**-tor-ee), **specialized**
Stratified squamous epithelium (**strat**-i-fide **skway**-mus ep-ee-**thee**-lee-um): **nonkeratinized** (non-**ker**-ah-tin-izd), **orthokeratinized** (or-tho-**ker**-ah-tin-izd), **parakeratinized** (pare-ah-**ker**-ah-tin-izd)

Stippling
Submucosa (sub-mu-**ko**-sah)
Taste pore
Tongue: black hairy, geographic

ORAL MUCOSA

Dental professionals must have a clear understanding of the basic histology of the **oral mucosa**, the regional differences, and any clinical considerations that might be related to this information. Only then will they be able to understand the clinical considerations involved in injury to the oral mucosa, such as injury that occurs with trauma, inflammation, infection, and cancer, as well as with aging. With this information, they then can promote the health of the oral mucosa.

CLASSIFICATION OF ORAL MUCOSA

Oral mucosa almost continuously lines the oral cavity. Oral mucosa is composed of **stratified squamous epithelium** overlying a **connective tissue proper**, or lamina propria, with possibly a deeper submucosa (Figure 9-1; see Chapter 8).

Even though the entire oral cavity has an epithelial covering, and connective tissue makes up the bulk of lamina propria, regional differences are noted throughout the oral mucosa. For example, the oral mucosa is perforated in various regions by the **ducts** of **salivary glands** (see Figures 11-3 and 11-6). This chapter discusses later these regional differences, except the gingival sulcular region is discussed in more detail in Chapter 10.

A **basement membrane** lies between the epithelium and connective tissue in the oral mucosa (see Figures 7-6 and 8-4). It serves not as a separation between the two tissue types but as a continuous structure linking the two. Studies are focusing on trying to understand the interactions between these two tissue types, and the basement membrane may hold these answers.

Three main types of oral mucosa are found in the oral cavity: lining, masticatory, and specialized mucosa (Table 9-1). This classification of mucosa is based on the general histological features of the tissue. The specific histological features of each oral region are discussed later.

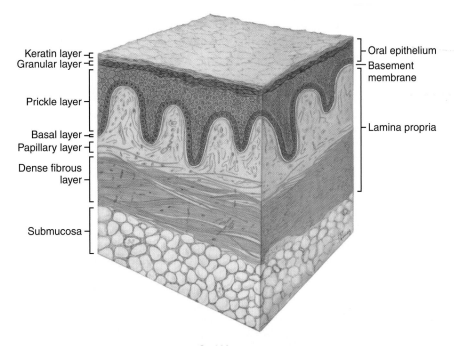

Keratin layer — Oral epithelium
Granular layer — Basement membrane
Prickle layer
Basal layer — Lamina propria
Papillary layer
Dense fibrous layer
Submucosa

Oral Mucosa
(and underlying tissues)

FIGURE 9-1 General histological features of an oral mucosa composed of stratified squamous epithelium overlying lamina propria. A deeper submucosa may be present as shown.

TABLE 9-1	Types of Oral Mucosa		
TYPES	**REGIONS**	**GENERAL CLINICAL APPEARANCE**	**GENERAL MICROSCOPIC APPEARANCE**
Lining mucosa	Buccal mucosa, labial mucosa, alveolar mucosa, ventral tongue surface, floor of the mouth, and soft palate	Softer surface texture, moist surface, and ability to stretch and be compressed, acting as a cushion	Nonkeratinized epithelium with smooth interface, few rete ridges, and CT papillae with elastic fibers in lamina propria and submucosa
Masticatory mucosa	Attached gingiva, hard palate, and dorsal tongue surface	Rubbery surface texture and resiliency, serving as firm base	Keratinized epithelium and interdigitated interface with many rete ridges and CT papillae with thin layer of submucosa or none
Specialized mucosa	Dorsal tongue surface	Associated with lingual papillae	Discrete structures of epithelium and lamina propria; some with taste buds (see Table 9-3)

CT = Connective tissue.

Overall, the clinical appearance of the tissue reflects the underlying histology, both in health and disease.

In addition, the oral cavity has sometimes been described as a mirror that reflects the health of the individual. Changes indicative of disease are seen as alterations in the oral mucosa lining the mouth, which can reveal systemic conditions, such as diabetes or vitamin deficiency, or the local effects of chronic tobacco or alcohol use.

LINING MUCOSA

Lining mucosa is a type of mucosa noted for its softer surface texture, moist surface, and ability to stretch and be compressed, acting as a cushion for the underlying structures. Lining mucosa includes the buccal mucosa, labial mucosa, alveolar mucosa, as well as the mucosa lining the ventral surface of the tongue, floor of the mouth, and soft palate.

Histologically, lining mucosa is a type that is associated with **nonkeratinized stratified squamous epithelium** (Figure 9-2). In contrast to masticatory mucosa (discussed next), the interface between the epithelium and the lamina propria is generally smoother, with fewer and less-pronounced rete ridges and connective tissue papillae. In addition to these factors, the presence of **elastic fibers** in the lamina propria also provides the tissue with a movable base.

A **submucosa** deep to the lamina propria is usually present, overlying muscle and allowing compression of the superficial tissue. These general histological features allow this type of mucosa to serve in regions of the oral cavity where a movable base is needed, as during speech, mastication, and swallowing. Surgical incisions in this tissue frequently require sutures for closure. Local anesthetic injections into these areas are easier to accomplish than in masticatory mucosa, with less discomfort and easy dispersion of the agent, but infections also spread rapidly.

MASTICATORY MUCOSA

Masticatory mucosa is noted for its rubbery surface texture and resiliency. Masticatory mucosa includes the hard palate, attached gingiva, and dorsal surface of the tongue.

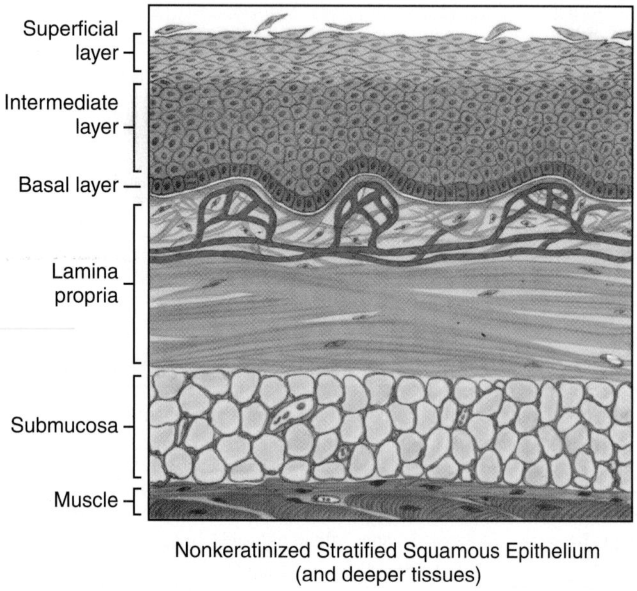

FIGURE 9-2 General histological features of a lining mucosa composed of nonkeratinized, stratified squamous epithelium (*with three layers*) overlying lamina propria. A deeper submucosa is usually present overlying muscle.

Histologically, masticatory mucosa is associated with **orthokeratinized stratified squamous epithelium,** as well as **parakeratinized stratified squamous epithelium** (Figures 9-3 to 9-5). Unlike lining mucosa discussed earlier, the interface between the epithelium and lamina propria in masticatory mucosa is highly interdigitated with numerous and more-pronounced rete ridges and connective tissue papillae, giving it a firm base. In addition, the submucosa is an extremely thin layer or is absent. When masticatory mucosa overlies bone, with or without submucosa, it increases the firmness of the tissue.

These general histological features allow this type of mucosa to function in the regions that need a firm base during mastication and speech. Sutures are rarely needed for this tissue after surgery. However, local anesthetic injections are more difficult and cause greater discomfort than those in lining mucosa, as well as when any swelling from an infectious source occurs.

SPECIALIZED MUCOSA

Specialized mucosa is found on the **dorsal surface of the tongue,** as well as the **lateral surface of the tongue**, in the form of the **lingual papillae** (discussed later). Lingual papillae are discrete structures composed of keratinized epithelium and lamina propria (see Figure 2-14).

EPITHELIUM OF ORAL MUCOSA

Three types of stratified squamous epithelium are found within the oral cavity: nonkeratinized, orthokeratinized, and parakeratinized (Table 9-2). Nonkeratinized epithelium is associated with lining mucosa. Orthokeratinized and parakeratinized epithelium are both associated with masticatory mucosa. All forms of epithelium act as a barrier to pathogenic invasion and mechanical irritation and offer protection against dryness. These protective features are accentuated in epithelium with keratin.

Histologists use the term *keratinocytes* for the epithelial cells in oral mucosa because they can produce keratin either naturally at normal levels if it is a keratinized tissue, or at higher levels when the tissue becomes traumatized, even in previously nonkeratinized tissue. Nonkeratinocytes, those cells that do not produce keratin, may be present in much smaller numbers in the epithelium (Table 9-3). These include melanocytes, discussed later with **melanin pigmentation,** as well as Langerhans and Granstein cells, both of which arise from the **bone marrow** and help the skin's immune responses by acting as antigenic markers. **White blood cells (WBCs)** are also present, with the **polymorphonuclear leukocyte (PMN)** being the most commonly occurring WBC in all forms of oral mucosa (see Figure 8-17).

NONKERATINIZED STRATIFIED SQUAMOUS EPITHELIUM

Nonkeratinized stratified squamous epithelium is in the superficial layers of **lining mucosa,** such as in the labial mucosa, buccal mucosa, and alveolar mucosa, as well as in the mucosa lining the floor of the mouth, the ventral surface of the tongue, and the soft palate (see Figure 9-2). Lining mucosa has similar epithelial histological traits, even though it has its own regional differences. Nonkeratinized epithelium is the most common form of epithelium in the oral cavity.

Each lining mucosa has at least three layers within the epithelium. A basal layer, or *stratum basale*, is the deepest of the three layers. The basal layer is a single layer of cuboidal epithelial cells overlying the basement membrane, which, in turn, is situated superior to the lamina propria. The basal layer produces the basal lamina of the basement membrane.

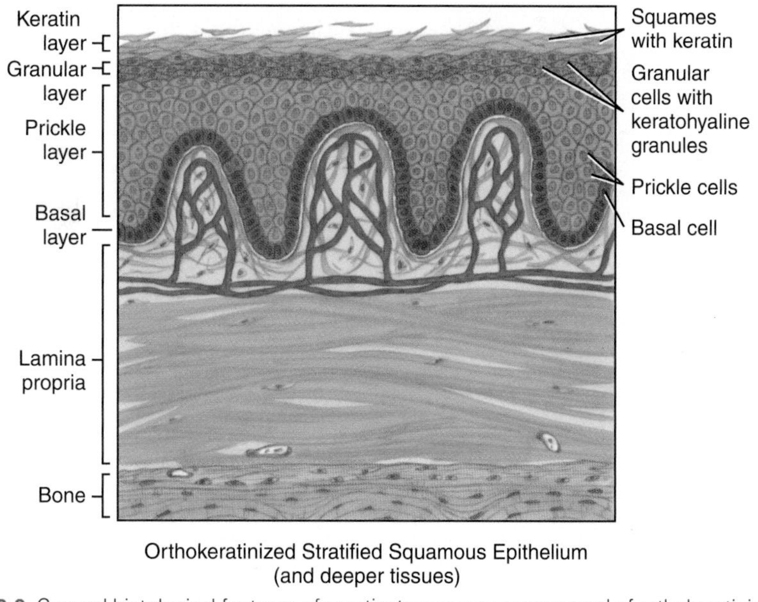

Keratin
layer
Granular
layer
Prickle
layer
Basal
layer
Lamina
propria
Bone

Squames
with keratin
Granular
cells with
keratohyaline
granules
Prickle cells
Basal cell

Orthokeratinized Stratified Squamous Epithelium
(and deeper tissues)

FIGURE 9-3 General histological features of masticatory mucosa composed of orthokeratinized stratified squamous epithelium (*with four layers*) overlying lamina propria. A deeper thin submucosa may or may not be present, as shown here, and may overlay bone. Note that the cells in the keratin layer have lost their nuclei and are filled with keratin. However, the artifact of the spiky look of the prickle layer has not been shown.

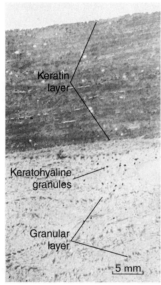

Keratin
layer

Keratohyaline
granules

Granular
layer

5 mm

FIGURE 9-4 Electron micrograph of keratinized epithelium showing both the granular and keratin layers. Small keratohyaline granules are visible in the granular layer; the cells of the keratin layer are flattened and contain keratin. However, it is hard to discern at this magnification whether this tissue is orthokeratinized or parakeratinized based on the presence of nuclei of the keratin layer. *(From Nanci A: Ten Cate's Oral Histology, ed 7, Mosby, St Louis, 2008.)*

intermedium. The intermediate layer is composed of larger, stacked, polyhedral-shaped cells. These cells appear larger or plumper than the basal layer cells, because they have larger amounts **cytoplasm**. The cells of the intermediate layer have lost the ability to undergo mitosis as they migrated. The intermediate layer makes up the bulk of nonkeratinized epithelium.

The most superficial level in nonkeratinized epithelium is termed the superficial layer, or *stratum superficiale.* It is hard to discern the exact division between the superficial layer and the intermediate layers in lining mucosa when viewing histological sections. This layer shows even larger similarly stacked polyhedral epithelial cells with the outer cells flattening into **squames**. The squames in these layers show shedding or loss as they age and die during the turnover of the tissue. Thus, **maturation** within this tissue is seen only as an increase in the size of cells as they migrate superficially.

ORTHOKERATINIZED STRATIFIED SQUAMOUS EPITHELIUM

Orthokeratinized stratified squamous epithelium demonstrates a keratinization of the epithelial cells throughout its most superficial layers (see Figures 9-3 and 9-4). Orthokeratinized epithelium is the least common form of epithelium found in the oral cavity. It is associated with the **masticatory mucosa** of the hard palate and the attached gingiva. It is also associated with the **specialized mucosa** of the **lingual papillae** on the dorsal surface of the tongue. As this tissue matures, it forms keratin within its superficial cells, showing a visible and physiological difference in the cells as they migrate superficially.

Like nonkeratinized epithelium, orthokeratinized epithelium has a single basal layer, or *stratum basale,* undergoing **mitosis**. This layer also produces the basal lamina of the adjacent basement membrane. Unlike nonkeratinized epithelium, however, orthokeratinized epithelium has more layers superficial to the basal layer: four separate layers with somewhat distinct divisions.

Superficial to the basal layer is the prickle layer, or the *stratum spinosum.* This layer is named for an artifact that occurs when the

The basal layer is also considered germinative because **mitosis** of the epithelial cells occurs within this layer; however, this cell division is seen only under higher magnification of the tissue (see Table 7-2). Future studies may show the existence of an epithelial stem cell in the basal layer that produces other stem and daughter cells, similar to the situation for blood cells in the bone marrow.

The layer of epithelium superficial to the basal layer in nonkeratinized epithelium is the intermediate layer, or *stratum*

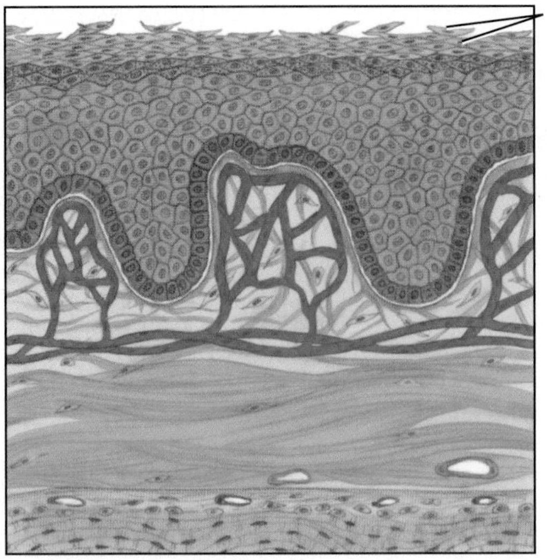

Parakeratinized Stratified Squamous Epithelium
(and deeper tissues)

FIGURE 9-5 General histological features of masticatory mucosa, which is composed of parakeratinized stratified squamous epithelium (*with three to four layers*) overlying lamina propria. A deeper thin submucosa may or may not be present, as shown here, and may overlay bone. Note that the cells in the keratin layer have retained their nuclei and are filled with keratin. However, the artifact of the spiky look of the prickle layer is not shown.

TABLE 9-2	Epithelium of Oral Mucosa	
TYPES OF EPITHELIUM	**ASSOCIATED TYPE OF MUCOSA**	**BASIC HISTOLOGICAL DESCRIPTION**
Nonkeratinized epithelium	Lining mucosa	Basal, intermediate, superficial layers
Orthokeratinized epithelium	Masticatory mucosa	Basal, prickle, granular, keratin layers (cells contain only keratin and no nuclei)
Parakeratinized epithelium	Masticatory mucosa	Basal, prickle, granular, keratin layers (cells contain keratin and nuclei)

TABLE 9-3	Types of Cells in Epithelium*	
TYPES	**FEATURES**	**FUNCTIONS**
Epithelial cell	Rapidly renewing cell that undergoes pathway of differentiation with desmosomes; can be derived from all three embryonic cell layers	Forms cohesive sheet that resists physical forces and serves as barrier to infection
Melanocyte	Dendritic cell of neural crest origin, forms a continuous network near basement membrane	Synthesis of melanin pigmentation with transfer to adjacent cells by injection (melanosomes)
Langerhans cell	Dendritic bone marrow–derived cell noted near basement membrane	Immune response with T-cell lymphocytes
Granstein cell	Similar to Langerhans cell	Same as Langerhans cell
Merkel cell	Neural cell noted near basement membrane	Sensory information

*White blood cells are not included in this table.

epithelial cells of this layer are dried for prolonged microscopic study; the cells shrink as a result of cytoplasm loss but still maintain their cellular junctions of **desmosomes** (see Figure 7-5). Thus, a prickly or spiky look results when the individual dehydrated epithelial cells are shrinking but still joined at their outer edges. Once they migrate to this superior a level in the tissue, cells of the prickle layer lose the ability to undergo mitosis, such as noted in the deeper basal layer. The prickle layer makes up the bulk of orthokeratinized epithelium.

Superficial to the prickle layer is the granular layer, or *stratum granulosum*. The epithelial cells in this layer are flat and stacked in a layer three to five cells thick. In their cytoplasm, each of the cells has a **nucleus** with prominent keratohyaline granules, which stain as dark spots. The keratohyaline granules form a chemical precursor for the keratin that is found in the more superficial layers.

The most superficial layer in orthokeratinized epithelium is the keratin layer, or *stratum corneum*, which shows variable thickness depending on the region. The cells in the keratin layer are flat and have no nuclei, and their cytoplasm is filled with **keratin**. This soft, opaque, waterproof material is formed from a complex of keratohyaline granules and intermediate filaments from the cells and stains as

a translucent dense material. The outer cells of the keratin layer, or **squames**, show increased flattening and also shedding or loss, because they are no longer viable.

In addition, parts of the keratin material are also shed as a result of the turnover of the tissue. However, these squames and their cornified cell envelope make up a major part of the epithelial barrier and are continuously being renewed. The epithelial barrier serves as protection from physical, chemical, and pathogenic attack, as well as dehydration and heat loss, that sometimes occur in the oral cavity environment.

PARAKERATINIZED STRATIFIED SQUAMOUS EPITHELIUM

Parakeratinized stratified squamous epithelium is associated with the **masticatory mucosa** of the attached gingiva, in higher levels than with orthokeratinization, and also the tongue's dorsal surface (see Figure 9-5). Most histologists believe that parakeratinized epithelium is an immature form of orthokeratinized epithelium. The presence of this form of keratinization on the skin is considered a disease state; therefore, parakeratinization is one of the unique histological features of the healthy oral cavity. Parakeratinized epithelium is also associated with the **specialized mucosa** of the **lingual papillae** on the dorsal surface of the tongue as well as the sulcular epithelium lining the sulcus.

Parakeratinized epithelium may have all the same layers of epithelium as orthokeratinized epithelium, such as the basal layer, prickle layer, granular layer, and keratin layer, although the granular layer may be indistinct or absent altogether.

The main difference between parakeratinized epithelium and orthokeratinized epithelium is in the cells of the **keratin layer**. In parakeratinized epithelium, the most superficial layer is still being shed or lost; however, these cells of the keratin layer contain not only **keratin** but also **nuclei**, unlike those of orthokeratinized epithelium. This distinction is sometimes difficult to discern under lower microscopic power in certain histological sections. Studies have shown that even though the epithelial cells have nuclei in the parakeratinized epithelium, they possibly are no longer viable, similar to the orthokeratinized epithelium.

LAMINA PROPRIA OF ORAL MUCOSA

All forms of epithelium, whether associated with lining, masticatory, or specialized mucosa, have a **lamina propria** located deep to the basement membrane (see Figure 9-1). The main fiber group in the lamina propria is collagen fibers, but elastic fibers are present in certain regions of the oral cavity. The lamina propria, like all forms of connective tissue proper, has two layers: papillary and dense (Figure 9-7).

The **papillary layer** is the more superficial layer of the lamina propria. It consists of loose connective tissue within the connective tissue papillae, along with blood vessels and nerve tissue. The tissue has an equal amount of fibers, cells, and intercellular substance. The **dense layer** is the deeper layer of the lamina propria. It consists of dense connective tissue with a large amount of fibers. Between the papillary layer and the deeper layers of the lamina propria is a capillary plexus, which provides nutrition for the all layers of the mucosa and sends capillaries into the connective tissue papillae.

A **submucosa** may or may not be present deep to the dense layer of the lamina propria, depending on the region of the oral cavity. If present, the submucosa usually contains **loose connective** tissue and may also contain **adipose connective tissue** or **salivary glands,** as well as overlying bone or muscle within the oral cavity.

Lining mucosa does not have prominent connective tissue papillae and alternating rete ridges. In addition, elastic fibers are present in the papillary layer, thus allowing the tissue to stretch and recoil during speech, mastication, and swallowing. In contrast to lining mucosa, masticatory mucosa has numerous and prominent connective tissue papillae, giving the mucosa a firm base, which is needed for speech and mastication.

The most common cell in the lamina propria, similar to all types of **connective tissue proper**, is the **fibroblast** (see Figure 8-5). Fibroblasts synthesize certain types of protein fibers and **intercellular substances**. Histologists believe that subpopulations of the fibroblast may exist and that controlling the beneficial productive groups, such as fibroblasts, may be the answer to periodontal disease and age-related changes that occur in the lamina propria and other components of the periodontium. Other cells present in the lamina propria in smaller

---

Clinical Considerations for Oral Mucosal Changes

Unlike keratinized epithelium, nonkeratinized epithelium normally has no superficial layers showing keratinization. Nonkeratinized epithelium may, however, readily transform into a keratinizing type in response to frictional or chemical trauma, in which case it undergoes **hyperkeratinization.**

This change to hyperkeratinization commonly occurs on the usually nonkeratinized buccal mucosa when the **linea alba** forms, a white ridge of calloused tissue that extends horizontally at the level where the maxillary and mandibular teeth come together and occlude (see Figure 2-3, *B*). Histologically, an excess amount of **keratin** is noted on the surface of the tissue, and the tissue has all the layers of an orthokeratinized tissue with its granular and keratin layers.

In patients who have habits such as **clenching** or grinding (**bruxism**) their teeth, a larger area of the buccal mucosa than just the linea alba becomes hyperkeratinized (Figure 9-6). This larger white, rough, raised lesion needs to be recorded so that changes may be made in the dental treatment plan regarding the patient's **parafunctional habits** (see **Chapter 20**). Even keratinized tissue can undergo further level of hyperkeratinization; an increase in the amount of keratin is produced as a result of chronic physical trauma to the region.

Changes such as hyperkeratinization are reversible if the source of the injury is removed, but it takes time for the keratin to be shed or lost by the tissue. Thus, to check for malignant changes, a baseline biopsy and microscopic study of any whitened tissue may be indicated, especially if in a high-risk cancer category, such with a history of tobacco or alcohol use or are HPV positive. Hyperkeratinized tissue is also associated with the heat from smoking or hot fluids on the hard palate in the form of **nicotinic stomatitis** (see Figure 11-11).

When a graft procedure is performed to reduce the amount of **gingival recession** on the root, keratinization is taken into consideration because the goal of grafting is to increase the amount of attached keratinized tissue. One type of graft, the free gingival graft, uses a thickness of both keratinized epithelium and lamina propria harvested from the hard palate and grafted to the root to form a new band of keratinized attached gingiva. This procedure generally is somewhat successful, but the graft tends to be lighter colored, and studies show that the epithelium does not survive the procedure, which means that the donor site requires extra time to heal and allow migration of the surrounding epithelium to cover the site.

In contrast, a subepithelial connective tissue graft consists only lamina propria that is taken from the surrounding keratinized attached gingiva and then grafted directly to the root. Epithelial cells from the surrounding tissue migrate to cover the graft and heal the area. This procedure is consistently successful: the new keratinized attached gingiva blends with the surrounding tissue, and healing of the donor site is rapid. Thus, the **induction** to form keratin may come from the deeper lamina propria and does not only involve the epithelium.

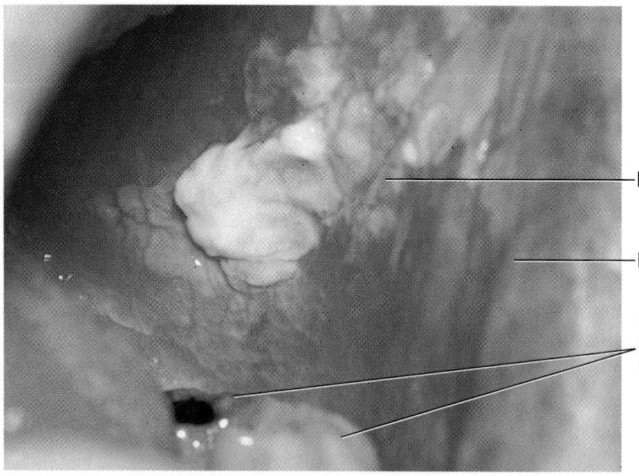

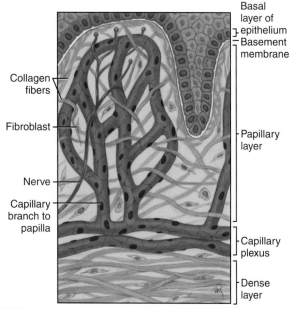

Hyperkeratosis

Buccal mucosa

Mandibular posterior teeth

FIGURE 9-6 Hyperkeratinization of the buccal mucosa shown by larger white, rough, raised calloused lesion. Buccal mucosa usually has nonkeratinized epithelium, but this tissue has undergone chronic physical injury to the area as a result of grinding, or bruxism, of the teeth. Thus, the epithelium has become keratinized in response. Other, more serious lesions of the oral cavity must be ruled out when diagnosing this lesion.

Basal layer of epithelium

Basement membrane

Collagen fibers

Fibroblast

Papillary layer

Nerve

Capillary branch to papilla

Capillary plexus

Dense layer

FIGURE 9-7 General histological features of the lamina propria (*with two layers*) of the oral mucosa and its relationship to the adjoining basement membrane and overlying epithelium.

numbers are WBCs, such as PMNs, macrophages, lymphocytes, and mast cells (see Table 8-4).

REGIONAL DIFFERENCES IN ORAL MUCOSA

Specific histological features are noted in the different regions of the oral cavity (Table 9-4). These specific histological features are the basis for the differences observed clinically, when these regions are examined. One way to integrate these two related concepts is to review the clinical appearance of the different regions of oral mucosa during an intraoral examination, when armed with the new knowledge of the specific underlying histological features.

Thus, the novice dental professional must look closely at the clinical photographs of the different regions of the oral cavity, as presented in Chapter 2, and compare these with the histological presentation discussed in this chapter, as well as in the descriptions of their clinical presentation. Next, practice finding these regional differences in the oral cavity using a mirror, and this textbook for review, in order to improve skills of examination. Later, locate them on peers and then on patients in a clinical setting.

LABIAL MUCOSA AND BUCCAL MUCOSA

CLINICAL APPEARANCE

The **labial mucosa** and **buccal mucosa** line the inner lips and cheeks (see Figures 2-2 and 2-3). Both of these regions appear clinically as an opaque pink, shiny, moist, compressible tissue that stretches easily. Areas of **melanin pigmentation** may be noted (discussed later). A variable number of **Fordyce's spots** are scattered throughout the tissue. These are a normal variant, visible as small, yellowish bumps on the surface of the mucosa. They correspond to deposits of sebum from misplaced sebaceous glands in the submucosa that are usually associated with hair follicles. The mucosa of the lips and cheeks is classified as a **lining mucosa**.

HISTOLOGICAL FEATURES

The **nonkeratinized stratified squamous epithelium** of the labial mucosa and buccal mucosa is extremely thick tissue that overlies and obscures a lamina propria with an extensive vascular supply, giving the overall mucosa an opaque and pinkish appearance (Figure 9-8). The lamina propria has irregular and blunt connective tissue papillae but contains some **elastic fibers** in addition to its collagen fibers, giving the tissue the ability to stretch and return to its original shape.

The lamina propria overlies a **submucosa** that contains **adipose connective tissue** and **minor salivary glands**, giving the tissue its compressibility and moisture, respectively. The submucosa is firmly attached to the underlying muscle in the region of the labial and buccal mucosa, thus preventing any of the tissue from interfering during mastication or speech because the mucosa and muscle function as one unit.

TABLE 9-4	Regional Differences in Oral Mucosa		
REGION/APPEARANCE	**EPITHELIUM**	**LAMINA PROPRIA**	**SUBMUCOSA**
Lining Mucosa			
Labial mucosa and buccal mucosa: opaque pink, shiny, moist; with possible areas of melanin pigmentation and Fordyce's spots	Thick nonkeratinized	Irregular and blunt CT papillae, some elastic fibers, extensive vascular supply	Present with adipose CT and minor salivary glands, with firm attachment to muscle
Alveolar mucosa: reddish-pink, shiny, moist, extremely mobile	Thin nonkeratinized	CT papillae sometimes absent, many elastic fibers, with extensive vascular supply	Present with minor salivary glands and many elastic fibers, with loose attachment to muscle or bone
Ventral tongue surface and floor of the mouth: reddish pink, moist, shiny, compressible, with vascular blue areas; mobility varies	Extremely thin nonkeratinized	Extensive vascular supply **Ventral tongue:** numerous CT papillae, some elastic fibers, minor salivary glands **Floor:** broad CT papillae	Present **Ventral tongue:** extremely thin and firmly attached to muscle **Floor:** adipose CT with submandibular and sublingual salivary glands, loosely attached to bone/muscles
Soft palate: deep pink with yellow hue and moist surface; compressible and extremely elastic	Thin nonkeratinized	Thick lamina propria with numerous CT papillae and distinct elastic layer	Extremely thin with adipose CT and minor salivary glands, with a firm attachment to underlying muscle
Masticatory Mucosa			
Hard palate: pink, immobile, and firm medial zone, with rugae and raphe; cushioned lateral zones	Thick orthokeratinized	Medial zone serving as mucoperiosteum to bone; features of rugae and raphe	Present only in lateral zones, with anterior part having adipose CT and posterior part having minor salivary glands; absent in medial zone, with rugae, and raphe
Attached gingiva: opaque pink, dull, firm, immobile; with areas of melanin pigmentation possible and varying amounts of stippling	Thick keratinized (mainly parakeratinized, some orthokeratinized)	Tall, narrow CT papillae, extensive vascular supply, and serves as mucoperiosteum to bone	Not present

CT = Connective tissue.

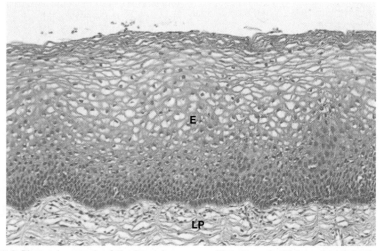

FIGURE 9-8 Photomicrograph of the buccal mucosa with extremely thick nonkeratinized epithelium (*E*) overlying an extensively vascular lamina propria (*LP*). However, the deeper submucosa usually overlying muscle is not shown. *(From Young B, Heath JW: Wheater's Functional Histology, ed 5, Churchill Livingstone, Edinburgh, 2006.)*

ALVEOLAR MUCOSA
CLINICAL APPEARANCE

The **alveolar mucosa** is a reddish-pink tissue with blue vascular areas (see Figures 2-2, 2-9, and 2-10). This shiny, moist region is extremely mobile and lines the **vestibules** of the oral cavity. Alveolar mucosa is classified as a **lining mucosa**.

HISTOLOGICAL FEATURES

The epithelium of the alveolar mucosa is extremely thin, **nonkeratinized stratified squamous epithelium** that overlies, but does not obscure, an extensive vascular supply in the lamina propria, making the mucosa redder than the labial mucosa or buccal mucosa. Connective tissue papillae are sometimes absent, and numerous **elastic fibers** are present in the lamina propria, thus allowing mobility of the tissue.

The **submucosa** associated with the alveolar mucosa has **minor salivary glands** and, again, numerous **elastic fibers** in a **loose connective tissue**, thus giving the tissue its moisture and additional mobility, respectively. The submucosa is loosely attached to the underlying muscle or bone, increasing the ability of the tissue to move because the tissue is located between the moving lips and the stationary attached gingiva.

VENTRAL TONGUE SURFACE AND FLOOR OF THE MOUTH
CLINICAL APPEARANCE

Both the **ventral surface of the tongue** and **floor of the mouth** appear as a reddish-pink tissue with vascular blue areas of veins (see Figures 2-16 and 2-17). The tissue is also moist, shiny, and compressible. Although the floor of the mouth has some mobility, the ventral surface of the tongue is firmly attached, yet allows some stretching along with the tongue muscles. The mucosa of both the ventral tongue surface and floor of the mouth is classified as a **lining mucosa**.

HISTOLOGICAL FEATURES

Both the ventral tongue surface and floor of the mouth have an extremely thin, **nonkeratinized, stratified, squamous epithelium** overlying, but not obscuring, a lamina propria with an extensive vascular supply, thus making both tissue redder and the veins, such as the deep lingual veins, more apparent.

The connective tissue papillae of the lamina propria of the tongue's ventral surface are numerous. Some **elastic fibers** and a few **minor salivary glands** provide the ability to stretch and supply moisture. The **submucosa** associated with the ventral surface of the tongue is extremely thin and firmly attached to the underlying tongue muscle. This arrangement allows the mucosa and muscles to function as one unit, thus reducing mobility during mastication and speech.

The connective tissue papillae of the lamina propria are also broad in the floor of the mouth. The **submucosa** deep to the lamina propria consists of loose connective tissue with **adipose connective tissue** and includes the **submandibular salivary gland** and **sublingual salivary gland**, giving the tissue its compressibility and moisture, respectively. The **submucosa** associated with the floor of the mouth is loosely attached to the underlying bone and muscles, thus giving the tissue its mobility when the attached tongue moves during mastication and speech.

SOFT PALATE
CLINICAL APPEARANCE

The posterior part of the palate, the **soft palate**, is deep pink with a yellowish hue and a moist surface (see Figures 2-11 and 2-12). The tissue is compressible and extremely elastic to allow speech and swallowing. The mucosa of the soft palate is classified as a **lining mucosa**.

HISTOLOGICAL APPEARANCE

The soft palate has a thin nonkeratinized epithelium overlying a thick lamina propria (Figure 9-9). The lamina propria has numerous connective tissue papillae and a distinct **elastic connective tissue** layer for increased mobility with its **elastic fibers**.

The **submucosa** associated with the mucosa of the soft palate is extremely thin and has a firm attachment to the underlying muscle to allow the mechanisms of speech and swallowing. Again, this arrangement allows the mucosa and muscles to function as one unit. **The submucosa** contains **adipose connective tissue**, which gives the tissue its yellow hue and compressibility, and having **minor salivary glands** gives the tissue its moisture.

HARD PALATE
CLINICAL APPEARANCE

The anterior zone of the palate, the **hard palate**, appears pink and is immobile and firm (see Figures 2-11 and 2-12). A cushioned feeling is noted in the more posterior lateral zones and a firmer feeling in the adjacent medial zone when the hard palate is palpated. The **palatine rugae** and the **median palatine raphe** are also firm to the touch. Palatine rugae are permanent and unique to each person, and can be used to establish identity through discrimination, like using fingerprints. The mucosa of the hard palate is classified as a **masticatory mucosa**.

HISTOLOGICAL FEATURES

The hard palate has a thick layer of **orthokeratinized stratified squamous epithelium** overlying a thick lamina propria (Figure 9-10). Only the lateral zones of the hard palate have a **submucosa**, giving the tissue here a cushioned feeling when palpated. The submucosa in the

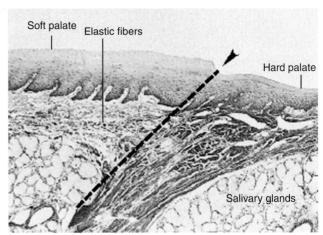

FIGURE 9-9 Junction of the soft palate and hard palate (see *arrow* and *dotted line*), which is also a junction between a lining mucosa and a masticatory mucosa, as well as a junction between nonkeratinized epithelium and keratinized epithelium. *(From Nanci A: Ten Cate's Oral Histology, ed 7, Mosby, St Louis, 2008.)*

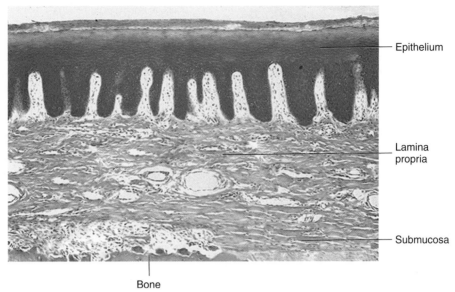

FIGURE 9-10 Photomicrograph of the lateral zone of the hard palate with orthokeratinized epithelium overlying lamina propria. Note the deeper thin submucosa overlying palatal bone. *(From Nanci A: Ten Cate's Oral Histology, ed 7, Mosby, St Louis, 2008.)*

anterior part of the lateral zone (from the canines to the premolars) contains **adipose connective tissue**. The submucosa in the posterior part of the lateral zone of the hard palate (around the molars) contains **minor salivary glands**. However, the amount of submucosa in these areas of the hard palate is thinner than that associated with lining mucosa, which becomes apparent when injections of local anesthetic are placed in the area, because they can produce more discomfort.

Submucosa is absent in the medial zone of the hard palate; thus the tissue has a firmer feeling when palpated. This firm feeling is enhanced as a result of the firmness with which the lamina propria is attached to the underlying bone; thus the **lamina propria** serves as a **periosteum** for the underlying palatal bone or mucoperiosteum. The anterior zone surface landmarks on the hard palate, the palatine rugae, and the median palatal raphe have histological features similar to those of the medial zone of the hard palate.

ATTACHED GINGIVA
CLINICAL APPEARANCE

Healthy **attached gingiva** is opaque pink, and areas of **melanin pigmentation** may be seen (discussed later) (see Figures 2-9 and 2-10). When dried, the tissue is dull, firm, and immobile. Stippling is observed clinically as small pinpoint depressions, which give the surface of the attached gingiva an orange-peel appearance. The amount of stippling varies even within healthy oral cavities. The attached gingiva that covers the **alveolar bone** of the **dental arches** is classified as a **masticatory mucosa**.

Also noted is the **mucogingival junction**, a sharply defined scalloped junction between the pinker attached gingiva and the redder alveolar mucosa. Other types of gingival tissue, such as those that face the tooth surface lining the gingival sulcus, are discussed in Chapter 10.

HISTOLOGICAL FEATURES

The attached gingiva has a thick layer of mainly **parakeratinized stratified squamous epithelium** that obscures the extensive vascular supply in the lamina propria, making the tissue appear opaque and pinkish (Figure 9-11). Again, the cells of the **keratin layer** that

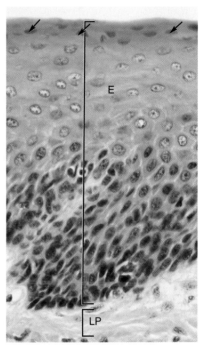

FIGURE 9-11 Photomicrograph of attached gingiva with a thick layer of mainly parakeratinized epithelium (*E*) overlying an extensively vascular lamina propria (*LP*) that acts as a mucoperiosteum. Note that the cells in the keratin layer have retained their nuclei and are filled with keratin (*arrows*), although it is hard to see at this lower level of magnification. The deeper alveolar bone is not shown. *(From Nanci A: Ten Cate's Oral Histology, ed 7, Mosby, St Louis, 2008.)*

have **nuclei** along with **keratin** may be difficult to see under low microscopic power in certain histological sections. However, minor amounts of **orthokeratinized stratified squamous epithelium** without nuclei in the keratin layer may still be found.

The lamina propria of the attached gingiva also has tall, narrow connective tissue papillae; its stippling is due to a strong attachment

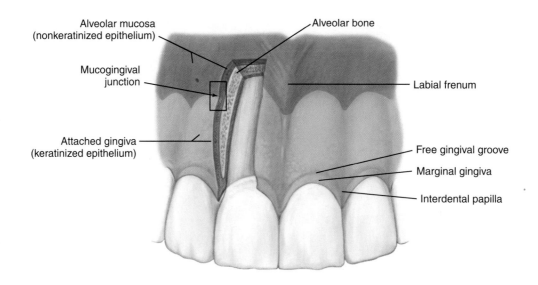

Alveolar mucosa (nonkeratinized epithelium)

Mucogingival junction

Attached gingiva (keratinized epithelium)

Alveolar bone

Labial frenum

Free gingival groove

Marginal gingiva

Interdental papilla

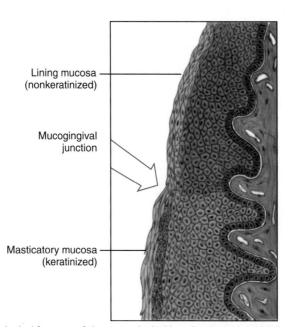

Lining mucosa (nonkeratinized)

Mucogingival junction

Masticatory mucosa (keratinized)

FIGURE 9-12 Histological features of the mucogingival junction (*arrow*), which is a junction between the alveolar mucosa and attached gingiva, as well between a lining mucosa (nonkeratinized) and masticatory mucosa (keratinized).

or pull of the epithelium toward the lamina propria in these areas, a process that is analogous to the button tufting on upholstery. No submucosa is present. The lamina propria is directly attached to the underlying jaws, making the attached gingiva firm and immobile. The **lamina propria** acts as a **periosteum** to the underlying jaws, and thus is termed a **mucoperiosteum.**

Histologically, the **mucogingival junction** can be seen as a dividing zone between the keratinized attached gingiva and the nonkeratinized alveolar mucosa, and thus is present between a masticatory mucosa and a lining mucosa (Figures 9-12 and 9-13). It is also a junction between a tissue with a thick epithelial layer in the pinkish attached gingiva and a tissue with a thin epithelial layer in the redder alveolar mucosa, even though both tissue types have a similar extensive vascular supply in the lamina propria.

TONGUE AND LINGUAL PAPILLAE

The V-shaped line, the **sulcus terminalis**, divides the **dorsal surface of the tongue** into the anterior two thirds, or **body of the tongue,** and the posterior one third, which is the **base of the tongue** (see Figure 2-14). The **tongue** is a mass of striated muscle in its core, covered by **oral mucosa** (Figure 9-14). In the mobile anterior, the striated muscle bundles are tightly packed, with relatively little intervening adipose connective tissue in the core. In the bulkier, less-mobile posterior, the adipose connective tissue is more abundant in the core. Collections of **minor salivary glands** are numerous in the **submucosa** and muscular core of the posterior part of the tongue, particularly close to the junction between the posterior and anterior parts.

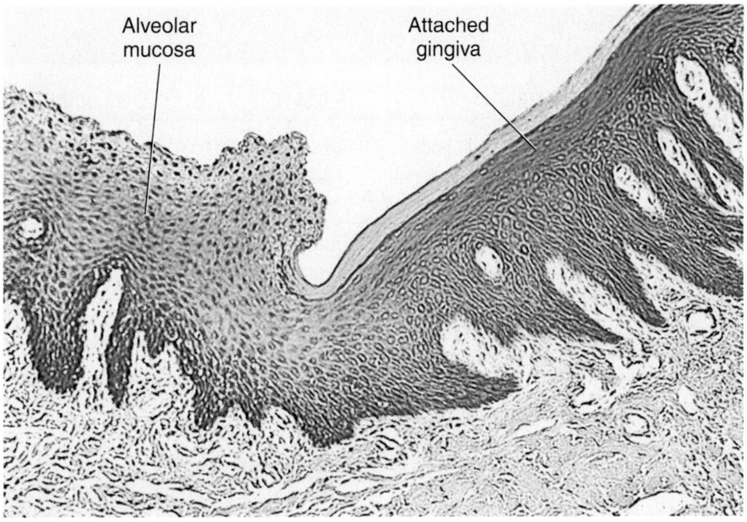

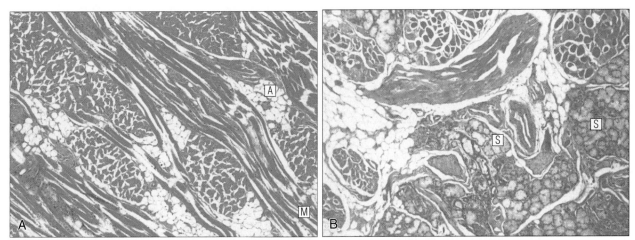

FIGURE 9-13 Photomicrograph of the mucogingival junction, which is a junction between the non-keratinized alveolar mucosa and the keratinized attached gingiva, as well as between a lining mucosa and a masticatory mucosa. *(From Nanci A: Ten Cate's Oral Histology, ed 7, Mosby, St Louis, 2008.)*

FIGURE 9-14 Photomicrographs of the muscular core of the tongue. **A:** In the mobile anterior, the striated muscle bundles (*M*) are tightly packed with relatively little intervening adipose connective tissue (*A*), unlike the less mobile posterior. **B:** Collections of salivary glands (*S*) are numerous in the submucosa and muscular core of the posterior tongue. *(From Stevens A, Lowe J: Human Histology, ed 3, Mosby, St Louis, 2005.)*

The dorsal surface has both a **masticatory mucosa** and **specialized mucosa** present. The masticatory mucosa, an **orthokeratinized stratified squamous epithelium**, generally covers the surface of the muscle associated with the tongue.

The specialized mucosa found on the dorsal surface, the **lingual papillae**, are small discrete structures or appendages of keratinized epithelium, with both orthokeratinized and parakeratinized are present, with a lamina propria (see Figures 2-14 and 2-15). Lingual papillae are also found on the **lateral surface of the tongue**. There are four types of lingual papillae: filiform, fungiform, foliate, and circumvallate (Table 9-5). The development of the lingual papillae and the tongue is discussed in Chapter 5.

Three types of lingual papillae are associated with taste buds: fungiform, foliate, and circumvallate. **Taste buds** are barrel-shaped organs of taste derived from the epithelium (Figure 9-15). They are composed of 30 to 80 spindle-shaped cells that extend from the basement membrane to the epithelial surface of the lingual papilla. The **turnover time** of the taste bud cells is a fairly rapid process of about 10 days.

The two types of taste bud cells are the *supporting cell*s and the *taste cells*. However, the difference between the two is hard to discern under lower power magnification of most histological sections, and immature forms are also noted. The supporting cells support the taste bud and are usually located on the outer part of the taste bud. The taste cells are usually located in the central part of the taste bud and have superficial taste receptors that are responsible for making contact with dissolved molecules of food and producing a taste sensation from the taste pore (see Figures 9-15 and 9-16).

Dissolved molecules of food contact the taste receptors at the taste pore, which is an opening in the most superficial part of the taste bud. Taste cells are also associated with sensory neuron processes in the inferior part of the taste bud among the cells. These sensory neuron processes receive messages of taste sensation through the receptors. This message is then sent by the nerve to the central nervous system, where it is identified as a certain type of taste.

Evidence suggests that the four fundamental taste sensations—sweet, sour, salty, and bitter—are different because of four slightly

TABLE 9-5	Comparison of Lingual Papillae			
COMPARISONS	**FILIFORM**	**FUNGIFORM**	**FOLIATE**	**CIRCUMVALLATE**
Clinical appearance	Most common on body; fine-pointed cones giving the tongue velvety texture	Lesser numbers on body; mushroom-shaped, small, red dots	About 4–11 vertical ridges on lateral surface of posterior tongue	About 7–15 large, raised, mushroom-shaped structures anterior to sulcus terminalis
Microscopic appearance	Pointed structure with thick layer of keratinized epithelium, overlying core of lamina propria; no taste buds	Mushroom-shaped structure with thin layer of keratinized epithelium overlying core of lamina propria, with taste buds in most superficial part	Leaf-shaped structure of keratinized epithelium overlying core of lamina propria, with taste buds in superficial lateral part	Mushroom-shaped structure with similar histology to fungiform but also sunken deep to tongue surface, taste buds in papilla base, and surrounded by a trough, with von Ebner's minor salivary glands in submucosa
Function	Possibly mechanical	Taste	Taste	Taste

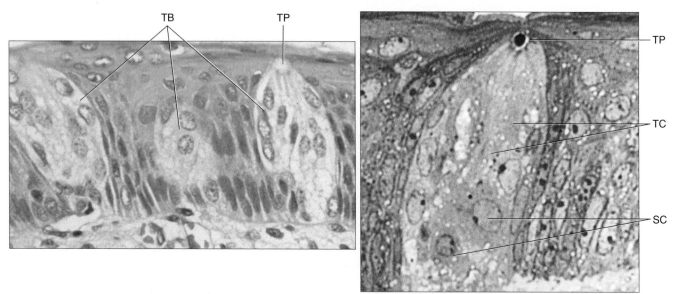

FIGURE 9-15 Histological sections of taste buds (*TB*), with supporting cells (*SC*) and taste cells (*TC*); immature forms are also present. However, it is hard to discern the associated nerves and differences between the two cell types at this lower level of magnification. Note taste pores (*TP*) at most superficial parts. *(From Stevens A, Lowe J:* Human Histology, *ed 3, Mosby, St Louis, 2005.)*

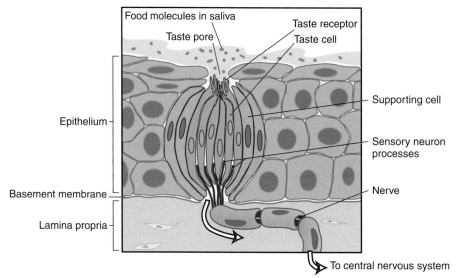

FIGURE 9-16 Events involved in taste sensation with a taste bud. Dissolved food contacts the taste receptors of the taste cells at the taste pore. Taste cells are also associated with sensory neuron processes in the inferior part of the taste bud, among the cells that receive messages of taste sensation from the taste receptors. This message is then sent by the nerve to the central nervous system, where it is identified as a certain type of taste.

differentiated taste cells. The tastes experienced are the result of the blending of the four fundamental taste sensations, the addition of other sensations by the tongue, and the interplay of smell and taste. In the past, the tongue was thought to have a specific mapping of taste sensations, but studies have proved this assumption false. Other taste categories include umami and fatty acid tastes.

FILIFORM LINGUAL PAPILLAE
CLINICAL APPEARANCE

The **filiform lingual papillae** are the most common lingual papillae located on the body of the dorsal surface of the tongue (see Figure 2-14). They are shaped like fine-pointed cones of 2 to 3 mm, with the tips naturally turned toward the **pharynx**, giving the dorsal surface of the tongue its velvety texture. They are sensitive to changes in the body and thus are associated with certain clinical considerations (discussed later).

HISTOLOGICAL FEATURES

A filiform is a pointed structure with a thick layer of orthokeratinized or parakeratinized epithelium overlying a core of lamina propria (Figure 9-17). An increased amount of **keratin** is noted also at the surface of each filiform, forming a snow-covered "Christmas tree" arrangement and whiter color for this lingual papilla. No taste buds are present in the epithelium. The filiform possibly have a rudimentary mechanical function as a result of their surface texture, which is related to the increased amount of surface keratinization present, and thus may aid in guiding food back to the **pharynx** for swallowing.

FUNGIFORM LINGUAL PAPILLAE
CLINICAL APPEARANCE

The **fungiform lingual papillae** are found in lesser numbers than are the filiform on the body of the dorsal surface of the tongue (see Figure 2-14). They appear as smaller reddish dots, which on closer inspection are slightly raised and mushroom-shaped with a 1-mm diameter. Fungiform are not found near the sulcus terminalis.

HISTOLOGICAL FEATURES

A fungiform is a smaller mushroom-shaped structure with a thin layer of orthokeratinized or parakeratinized epithelium overlying a highly vascularized core of lamina propria, thus producing the redder appearance of this lingual papilla (see Figure 9-17). A variable number of **taste buds** are located in the most superficial part of the epithelial layer; however, taste buds are not located near the base of the structure. Thus, the function of the fungiform is taste sensation.

FOLIATE LINGUAL PAPILLAE
CLINICAL APPEARANCE

The **foliate lingual papillae** appear as 4 to 11 vertical ridges parallel to one another on the **lateral surface of the tongue** in its most posterior part (see Figure 2-15).

HISTOLOGICAL FEATURES

The foliate are leaf-shaped structures with a layer of orthokeratinized or parakeratinized epithelium overlying a core of lamina propria (Figure 9-18). **Taste buds** are located in the epithelial layer on the lateral parts of the leaf-shaped structure. Thus, the function of the foliate is taste sensation. Some histologists believe that the foliate are not true lingual papillae because of their rudimentary appearance, developmental background, and location.

CIRCUMVALLATE LINGUAL PAPILLAE
CLINICAL FEATURES

When the tongue is arched and extended, the **circumvallate lingual papillae** appear as 7 to 15 raised, large, mushroom-shaped structures just anterior to the **sulcus terminalis** (see Figure 2-14). With the tongue in a

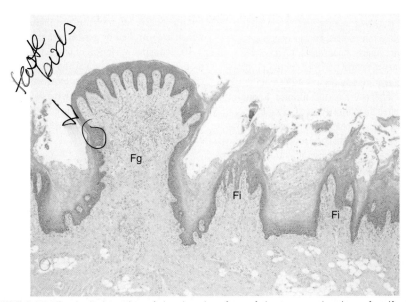

FIGURE 9-17 Histological section of the dorsal surface of the tongue showing a fungiform lingual papilla (*Fg*) and filiform lingual papillae (*Fi*). Note the mushroom shape of the fungiform and the tree shape of the filiform. However, the taste buds at the superficial surface of fungiform are difficult to discern at this low level of magnification. (*From Young B, Heath JW:* Wheater's Functional Histology, *ed 5, Churchill Livingstone, Edinburgh, 2006.*)

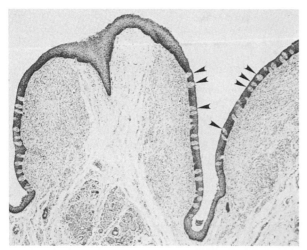

FIGURE 9-18 Histological section of the lateral surface of the tongue showing the foliate lingual papillae. Taste buds (*arrows*) are located in the epithelial layer on the lateral parts of the leaf-shaped structure. *(From Nanci A: Ten Cate's Oral Histology, ed 7, Mosby, St Louis, 2008.)*

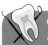
Clinical Considerations with the Tongue and Its Structures

Two commonly found lesions are associated with the dorsal surface of the tongue and involve the lingual papillae. Neither lesion is serious, but both should be recorded on the patient record if such lesions are present. One of these tongue lesions is a **geographic tongue**, which appears as red and then paler pink to white patches on the body of the tongue. These patches change shape with time, resembling a geographic map (Figure 9-20). This lesion is found in all age groups and is a type of normal variation that shows the sensitivity of the **filiform lingual papillae** to changes in their environment.

These red and white surface patches of geographic tongue correspond to groups of filiform undergoing changes from parakeratinized epithelium, which appears redder, to orthokeratinized epithelium, which appears whiter. This lesion is sometimes associated with soreness or slight burning on the surface of the tongue. However, no treatment is needed for geographic tongue, although dental professionals should reassure the patient and rule out any other more serious tongue lesion.

A less common change, and not a normal variation, noted on the dorsal tongue surface is **black hairy tongue** (Figure 9-21). With this disturbance, normal shedding of epithelium of the **filiform lingual papillae** does not occur. As a result, a thick layer of dead cells and keratin builds up on the tongue surface, which becomes extrinsically stained by tobacco, medications, or chromogenic (colored) oral bacteria. Studies show that this condition, in some cases, might be an effect of fungal overgrowth, possibly as a result of high doses of antibiotics or radiation therapy. Brushing the tongue is recommended in this case to promote tissue shedding and remove debris.

Generally, brushing the **dorsal surface of the tongue** is important for overall homecare of the oral cavity and to reduce bad breath (or malodor, halitosis) because microbial colonization on the tongue's surface is an important factor in its development.

more relaxed and natural position, the circumvallate are sunken as deep as the tongue surface because they are surrounded by a circular trough or trench. They are lined up in an inverted V-shaped row facing the **pharynx**, mimicking the shape of the sulcus terminalis. The circumvallate have a larger diameter than the fungiform, measuring from 3 to 5 mm.

HISTOLOGICAL FEATURES

The circumvallate are larger mushroom-shaped structures with orthokeratinized or parakeratinized epithelium overlying a core of lamina propria (Figure 9-19). Hundreds of **taste buds** are located in the epithelium surrounding the entire base of each papilla, opposite the circular trough lined by the surrounding tongue surface tissue.

It is important to note that **von Ebner's salivary glands** are also present in the submucosa deep to the lamina propria of the circumvallate. These are **minor salivary glands** with only **serous cells** present (with ducts that open into the trough), flushing the area near the **taste pores** so as to introduce new taste sensations from several sequential food molecules (see Chapter 11). Thus, the function of the circumvallate is taste sensation.

PIGMENTATION OF THE ORAL MUCOSA

The oral mucosa can range in color from pink to reddish pink (see Chapter 2). The presence of **melanin pigmentation** in the epithelium may give rise to localized flat areas of the oral mucosa that range in color from brown to brownish black (Figure 9-22). This condition is distinct from the nevus or mole that is a benign tumor of melanin, which appears in the oral cavity usually as one small macule or papule.

Melanin is a pigment formed by melanocytes, which are derived from the **neural crest cells**. Melanocytes are clear cells that occupy a position in the basal layer of the stratified squamous epithelium between the dividing epithelial cells (Figure 9-23). The melanocytes have small cytoplasmic granules, or inclusions, called *melanosomes*, which store the melanin pigment. They inject these melanosomes into the neighboring newly formed epithelial cells of the basal layer.

As the tissue ages, the injected cells migrate to the surface of the oral mucosa and appear clinically as a group of localized, flat, pigmented areas or macules. Because melanocytes are evenly distributed throughout the oral mucosa, clinical signs of pigmentation are based on the degree of melanin-producing activity of the melanocytes, which is controlled by genetic programming.

If the normal variation of pigmentation is present in the oral cavity, it appears most abundant at the base of the **interdental gingiva** associated with both dentitions. However, the pigmentation of both the oral mucosa and skin may increase with certain endocrine diseases. Additionally, if dramatic localized pigment changes are recently noted in the oral cavity, biopsy and histological study are recommended to rule out any malignancies.

TURNOVER TIME, REPAIR, AND AGING OF THE ORAL MUCOSA

Overall, the **turnover time** for the oral mucosa is higher than for the skin (see Chapter 8). Regional differences in the turnover times, however, do exist within the oral cavity (Table 9-6). The gingival epithelium that attaches to the tooth surface (**junctional epithelium**) has the highest turnover time, 4 to 6 days, of all the oral tissue (see Chapter 10). One of the lowest turnover times is for the **hard palate**, at 24 days. All other oral mucosal regions' turnover times fall between these two end points, thus between 4 to 24 days. Regional differences in the pattern of epithelial maturation or keratinization appear to be associated with different turnover times; nonkeratinized **buccal**

mucosa turns over faster than keratinized **attached gingiva**—about 1.5 times faster; thus, lining mucosa turns over faster than masticatory mucosa.

Generally, the **epithelium** of any region of **oral mucosa** has a higher turnover time than cells of the **lamina propria**, although the turnover time of its matrix, both fibers and intercellular substance, is quite rapid in response. All regions of the oral cavity have a higher turnover time than the skin, which has a turnover time of 27 days. Such differences noted in turnover times for oral mucosal regions can have important implications for healing and rate of recovery time from damage. Skin regions also have varying levels of turnover times (face faster than legs).

The repair process of the oral mucosa is similar to that of the skin (see Figure 8-3). After an injury to the oral mucosa, a moist clot from blood products forms in the area, and the inflammatory response is triggered with its white blood cells. In the next days, as tissue repair begins, the epithelial cells at the periphery of the injury will lose their desmosomal junctions and migrate to form a new epithelial surface

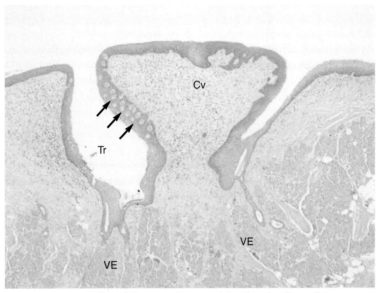

FIGURE 9-19 Histological section of the posterior part of the dorsal surface of the tongue showing a circumvallate lingual papilla (*Cv*), with taste buds (*arrows*) within the epithelial layer and surrounded by a circular trough (*Tr*). Note von Ebner's salivary glands (*VE*), which flush the trough between tastes. *(From Young B, Heath JW:* Wheater's Functional Histology, *ed 5, Churchill Livingstone, Edinburgh, 2006.)*

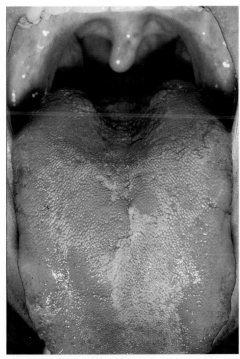

FIGURE 9-20 Geographic tongue showing its sensitivity of the filiform lingual papillae. This normal variation results in redder to paler pink and to white patches appearing on the body of the tongue over time.

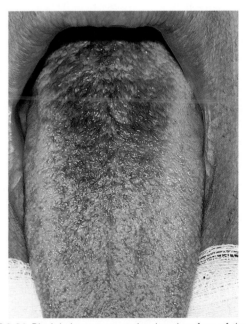

FIGURE 9-21 Black hairy tongue on the dorsal surface of the tongue where normal shedding of epithelium of the filiform lingual papillae is lacking. This results in the formation of a thick layer of dead cells and keratin, which becomes stained.

layer beneath the clot. Thus, the clot is highly important in repair of the epithelium and must be retained in the first days of repair because it acts as a guide to form a new surface. Instructions are given to patients before tooth extractions outlining behaviors to avoid in order not to disturb the clot, thus preventing *dry socket*, a postextraction infection. Later, after the epithelial surface is repaired, the clot breaks down through enzymatic activity, because it is no longer needed.

At the same time, **fibroblasts** migrate to produce an immature connective tissue in the injured lamina propria deep to the clot and newly forming epithelial surface. This immature connective tissue is considered **granulation tissue** and has fewer fibers and an increased number of blood vessels. Granulation tissue appears as a soft, bright red tissue that bleeds easily. This tissue may become abundant and may actually interfere with the repair process. Surgical removal of excess granulation tissue may be necessary to allow for optimal repair, such as in a tooth extraction or certain periodontal surgical techniques.

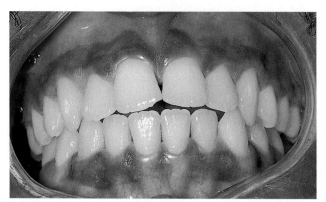

FIGURE 9-22 Pigmentation of the attached gingiva associated with the permanent dentition that is most abundant at the base of the interdental gingiva.

This temporary granulation tissue is later replaced by firmer and paler scar tissue in the affected area. Replacement tissue is characterized by an increased amount of fibers and fewer blood vessels. The amount of scar tissue varies depending on the type and size of the wound, amount of granulation tissue, and movement of tissue after injury. The oral mucosa shows less scar tissue, either clinically or histologically, after repair than does the skin, because fewer fibers are located in this area than in the skin when it undergoes a similar injury. The minimal scar tissue formation in oral mucosa after repair is similar to fetal tissue repair.

This difference in a lesser amount of scar tissue formation in the oral mucosa is useful both esthetically and functionally when oral or periodontal surgery is performed. Histologists believe it may be linked to the different embryological origins of the fibroblasts from the two tissue types; skin fibroblasts are derived from the mesoderm, and oral mucosal fibroblasts are derived from neural crest cells.

After the source of injury is removed, the repair of the oral mucosa generally follows a timeframe similar to its turnover time. Studies show that epithelial cells possess receptors for growth factors and respond also to chemical mediators of the inflammatory process; the future may show a way to speed repair and also prevent aging in the oral mucosa. Aging of the oral mucosa mirrors some of the changes observed in the skin, lips, and mucosa of other areas of the body (Figure 9-24). Unlike skin and lips, the oral mucosa is protected from changes due to UV radiation. And similar to skin, it is important to remember that it is sometimes difficult to distinguish changes caused by aging in the oral mucosa from those changes caused by chronic disease.

Aging of the oral mucosa is seen clinically as a reduction of stippling on the attached gingiva, an increase in Fordyce's spots in the labial and buccal mucosa, and enlargement of the lingual veins to form lingual varicosities on the ventral surface of the tongue. The number of lingual papillae, especially the foliate lingual papillae, and associated taste buds is also reduced and may be related to changes in

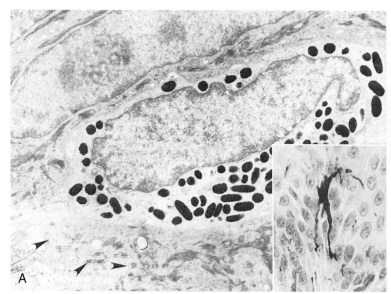

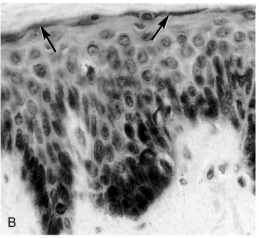

FIGURE 9-23 Pigmentation process. **A:** Electron micrograph of a melanocyte in the basal layer of pigmented oral epithelium, where the dense melanosomes are abundant near the basement membrane (*arrowheads*). Inset: Photomicrograph showing a melanocyte, which appears dark because it has been stained to reveal the presence of melanin. **B:** Photomicrograph of the attached gingiva, showing the pigmentation process within the oral mucosa. Note the granular layer (*arrows*) and the deposits of melanin, particularly in the basal layer. (**A** *from Nanci A:* Ten Cate's Oral Histology, *ed 7, Mosby, St Louis, 2008;* **B** *courtesy of TS Leeson, Professor Emeritus, Cell Biology and Anatomy, Medicine and Oral Health, University of Alberta, Alberta, Canada.*)

taste perception. Many of the changes in the oral cavity may be due to changes in the salivary glands that result in less production of saliva (hyposalivation); these changes make the oral mucosa drier (xerostomia) and thus less protective. However, the changes are not directly due to aging but mainly due to medications taken by older individuals or concurrent disease processes (see Figure 11-8).

Histologically, the thickness and number of rete ridges in the epithelium diminish as the oral mucosa ages. The mitosis in the epithelium is reduced, as is the surface area of the epithelium. In addition, the degree of keratinization of the masticatory mucosa declines, especially in the attached gingiva. Cell division at the basal layer of the epithelium does not slow down, but studies show that the turnover times do slow down for all regions of the oral cavity.

Exposure of the dental tissue from gingival recession of attached gingiva in the aged population is argued to be more a sign of disease than of age (see Figure 10-4). Also thought to be a sign of disease in the aged is creasing, and then cracking at the labial commissures, which possibly results from a loss of vertical dimension of the dentition and jaws (see Figure 14-22, Chapter 20).

Histologically, changes also occur in the composition of the matrix of the lamina propria and in a less-defined division between the papillary and dense layers in older oral mucosa. Collagen fibers appear thickened and are arranged into dense bundles resembling those found in tendons or ligaments. Elastic fibers, if present in the lamina propria, appear changed, even though more of them are present. This change in elastic fibers may explain the loss of resiliency found in aged oral mucosa.

The fibroblasts decrease in quantity, appear smaller, and are less active in older oral mucosa. The entire lamina propria has a slower collagen turnover time. Overall, with aging, the ability of the oral mucosa to repair itself is reduced and the length of the repair time is increased, just as turnover time is increased.

TABLE 9-6	Mean Turnover Time for Oral Tissue*
Hard palate	24 days
Floor of mouth	20 days
Buccal and labial mucosa	14 days
Attached gingiva	10 days
Taste buds	10 days
Junctional epithelium (attached to tooth)	4–6 days

*Note that for comparison, the turnover time for the skin is 27 days.

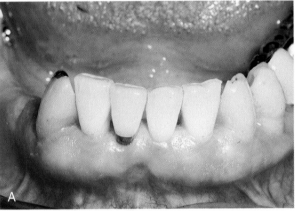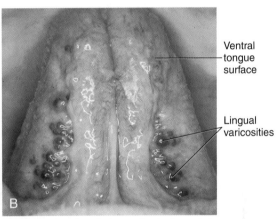

Ventral tongue surface

Lingual varicosities

FIGURE 9-24 Various changes resulting from aging in the oral cavity. **A:** Loss of stippling of the attached gingiva. **B:** Lingual varicosities on the ventral surface of the tongue.

 Clinical Considerations Concerning Oral Mucosa Turnover Time

Dental professionals must consider the shorter **turnover time** for oral regions when diagnosing lesions of the **oral mucosa**. Should the lesion be traumatic, complete healing takes up to approximately 2 weeks, depending on the region involved and if the source of the injury is first removed. Although possible sources of injury to the oral mucosa may be physical, chemical, or infectious, assumptions should never be made about the source of any lesion of the oral mucosa. Biopsy, followed with histological study, is the only way, actually, to effectively diagnose any lesion.

Thus, a delay of approximately 2 weeks, to allow a lesion to undergo healing before obtaining a referral or instigating a more serious clinical plan, does not adversely affect a patient's health. However, a longer delay (e.g., until the next maintenance visit of 6 months) before the lesion is checked is not in the best interests of a patient because malignant changes in a worst-case scenario do not heal but grow in size and may metastasize. Now, the larger lesion with metastasis gives the patient a poorer prognosis, if the lesion is later determined to be malignant after histological study.

Turnover times also have implications during the treatment of cancer by surgical, chemical, and radiologic means, because these methods can damage the oral mucosa while they are used to halt or reduce the cancerous growth. This forced healing also varies according to the original turnover times of the tissue, even if it takes longer due to the trauma of therapy. Thus, the buccal mucosa heals faster than the hard palate when subjected to cancer therapy methods.

With the increasing age of the patient base, dental professionals must consider the associated effects of aging on the oral mucosa during dental treatment; one being longer times for healing. Age-associated changes such as lingual varicosities and loss of stippling should be distinguished from conditions resulting from oral or systemic disease.

In the future, many changes associated with aging may be prevented. With present knowledge, gingival recession might be prevented by correct toothbrushing techniques, placement of a protective mouthguard against occlusal forces, or institution of crown-lengthening procedures. Other changes, such as a drier mouth (xerostomia) and loss of resiliency, should be considered and complications prevented when treatment is performed on older patients.

CHAPTER 10

Gingival and Dentogingival Junctional Tissue

●●●LEARNING OBJECTIVES

- Define and pronounce the key terms in this chapter.
- List and describe each of the types of gingival tissue.
- Describe the histological features of the different types of gingival tissue.
- Describe the composition and discuss the development of the dentogingival junctional tissue.
- Discuss turnover of the dentogingival junction tissue.
- Integrate the knowledge of the histology into an understanding of the promotion of the health of the dentogingival junction tissue and any the related pathology that may occur within it.

●●●NEW KEY TERMS

Basal lamina (bay-sal lam-i-nah): external, internal
Col (kohl)
Dentogingival junction (den-to-jin-**ji**-val), **junctional tissue** (jungk-shun-al)
Epithelial attachment (ep-ee-**thee**-lee-al)

Epithelium (ep-ee-**thee**-lee-um): **junctional (jungk**-shun-al), **pocket, sulcular (sul**-ku-lar)
Free gingival crest (jin-ji-vah)**, groove**
Gingival crevicular fluid (jin-**ji**-val kre-**vik**-koo-ler)**, hyperplasia** (hi-per-**play**-ze-ah)**, recession** (re-**sesh**-un)

Gingivitis (jin-ji-vie-tis)
Periodontal pocket
Periodontitis (pare-e-oh-*don*-**tie**-tis)

GINGIVAL TISSUE

Gingival tissue in the oral cavity is the most important tissue of the orofacial region for dental professionals to know and understand, and the most interesting as well. All the periodontal therapy performed, and homecare instruction given, are for the purpose of creating a healthy environment for the gingival tissue. Even with restorative care, the impact on the gingival tissue must be considered. When healthy, it presents an effective barrier to the barrage of periodontal insults to deeper tissue. Thus, the dental professional must have a clear understanding of the histology of the healthy, normal gingival tissue. This helps in understanding the pathological changes that occur during the disease states involving the gingival tissue. Overall, the clinical appearance of the tissue reflects the underlying histology, both in health and disease.

When the gingival tissue is not healthy, it can provide a gateway for periodontal disease to advance into the deeper tissue of the **periodontium**, leading to a poorer prognosis for long-term retention of the teeth. Thus, both the type of periodontal therapy and homecare instructions given to patients by dental professionals and restorative care are based on the clinical conditions of the tissue.

ANATOMY OF GINGIVAL TISSUE

Surrounding the maxillary and mandibular teeth in the alveoli and covering the alveolar processes is gingival tissue (Figure 10-1). When looking at the gingival tissue in a clinical setting, different types are noted in the oral cavity. The gingival tissue that tightly adheres to the bone around the roots of the teeth is the **attached gingiva.** The gingival tissue between adjacent teeth is an extension

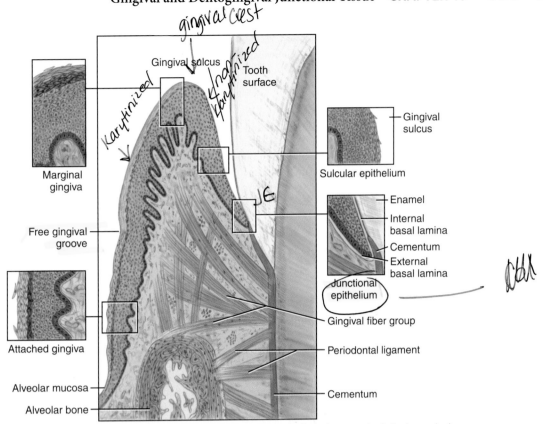

FIGURE 10-1 Gingival and dentogingival junctional tissue: marginal gingiva, attached gingiva, sulcular epithelium, and junctional epithelium.

of attached gingiva and is the interdental gingiva, forming the **interdental papillae**.

The attached gingiva is a **masticatory mucosa** (see Chapter 9). Healthy attached gingiva is pink in color, with some areas of **melanin pigmentation** possible (see Figures 2-10 and 9-22). The tissue when dried is dull, firm, and immobile, with varying amounts of **stippling**. The width of the attached gingiva varies according to its location. However, certain levels of attached gingiva may be necessary for the stability of the underlying root of the tooth.

The interdental papillae fill in the area between the teeth apical to their contact areas to prevent food impaction. The interdental papillae assume a conical shape for the anterior teeth and a blunted shape buccolingually for the posterior teeth.

At the gingival margin of each tooth is the free gingiva, or **marginal gingiva**, which is continuous with the attached gingiva. The gingival tissue that faces the tooth, the dentogingival junctional tissue, is discussed later.

Both the attached gingiva and the marginal gingiva are easily seen in the oral cavity, whether the gingival tissue is healthy or not. The gingival margin, or free gingival crest, at the most superficial part of the marginal gingiva, is also easily seen clinically, and its location should be recorded on a patient's chart.

A free gingival groove separates the attached gingiva from the marginal gingiva. This slight depression on the outer surface of the gingiva does not correspond to the depth of the gingival sulcus but instead to the apical border of the junctional epithelium. This outer groove varies in depth according to the area of the oral cavity; the groove is very prominent on mandibular anteriors and premolars.

The marginal gingiva varies in width from 0.5 to 2.0 mm from the free gingival crest to the attached gingiva. The marginal gingiva follows the scalloped pattern established by the contour of the **cementoenamel junction (CEJ)** of the teeth. The marginal gingiva has a more translucent appearance than the attached gingiva, yet has a similar clinical appearance, including pinkness, dullness, and firmness. In contrast, the marginal gingiva lacks the presence of stippling, and the tissue is mobile or free from the underlying tooth surface, as can be demonstrated with a periodontal probe.

Apical to the contact area, the interdental gingiva assumes a nonvisible concave shape between the facial and lingual gingival surfaces forming the gingival col. The col varies in depth and width, depending on the expanse of the contacting tooth surfaces. The epithelium covering the col consists of the marginal gingiva of the adjacent teeth, except that it is nonkeratinized. It is mainly present in the broad interdental gingiva of the posterior teeth, and generally is not present with those interproximal tissue associated with anterior teeth because the latter tissue is narrower. In the absence of contact between adjacent teeth, the attached gingiva extends uninterrupted from the facial to the lingual aspect. The col may be important in the formation of periodontal disease but is visible clinically only when teeth are extracted.

HISTOLOGY OF GINGIVAL TISSUE

The attached gingiva and the marginal gingiva have some similar histology, yet each has features specific to the tissue (Figure 10-2). The attached gingiva has a thick layer of mainly **parakeratinized stratified squamous epithelium**, which obscures its extensive vascular supply in the **lamina propria**, making the tissue pinkish (see Figure 9-11). The lamina propria also has tall, narrow **connective tissue papillae** and **rete ridges**, giving the tissue its varying amounts of stippling. Thus, the interface between the epithelium and lamina propria is highly interdigitated. The lamina propria is directly attached to the underlying jaws, making the attached gingiva firm and immobile, and thus serves as a **mucoperiosteum**.

Similar to the attached gingiva, the marginal gingiva is a **masticatory mucosa** but mainly has a surface layer of **orthokeratinized**

stratified squamous epithelium. The associated lamina propria also has tall, narrow papillae, but this lamina propria is continuous with the lamina propria of the gingival tissue that faces the tooth. Unlike the attached gingiva, the marginal gingiva is not attached to the underlying jaws, making this tissue firm but mobile.

Note that the **gingival fiber group** is found in the lamina propria of the marginal gingiva (see Figure 14-32). Some histologists consider the gingival fiber group part of the periodontal ligament, but this fiber group supports only the gingival tissue and not the tooth in relationship to the jaws. The lamina propria of the marginal gingiva is also continuous with the adjacent connective tissue, which includes the lamina propria of the attached gingiva, as well as the periodontal ligament.

DENTOGINGIVAL JUNCTIONAL TISSUE

The dentogingival junction is the junction between the tooth surface and the gingival tissue. Together, the sulcular epithelium and junctional epithelium form the dentogingival junctional tissue. Both the sulcular epithelium and junctional epithelium are difficult to see in clinical examination of healthy gingival tissue.

The crevicular epithelium, or sulcular epithelium, stands away from the tooth, creating a **gingival sulcus**, or space that is filled with gingival crevicular fluid (GCF) (see Figure 10-1). The depth of the healthy gingival sulcus varies from 0.5 to 3 mm, with an average of 1.8 mm. A normal GCF flow rate is quite slow and has been calculated at 1 to 2 microliters per tooth per hour. Thus, the amount of GCF is minimal in the healthy state.

The GCF seeps between the epithelial cells and into the gingival sulcus. It allows the components of the blood to reach the tooth surface through the junctional epithelium from the blood vessels of the adjacent lamina propria. The GCF contains both the immunological components and cells of the **blood**, although in lower amounts and in different proportions. It also contains sticky **plasma** proteins in the sulcus that serve as adhesive for its lining tissue, keeping it intact.

The GCF also includes **white blood cells (WBCs)**, especially the **polymorphonuclear leukocytes (PMNs)**, as well as the **immuno-globulins** of IgG, IgM, and serum IgA from **plasma cells,** which all have a role in the specific defense mechanism against disease. Thus, any immunological reactions in the blood are directly relevant to those found in the GCF and may affect the health of the tooth and associated gingival tissue. It also supplies complement factors that serve to initiate both vascular and cellular inflammatory responses that can damage the periodontium. Later, the GCF passes from the gingival sulcus into the oral cavity, where it mixes with **saliva**.

A deeper extension of the sulcular epithelium is the junctional epithelium (JE), which lines the floor of the gingival sulcus and is attached to the tooth surface. The JE is attached to the tooth surface by way of an epithelial attachment (EA). The attachment of the JE to the tooth surface can occur on enamel, cementum, or dentin. The position of the EA on the tooth surface is initially on the cervical half of the **anatomical crown** when the tooth first becomes functional after eruption (discussed later).

The probing depth of the **gingival sulcus** is measured by a calibrated periodontal probe. In a healthy-case scenario, the probe is gently inserted, slides by the sulcular epithelium, and is stopped by the EA. However, the probing depth of the gingival sulcus may be considerably different from the true histological gingival sulcus depth.

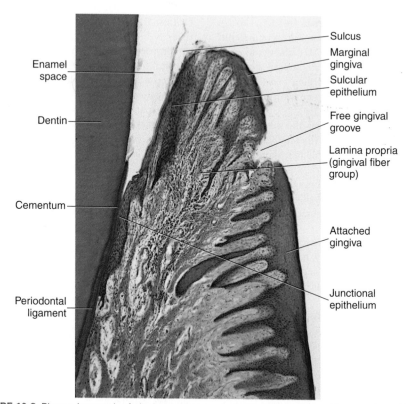

FIGURE 10-2 Photomicrograph of gingival and dentogingival junctional tissue. Deep to the epithelium is the underlying lamina propria, which is continuous with the periodontal ligament, which is adjacent to the hard tissue of the tooth: cementum, dentin, and enamel. *(Courtesy of James McIntosh, PhD, Assistant Professor Emeritus, Department of Biomedical Sciences, Baylor College of Dentistry, Dallas, TX.)*

Clinical Considerations of Gingival Tissue

With active periodontal disease, both the marginal gingiva and attached gingiva can become enlarged, especially the **interdental papillae** (Figure 10-3). This enlargement results from edema occurring in the lamina propria of the tissue caused by the inflammatory response (see later discussion of gingivitis).

Tissue fluid from the **capillary plexus** of the lamina propria flows out to flush the area of its injurious agents (see Figure 9-7). The gingival tissue can also become redder with active periodontal disease, because hyperemia, or increased blood flow, occurs in the capillaries of the lamina propria. The **stippling** may also be lost, because the inflammatory edema reduces the strong attachment between the epithelium and lamina propria. The location of the free gingival crest can also change with periodontal disease. When the tissue becomes inflamed, the gingival margin can become more coronal.

In contrast, with gingival recession the gingival margin can become more apical, which can also result from periodontal disease, tooth position, abrasion by incorrect toothbrushing methods, abfraction from occlusal stresses (such as **parafunctional habits)**, aging process, and possibly tight frenal attachments (Figure 10-4). The width of the attached gingiva may also decrease with periodontal disease, reducing the underlying support for the tooth, and should be recorded as well. All changes in the gingival tissue should be recorded in the patient record.

Within the gingival tissue, gingival hyperplasia can affect both the epithelium and lamina propria. This is an overgrowth of the interproximal gingiva resulting from the intake of drugs for seizure control (phenytoin sodium), certain antibiotics, and specific heart medications (Figure 10-5). According to some theories, these drugs either increase the output or even populations of certain types of **fibroblasts**. The amount of gingival overgrowth is related to the drug dose, as well as the amount of inflammation induced by dental biofilm. In fact, gingival overgrowth can interfere with proper homecare, and thus may need to be periodically removed by surgery. Hyperplasia of the gingival tissue is also a hallmark of periodontal disease within the tissue (discussed later).

The gingival contours form a silhouette around the cervical section of a tooth, a fact that should be acknowledged when considering smile design. The cervical peak of the gingival contour is referred to as the *gingival apex of the contour*. The apex of maxillary central incisors and canines is distal to a line drawn through the midline or long axis of the tooth. The maxillary lateral incisor apex is equal to the midline or long axis of the tooth. The gingival apex of a lateral incisor is also 1 mm short of the central incisor and canine's apex heights. The canine and central incisor gingival apices are equal in height.

The gingival contour is also related to its position in regard to the lip line. Some cases of a "gummy smile," or an excessive display of gingival tissue, are not ideal, such as when the maxillary central incisors and canines barely touch the lip line or border of the upper lip. The lateral incisor may touch the lip line or be 1- to 2-mm coronal to the lip line, revealing some gingival tissue. In most cases, orthodontic therapy, in conjunction with esthetic periodontal surgery, can alter the gingival contours for a more pleasing smile.

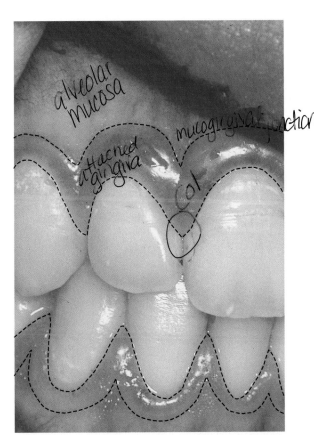

FIGURE 10-3 Extensive tissue enlargement (*dashed lines*) in both the marginal gingiva and the attached gingiva, which is due to the edema from the acute inflammation as a result of the active periodontal disease of gingivitis.

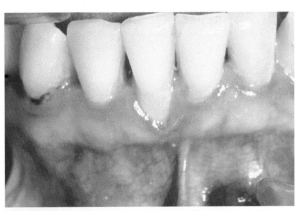

FIGURE 10-4 Gingival recession of an anterior tooth, possibly due to an adjacent tight frenal attachment.

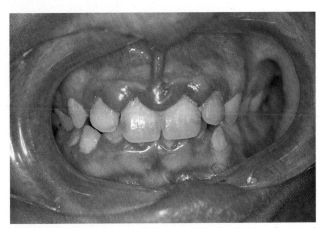

FIGURE 10-5 Gingival hyperplasia caused by the intake of a certain drug and poor homecare.

Probing measurements are subject to variations depending on the clinician's insertion pressure, the accuracy of the readings, and the ability of the probe tip to easily penetrate tissue that is ulcerated or inflamed; digital probes are available for more consistent results between clinicians. Studies show that probing both teeth and implants does not seem to cause irreversible damage to the soft tissue as it quickly heals itself (discussed later).

HISTOLOGY OF DENTOGINGIVAL JUNCTIONAL TISSUE

Histologically, the sulcular epithelium consists of **stratified squamous epithelium** similar to the epithelium of the attached gingiva and adjacent outer marginal gingiva (Figure 10-6). In contrast, the sulcular epithelium is either **nonkeratinized stratified squamous epithelium** or **parakeratinized stratified squamous epithelium,** with its cells tightly packed, unlike the keratinized marginal gingiva and attached gingiva. In addition, the interface between the sulcular epithelium and the lamina propria that it shares with the outer gingival tissue is relatively smooth compared with the others' strongly interdigitated interface.

The deeper interface between the JE and the underlying lamina propria is also relatively smooth, without rete ridges or connective tissue papillae (Figures 10-7 and 10-8). The JE cells are loosely packed, with fewer **intercellular junctions** with **desmosomes** between cells, as compared with other types of gingival tissue (see Figure 7-5). The number of **intercellular spaces** between the epithelial cells of the JE is also more

than other types of gingival tissue and all are filled with **tissue fluid.** Overall, the JE is more permeable than other gingival tissue due to its fewer desmosomal junctions and increased intercellular spaces.

This increased permeability allows for emigration of large numbers of mobile WBCs from the blood vessels in the deeper lamina propria into the JE, even in healthy tissue. This mainly involves the **PMNs,** with those cells actively undergoing **phagocytosis** (see Figure 8-17). The PMNs also enter the **GCF** in the **gingival sulcus** in healthy mouths. In the absence of clinical signs of inflammation, approximately 30,000 PMNs migrate per minute through the JE into the oral cavity. The presence of these WBCs may keep the tissue healthy by protecting it from microorganisms, within the dental biofilm, and associated toxins that continually form on the exposed tooth surface in the vicinity. Antigen-presenting cells present may be involved as well (see Chapter 8). The JE, particularly its basal cell layers, is well innervated by sensory nerve fibers.

In addition, the JE is also thinner than the sulcular epithelium, ranging coronally from only 15 to 30 cells thick at the floor of the gingival sulcus, and then tapering to a final thickness of 3 to 4 cells at its apical part. The superficial, or suprabasal, cells of the JE serve as part of the EA of the gingiva to the tooth surface.

These superficial, or suprabasal, epithelial cells of the JE provide the **hemidesmosomes** and an internal basal lamina that create the EA, because this is a cell-to-noncellular type of **intercellular junction** (see Figure 7-6). The structure of the EA is similar to that of the junction between the epithelium and subadjacent connective tissue; the internal basal lamina consists of a lamina lucida and lamina densa (Figures 10-8 and 10-9).

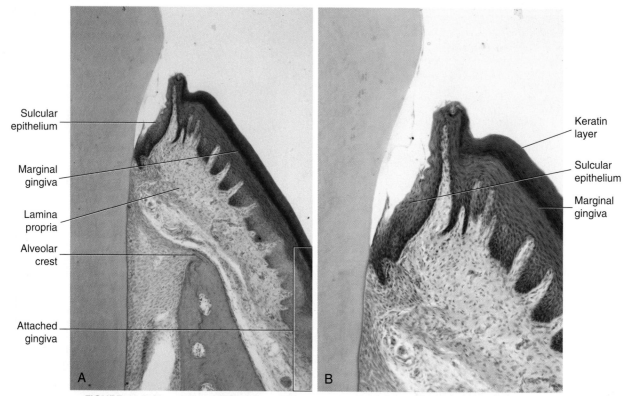

Sulcular epithelium

Marginal gingiva

Lamina propria

Alveolar crest

Attached gingiva

Keratin layer

Sulcular epithelium

Marginal gingiva

FIGURE 10-6 Photomicrographs of the sulcular epithelium. **A:** Deep to the sulcular epithelium is the lamina propria for both the marginal gingiva and the attached gingiva, as well as the alveolar crest. **B:** Close-up view showing the nonkeratinized epithelium. Note the relatively smooth interface between it and the lamina propria shared with the outer keratinized marginal gingiva, as compared with the other's strongly interdigitated interface. *(Courtesy of James McIntosh, PhD, Assistant Professor Emeritus, Department of Biomedical Sciences, Baylor College of Dentistry, Dallas, TX.)*

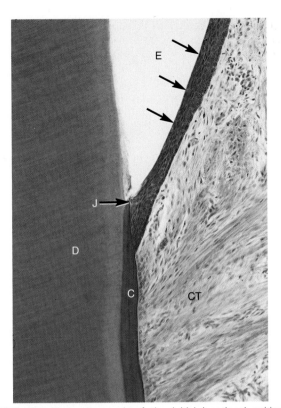

FIGURE 10-7 Photomicrograph of the initial junctional epithelium before eruption *(arrows)* overlying the enamel *(E)*, which is a space created by fixation. Note the cementoenamel junction *(J)*, the cementum *(C)*, and dentin *(D)*. Deep to the junctional epithelium is the underlying connective tissue *(CT)* of the both lamina propria and overlapping periodontal ligament. *(Courtesy of James McIntosh, PhD, Assistant Professor Emeritus, Department of Biomedical Sciences, Baylor College of Dentistry, Dallas, TX.)*

This internal basal lamina of the EA is continuous with the external basal lamina between the junctional epithelium and the lamina propria at the apical extent of the JE. The EA is very strong in a healthy state, acting as a type of seal between the soft gingival tissue and the hard tooth surface.

The deepest layer of the JE, or basal layer, undergoes constant and rapid cell division, or **mitosis**. This process allows a constant coronal migration as the cells die and are shed into the gingival sulcus. The few layers present in the JE—from its basal layer to the suprabasal, or superficial, layer—does not show any change in cellular appearance related to **maturation**, unlike other types of gingival tissue. Thus, the JE does not mature like keratinized tissue, such as the marginal gingiva or attached gingiva, which fills its matured superficial cells with **keratin**. Nor does JE mature on a lesser level like nonkeratinized tissue of the sulcular gingiva and throughout the rest of the oral cavity, which enlarges its cells as they mature and migrate superficially. The JE cells do not mature and form into a **granular layer** or **intermediate layer**.

Without a keratinizing superficial layer at the free surface of the JE, there is no physical barrier to microbial attack. Other structural and functional characteristics of the JE must compensate for the absence of this barrier. The JE fulfills this difficult task with its special structural framework and the collaboration of its epithelial and nonepithelial cells that provide very potent antimicrobial mechanisms, such as the WBCs. However, these defense mechanisms do not preclude the development of extensive inflammatory lesions in the gingival tissue, and, occasionally, the inflammatory lesion may eventually progress to the loss of bone and the connective tissue attachment to the tooth (discussed later).

The JE cells have many **organelles** in their **cytoplasm**, such as rough endoplasmic reticulum, Golgi complex, and mitochondria, indicating a high metabolic activity. However, the JE cells remain immature or undifferentiated until they die and are shed or lost in the gingival sulcus. The key to this state of cellular immaturity of the JE may be found in future studies of the adjoining lamina propria; this lamina propria appears to be functionally different from the connective tissue

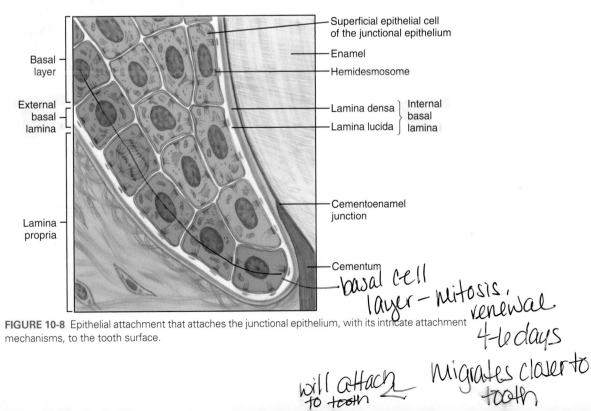

FIGURE 10-8 Epithelial attachment that attaches the junctional epithelium, with its intricate attachment mechanisms, to the tooth surface.

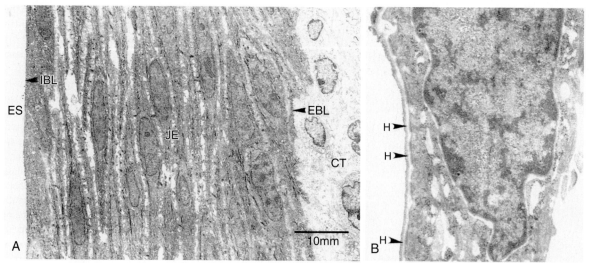

FIGURE 10-9 Electron micrographs of junctional epithelium *(JE)* and its epithelial attachment. **A:** Attachment of the JE to the enamel surface (space, *ES)* at the internal basal lamina *(IBL)* and to the connective tissue *(CT)* of the lamina propria by the external basal lamina *(EBL).* Note the lack of differentiation of the epithelium and the wide intercellular spaces. **B:** Structure of the attachment of a single JE cell to the enamel surface by the internal basal lamina and hemidesmosomes *(H).* *(**A** and **B** from Nanci A:* Ten Cate's Oral Histology, *ed 7, Mosby, St Louis, 2008.)*

underlying the other types of oral epithelium that do mature. **Lysosomes** are also found in large numbers in JE epithelial cells; enzymes contained within these lysosomes participate in the destruction of bacteria contained in dental biofilm.

DEVELOPMENT OF DENTOGINGIVAL JUNCTIONAL TISSUE

Before the eruption of the tooth and after enamel maturation, the **ameloblasts** secrete a **basal lamina** on the tooth surface that serves as a part of the primary EA. As the tooth actively erupts, the coronal part of the fused **reduced enamel epithelium (REE)** and surrounding epithelium peels back off the crown (see Figure 6-25, *D).* The ameloblasts also develop hemidesmosomes for the primary EA and become firmly attached to the enamel surface (see Figure 10-7).

However, the cervical part of the fused tissue remains attached to the neck of the tooth by the primary EA. This fused tissue, which remains near the cementoenamel junction after the tooth erupts, serves as the initial JE of the tooth, creating the first tissue attached to the tooth surface.

This tissue is later replaced by a definitive JE as the root is formed (see Figures 10-8 and 10-9).

The definitive JE is formed from all the cell types present in the REE as a result of **mitosis** of the cells, except for the ameloblasts, which are forever lost. This proliferating tissue now can provide both the **basal lamina** and **hemidesmosomes** for the secondary EA to the tooth surface. After eruption of the tooth, 3 or 4 years may pass before the initial tissue becomes the definitive JE, a multilayer nonkeratinizing squamous epithelium. Although controversial, studies now show that the ameloblasts undergo cellular changes that

make them indistinguishable from the other newly formed JE cells, with these transformed ameloblasts eventually replaced by these new cells.

In contrast, the superior tissue around implants always originates from epithelial cells of the **oral mucosa,** as opposed to the **JE** located around natural teeth, which originates from the REE (see Figure 14-23). Structurally, the periimplant epithelium closely resembles a long JE and is discussed as such by many clinicians, although dissimilarities have also been reported. Such an adaptive potential is also observed in the regenerating JE around teeth following gingivectomy—performed to surgically reduce pocket depths by removal of the soft tissue pocket wall, with a completely new JE forming within 20 days.

TURNOVER TIME OF DENTOGINGIVAL JUNCTIONAL TISSUE

In both the **sulcular epithelium** and epithelium of the marginal gingiva, the turnover process occurs in a manner similar to that of the epithelium of the attached gingiva; the basal cells migrate superficially after **mitosis,** undergo **maturation,** and take the place of the superficial cells, which are shed or lost in the oral cavity as they die.

In the **JE,** even though it does not undergo cellular maturation, its basal cells still migrate superficially upon dividing and continuously replace the dying suprabasal or superficial cells that are desquamated into the gingival sulcus at a fast pace. The migratory route of the cells, as turnover takes place in the JE, is in a coronal direction, parallel to the tooth surface. Such cells continuously dissolve and reestablish their attachments by **hemidesmosomes** on the tooth surface. The JE has the highest **turnover time** in the entire oral cavity, which is 4 to 6 days (see Table 9-6).

Clinical Considerations for Dentogingival Junctional Epithelium

The increased permeability of the **JE** that allows emigration of the PMN type of WBC also allows microorganisms from the dental biofilm, and associated toxins from the exposed tooth surface, to enter this tissue from the deeper lamina propria (Figure 10-10). When these damaging agents can enter the JE, the **gingival tissue** undergoes the initial signs of active periodontal disease with gingivitis. These signs include acute inflammation, epithelial ulceration, or tissue thinning and an increased number of **WBCs**. This ulceration of the JE allows even more damaging agents to enter the even deeper periodontium, thus advancing the disease. The interface between the dentogingival junctional tissue and the lamina propria with inflammation shows the formation of **rete ridges** and **connective tissue papillae**. The lamina propria also shows breakdown of the **collagen fibers** as the disease advances.

Bleeding after probing (BoP), even with a gentle touch, can also occur in this situation. It is due to the periodontal probe damaging the increased blood vessels in the **capillary plexus** of the **lamina propria,** which are close to the surface because of the ulceration of the JE (Figure 10-11). Bleeding can also occur with flossing. The presence of bleeding is one of the first clinical signs of active periodontal disease in uncomplicated cases and should be recorded per individual tooth and tooth surface in the patient record. However, in patients who smoke, the gingival tissue rarely bleeds because of unknown factors that do not seem related to dental biofilm and calculus formation.

Periodontal inflammation is also accompanied by an increase in the amount of **GCF** in order to fight the microbial attack, either of a serous (clear) or suppurative nature, distending the tissue further. Thus, relatively large amounts of fluid pass through the more permeable epithelial wall. This is noted clinically only when it involves visible whiter suppuration, or pus, resulting from the presence of cellular debris and extensive populations of **PMNs.**

Current clinical practice does not allow measurement of these increased fluid levels. In the future, however, this measurement may be possible in a dental setting; it is now used in research to show the level of activity of the disease. It is important to keep in mind that GCF also supplies the minerals for subgingival calculus formation, as well as a moist environment needed for dental biofilm growth.

Studies have shown that the JE cells themselves may play a much more active role in the innate defense system than previously assumed, by synthesizing a variety of molecules involved in the combat against bacteria and their products. In addition, they express molecules that mediate the migration of PMNs toward the bottom of the **gingival sulcus**.

When the deeper tissue of the **periodontium** are affected by periodontal disease, further damage can occur, and the disease can become chronic in nature; this condition is periodontitis. With the advancement of periodontal disease, the prognosis for retention of the tooth becomes risky, then guarded, as **alveolar bone** is lost and the **lamina propria** and adjacent **periodontal ligament** become increasingly disorganized, with collagen fibers breaking down. As the disease progresses, exposed **furcations** (areas between the roots) are noted around the posterior teeth and the teeth become mobile (see Figure 17-35).

True apical migration of the EA also occurs with advanced periodontal disease, causing a deepened gingival sulcus that is now lined by pocket epithelium (PE) instead of JE. In addition, this deepened **gingival sulcus** is now considered a periodontal pocket (see Figure 10-10). The depth of the periodontal pockets must be recorded in the patient record for proper monitoring of periodontal disease. Unlike in clinically healthy situations, parts of the sulcular epithelium can sometimes be seen in periodontally involved gingival tissue if air is blown into the periodontal pocket, exposing the newly denuded roots of the tooth.

Periodontopathogens, such as *Aggregatibacter actinomycetemcomitans* (Aa) or, in particular, *Porphyromonas gingivalis* (Pg), have developed sophisticated methods to disturb the structural and functional integrity of the JE, including the production of gingipains or cysteine proteinases. These virulence factors may specifically degrade components of the cell-to-cell contacts of the JE, furthering the progression of disease.

And an increased number of mononuclear WBCs, such as the **T-cell and B-cell lymphocytes** and **monocytes/macrophages**, together with **PMNs,** are also considered as factors that contribute to the focal disintegration of the JE as it forms into PE. Its most prominent histological characteristics are the presence of ulceration and gingival hyperplasia with the formation of rete ridges and connective tissue papillae. In addition, the PE has a wrinkled papillary relief, increased levels of exfoliation of epithelial cells, WBC migration, and bacterial internalization, as well as internalization-induced programmed epithelial cell death.

A periodontal pocket can become an infected space and may result in an abscess formation with a papule on the gingival surface. Incision and drainage of the abscess may be necessary, as well as systemic antibiotics; placement of local antimicrobial delivery systems within the periodontal pocket to reduce localized infections may also be considered.

Endoscopic photographic evaluation is also becoming available; it can facilitate subgingival visual examination without reliance on tactile sense and without surgical flap access. The clinician views a video monitor that displays the magnified image transmitted by a fiberoptic bundle attached to a subgingival instrument. This direct, real-time visualization of the hard and soft tissue within the gingival sulcular region may aid the clinician in diagnosis and therapy of periodontal disease. Techniques for identification and interpretation of the hard and soft tissue images, as well as the location of root deposits and caries, are being developed.

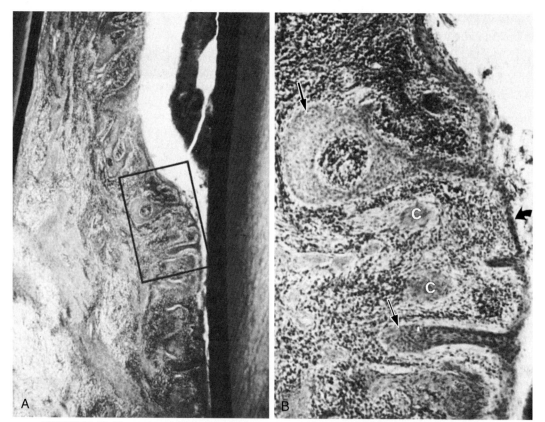

FIGURE 10-10 Photomicrographs of the advancement of chronic periodontal disease or periodontitis. A: Disease moves in an apical direction; note the alveolar crest bone loss across from the ulcerated junctional epithelium that has become pocket epithelium *(box)* with its true apical migration of the EA, causing a deepened gingival sulcus or periodontal pocket. B: Higher magnification of the newly formed pocket epithelium *(curved arrow to right)*, increased numbers of blood vessels in the lamina propria, and formation of rete ridges and connective tissue papillae at the interface between the dentogingival junctional tissue and the lamina propria *(straight arrows to left)*, as well as the breakdown of the collagen fibers *(C)* of the lamina propria and adjacent and overlapping periodontal ligament. *(From Newman MG, Takei HH, Carranza FA, Clinical Periodontology, ed 10, WB Saunders, Philadelphia, 2006.)*

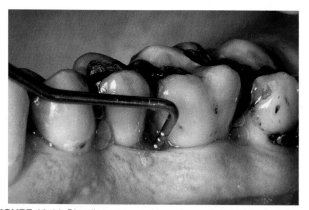

FIGURE 10-11 Bleeding upon probing of a periodontal pocket due to increased blood vessels in the lamina propria, which are closer to the surface because of ulceration of the junctional epithelium caused by periodontal inflammation.

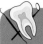 **Clinical Considerations with Dentogingival Junctional Tissue Turnover Time**

Given that the **turnover time** of the **JE** is approximately 1 week, evaluation of periodontal therapy must occur after this time to allow full healing of the area. Thus, scheduling of patients should follow this biological temporal factor of turnover time. In addition, patients must have the information and skills necessary to enact a change in their homecare to allow optimal healing during this period.

Finally, if, in a patient with periodontal tissue damage, methods could be devised to allow a more coronal reattachment of the **EA** of the JE and total periodontal regeneration, changes would also occur in the way periodontal treatment is performed and homecare instructions are given. Thus, practicing dental professionals must keep up with changes in this area of information to remain current in periodontal treatment and homecare instruction.

Head and Neck Structures

●●● CHAPTER OUTLINE

●●● LEARNING OBJECTIVES

- Define and pronounce the key terms in this chapter.
- Describe the location of each head and neck structure.
- Discuss the histological features and describe the embryological development of each head and neck structure.

- Integrate the knowledge of the histology of head and neck structures with the related pathology that may occur as well as the ways to promote their health.

●●● NEW KEY TERMS

Acinus (plural, **acini**) (**as**-i-nus, **as**-i-ny): serous (**sere**-us), mucoserous (mu-ko-**sere**-us), mucous (**mu**-kis)
Capsule (**kap**-sule)
Cells: goblet, mucous (**mu**-kis), myoepithelial (my-oh-epee-**thee**-lee-al), secretory (sek-**kre**-tory)
Colloid (**kol**-oid)
Duct: excretory (ex-**kreh**-tor-ee), intercalated (in-**turk**-ah-lay-ted), striated (**stri**-ate-ed), thyroglossal (thy-ro-**gloss**-al)
Erectile tissue (e-**rek**-tile)
Follicles (**fol**-i-kls)
Germinal center (**jurm**-i-nil)
Gland: endocrine (**en**-dah-krin), exocrine (**ek**-sah-krin)
Goiter (**goy**-ter)
Hilus (**hi**-lus)

Hyposalivation (hi-po-sal-i-**vay**-shen)
Lobes
Lobules (**lob**-ules)
Lumen (**loo**-men)
Lymph (limf)
Lymphadenopathy (lim-fad-uh-**nop**-ah-thee)
Lymphatic ducts (lim-**fat**-ik), **nodules** (**nah**-jools), **vessels**
Lymphatics (lim-**fat**-iks)
Mucosa: olfactory (**ol**-fak-tor-e), respiratory
Mucocele (**mu**-kah-sele)
Nasal cavity (**nay**-zil **kav**-it-ee), **conchae** (**kong**-kay)
Nicotinic stomatitis (nik-ah-**tin**-ik sto-mah-**ti**-tis)
Paranasal sinuses (pare-ah-**na**-zil **sy**-nuses)
Pharyngeal tonsils (fah-**rin**-je-il)

Ranula (**ran**-u-lah)
Saliva (sah-**li**-vah)
Salivary glands (**sal**-i-ver-ee): major, minor
Septum (plural, **septa**) (**sep**-tum, **sep**-tah)
Serous cells (**sere**-us), **demilune** (dem-ee-lune)
Sinusitis (sy-nu-**si**-tis)
Thyroxine (thy-**rok**-sin)
Tonsillar tissue
Trabeculae (trah-**bek**-u-lay)
Vessels: afferent (**af**-er-int), efferent (**ef**-er-ent)
von Ebner's salivary glands (von **eeb**-ners **sal**-i-ver-ee)
Xerostomia (zer-oh-**sto**-me-ah)

HEAD AND NECK STRUCTURES

Dental professionals must have a clear understanding of the histology and prenatal development concerning not only the oral cavity but also of the associated head and neck structures. The clinical functioning of the head and neck structures is related to the underlying histology. In addition, many pathological lesions that are encountered in the oral cavity can be associated with changes in these associated structures of the head and neck, and thus are reflected in changes in their underlying histology. The head and neck structures to be discussed include the salivary glands, thyroid gland, lymphatics, nasal cavity, and paranasal sinuses.

GLANDS

A **gland** is a structure that produces a secretion necessary for normal body functioning. An **exocrine gland** is a gland having a duct associated with it. A **duct** is a passageway that allows the glandular secretion to be emptied directly into the location where the secretion is to be used. An **endocrine gland** is a ductless gland with its secretions conveyed directly into the blood, and then carried to some distant location to be used. Motor nerves associated with both types of glands help regulate the flow of the secretion. Sensory nerves are also present in the gland.

SALIVARY GLANDS

The **salivary glands** produce saliva, or "spit." Saliva contains **immunoglobulins** (secretory IgA), minerals, electrolytes, buffers, enzymes, and metabolic wastes. The secretion by these glands is controlled by the autonomic nervous system. Saliva lubricates and cleanses the oral mucosa, protecting it from dryness and potential carcinogens. This secretory product also helps in digestion of food by enzymatic activity. Additionally, it serves as a buffer, protecting the oral mucosa against acids from food and dental biofilm; it is also involved in antibacterial activity.

Finally, saliva helps maintain tooth integrity, because it is involved in remineralization of the tooth surface. However, because it contributes to the formation of the pellicle on the tooth and mucosal surfaces, saliva is also involved in the first step in dental biofilm formation. It also supplies the minerals for supragingival calculus formation.

Salivary glands are classified as either major or minor, depending on their size, but both types have similar histological features. Further, both the major and minor salivary glands are **exocrine glands,** and thus have associated ducts that help convey the saliva directly into the oral cavity, where it is used.

HISTOLOGY OF SALIVARY GLANDS

Both major and minor salivary glands are composed of both **epithelium** and **connective tissue** (Figure 11-1). Epithelial cells both line the **ducts** and produce the saliva. Connective tissue surrounds the epithelium, protecting and supporting the gland. The connective tissue of the gland is divided into the capsule, which surrounds the outer part of the entire gland, and the septa. Each septum (plural, septa) helps divide the inner part of the gland into the larger lobes and smaller lobules. Both the capsule and septa carry nerves and blood vessels that serve the gland.

SECRETORY CELLS AND ACINI

Epithelial cells that produce the saliva are the secretory cells (Figure 11-2). The two types of secretory cells are classified as either mucous or serous cells, depending on the type of secretion produced. Mucous cells have a cloudier-looking cytoplasm and produce mucous secretory product. In contrast, serous cells have a clear cytoplasm and produce serous secretory product. A combination of secretory cells present in the gland can produce a mixed secretory product. In some glands, one type of cell predominates so that the product is either more mucous or more serous than if it had a range of both cell types.

Secretory cells are found in a group, or acinus (plural, acini), which resembles a cluster of grapes. Each acinus is located at the terminal part of the gland connected to the ductal system, with many acini within each lobule of the gland. Each acinus consists of a single layer of cuboidal epithelial cells surrounding a lumen, a central opening where the **saliva** is deposited after being produced by the secretory cells.

The three forms of acini are classified in terms of the type of epithelial cell present and the secretory product being produced. The major and minor salivary glands have different types of acini (Table 11-1). However, the different types of acini are often difficult to classify on histological sections of the glands.

Serous acini are composed of serous cells producing serous secretory product and have a narrow lumen (Figure 11-3). In contrast, mucous acini are composed of mucous cells producing mucous secretory product, and their lumen is wider. Mucoserous acini have both a group of mucous cells surrounding the lumen and a serous demilune, or "bonnet" of serous cells superficial to the group of mucous secretory cells (Figures 11-4 and 11-5). Because the mucoserous acini contain both types of secretory cells, they produce a mixed secretory product. However, the major distinctions between serous and mucous cells have become less important with additional studies of their cellular functioning.

To facilitate the flow of **saliva** out of each lumen into the connecting ducts, myoepithelial cells are located on the surface of some of the **acini,** as well as on parts of the ductal system, the **intercalated ducts** (Figure 11-6). Each myoepithelial cell consists of a cell body with four to eight cytoplasmic processes radiating outward. They are specialized cells of **epithelium** that resemble an octopus on a rock; they are situated on the surface of the acini and have a contractile nature.

When these cells contract, they squeeze the acinus, forcing the saliva out of the lumen and into the connecting duct. When associated with the ducts, the cells orient themselves lengthwise and contract to shorten or widen the ducts to keep them open, and more than one myoepithelial cell can sometimes be found on a single acinus. Studies show additional functions, such as signaling the secretory cells and protecting the salivary gland tissue.

DUCTAL SYSTEM

The ductal system of salivary glands consists of hollow tubes connected initially with the **acinus,** and then with other **ducts,** as the ducts progressively grow larger from the inner to the outer parts of the gland (see Figure 11-6). Each type of duct is lined by different epithelium, depending on its location in the gland (see Table 8-2). In comparison, each **major salivary gland** displays differences in the length or types of ducts present (see Table 11-1); minor salivary glands do not show these differences due to the shortness of their ductal system. It is important to note that the ductal system does not serve just as a pipeline for the passageway of saliva; it also actively participates in the production and modification of **saliva.**

The duct associated with an acinus or terminal part of the gland is the intercalated duct. Thus, this duct is attached to the **acinus,** much as a stalk is attached to a cluster of grapes. The intercalated duct consists of a hollow tube lined with a single layer of cuboidal epithelial cells. Many are found in each **lobule** of the gland. These ducts not only serve as a passageway for saliva, but they also contribute many macromolecular components to the saliva. These include lysozyme and lactoferrin, which are stored in the secretory granules of ductal cells.

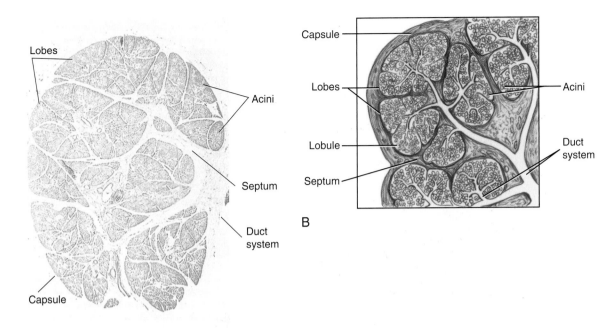

FIGURE 11-1 Composition of a salivary gland. **A:** Micrograph. **B:** Diagram. (**A** *from Nanci A:* Ten Cate's Oral Histology, *ed 7, Mosby, St Louis, 2008.)*

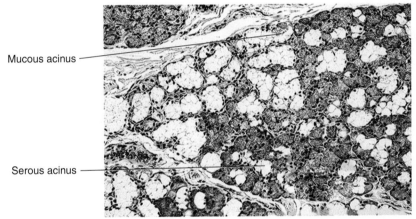

FIGURE 11-2 Microscopic section of a lobule showing two types of acini: mucous acinus and serous acinus. *(From Nanci A:* Ten Cate's Oral Histology, *ed 7, Mosby, St Louis, 2008.)*

TABLE 11-1	Comparison of Major Salivary Glands		
	PAROTID	**SUBMANDIBULAR**	**SUBLINGUAL**
Size	Largest, encapsulated	Intermediate, encapsulated	Smallest, no capsule
Location	Behind mandibular ramus, anterior and inferior to ear	Beneath the mandible	Floor of the mouth
Excretory ducts	Parotid duct (Stenson's): opens opposite maxillary second molar on buccal mucosa	Submandibular duct (Wharton's): opens near lingual frenum on floor of mouth	Sublingual duct (Bartholin's): opens at same area as submandibular duct; may have additional ducts at submandibular folds
Striated ducts	Short	Long	Rare or absent
Intercalated ducts	Long	Short	Absent
Acini	Mainly serous	Serous and mucoserous	Mainly mucous, with some mucoserous

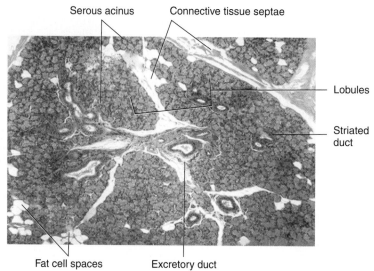

Serous acinus · Connective tissue septae · Lobules · Striated duct · Fat cell spaces · Excretory duct

FIGURE 11-3 Photomicrograph of the parotid salivary gland showing connective tissue septae dividing the serous acini into lobules to produce a mainly serous secretory product. Note the excretory duct. (*From Nanci A:* Ten Cate's Oral Histology, *ed 7, Mosby, St Louis, 2008.*)

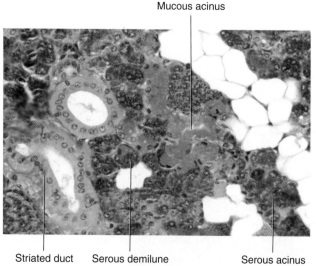

Mucous acinus · Striated duct · Serous demilune · Serous acinus

FIGURE 11-4 Microscopic magnification of the submandibular salivary gland showing mucous acinus with a serous demilune. Note the striated duct and serous acinus because the gland produces a mixed salivary product. (*From Nanci A:* Ten Cate's Oral Histology, *ed 7, Mosby, St Louis, 2008.*)

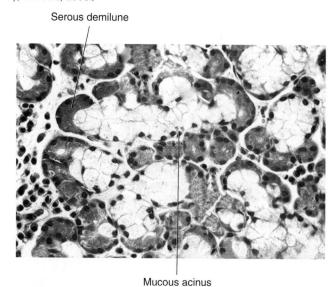

Serous demilune · Mucous acinus

FIGURE 11-5 Seromucous demilunes capping mucous cells of a mucous acinus in the sublingual salivary gland, which produces a mixed secretory product in which the mucous component predominates. (*From Nanci A:* Ten Cate's Oral Histology, *ed 7, Mosby, St Louis, 2008.*)

The **striated duct** is a part of the ductal system that is connected to the intercalated ducts in the **lobules** of the gland. The overall diameter of this duct is greater than that of each acinus, and its lumen is larger than those of both the acini and intercalacted ducts. The striated duct consists of a hollow tube lined with a single layer of columnar epithelial cells characterized by what appear to be *basal striations*. These basal striations are due to the presence of numerous elongated **mitochondria** in narrow cytoplasmic partitions separated by highly folded and interdigitated cell membranes. Not only does the striated duct serve as a passageway for saliva, but it is also involved in the modification of saliva. Its ductal cells actively resorb and secrete electrolytes into the saliva from the adjacent blood vessels near the striated regions.

The final part of the salivary gland ductal system is the **excretory duct**, or secretory duct, which is located in the **septum** of the gland. These ducts are larger in diameter than the hstriated ducts. Saliva exits by this duct into the oral cavity. The excretory duct is a hollow tube

lined with a variety of epithelial cells. The cells lining the excretory duct initially consist of **pseudostratified columnar epithelium**, which then undergoes a transition to stratified cuboidal epithelium as the duct moves to the outer part of the gland.

On the outer part of the ductal system that empties into the oral cavity, the excretory duct lining becomes **stratified squamous epithelium**, blending with surrounding oral mucosa at the ductal opening. Thus, the excretory duct serves as a passageway for saliva; however, it may have more functions as it is studied further.

MAJOR SALIVARY GLANDS

The **major salivary glands** are three, large, paired glands that have ducts named for them (Figure 11-7, see Table 11-1 and Figure 1-5). These major salivary glands are the parotid, the submandibular, and the sublingual glands. The submandibular and sublingual glands can

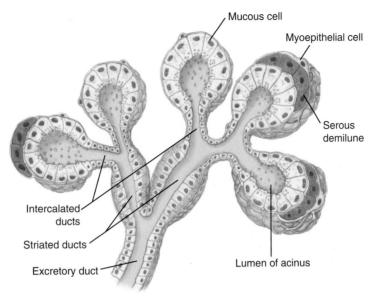

FIGURE 11-6 Salivary gland and its ductal epithelium. Note the myoepithelial cell on top of an acinus.

be palpated as nontender, firm masses in a healthy patient, but only a part of the parotid gland can be similarly palpated because part of the gland is deep to the overlying musculature and skin.

Although the **parotid salivary gland** is the largest encapsulated major salivary gland, it provides only 25% of the total salivary volume. It is located in an area behind the mandibular ramus, anterior and inferior to the ear. The **serous cell** predominates in the parotid, making the gland secrete a mainly serous secretory product (see Figure 11-3). The duct associated with the parotid gland is the **parotid duct** (or Stenson's duct). This long duct emerges from the gland and then opens up into the oral cavity on the inner surface of the buccal mucosa, usually opposite the maxillary second molar, at the **parotid papilla** (see Figure 2-2).

The **submandibular salivary gland** is the second-largest encapsulated major salivary gland, but it provides 60% to 65% of the total salivary volume. It lies beneath the mandible in the submandibular fossa, posterior to the sublingual salivary gland. Because the secretory cells in the submandibular gland are both **serous cells** and **mucous cells**, the gland secretes a mixed secretory product (see Figure 11-4). The gland also contains serous demilunes. The duct associated with the submandibular gland is the **submandibular duct** (or Wharton's duct). This long duct travels anteriorly on the floor of the mouth and opens into the oral cavity at the **sublingual caruncle** (see Figure 2-17).

The **sublingual salivary gland** is the smallest, most diffuse, and the only unencapsulated major salivary gland. It provides only 10% of the total salivary volume. It is located in the sublingual fossa, anterior to the submandibular salivary glands, in the floor of the mouth. The secretory cells in the sublingual gland are both serous and mucous, but the **mucous cells** are in the majority. Thus, the gland secretes a mixed secretory product, but with a predominately mucous component (see Figure 11-5). The short ducts associated with the sublingual gland sometimes combine to form the **sublingual duct** (or Bartholin's duct). The sublingual duct then opens directly into the oral cavity through the same opening as the submandibular duct, the **sublingual caruncle** (see Figure 2-17). Some other smaller ducts of the sublingual gland may open along the **sublingual fold**.

MINOR SALIVARY GLANDS

The minor salivary glands are much smaller than the major salivary glands but are more numerous. The minor salivary glands are also **exocrine glands**, but their unnamed **ducts** are shorter than those of any of the major salivary glands. These short ducts open directly onto the mucosal surface. These glands are scattered in the tissue of the buccal, labial, and lingual mucosa, as well as the soft palate, lateral zones of the hard palate, and the floor of the mouth. Most minor salivary glands have mostly **mucous cells**, with a few serous cells. As a result, most minor salivary glands secrete a mainly mucous secretory product, with some serous influence.

There are also minor salivary glands, von Ebner's salivary glands, associated with the larger **circumvallate lingual papillae**, on the posterior part of the **dorsal surface of the tongue** (see Figure 9-19). These glands are the exception to minor salivary glands, mainly having mucous cells, because these contain only **serous cells** and thus secrete only a serous secretory product.

DEVELOPMENT OF SALIVARY GLANDS

Between the sixth and eighth weeks of prenatal development, the three major salivary glands begin as epithelial proliferations, or buds, from the ectoderm lining of the primitive mouth. The rounded terminal ends of these epithelial buds grow into the underlying mesenchyme, producing the secretory cells, or glandular acini, and the ductal system.

The parts of the glands that contain supporting connective tissue, such as the outer capsule and inner septa, are produced from the mesenchyme, which is influenced by neural crest cells. It is important to note that interaction between the developing components of the epithelium, mesenchyme, nerves, and blood vessels is necessary for complete development of the salivary glands.

The parotid salivary glands appear early in the sixth week of prenatal development and are the first major salivary glands formed. The epithelial buds of these glands are located on the inner part of the cheek, near the labial commissures of the primitive mouth. These buds will grow posteriorly toward the otic placodes of the ears and branch to form solid cords with rounded terminal ends near the developing facial nerve.

Later, at approximately 10 weeks of prenatal development, these cords are canalized and form ducts, with the largest becoming the parotid duct for the parotid gland. The rounded terminal ends of the cords form the acini of the glands. Secretion by the parotid glands via the parotid duct begins at approximately 18 weeks of gestation. Again, the supporting connective tissue of the gland develops from the surrounding mesenchyme.

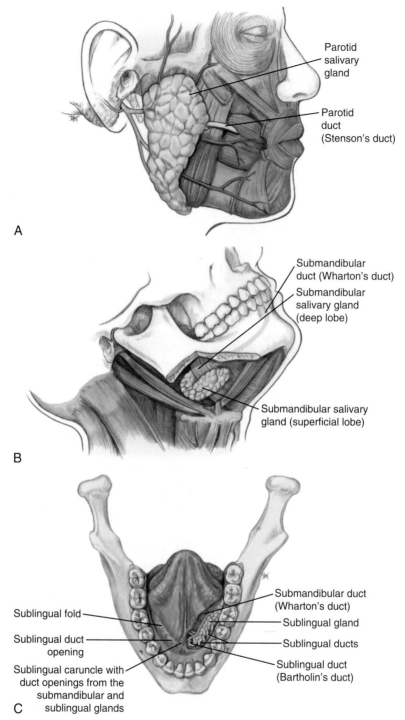

A

B

C

FIGURE 11-7 Major salivary glands. **A:** Parotid. **B:** Submandibular. **C:** Sublingual, with the tongue elevated and the floor of mouth sectioned. (***A*** and ***B*** from Fehrenbach MJ, Herring SW: Illustrated Anatomy of the Head and Neck, *ed 3, WB Saunders, Philadelphia, 2007.*)

The submandibular salivary glands develop later than the parotid glands and appear late in the sixth week of prenatal development. They develop bilaterally from epithelial buds in the sulcus surrounding the sublingual folds on the floor of the primitive mouth. Solid cords branch from the buds and grow posteriorly, lateral to the developing tongue.

The cords of the submandibular gland later branch further and then become canalized to form the ductal part. The submandibular gland acini develop from the cords' rounded terminal ends at 12 weeks,

and secretory activity via the submandibular duct begins at 16 weeks. Growth of the submandibular gland continues after birth with the formation of more acini. Lateral to both sides of the tongue, a linear groove develops and closes over to form the submandibular duct.

The sublingual salivary glands appear in the eighth week of prenatal development, later than the other two major salivary glands. They develop from epithelial buds in the sulcus surrounding the sublingual folds on the floor of the mouth, lateral to the developing submandibular gland. These buds branch and form into cords that canalize to form

Clinical Considerations for Salivary Glands

Certain medications, disease processes, or destruction of salivary tissue by radiation may result in decreased production of **saliva** by **salivary glands**. The decreased production of saliva is considered **hyposalivation** and can result in **xerostomia**, or dry mouth, also known appropriately as *cotton mouth*. Xerostomia can result in increased trauma to a nonprotected oral mucosa, increased cervical caries, problems in speech and mastication, and bad breath (halitosis) (Figure 11-8).

Thus, important changes must be made in the dental treatment plan of patients with hyposalivation and xerostomia after checking that the source of the disturbance is not related to any disease processes such as diabetes that must first be dealt with directly. Such alterations in care include the recommendation of sipping water, artificial saliva use, remineralization products such as fluoride and casein phosphopeptide-amorphous calcium phosphate (CPP-ACP), avoidance of alcohol-containing products, and increased recare visits. Medications that stimulate salivary production are available for nondrug-related hyposalivation, and transplanting lost salivary tissue is now being performed. Aging does not seem to influence the production of resting saliva, or unstimulated saliva production, but studies show that stimulated saliva production may be less than normal in older individuals.

The salivary glands may also become blocked, stopping the drainage of saliva from the duct. This blockage can cause glandular enlargement and tenderness resulting from retention of saliva in the gland. The blockage of the duct can result from either stone (or sialolith) formation or trauma to the duct opening.

This retention of **saliva** in the **salivary gland** can result in a **mucocele**, if it involves a minor salivary gland, or in a **ranula**, if it involves the submandibular salivary gland (Figures 11-9 and 11-10). These two salivary gland lesions are treated by removal of the stone or surgical removal of the entire gland. The tortuous travel of the **submandibular duct** to its ductal opening for a considerable upward distance may be the reason this gland is the one most commonly involved in stone formation.

Another oral lesion associated with salivary glands is **nicotinic stomatitis** (Figure 11-11). With this lesion, the **hard palate** is whitened by **hyperkeratinization** caused by the heat from tobacco use or hot liquid consumption (see **Chapter 9**). This heat also causes inflammation of the **duct** openings of the **minor salivary glands** of the palatal area, and thus they become dilated. This inflammation of the ductal epithelium is seen clinically in the red macules scattered on the whiter background of the palatal mucosa.

Saliva is also being used, similarly to the secretions of urine and blood, to test for drug usage, systemic diseases, and changes in physiological and psychological states, as well as oral cancer. Unlike the other bodily secretions, using saliva is very successful as a screening test because of the ease and low cost with which the sample can be obtained.

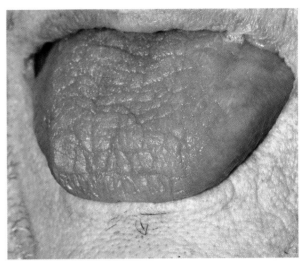

FIGURE 11-8 Xerostomia (dry mouth) due to hyposalivation (reduced saliva) causing inflammation of the oral mucosa including the tongue and lips.

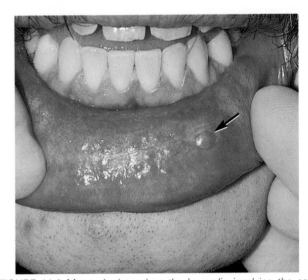

FIGURE 11-9 Mucocele *(arrow)* on the lower lip involving the severance of the associated minor salivary gland duct and resulting in enlargement of the gland.

the sublingual ducts associated with the gland. The rounded terminal ends of the cords form acini.

Much like the major salivary glands, the minor salivary glands arise from both the ectoderm and endoderm associated with the primitive mouth, similar to the major glands. They remain as small, isolated acini and ducts within the oral mucosa or submucosa lining the mouth.

The contractile myoepithelial cells, which are important in the secretion of saliva from each acinus, arise from neural crest cells, and thus are ectodermal in origin. They surround the developing acini, as well as parts of the ductal system, and become active between the 24th and 25th week of prenatal development.

THYROID GLAND

The **thyroid gland** is the largest **endocrine gland** and is located in the anterior and lateral regions of the neck, inferior to the **thyroid cartilage** (see Figure 1-13). Because it is ductless, the thyroid gland produces and secretes its products or hormones directly into the blood, such as thyroxine. Thyroxine is a hormone that stimulates the metabolic rate. The gland consists of two lateral lobes connected anteriorly by an isthmus. In a healthy patient, the gland is not visible but can be palpated and should be mobile, moving superiorly when a person swallows.

The **parathyroid glands** typically consist of 4 to 8 small endocrine glands, two on each side, usually close to the thyroid gland, or even inside it on its posterior surface. These glands are not visible or palpable during an extraoral examination of a patient. However, the parathyroid glands may alter the thyroid gland because of their involvement in a disease process.

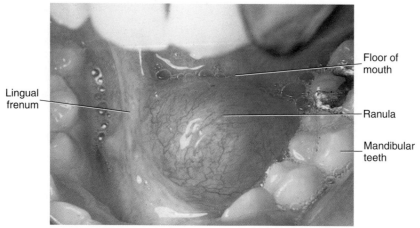

FIGURE 11-10 Ranula on one side of the floor of the mouth involving blockage of the submandibular salivary gland duct from stone formation resulting in enlargement of the gland.

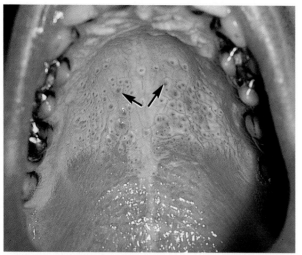

FIGURE 11-11 Nicotinic stomatitis with hyperkeratinization of the palatal mucosa and ductal inflammation of the minor salivary glands *(arrows)*. This lesion can be from smoking or hot liquid consumption.

HISTOLOGY OF THYROID GLAND

The thyroid gland is covered by a connective tissue **capsule**, which extends into the gland by way of septa (Figure 11-12). The **septa** divide the gland into larger **lobes** and smaller **lobules**. Each lobule is composed of **follicles**, irregularly shaped spheroidal masses that are embedded in a meshwork of **reticular fibers**. Each follicle consists of a layer of simple cuboidal epithelium enclosing a cavity that is usually filled with colloid, a stiff material, which is reserved for the future production of thyroxine.

DEVELOPMENT OF THYROID GLAND

The thyroid gland is the first endocrine gland to appear in embryonic development and develops from endoderm invaded by mesenchyme. At approximately the 24th day of prenatal development, the thyroid gland develops. It forms from a median downgrowth at the base of the tongue, connected by a thyroglossal duct, a narrow tube that later becomes obliterated (Figure 11-13).

The **foramen cecum**, which is the opening of the thyroglossal duct, is a small, pitlike depression located where the **sulcus terminalis** points backward toward the **oropharynx**. This duct shows the origin of the thyroid and the migration pathway of the thyroid gland into the neck region.

🦷 Clinical Considerations for the Thyroid Gland

During a disease process involving the **thyroid gland**, the gland may become enlarged and possibly may be viewed during an extraoral examination. This enlarged thyroid gland is considered a goiter (Figure 11-14). A goiter may be firm and tender when palpated and may contain hard masses. Any patient who has any undiagnosed changes in the thyroid gland or complains of related symptoms should be referred to a physician.

LYMPHATICS

The lymphatics are a part of the immune system and help fight disease processes. They also serve other functions in the body. The lymphatic system consists of a network of lymphatic vessels linking **lymph nodes** throughout most of the body. **Tonsillar tissue** located in the oral cavity and pharynx is part of the lymphatic system. This chapter describes only the intraoral tonsillar tissue in detail; the tubal tonsillar tissue is not discussed.

The lymphatic vessels are a system of endothelial-lined channels that are mostly parallel to the venous blood vessels in location but are more numerous. **Tissue fluid** drains from the surrounding region into the lymphatic vessels as lymph. Lymph is similar in composition to tissue fluid and plasma (see Chapters 7 and 8).

Each lymphatic vessel drains its particular region, and all of these vessels communicate with one another. Lymphatic vessels are lined with **endothelium** similar to blood vessels, but the lymphatic vessels are larger and thicker in diameter than capillaries of the blood system. Lymphatic vessels are found within most of the oral tissue, even within the tooth's pulp.

Smaller lymphatic vessels containing lymph converge into the larger endothelial-lined lymphatic ducts, which empty into the venous system of the blood in the chest area. The drainage pattern of the lymphatic vessels into the lymphatic ducts depends on the side of the body involved, either the right or left, because the lymphatic ducts are different on each side.

LYMPH NODES

The **lymph nodes** are bean-shaped bodies grouped in clusters along the connecting **lymphatic vessels,** positioned to filter toxic products from the lymph to prevent their entry into the blood system (Figure 11-15, A). They are located in various regions of the head and neck area (see Figures 1-2 and 1-12).

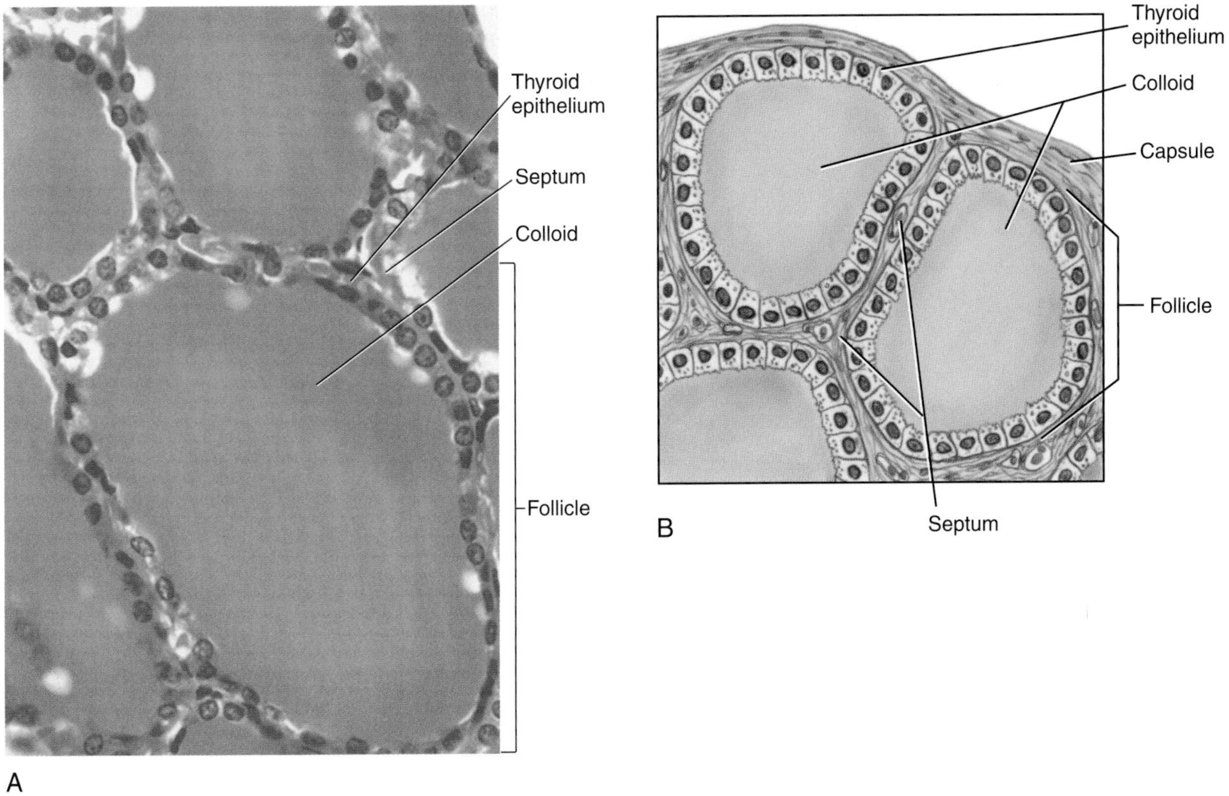

FIGURE 11-12 Histology of the thyroid gland. **A:** Photomicrograph. **B:** Diagram. (***A** from Young B, Heath JW: Wheater's Functional Histology, ed 5, Churchill Livingstone, Edinburgh, 2006.*)

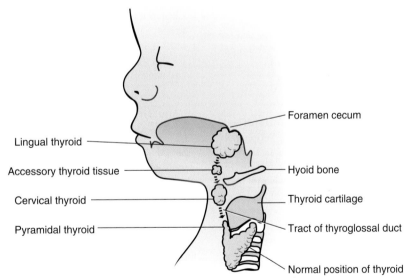

FIGURE 11-13 Development of the thyroid gland from a median downgrowth of the tongue (*broken line*), connected by a thyroglossal duct. Remnants of thyroid tissue can remain at these original sites and become cystic.

In healthy patients, lymph nodes are usually small, soft, and free or mobile in the surrounding tissue. They can be superficial in position, with the superficial veins, or deep in the tissue, with the deep blood vessels. Normally, lymph nodes cannot be seen or palpated during an extraoral examination of a healthy patient.

The lymph flows into the lymph node through many **afferent vessels**. On one side of the node is a depression, or **hilus**, where the lymph flows out of the node through fewer vessels, or even a single **efferent vessel**. Lymph nodes can be classified as either primary or secondary nodes. Lymph from a particular tissue region drains into primary nodes or regional nodes. Primary nodes, in turn, drain into secondary nodes or central nodes.

HISTOLOGY OF LYMPH NODES

Each lymph node is composed of organized lymphoid tissue and contains **lymphocytes** that actively filter toxic products from the lymph (see Figure 8-16). The node itself is surrounded by **capsule** and bands of

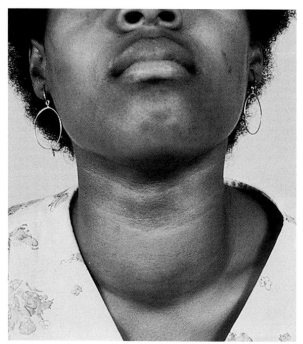

FIGURE 11-14 Goiter or enlarged thyroid gland caused by an endocrine disorder.

connective tissue, the trabeculae, extending from the capsule into the node (Figure 11-16, *B*). The trabeculae separate the node into masses of lymphocytes, the lymphatic nodules, or follicles. The **lymph** flows between the lymphatic nodules and other tissue spaces or sinuses.

Each lymphatic nodule has a germinal center containing many immature lymphocytes. As they mature, these lymphocytes enter either the area of the nodule surrounding the germinal center or the lymph. These mature **lymphocytes** are of the **B-cell** type and are mainly involved in the humoral immune response with **immunoglobulin** production by the **plasma cells** (see Figure 8-16).

DEVELOPMENT OF LYMPH NODES

Lymphatic vessels develop from the blood vessels by a process of budding and fusion of isolated cell groups of mesenchyme. Peripherally located mesenchymal cells form the lymphatic nodules in the connective tissue associated with the developing lymphatic vessels. The nodules become surrounded by sinuses, completing the lymph node. Later, a capsule and trabeculae will form around the developing lymphatic nodules from the surrounding mesenchyme.

INTRAORAL TONSILLAR TISSUE

Intraoral tonsillar tissue consists of nonencapsulated masses of lymphoid tissue located in the **lamina propria** of the **oral mucosa**. It is covered by **stratified squamous epithelium** that is continuous with the surrounding oral mucosa. Tonsils, like lymph nodes, contain **lymphocytes** that remove toxic products and then move to the epithelial surface as they mature. Unlike lymph nodes, tonsillar tissue is not located along lymphatic vessels but is situated near airway and food passages to protect the body against disease processes from the related toxic.

The **palatine tonsils** are two rounded masses of variable size located between the **anterior faucial pillar** and **posterior faucial pillar** (see Figure 2-11). Histologically, each mass contains fused-together lymphatic nodules that generally have germinal centers (Figure 11-16).

Each tonsil also has 10 to 20 epithelial invaginations, or grooves, which penetrate deeply into the tonsil to form tonsillar crypts. These crypts contain shed epithelial cells, mature lymphocytes, and oral bacteria.

The **lingual tonsil** is an indistinct layer of diffuse lymphoid tissue located on the base of the **dorsal surface of the tongue**, posterior to the **circumvallate lingual papillae** (see Figure 2-14). The lymphoid tissue consists of many lymphatic nodules, usually each with a germinal center and only one associated tonsillar crypt.

Behind the **uvula**, on the superior and posterior walls of the **nasopharynx**, are the pharyngeal tonsils, forming an incomplete ring of tissue, Waldeyer's ring. When they become enlarged, as is common in children, they are considered the *adenoids*.

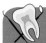
Clinical Considerations for Lymph Nodes and Intraoral Tonsillar Tissue

When a patient has an active disease process, such as cancer or infection, in a specific region, the region's **lymph nodes** respond. The resultant increase in size and change in consistency of the lymphoid tissue is termed **lymphadenopathy**. Lymphadenopathy results from an increase in both the size of each individual lymphocyte and the overall cell count in the lymphoid tissue. With more and larger lymphocytes, the lymphoid tissue is better able to fight the disease process.

This lymphadenopathy allows the node to now be more easily noted during an extraoral examination. More important, changes in consistency from firm to bony hard allow the lymph node to be palpated during the extraoral examination. Palpation of an involved node may be painful, and the node can become fixed and attached to the surrounding tissue.

Lymphadenopathy can also occur in the intraoral **tonsillar**, causing tissue enlargement that can be viewed on an intraoral examination (Figure 11-17). The intraoral tonsils may also be tender when palpated. This situation may cause airway obstruction with its complications and lead to infection of the tonsillar tissue. If any lymph nodes are palpable, or if there is an enlargement or infection of intraoral tonsillar tissue, these findings should be recorded in the patient record and appropriate physician referrals should be made.

NASAL CAVITY

The nasal cavity is the inner space of the nose (Figure 11-18). It communicates with the exterior by two **nares**. The nares are separated by the midline **nasal septum**, which consists of both bone and cartilage (see Figure 1-4). The nasal septum also divides the internal nasal cavity into two parts.

Each lateral wall of the nasal cavity has three projecting structures, or nasal conchae, which extend inward. Beneath each concha are openings through which the **paranasal sinuses** or nasolacrimal ducts communicate with the nasal cavity. The posterior part of the nasal cavity communicates with the **nasopharynx** and then with the rest of the respiratory system. The development of the nasal septum and cavity is described in Chapter 5.

HISTOLOGY OF NASAL CAVITY MUCOSA

The nasal cavity is lined by a respiratory mucosa, like the rest of the respiratory system (see Chapter 8). Respiratory mucosa is different from oral mucosa lining the oral cavity but similar to that lining the trachea and bronchi. It consists of ciliated **pseudostratified columnar**

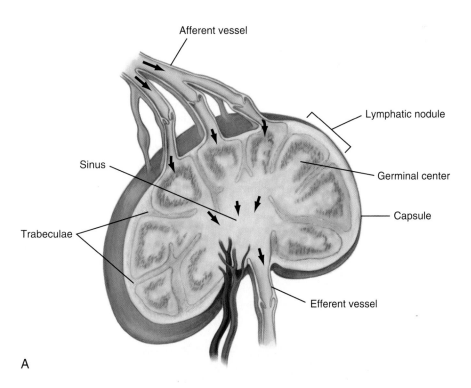

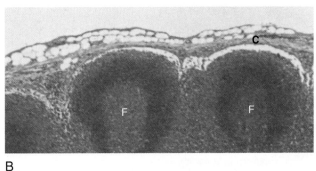

FIGURE 11-15 Lymph node and its features. **A:** Diagram showing entering of lymph by the afferent vessels and exiting by way of the efferent vessel *(arrows)*. **B:** Photomicrograph showing the lymphatic nodule or follicle with its germinal center *(F)* and capsule *(C)*. *(**A** and **B** from Fehrenbach MJ, Herring SW: Illustrated Anatomy of the Head and Neck, ed 3, WB Saunders, Philadelphia, 2007; **B** from Young B, Heath JW: Wheater's Functional Histology, ed 5, Churchill Livingstone, Edinburgh, 2006.)*

epithelium (Figure 11-19). Within the epithelium, and surrounded by mucous and serous glands, are goblet cells, which rest on the basement membrane. Fluids or mucus from the goblet cells and glands keep this mucosa moist, provide humidity, and trap any foreign materials from the inspired air.

The moist mucus forms a superficial coating on the respiratory mucosa. This coating is moved by ciliary action posteriorly to the nasopharynx, where it is either expectorated or swallowed. In this manner, foreign materials are trapped and removed. Because the **lamina propria** of the mucosa is extremely vascular, it also warms the air. In the roof of each part of the nasal cavity is a specialized area containing the olfactory mucosa, which carries the receptors for the sense of smell.

Overlying the conchae is an extensive, superficial plexus of large, thin-walled vessels termed erectile tissue. This tissue is capable of considerable engorgement. This engorgement happens at periodic intervals of 30 to 60 minutes, thus closing off the involved side of the nasal cavity to enable the respiratory mucosa to recover from the effects of dryness during respiration. The deepest parts of the lamina

propria are continuous with the **periosteum** of the nasal bone or **perichondrium** of the nasal cartilage.

The respiratory mucosa of the nasal cavity and septum is continuous and similar to that of the nasopharynx (see Figure 2-18). The respiratory mucosa of the nasopharynx gives way to the stratified squamous epithelium of the **oropharynx**. The stronger stratified squamous epithelium of the oropharynx, with its soft palate and posterior wall of the **pharynx**, allows the mechanical stress of swallowing.

PARANASAL SINUSES

The paranasal sinuses are paired, air-filled cavities in bone that include the frontal, sphenoidal, ethmoidal, and maxillary sinuses (Figure 11-20). The sinuses communicate with the **nasal cavity** through small openings in the lateral nasal wall. The openings mark the outpouchings from which the paranasal sinuses develop. The sinuses serve to lighten the skull bones, act as sound resonators, and provide mucus for the nasal cavity.

HISTOLOGY OF PARANASAL SINUS MUCOSA

The sinuses are lined with **respiratory mucosa** consisting of ciliated **pseudostratified columnar epithelium** continuous with the epithelial lining of the nasal cavity (see Figures 11-20 and 8-2). The epithelium of the sinuses, although it is similar to that of the nasal cavity, is thinner and contains fewer goblet cells. The respiratory mucosa of the sinuses also shows a thinner underlying lamina propria that is continuous with the deeper periosteum of the bone. It also has fewer associated glands, and no erectile tissue is present in the sinuses.

DEVELOPMENT OF PARANASAL SINUSES

Certain sinuses develop during late fetal life; the rest develop after birth. They form as outgrowths of the wall of the nasal cavity and become air-filled extensions in the adjacent bones. The original openings of the outgrowths persist as orifices of the adult sinuses.

The maxillary sinuses are small at birth, and only a few of the ethmoidal sinuses are present. The maxillary sinuses grow until puberty, and thus are not fully developed until all the permanent teeth have erupted in early adulthood. The ethmoidal sinuses do not start to grow until 6 to 8 years of age.

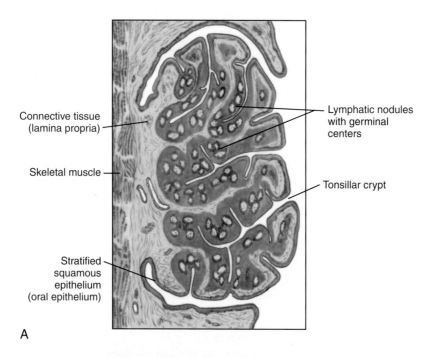

Connective tissue (lamina propria)

Skeletal muscle

Stratified squamous epithelium (oral epithelium)

Lymphatic nodules with germinal centers

Tonsillar crypt

A

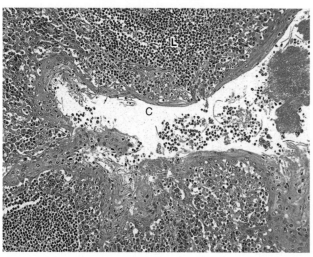

B

FIGURE 11-16 Histological features of the palatine tonsillar tissue. **A:** Diagram. **B:** Photomicrograph showing lymphatic nodule *(L)* and the crypt *(C)* lined by epithelium. Note that the crypt normally contains oral bacteria. *(B From Stevens A, Lowe J: Human Histology, ed 3, Mosby, St Louis, 2005.)*

The frontal sinuses and sphenoidal sinuses are not present at birth. At approximately 2 years of age, the two anterior ethmoidal sinuses grow into the frontal bone, forming the frontal sinus on each side, and are visible on radiographs by the seventh year. At the same time, the two posterior ethmoidal sinuses grow into the sphenoid bone and form the sphenoidal sinuses. Growth of sinuses in the size and shape of the face is important during infancy and childhood and adds resonance to the voice during puberty.

Clinical Considerations for the Nasal Cavity and Paranasal Sinuses

The **respiratory mucosa** of the **nasal cavity** and **paranasal sinuses** can become inflamed and the space congested with mucus as a result of allergies or respiratory tract infection. This inflammation can lead to a stuffed-up feeling in the nasal cavity and **sinusitis** in the sinus. The symptoms for both are discomfort caused by the pressure of the increased mucus production with nasal or pharyngeal discharge.

With blocked nasal passages and with sinusitis, medications are used to produce vasoconstriction in the blood vessels while reducing the amount of mucus produced. In cases of chronic sinusitis, surgical treatment may be needed. Patients undergoing these respiratory difficulties may not be able to use nitrous oxide adequately, may feel uncomfortable with the use of a rubber dam, and may breathe through the mouth, causing chronic gingivitis of the maxillary anterior teeth.

Because the maxillary **posterior teeth** are in close proximity to the **maxillary sinus**, maxillary sinusitis can sometimes result as infection spreads from a periapical abscess associated with a maxillary posterior tooth (Figure 11-21). As the infection spreads, the sinus floor is perforated, and the sinus mucosa becomes involved in the infection. During an extraction, a contaminated tooth or root fragments can also be surgically displaced into the maxillary sinus. In addition, the pain from a maxillary sinusitis can sometimes be mistakenly misinterpreted by the patient as involving the maxillary teeth, because of their close proximity (see **Chapter 17**). Differential diagnosis of the symptoms and radiographs can aid in determining the correct cause of this facial pain.

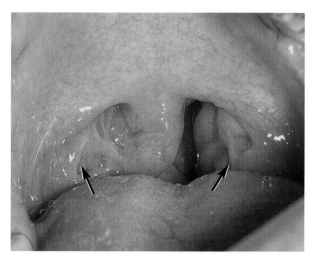

FIGURE 11-17 Lymphadenopathy of the palatine tonsils (*arrows*) showing enlargement. *(From Fehrenbach MJ, Herring SW: Illustrated Anatomy of the Head and Neck, ed 3, WB Saunders, Philadelphia, 2007.)*

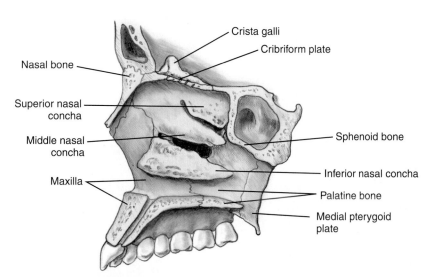

FIGURE 11-18 Nasal cavity and its nasal conchae. *(From Fehrenbach MJ, Herring SW: Illustrated Anatomy of the Head and Neck, ed 3, WB Saunders, Philadelphia, 2007.)*

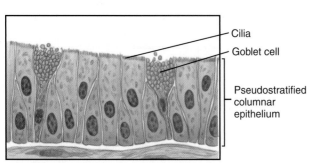

FIGURE 11-19 Histological features of the respiratory mucosa of the nasal cavity.

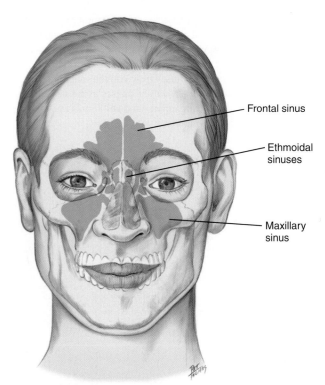

FIGURE 11-20 Paranasal sinuses: frontal, ethmoidal, maxillary; sphenoidal sinus is not shown in this view because it is deep to the ethmoidal sinus. *(From Fehrenbach MJ, Herring SW: Illustrated Anatomy of the Head and Neck, ed 3, WB Saunders, Philadelphia, 2007.)*

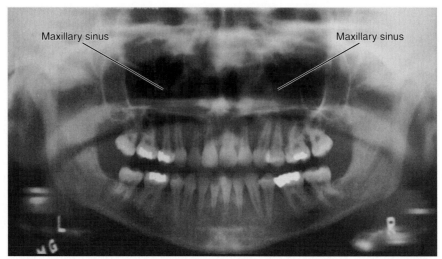

FIGURE 11-21 Panoramic radiograph showing the maxillary posterior teeth are in close proximity to the maxillary sinuses.

Enamel

●●● LEARNING OBJECTIVES

- Define and pronounce the key terms in this chapter.
- Describe the properties of enamel.
- Discuss the apposition and maturation of enamel.
- Indicate and discuss the microscopic features of enamel.
- Integrate the knowledge of the histology with the clinical considerations involved with enamel in order to preserve its integrity.

●●● NEW KEY TERMS

Abfraction (ab-**frak**-shen)
Abrasion (uh-**brey**-zhun)
Attrition (ah-**trish**-un)
Enamel (ih-**nam**-l) **caries, dysplasia** (dis-**play**-ze-ah)**, lamellae** (lah-**mel**-ay)**, rod, spindles, tufts**

Erosion (e-**ro**-zhun)
Imbrication lines (im-bri-**kay**-shun)
Interprismatic region (in-ter-**priz**-mat-ik)
Lines of Retzius (ret-**zee**-us)

Neonatal line (ne-oh-**nate**-l)
Perikymata (per-ee-**ki**-maht-ah)
Pit and groove patterns

ENAMEL

Preservation of the **enamel** of every tooth during a patient's lifetime is one of the goals of every dental professional. Dental professionals must take into consideration the histology of enamel, as well as the properties of enamel, when deciding the caries risk for patients, counseling patients and communities on fluoride use, applying enamel sealants, and using and recommending polishing or toothpaste agents (discussed later).

MATURE ENAMEL

Mature enamel is a crystalline material that is the hardest mineralized tissue in the human body (see Table 6-2). Enamel can endure crushing pressure of around 100,000 pounds per square inch; a layering of the deeper dentin and surrounding periodontium, coupled with the hardness of the enamel, produces a cushioning effect of the tooth's differing structures enabling it to endure the pressures of **mastication**.

In its mature state, it is noted for its almost total absence of the softer organic matrix. Enamel in a healthy state, precluding trauma or disease, can be removed only by rotary cutting instruments or rough files such as those used in dental practice. Enamel is avascular and has no nerve supply within it. Although enamel is the hardest mineralized tissue in the body, it can be lost forever because it is nonvital and therefore not a renewable resource. However, it is not a static tissue, because it can undergo mineralization changes (discussed later).

Thus, mature enamel is by weight 96% inorganic material (or mineralized) 1% organic material, and 3% water. This crystalline formation of mature enamel consists of mainly **calcium hydroxyapatite** with the chemical formula of $Ca_{10}(PO_4)_6(OH)_2$. The calcium hydroxyapatite is similar to that found in lesser percentages in dentin, cementum, and alveolar bone. On radiographs, the differences in the mineralization of different parts of the tooth and surrounding periodontium can be noted. Enamel appears more radiopaque (or lighter) than either dentin or pulp because it is denser than the latter structures, both of which appear more radiolucent (or darker).

Other minerals, such as carbonate, magnesium, potassium, sodium, and fluoride, are also present in smaller amounts. Studies have challenged this composition of enamel, and, instead, maintain that it is mainly carbonated hydroxyapatite because of its relationship with fluoride uptake. Whatever the true formation, the crystals of enamel are set at different angles throughout the crown area. Discussion of the elegant crystalline nature of enamel is awkward at best, but this chapter is an attempt to do justice to this beautiful, jewel-like material.

Enamel is usually the only part of a tooth that is seen clinically in a healthy oral cavity because it covers the **anatomical crown** (see Figure 15-8). Enamel provides a hard surface for mastication and speech; it is able to withstand the masticatory impact of 20 to 30 pounds of pressure per tooth. It shows a thin layer in the cervical areas and is thicker in masticatory areas, such as at the **incisal edges** and **cusps,** where impact can be greater.

Enamel also provides the pleasing whiteness of a healthy smile. Enamel alone is various shades of bluish white, which is seen on the **incisal ridge** of newly erupted incisors, but it turns various shades of yellow-white elsewhere because of the underlying dentin (see Figure 6-18). The enamel on **primary teeth** has a more opaque crystalline form, and thus appears whiter than on **permanent teeth**.

Because the overall shade of enamel varies in each person and possibly within a dentition, a shade value is taken when integrating tooth-colored

Clinical Considerations about Enamel Pathology

One way that enamel and other hard tissue of the tooth are lost is through **attrition**, which is the wearing away of hard tissue as a result of tooth-to-tooth contact (Table 12-1). Tooth wear from attrition increases with age. Permanent first molars wear more than seconds; seconds more than thirds. Attrition is discussed in **Chapter 20** with regard to **parafunctional habits** (see also Figures 16-8, 16-17, 16-25, 20-8). The relationship between the loss of the **vertical dimension of the face** and **alveolar bone** loss is discussed in **Chapter 14**. Enamel loss may also result from friction caused by excessive toothbrushing and abrasive toothpaste. This wear is considered **abrasion**.

Enamel can also be lost by **erosion** through chemical means. Erosion is particularly apparent in patients with the eating disorder of bulimia, in which patients force themselves to vomit to remove their stomach contents in pursuit of weight loss (Figure 12-1). The lingual surface of the anterior teeth and the occlusal surface of all the teeth are eroded by the acid content of the vomit. The yellow underlying **dentin** is thereby exposed and can undergo attrition, because it is less mineralized than enamel. Treatment of bulimia is multifactorial and includes behavior changes. Similar erosion can be caused by gastric reflux, as well as certain recreational drug use ("meth mouth"). If facial enamel lesions of the anterior teeth are evident, the patient may be overusing acid-containing carbonated soft drinks and sport or health drinks (especially diet formulations and those containing enamel-eroding citric acid).

Another way that enamel and other hard tissue of the tooth can be lost is by **enamel caries**. Caries is a process through which a cavity is created by demineralization, or loss of minerals. This demineralization is due to acid production by cariogenic bacteria (discussed later) and occurs to enamel when the pH is less than 5.5 (see later discussion).

Finally, enamel can be lost as a result of **abfraction** (see Figure 12-1, *B*). Abfraction is thought to be caused by tensile and compressive forces during tooth flexure, which possibly occurs during parafunctional habits with their occlusal loading (see **Chapter 20**). It consists of cervical lesions that cannot be attributed to any particular cause, such as erosion or toothbrush abrasion; abfraction causes the enamel to pop off, starting at the cervical region, thus exposing the area to possible further wear, dentinal hypersensitivity, or caries.

TABLE 12-1	Hard Tissue Loss	
TERM	**DEFINITION**	**CLINICAL APPEARANCE**
Attrition	Loss through tooth-to-tooth contact (mastication or parafunctional habits)	• Matching wear on occluding surfaces • Shiny facets on amalgam contacts • Enamel and dentin wear at the same rate • Possible fracture of cusps or restorations
Abrasion	Loss through friction from toothbrushing and/or toothpaste	• Usually located at facial cervical areas • Lesions more wide than deep • Canines commonly affected because of tooth position
Erosion	Loss through chemical means (acid) not involving bacteria	• Broad concavities within smooth surface enamel • Cupping of occlusal surface (incisal grooving) with dentin exposure (possible dentinal hypersensitivity) • Increased incisal translucency • Wear on nonoccluding surfaces (location depends on acid intake–type) • Raised and shiny amalgam restorations • Preservation of enamel cuff in gingival crevice common • Pulp exposure and loss of surface characteristics of enamel in primary teeth
Caries	Loss through chemical means (acid) from cariogenic bacteria by way of dental biofilm	• All surfaces can be affected • Occlusal surfaces more commonly affected, especially in pits and grooves • Possibly rapid progression of interproximal lesions if progress goes unchecked • Cervical lesions sometimes secondary to other forms of hard tissue loss or gingival recession
Abfraction	Possible loss through tensile and compressive forces during tooth flexure (parafunctional habits)	• Can affect both facial and lingual cervical areas • Deep, narrow V-shaped notch • Commonly affects single teeth that have occlusal loads

restorative materials or artificial teeth or crowns within an individual dentition. The goal is to match, as closely as possible, the color of the patient's other teeth. This shade value is selected by comparing the patient's natural teeth to a shade guide of plastic model crowns that have been moistened and are viewed in natural light. These shade guides are provided by various manufacturers. New technology allows a digital read-out of the color of the enamel (whitening process is discussed later.)

APPOSITION OF ENAMEL MATRIX

Amelogenesis is the process of **enamel matrix** formation that occurs during the stage of apposition of tooth development. The exact time of the stage of **apposition** or secretory phase varies according to the tooth that is undergoing development. Many factors can affect amelogenesis (see Figures 6-13 through 6-15).

Enamel matrix is produced by **ameloblasts** (Figure 12-2). Each ameloblast is approximately 4 micrometers in diameter, 40 micrometers in length, and hexagonal in cross section. The ameloblasts are columnar cells that differentiate during the stage of apposition in the crown area. Ameloblasts are not differentiated in the root area; thus, the enamel is normally just confined to the **anatomical crown**.

The enamel matrix is secreted from each ameloblast from its own **Tomes' process** with its microscopic "picket-fence" appearance (see Figure 12-2, *B*). Tomes' process is not a true process, but, instead, it is a six-sided projection of the basal or secretory end of each ameloblast that faces the **dentinoenamel junction (DEJ)** (see Figure 6-12). This is unlike the process associated with the odontoblast, which is a true cytoplasmic process from a cell body.

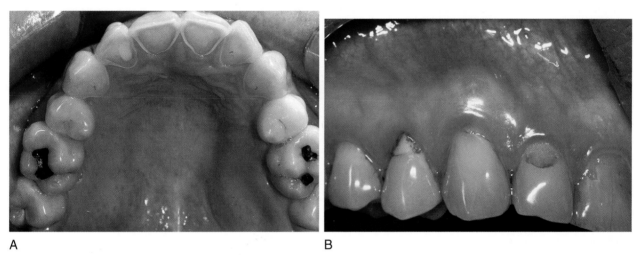

A   B

FIGURE 12-1 Examples of the loss enamel. **A:** Lingual erosion in a patient with a past history of bulimia. Note that the facial surface of the permanent maxillary central incisors have been covered using a veneer restoration because of the amount of hard tissue loss, which caused the teeth to look more transparent and gray. **B:** Abfraction of the upper right quadrant, especially on the maxillary right incisor. The first premolar has been repaired with restorative materials but has secondary enamel caries around the margins.

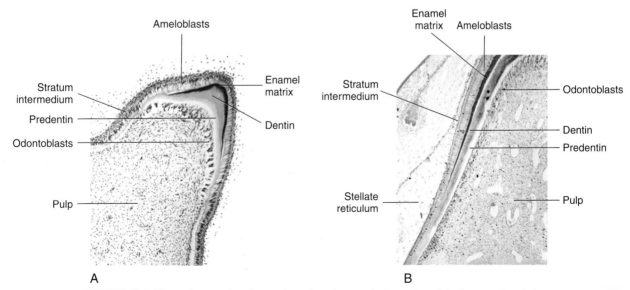

A   B

FIGURE 12-2 Photomicrographs of a tooth undergoing matrix formation of both enamel and dentin, with dentin already showing maturation **(A).** The close-up view **(B)** shows ameloblasts producing enamel matrix from their Tomes' processes. *(From Nanci A:* Ten Cate's Oral Histology, *ed 7, Mosby, St Louis, 2008.)*

Tomes' process is responsible for the way the enamel matrix is laid down; thus, it is the guiding factor similar to a snowplow going through a snowy parking lot. The body of the cell between the processes first deposits enamel matrix between the ameloblasts, which will become the periphery of the enamel rods, or its outside mold (the **interprismatic region,** discussed later with rods). Then, the Tomes' process will infill the future main body of the enamel rod; thus, more than one ameloblast contributes to a single rod.

Enamel matrix is an ectodermal product, because ameloblasts are derived from the **inner enamel epithelium** of the enamel organ, which was originally derived from the **ectoderm** of the **embryo**. Enamel matrix initially is composed of proteins, carbohydrates, and only a small amount of calcium hydroxyapatite crystals. Unlike dentin, cementum, and alveolar bone, which are mesodermal products, enamel does not contain collagen protein. Instead, it has two unique classes of proteins, amelogenins and enamelins.

Because it only has a small amount of calcium, the initial enamel matrix is therefore only partially mineralized, as compared with fully matured enamel (discussed later). Ameloblasts are also responsible for this partially mineralized state of the enamel matrix, because they actively pump calcium hydroxyapatite into the forming enamel matrix as it is secreted by Tomes' processes.

Enamel matrix is first formed in the incisal/occlusal part of the future crown near the forming DEJ (Figure 12-3). This is the first wave of enamel apposition, which moves to the future outer enamel surface. The second wave of enamel apposition overlaps the first wave, and this entire process then moves cervically to the **cementoenamel junction (CEJ).** The morphology of the CEJ is discussed further in Chapter 14.

MATURATION OF ENAMEL MATRIX

During the **maturation** stage of tooth development, enamel matrix completes its mineralization process after the apposition of enamel matrix when it is only approximately 30% mineralized. Thus, mineralization of enamel matrix to a fully matured tissue covers two stages of tooth development, the stages of apposition and maturation. Enamel mineralization also continues after eruption of the tooth (discussed next).

🦷 Clinical Considerations with Enamel Structure

Certain developmental disturbances, such as an **enamel pearl** and **enamel dysplasia,** can occur in enamel during the stage of apposition (see Table 6-3, *H* and *J*). Another common developmental disturbance is the deepened **pit and groove patterns** on the occlusal surface of posterior teeth and lingual surface of anterior teeth (see **Chapters 16** and **17**; Figures 16-9 and 17-7). These are created when **ameloblasts** back into one another during the stage of apposition, cutting off their source of nutrition. This loss of nutritional support causes incomplete maturation of **enamel matrix**, making it weak or even absent in that area.

These weak areas of pits and grooves are target areas for **enamel caries** (Figure 12-4). Dental biofilm can become sheltered in these irregular areas (or niches) and cannot be reached by careful oral hygiene. The dental biofilm produces acids that slowly demineralize the weak enamel areas, producing caries. There is a "tug-of-war" between demineralization and remineralization at the enamel surface; thus, when demineralization outweighs remineralization, enamel caries results. Remineralization is the deposition of minerals into enamel from salivary minerals and fluoride or other therapies (discussed later). However, with the cariogenic process, the surface enamel of the pit or groove remains intact as the subsurface zones become further demineralized. Thus, enamel caries remains in the subsurface, working its way to the dentin/pulp area to form dental caries, or pulpitis, if the acidic and/or bacterial assault continues.

Protection against enamel caries is provided by the use of enamel sealants that cover the deepened **pit and groove patterns** on the teeth (see **Chapters 16** and **17**). Educating patients about the importance of enamel sealants in caries prevention is an important responsibility for dental professionals. Many clinicians are even recommending these sealants for adults, because of the risk of future caries at these sites.

Similar to the caries that occurs in pits and grooves, smooth surface caries, which occurs interproximally, does not involve the breakdown or demineralization of the surface layers of enamel (see Figure 12-4). Zones are also present with smooth surface caries, as they are with caries of pits and grooves. In the past, tooth caries predominated on smooth surfaces (on interproximal surfaces). With the widespread use of fluoride, the very nature of tooth decay has changed; the outer surfaces of teeth are strengthened and more resistant, and thus pit and groove cavities are more prevalent than smooth surface cavities. Pit and groove caries are traditionally the most difficult to detect using radiographs due to the direction from which the images are taken.

Both incipient caries in the pits and grooves and on smooth surfaces are first noted in many cases, clinically, as a white-spot lesion, with the involved enamel appearing whiter and rougher as a result of slight surface demineralization of the enamel. However, this initial lesion may also be detected through the use of a "sticky" explorer for both types of caries. Thus, the enamel surface is finally undermined, and the explorer falls into already destroyed subsurface.

It is important to remember that early subsurface lesions cannot be detected on radiographs until they spread at least 200 micrometers into the dentin, a process that can take more than 3 to 5 years. Light-induced devices that measure changes in laser fluorescence of hard tissue allow dental professionals to better diagnose early carious lesions involving the enamel in a pit and groove, before involving the deeper and more extensive dentin layers. However, clinicians should not rely on readings alone to determine the extension of incipient pit and groove caries.

If caries is only present in the enamel, it does not cause pain to the patient because the enamel has no nerves within it. For the same reason, initial cavity preparation during removal of enamel only is usually painless. Pain occurs only when the deeper layers of dentin, and then the associated pulp tissue, are involved (see Figure 13-8). Thus, it is important to emphasize to patients the need for recall examinations for early detection of decay before pain is involved. Pain is a late finding in caries, and the risk of tooth loss increases while waiting for this symptom to appear.

The type of polishing agent used by dental professionals, and by patients at home, is also a very important consideration. Older toothpastes and professional polishing agents abraded the enamel surface, removing valuable tooth layers to obtain temporary esthetic results. Selective polishing methods are now used only to remove extrinsic stain on natural enamel surfaces; many clinicians use ultrasonic devices for removal, instead, because it is faster and prevents overall enamel removal. However, the use of less abrasive professional and home-care polishing agents, such as with the newer air polishing agents, helps preserve the limited enamel on the crowns. It is also not necessary to polish the teeth to remove dental biofilm before topical fluoride application or, in many cases, before enamel sealant placement.

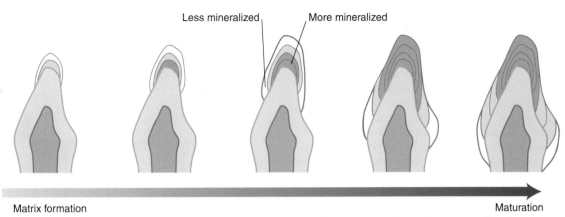

FIGURE 12-3 Wave patterns in the crown from the time of enamel matrix formation to maturation of enamel.

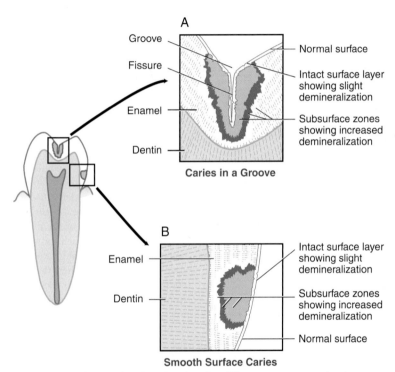

FIGURE 12-4 Process of enamel caries showing the different zones occurring in a groove **(A)** or smooth surface caries **(B).** Note that both types have an intact surface layer and demineralization is in the subsurface zones.

During the maturation of enamel matrix, **ameloblasts** move from production to actively transporting materials into the already partially mineralized enamel, such as proteins and minerals. Thus, ameloblasts are specifically responsible for maturation of enamel matrix into mature enamel.

Two waves of maturation in the tooth follow the same pattern as enamel matrix formation (see Figure 12-3). The first wave of enamel mineralization occurs in the occlusal part of the future crown near the forming DEJ and moves to the future outer enamel surface. The second wave of enamel mineralization overlaps the first wave as the process moves cervically to the forming CEJ.

After the ameloblasts are finished with both enamel apposition and maturation, they become part of the **reduced enamel epithelium (REE),** along with the other tissue types of the compressed enamel organ (see Figures 6-23 and 6-24). The REE fuses with the **oral mucosa,** creating a canal to allow the enamel cusp tip to erupt through the oral mucosa into the oral cavity (see Figure 6-25). Unfortunately, the ameloblasts are lost forever as the fused tissue disintegrates during tooth eruption, preventing any further enamel apposition. The tissue later becomes part of **Nasmyth's membrane** (see Figure 6-29).

Enamel is not a renewable resource, because there is no way to retrieve the lost ameloblasts. Research involves the study of amelogenins, the principal extracellular matrix protein component involved in this process of mineralizing enamel; amelogenins may play a substantial role in controlling the growth and organization of enamel crystals.

After the tooth erupts into the oral cavity, however, the mineralization of enamel continues. This posteruptive maturation is due to the deposition of minerals, such as fluoride and calcium, from saliva into hypomineralized areas of enamel (see discussion of fluoride next).

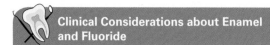

Fluoride can enter the enamel systemically through the blood supply of developing teeth by ingestion of fluoride in drops, tablets, or treated water, all of which are considered preeruptive methods. It can also enter topically by direct contact on exposed teeth surfaces by ingestion of fluoridated water or professional application, or by directed use of pre-scription or over-the-counter rinses, gels, foams, chewable tablets, and fluoridated toothpastes, all of which are considered posteruptive meth-ods. Fluoride in prophylaxis pastes provides only brief action and must not take the place of topical fluoride applications.

A theory of systemic fluoride action proposes that fluoride enters the crystalline formation of enamel during tooth development. This action may produce differences in the **morphology** of the teeth, resulting in more caries-resistant teeth, which are slightly smaller in their **occlusal surfaces** and have shallower **pit and groove patterns**; further studies in this area are necessary for a more complete understanding.

In contrast, studies have shown that topical (as opposed to systemic) uses of fluoride have a more important role in caries control than pre-viously thought. Topical use results in an increased level of remineral-ization of any demineralized regions at the surface, which can actually reverse the carious process. Remineralization is the deposition of miner-als into enamel in a way that resembles that of posteruptive maturation, although the minerals are now being deposited into previously deminer-alized enamel. This remineralization may produce an enamel crystal that is larger, and thus more resistant to acid attack.

In addition to its direct mineralizing effect on enamel, fluoride may affect oral bacteria by interfering with the actual microbial acid produc-tion, reducing potential enamel destruction. Thus, the need for daily topi-cal fluoride exposure, through a combination of fluoride therapies, has been demonstrated for all age groups. In addition, other non-invasive caries management system therapies such as casein phosphopeptide–amorphous calcium phosphate (CPP-ACP) is being used for tooth remineralization.

Just as important, clinically, to situations with reduced fluoride levels, is that of excess systemic fluoride during tooth development, which can occur in areas where the water naturally has a higher than normal level of fluoride. This can cause a type of enamel dysplasia, *dental fluorosis*, with intrinsic staining, giving affected teeth a mottled discoloration (see **Chapter 6**; Figure 12-5). It can also occur with younger children who ingest too much sweetly flavored fluoridated toothpaste or inappropriate prescription of fluoride.

MICROSCOPIC FEATURES OF MATURE ENAMEL

The enamel rod (or enamel prism) is the crystalline structural unit of enamel; thus, enamel is composed of millions of enamel rods (Figure 12-6). Enamel rods and associated structures should be viewed under a microscope to best understand them. Generally, each enamel rod is cylindrical in longitudinal section. In most areas of enamel, the rod is also 4 micrometers in diameter, with head and tail ends. However, there seems to be less of an emphasis on the classical model in cross section, with its keyhole or fish-scale shape, because there are so many variations in the structural arrangement of the enamel components and the crystals within each enamel rod are highly complex. Both **ameloblasts** and their **Tomes' processes** affect the crystals' pattern. Enamel crystals in rod head are oriented parallel to the long axis of

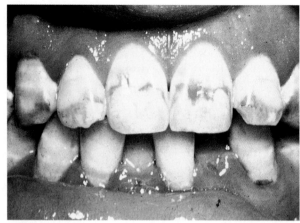

FIGURE 12-5 Dental fluorosis with its intrinsic staining caused by ingestion of excess amounts of fluoride that occurred naturally in the water system.

the rod. When found in the rod tail, the crystals' orientation diverges slightly from the long axis.

In addition, the prisms in the rod groups bend to the right or left at a slightly different angle than do adjacent groups, increasing their masticatory strength (see Figure 12-6). This is shown in the Hunter-Schreger light to dark bands noted in certain sections of enamel (see Figure 12-8).

The arrangement of enamel rods is understood more clearly than their internal structure. Enamel rods are found in rows along the tooth, and within each row, the long axis of the enamel rod is generally perpendicular to the underlying dentin. However, in permanent teeth the enamel rods near the CEJ tilt slightly toward the root of the tooth.

Most rods extend the width of the enamel from the DEJ to the outer enamel surface. Thus, each rod varies in length because the width of enamel varies in different locations of the crown area. Those near the cusps or incisal edges, where the enamel is the thickest, are quite long compared with those near the CEJ. However, the course of the rods from these two end points is not an overall straight course. Rather, the rods show varying degrees of curvature from the DEJ to the outer enamel surface. This curved course of the enamel rods reflects the movements of the ameloblasts during enamel production.

Surrounding the outer part is the interprismatic region (or inter-rod enamel). This interprismatic region appears different from the rod core on cross sections because of its different crystalline orientation. Whether an organic rod sheath, or lesser-mineralized interprismatic substance, exists between the enamel rods remains controversial.

The **DEJ** between mature enamel and dentin appears scalloped on a cross section of a tooth (Figure 12-7). The convex side of the DEJ is toward the dentin, and the concave side is toward the enamel. This difference in the length of the enamel rods and corresponding den-tinal tubules occurs during the apposition of the two tissue types (see Chapter 6). The DEJ was formerly the **basement membrane** between the enamel organ and the dental papilla. In reality, the DEJ is simply a ridge between the two tissue types that allows increased adherence between them, adding to the strength of the junction when the teeth are in function during **mastication**. Thus, the presence of the DEJ is most pronounced in the coronal region, where occlusal forces are the greatest.

The lines of Retzius appear as incremental lines (or striae) that appear brown in a stained section of mature enamel (Figure 12-8). These lines are composed of bands or cross striations on the enamel rods that, when combined in longitudinal sections, seem to traverse

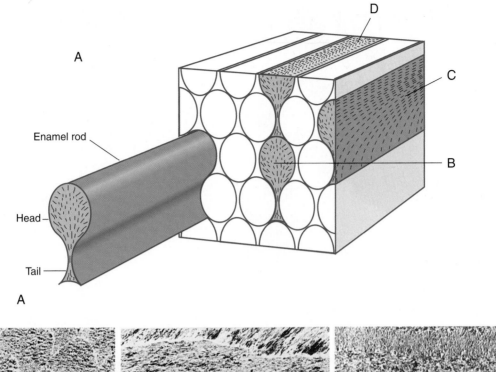

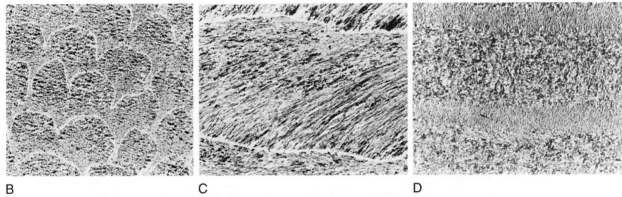

FIGURE 12-6 Enamel rods. **A:** Diagram of an enamel rod and its integration with other adjacent rods in a block of enamel. **B:** Electron micrograph of the rod in cross section. **C** and **D:** Crystal orientation along the other two cut faces of the block of enamel, showing the bending of adjacent prisms of rod groups, which produces Hunter-Schreger bands. *(From Nanci A: Ten Cate's Oral Histology, ed 7, Mosby, St Louis, 2008.)*

the enamel rods. On transverse sections of enamel, the lines of Retzius appear as concentric rings, similar to the growth rings in a tree.

Associated with the lines of Retzius are the raised imbrication lines and grooves of perikymata noted clinically on the nonmasticatory surfaces of some teeth in the oral cavity. The imbrication lines and perikymata are usually lost through tooth wear, except on the protected cervical regions of some teeth, especially the permanent maxillary central incisors, canines, and first premolars, and may be confused as calculus.

The exact mechanism that produces these lines is still being debated. Some researchers hypothesize that the lines are a result of the diurnal, or 24-hour, metabolic rhythm of the **ameloblasts** producing the **enamel matrix**, which consists of an active secretory work period followed by an inactive rest period during tooth development. Thus, each band on the enamel rod demonstrates the work/rest pattern of the ameloblasts that generally occurs over a span of a week.

The neonatal line is a pronounced **incremental line of Retzius** (Figure 12-9). The neonatal line marks the stress or trauma experienced by the ameloblasts during birth, again illustrating the sensitivity

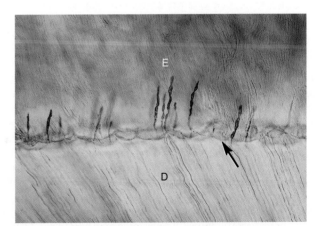

FIGURE 12-7 Microscopic view of the dentinoenamel junction *(arrow)* showing its scalloped interface with its concave side toward the enamel *(E)*, and convex side toward the dentin *(D)*. *(Courtesy of James McIntosh, PhD, Assistant Professor Emeritus, Department of Biomedical Sciences, Baylor College of Dentistry, Dallas, TX.)*

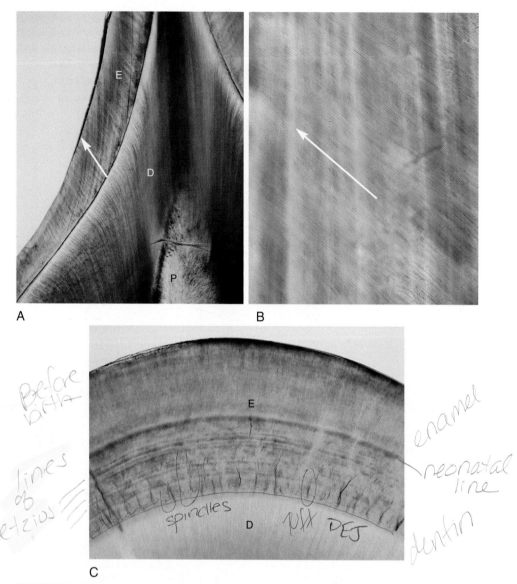

FIGURE 12-8 Microscopic views of the lines of Retzius that traverse the enamel rods *(E)*. **A:** Long section of rods (direction, *arrow*) overlying dentin *(D)* and pulp *(P)* in the crown. **B:** Close-up view of long section of rods (direction, *arrow*), with the lines of Retzius; note the light to dark Hunter-Schreger bands. **C:** Cross section of rods overlying dentin *(D)*, with the lines of Retzius resembling growth rings of a tree. *(Courtesy of James McIntosh, PhD, Assistant Professor Emeritus, Department of Biomedical Sciences, Baylor College of Dentistry, Dallas, TX.)*

of the ameloblasts as they form enamel matrix. Microscopically, the darker neonatal line marks the border between the enamel matrix formed before and after birth. As one would expect, the neonatal line is found in all the enamel of the primary teeth and in the larger cusps of the permanent first molars. They contain irregular structures of enamel prisms with disordered crystal arrangements, basically formed by the abrupt bending of the prisms toward the root; usually, the prisms gradually bend back again to regain their previous orientation.

Enamel spindles are another microscopic feature of mature enamel and represent short **dentinal tubules** near the DEJ (Figure 12-10). Enamel spindles result from odontoblasts that crossed the basement membrane before it mineralized into the DEJ. Thus, these dentinal tubules become trapped during the apposition of enamel matrix, and enamel becomes mineralized around them. Enamel spindles are especially noted beneath the cusps and incisal tips of the teeth. Clinical

implications of enamel spindles are unknown at this time, and it is doubtful that these dentinal tubules contain any live odontoblastic processes, as noted in the tubules in dentin.

Enamel tufts are another microscopic feature and are noted as small, dark brushes with their bases near the DEJ (Figure 12-11). Enamel tufts are found in the inner one third of enamel and represent areas of less mineralization. They are an anomaly of crystallization and seem to have no clinical importance. Enamel tufts are best seen on transverse sections of enamel.

Enamel lamellae are partially mineralized vertical sheets of enamel matrix that extend from the DEJ near the tooth's cervix to the outer occlusal surface (see Figure 12-11). Enamel lamellae are narrower and longer than enamel tufts. This is another anomaly of crystallization that has unknown clinical importance. Enamel lamellae are best seen on transverse sections of enamel. Both enamel tufts and lamellae may be likened to geologic faults within mature enamel.

Clinical Considerations with the Microscopic Features of Enamel

These microscopic features must be taken into consideration during clinical treatment involving enamel. Enamel resembles a steel product with a moderate level of hardness, which also makes it brittle; therefore, an underlying layer of more break-resistant dentin must be present to preserve its integrity. This property, along with the direction of the **enamel rods**, is taken into consideration during cavity preparation, as well as the **dentinal tubules** direction (discussed later). The decay and adjacent parts of the enamel are removed in a way that allows all the enamel rods to remain supported by other rods and the underlying dentin. An isolated enamel rod is extremely brittle and breaks away easily. If enamel rods are undercut during cavity preparation, they may break, thus rendering the margin of restoration possibly leaky, and thus defective. This brittleness of unsupported enamel also is noted during the progression of caries: The enamel breaks away easily, as the dentin is undermined beneath it.

In some cases, an acid etch is briefly used to remove some of the organic parts of the enamel crystals in the **interprismatic region**, enabling an enamel sealant or other dental biomaterial to flow into the newly created gaps, and thus offer more surface area for better adherence (Figure 12-12). This demineralization by acid etching is seen clinically as the surface of enamel whitens. When placing certain enamel sealants (hydrophobic),

dental professionals must be careful to protect the demineralized enamel surface from being contaminated and remineralized by saliva, thereby reducing sealant uptake; luckily, new sealants are more resistant to this situation. Acid etch is also used to prepare the enamel surface for other restorative procedures.

Whitening (bleaching) of the teeth to remove staining that has occurred due to lifestyle choices (e.g., ingestion of dark drinks and foods, as well as tobacco use) is of increased importance to the dental profession (see **Chapter 13** on dentin staining). Studies show that patients who have whitened their teeth take better care of them. Staining occurs in the **interprismatic region** internally on the enamel, which causes the tooth to appear darker or more yellow overall.

In a perfect state, enamel is colorless, but it does reflect underlying tooth structure with its stains because light reflection properties of the tooth are low. Oxygen radicals from the peroxide in the whitening agents contact the stains in the interprismatic spaces within the enamel layer. When this occurs, stains will be bleached, and the teeth now appear lighter in color. Teeth not only appear whiter but also reflect light in increased amounts, which makes the teeth appear brighter as well. Studies show that whitening does not produce any ultrastructural or microhardness changes in the dental tissue.

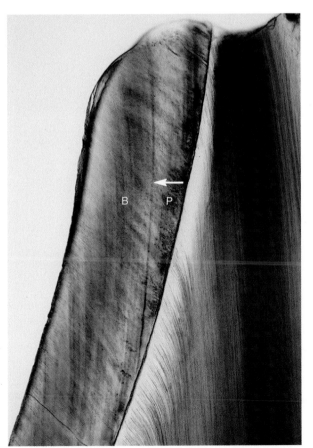

FIGURE 12-9 Microscopic view of the neonatal line *(arrow)*, a pronounced line of Retzius that corresponds to the birth of the individual. Thus, it demarcates the enamel formed prenatally *(P)* and after birth *(B)*. *(Courtesy of James McIntosh, PhD, Assistant Professor Emeritus, Department of Biomedical Sciences, Baylor College of Dentistry, Dallas, TX.)*

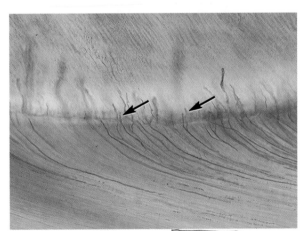

FIGURE 12-10 Microscopic view of enamel spindles *(arrows)* within the enamel and near the dentinoenamel junction. *(Courtesy of James McIntosh, PhD, Assistant Professor Emeritus, Department of Biomedical Sciences, Baylor College of Dentistry, Dallas, TX.)*

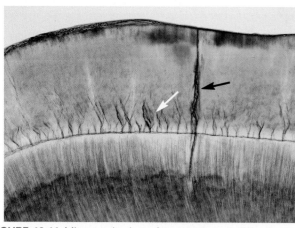

FIGURE 12-11 Microscopic view of a transverse section of enamel showing enamel tufts *(white arrow)* and enamel lamella *(black arrow)*. *(Courtesy of James McIntosh, PhD, Assistant Professor Emeritus, Department of Biomedical Sciences, Baylor College of Dentistry, Dallas, TX.)*

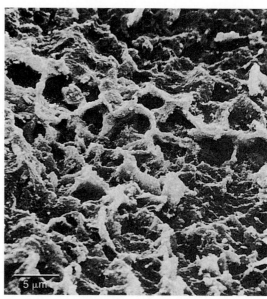

FIGURE 12-12 Photomicrograph showing the enamel rods after acid etching, which demineralizes the interprismatic region to allow the flow of the enamel sealant or other restorative materials into the enamel for greater strength. *(From Nanci A:* Ten Cate's Oral Histology, *ed 7, Mosby, St Louis, 2008.)*

Dentin and Pulp

●●● LEARNING OBJECTIVES

- Define and pronounce the key terms in this chapter.
- Discuss the dentin-pulp complex and describe the properties of dentin and pulp.
- Describe the processes of the apposition and the maturation of dentin.
- Outline the types of dentin.
- Label the anatomical components of pulp.

- Indicate and discuss the microscopic features of dentin and pulp.
- Describe the aging of dentin and pulp and discuss future concerns.
- Integrate the knowledge of the histology with the clinical considerations involved in dentin and pulp and promote their health.

●●● NEW KEY TERMS

Accessory canals
Apical foramen (ay-pi-kl for-ay-men)
Contour lines of Owen
Dentin: circumpulpal (serk-um-**pul**-pal),
  globular, interglobular, intertubular
  (in-ter-**tube**-u-lar), **mantle,**

peritubular (pare-i-**tube**-u-lar),
  primary, secondary, tertiary
Dentinal caries (**den**-tin-al), **fluid,**
  hypersensitivity (hi-per-**sen**-si-**tiv**-it-ee)
Imbrication (im-bri-**kay**-shun) **lines of**
  von Ebner (**eeb**-ner)

Pulp chamber, horns, stones
Pulp: coronal, radicular (rah-**dik**-u-lar)
Pulpitis (pul-**pie**-tis)
Tomes' granular layer (tomes)

DENTIN-PULP COMPLEX

Unlike enamel, both **dentin** and **pulp** cannot be viewed clinically if the teeth and associated periodontium are healthy. That is because both dentin and pulp make up the inner parts of the tooth and are not exposed to the oral environment except when certain dental pathology exists. In addition, because of their shared embryological background, close proximity, and interdependence, dentin and pulp form a dentin-pulp complex. Thus, this chapter discusses these two tissues together as one developmental and functioning unit.

Dental professionals must have a clear understanding of the histology of these two tissues. In the past, these two inner dental tissues were thought of as being analogous to a "black box" that was possibly opened only during restorative procedures and thus hidden the rest of the time. With the advent of expanded responsibilities and increased preventive concerns for patients, all dental professionals must be able to know about these two interesting and challenging dental tissues.

DENTIN

Mature dentin is a crystalline material that is less hard than enamel (see Table 6-2). Mature dentin is by weight 70% inorganic or mineralized material, 20% organic material, and 10% water. This crystalline formation of mature dentin consists of mainly **calcium hydroxyapatite** with the chemical formula of $Ca_{10}(PO_4)_6(OH)_2$. The calcium hydroxyapatite found in dentin is similar to that found in a higher percentage in enamel and in lower percentages in both cementum and bone tissue, such as alveolar bone. In addition, the crystals in dentin are platelike in shape and smaller in size than those in enamel.

Small amounts of other minerals, such as carbonate and fluoride, are also present. Dentin is covered by enamel in the crown and cementum in the root, as well as enclosing the innermost pulp tissue. Thus, dentin makes up the bulk of the tooth and protects the pulp.

Because of the translucency of overlying enamel, the dentin of the tooth gives the white enamel crown its underlying yellow hue, which is a deeper color in permanent teeth. If the outer coverings of either enamel or cementum are lost (discussed later), the exposed dentin on either the crown or root is various shades of yellow-white and appears rougher in surface texture than enamel. Yet, dentin is softer than enamel when instruments are used, allowing improper removal with hand instruments even in a healthy state, unlike enamel.

On a radiograph, the differences in the mineralization levels of different parts of the tooth can be noted. Dentin appears more radiolucent (or darker) than enamel because it is less dense, but is more radiopaque (or lighter) than pulp, which has the least density of the three dental tissues.

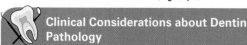

avascular

Clinical Considerations about Dentin Pathology

Attrition, which is the wearing away of a tooth surface through tooth-to-tooth contact, can also occur in dentin (see Figures 16-8, 16-17, 16-25, 20-8). In contrast to hard enamel, this attrition can occur at a more rapid rate when dentin is exposed, because its mineralized content is lower.

Coronal dentin can be exposed after attrition of the enamel, and also with certain enamel dysplasias. Coronal dentin can also become exposed when a patient asks to have the **incisal edge** "filled" with tooth-colored restorative materials on anteriors when trauma causes it to become chipped or worn.

Root dentin can be exposed when the thin layer of cementum is lost due to **gingival recession**, with its lower margin of the **free gingival crest** (Figure 13-1) (see **Chapter 10**). Dentin that is lost externally is not fully replaced by the possible addition of secondary dentin on the inside of the tooth along the outer pulpal wall (discussed later).

Another way that dentin can become exposed and then lost is through dentinal caries, the demineralization resulting from cariogenic bacteria (discussed later). Dentin demineralizes when the pH is less than 6.8. Finally, cavity preparation during restorative treatment exposes and then removes carious dentin in order to prevent further decay.

Newly exposed dentin is already more yellow than the whitish enamel. When dentin remains exposed, it can also pick up food and tobacco stains over time, becoming more yellow or even brown to black (see Figure 13-1). It absorbs these stains because it is more permeable, or porous, than intact enamel. Dentin is permeable from both its high organic content and the presence of **dentinal tubules**, acting as a sponge to contain these staining products and causing esthetic concerns for patients.

Removal of these extrinsic stains by hand instrumentation or air-polishing device can remove even more dentin; thus ultrasonic devices, which remove no hard tooth products when used correctly, may be the better choice for stain removal. **Dentinal hypersensitivity** that can occur when instruments expose dentin, such as on root surfaces, can be prevented with certain mineralizing products or temporarily reduced with the use of local anesthetic (discussed later). Vital whitening (bleaching) of the teeth may also be performed either at the office or in the home; however, whitening at home must be done with appropriate supervision, because it may also lead to dentinal hypersensitivity. Whitening is discussed in **Chapter 12**. Studies show that whitening does not produce ultrastructural changes in the dental tissues.

APPOSITION OF DENTIN MATRIX

Dentinogenesis is the process of **predentin** formation that produces the initial dentin matrix during the stage of apposition of tooth development. The exact time of the stage of **apposition** varies according to the tooth that is undergoing development. Many factors can affect dentinogenesis when it is occurring (see **Chapter 6**).

Predentin is the initial material laid down by the **odontoblasts** (Figure 13-2). It is a mesenchymal product consisting of nonmineralized **collagen fibers**. Odontoblasts were originally the **outer cells of the dental papilla**. Thus, dentin and pulp tissue have similar embryological backgrounds, because both are originally derived from the **dental papilla** of the **tooth germ**. These newly formed odontoblasts are induced by the equally newly formed ameloblasts to produce predentin in layers, moving away from the **dentinoenamel junction (DEJ)**. Unlike cartilage and bone, as well as cementum, the odontoblast's cell body does not become entrapped in the product; rather, one long, cytoplasmic attached extension remains behind in the formed dentin. Odontoblasts form approximately 4 μm of predentin daily during tooth development.

Apposition of dentin, unlike enamel, occurs throughout the life of the tooth (discussed later). Although ameloblasts are lost after the eruption of the tooth and enamel production ceases, production of dentin continues because of the retention of the odontoblasts within the tooth, along the outer pulpal wall.

MATURATION OF DENTIN

Maturation of dentin or mineralization of predentin occurs soon after its apposition. The process of dentin maturation takes place in two phases: primary and secondary (Figure 13-3). Initially, the calcium

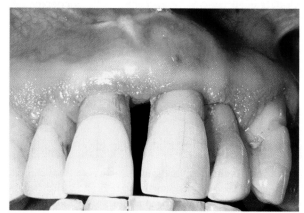

FIGURE 13-1 Clinical view of gingival recession. Note the difference in color between the whitish enamel and the yellowish dentin, which has undergone additional staining due to exposure.

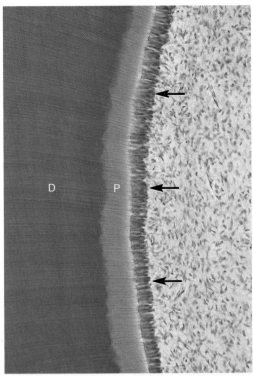

FIGURE 13-2 Microscopic view of odontoblasts *(arrows)* producing predentin *(P)* that will mature into dentin *(D)*. *(Courtesy of James McIntosh, PhD, Assistant Professor Emeritus, Department of Biomedical Sciences, Baylor College of Dentistry, Dallas, TX.)*

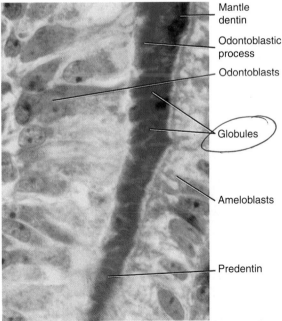

Mantle dentin

Odontoblastic process

Odontoblasts

Globules

Ameloblasts

Predentin

FIGURE 13-3 Photomicrograph of dentin maturation showing the odontoblasts producing predentin, which contains odontoblastic processes, with the ameloblasts located on the opposite side. The predentin matures by forming globules, which undergo mineralization in mantle dentin, because it is adjacent to the dentinoenamel junction. *(From Nanci A:* Ten Cate's Oral Histology, *ed 7, Mosby, St Louis, 2008.)*

hydroxyapatite crystals form as globules, or calcospherules, in the **collagen fibers** of the **predentin**, which allows for both the expansion and fusion during the primary mineralization phase. This process is analogous to the wash of watercolor paint placed on wet paper for a background, as the blobs of color run into each other—although, within dentin, it is a three-dimensional process.

Later, new areas of mineralization occur as globules form in the partially mineralized predentin during the secondary mineralization phase. These new areas of crystal formation are more or less regularly layered on the initial crystals, allowing them to expand, although they fuse incompletely. This process is analogous to additional blobs of paint placed in specific areas over a fuzzy painted background, but the colors of this additional layer do not run into each other to cover the page because the paper is no longer wet.

This incomplete fusion during the secondary mineralization phase results in differences noted in the microscopic features of the crystalline form of dentin. In areas where both primary and secondary mineralization have occurred with complete crystalline fusion, these appear as lighter rounded areas on a stained section of dentin and are considered globular dentin (Figure 13-4).

In contrast, the darker arclike areas in a stained section of dentin are considered interglobular dentin. In these areas, only primary mineralization has occurred within the predentin, and the globules of dentin do not fuse completely. Thus, interglobular dentin is slightly less mineralized than globular dentin. Interglobular dentin is especially evident in coronal dentin, near the DEJ, and in certain dental anomalies, such as in **dentin dysplasia** (see Figure 6-17).

COMPONENTS OF MATURE DENTIN

Within mature dentin, certain components, such as dentinal tubules and their contents, are noted (Figures 13-5 and 13-6). **Dentinal tubules** are long tubes in the dentin that extend from the **DEJ** in the crown area, or **dentinocemental junction (DCJ)** in the root area, to the outer wall of the pulp. After apposition of predentin and maturation into dentin, the cell bodies of the **odontoblasts** remain in the pulp inside the tooth, along its outer wall (discussed later).

Like enamel, dentin is avascular. Nutrition for odontoblasts within the dentin comes through the dentinal tubules from tissue fluid that originally traveled from the blood vessels located in the adjacent pulp tissue. Within each dentinal tubule is a space of variable size containing dentinal fluid, an odontoblastic process, and possibly an afferent axon.

The dentinal fluid in the tubule presumably also includes the tissue fluid surrounding the cell membrane of the odontoblast, which is continuous from the cell body in the pulp. The **odontoblastic process** is a long cellular extension located within the **dentinal tubule** that is still attached to the cell body of the odontoblast within the pulp. In a stained section of a tooth, odontoblastic processes within the dentinal tubule sometimes are not found at the periphery of dentin near the DEJ or DCJ. This absence may or may not be an artifact, given that live cell structures are difficult to preserve in dead mineralized tissues.

Studies suggest that the process occupies the full length of the tubule from the DEJ or DCJ to the pulp during only the early stages of odontogenesis. In mature dentin, however, the process may or may not run the full length of the dentinal tubule to extend near either the outlying DEJ or DCJ.

A sensory, or afferent axon, is associated with part of the odontoblastic process in some dentinal tubules. The myelinated axon may not extend farther than the process, and thus may not be located along either the DEJ or DCJ. Yet, the nerve cell body associated with the axon is located in the pulp along with the odontoblastic cell body. This axon is involved in registration of the sensation of pain only, and not

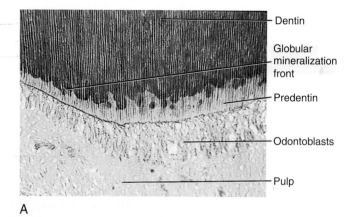

Dentin

Globular mineralization front

Predentin

Odontoblasts

Pulp

A

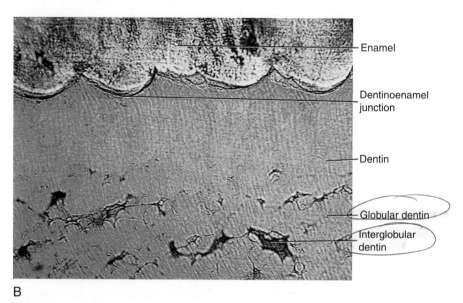

Enamel

Dentinoenamel junction

Dentin

Globular dentin

Interglobular dentin

B

FIGURE 13-4 Views of globular and interglobular dentin. **A:** Section of the globular mineralized front near the outer pulpal wall during primary mineralization. **B:** Ground section near the dentinoenamel junction, with its highly mineralized globular dentin (lighter) and less mineralized interglobular dentin (darker) after both primary and secondary mineralization. *(From Nanci A:* Ten Cate's Oral Histology, *ed 7, Mosby, St Louis, 2008.)*

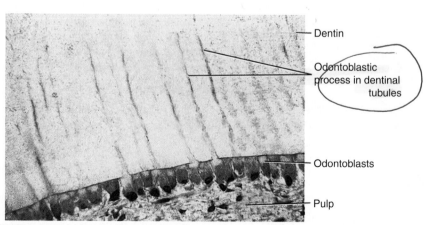

Dentin

Odontoblastic process in dentinal tubules

Odontoblasts

Pulp

FIGURE 13-5 Dentinal tubules in dentin (*section top*), with the odontoblastic processes entering the tubules from the pulp tissue. The pulp tissue contains an outer layer of the cell bodies of odontoblasts to which the odontoblastic processes are still attached. *(From Nanci A:* Ten Cate's Oral Histology, *ed 7, Mosby, St Louis, 2008.)*

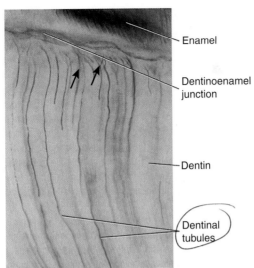

FIGURE 13-6 Microscopic view of the components of the dentinal tubule. The dentinal tubules contain odontoblastic processes *(arrows)*, as well as dentinal fluid. *(From Nanci A: Ten Cate's Oral Histology, ed 7, Mosby, St Louis, 2008.)*

any other sensations, even when triggered by other sensations (discussed later).

The direction of the tubule reflects the pathway of the odontoblast during apposition of predentin. There are two types of curvature established by the direction of the dentinal tubules: primary and secondary (Figure 13-7). The *primary curvature* of the dentinal tubules reflects the overall tubule course over time, which resembles a large S-shaped curve. The *secondary curvature* of the tubule consists of small, delicate curves noted in the primary curvature, reflecting the smaller daily changes in odontoblast direction during apposition. Dentinal tubules are not interrupted by the formation of the interglobular areas of dentin but pass right through them. Tubules can branch at any point along the way from the DEJ or DCJ to the pulp. Dentinal tubules are crowded near the pulp because of the narrowing of this region (see Figure 13-5).

TYPES OF DENTIN

Dentin is not a uniform tissue in the tooth but differs from region to region (Table 13-1). Different types of dentin can be designated by their relationship to the **dentinal tubules** (Figure 13-10; see also Figure 13-5). Dentin that creates the wall of the dentinal tubule is peritubular dentin. Peritubular dentin is highly mineralized after dentin maturation. The dentin that is found between the tubules is intertubular dentin. Intertubular dentin is highly mineralized, but less so than peritubular dentin.

Dentin can also be categorized by its relationship to the DEJ and pulp (Figure 13-11). Mantle dentin is the first **predentin** that forms and matures within the tooth. Mantle dentin shows a difference in the direction of the mineralized collagen fibers compared with the rest of the dentin, having fibers that are perpendicular to the DEJ. Mantle dentin also has more peritubular dentin than the inner dentin, and thus has higher levels of mineralization.

Deep to the mantle dentin, is the layer of dentin around the outer wall of pulp, the circumpulpal dentin, which makes up the bulk of the dentin in a tooth. This type forms and matures after mantle dentin. The collagen fibers of circumpulpal dentin are mainly parallel to the DEJ, compared with those of mantle dentin.

Dentin can also be categorized according to the time that it was formed within the tooth (Figure 13-12). Primary dentin is formed in a tooth before the completion of the **apical foramen(s)** of the root,

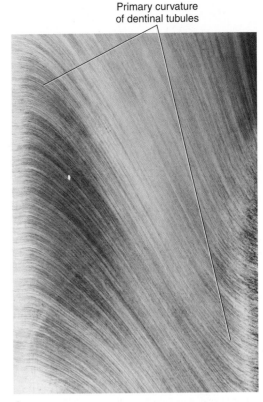

A

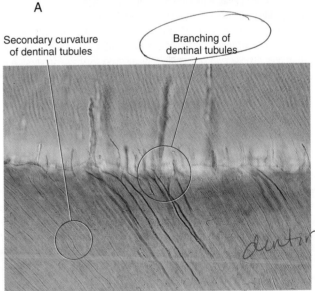

B

FIGURE 13-7 Curvature of the dentinal tubules in dentin. **A:** Primary curvature. **B:** Secondary curvature (*smaller circle*), with branching noted near the dentinoenamel junction (*larger circle*). *(Courtesy of James McIntosh, PhD, Assistant Professor Emeritus, Department of Biomedical Sciences, Baylor College of Dentistry, Dallas, TX.)*

which is the opening in the root's pulp canal. Primary dentin is characterized by its regular pattern of dentinal tubules.

Secondary dentin is formed after the completion of the apical foramen(s) and continues to form throughout the life of the tooth. Secondary dentin is formed more slowly than primary dentin and is less mineralized. Secondary dentin fills in along the outer pulpal wall as it is made by the odontoblastic layer that lines the dentin–pulp

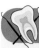

The dentinal tubules can serve as an entry mechanism for cariogenic microorganisms when the carious process begins to extend from the enamel to form **dentinal caries** (Figure 13-8). Microscopically, the microorganisms can be seen actually using the **dentinal tubules** as chutes that allow them to move toward the inner pulp, due to their connection with the odontoblasts in the outer pulpal wall. When caries extends into the dentin from enamel (enamel caries in **Chapter 12**), the carious process moves more rapidly because of the increased organic composition of dentin as compared with enamel. In addition, because of the primary curvature of the dentinal tubules, the pulp may be affected at a more apical level than the level at which the external injury (such as caries) occurred. The cavity preparation process during restorative treatment considers this curvature of the tubules when carious dentin is removed. Light-induced devices that measure changes in laser fluorescence of hard tissue allow dental professionals to better diagnose early lesions.

When dentin is exposed as a result of caries, cavity preparation, gingival recession, or attrition, the open dentinal tubules may be painful for the patient as discussed earlier, causing **dentinal hypersensitivity.** However, many times it is the microscopic anatomy of the tooth that is the culprit; the enamel and cementum do not meet, leaving a gap with dentin exposed at the CEJ interface area a third of the time (see Figure 14-3). In addition, the protective layers of both cementum and dentin can be inadvertently removed as a result of scaling with hand instruments, initiating sensitivity that may or may not be temporary.

Certain additional situations may additionally trigger the short, sharp pain of dentinal hypersensitivity. This includes stimuli such as thermal changes (cold water spray or ice), mechanical irritation (vibrations from instrumentation, dental handpieces, or ultrasonics), dehydration (stream of air or heat during cavity preparation), or chemical exposure (foods such as thick or hypertonic sweet, salty, or sour fluids; tooth-colored restorative materials; or vital whitening agents). By contrast, the pain from other tooth-related situations, such as from caries and pulpal or gingival infections, is usually dull and chronic in nature.

However, dentinal hypersensitivity is often a type of diffuse pain, making localization to a specific tooth difficult for the dental professional, as well as for the patient. This pain may wrongly be interpreted as caries, pulpal or gingival infections, or soft tissue inflammation. Because of the chronic nature of attrition and gingival recession, the pain present may not be as painful as other forms of dentinal exposure because both of these are gradual processes, allowing time for subtle changes to occur in the dentinal tubules, to close them off from the stimulation (discussed later). Dentinal hypersensitivity can occur with all teeth and all their surfaces but is especially evident in premolars and canines, usually on the facial and cervical regions.

The strongest held theory of dentinal hypersensitivity suggests that it is due to changes in the **dentinal fluid** associated with the processes, a type of hydrodynamic mechanism (Figure 13-9). This mechanism may be due to one or more of the following: evaporation and loss of dentinal fluid, movement of the fluid, and ionic changes in the fluid. These changes in the dentinal fluid are then transmitted to the afferent axon present in some tubules near the dentin–pulp interface, thus sending a painful message to the pulp and then on to the brain. Possibly, that is the reason the previously mentioned painful stimuli are involved in dentinal hypersensitivity: because they are involved with dentinal fluid movement within the tubule, and because local anesthetics do not block sensation when they are placed on the surface of exposed dentin, as they would with a fully innervated tissue. However, in the future, more than one theory may be used to fully explain surface dentinal pain.

Dentinal hypersensitivity can be treated somewhat successfully with solutions applied either by professionals or within over-the-counter dentifrices to patients. These desensitizing agents either temporarily block the exposed open ends of the dentinal tubules, similar to the process of tooth staining, or interfere with nerve transmission. However, restorations sometimes are the only permanent method to reduce hypersensitivity of the exposed dentinal surface in severe cases. Methods that will fully seal the dentinal tubules, and thus prevent any dentinal hypersensitivity, are being studied.

interface. This secondary dentinogenesis is noted for its regular pattern of tubules. Microscopically, a dark line shows the junction between the primary and secondary dentin that results from an abrupt change in the course of the odontoblasts during apposition as the tooth's apex or apices are completed. Certain medications placed during cavity preparation with restorative treatment can promote its formation and thus help protect the underlying pulp tissue after outer dentin is lost.

Reparative, reactive, or tertiary dentin is formed quickly in localized regions in response to a localized injury to the exposed dentin (see Figure 13-12). Tertiary dentin thus forms underneath the exposed dentinal tubules along the outer pulpal wall. The injury could be caries, cavity preparation, attrition, or recession. Odontoblasts in the area of the affected tubules might perish because of the injury, but neighboring undifferentiated mesenchymal cells of the pulp move to the area and become odontoblasts. Tertiary dentin tries to seal off the injured area, thus the term *reparative dentin*. Due to the more rushed timetable, the tubules in tertiary dentin assume a more irregular course than in secondary dentin.

A certain type of tertiary dentin, *sclerotic dentin,* is often found in association with the chronic injury of caries and is noted in increased amounts as the tooth ages. In this type of dentin, the odontoblastic processes die and leave the dentinal tubules vacant. These hollow dentinal tubules then become retrofilled and, finally, occluded by a mineralized substance similar to peritubular dentin. This type of dentin may be involved, in fact, with prolonging pulp vitality, because it reduces the permeability of dentin. Clinically, this is noted with presence of arrested caries and appears as dark, smooth, and shiny areas, which is usually noted in older dentitions.

MICROSCOPIC FEATURES OF MATURE DENTIN

When mature dentin is examined microscopically, certain features, such as dentinal tubules and most types of dentin, are easily noted. However, the dentinal process within tubules is hard to discern microscopically. Other microscopic features are also noted and will be discussed further. These features can occur in both primary and secondary dentin.

The imbrication lines of von Ebner are incremental lines or bands that stain darkly in a section of dentin and can be likened to the growth rings of trees, and are also similar to the incremental lines of Retzius noted in enamel (Figure 13-13). These lines show the incremental nature of dentin during the **stage of apposition** of tooth development, and run at right angles to the dentinal tubules. With each

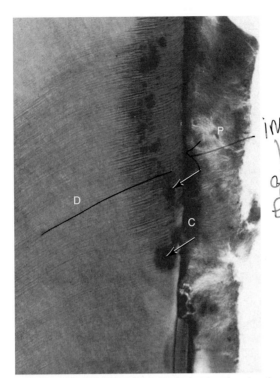

imb.
lines
of Von
Ebner

FIGURE 13-8 Photomicrograph of the dentinal caries showing the cariogenic microorganisms entering the deeper dentin *(D)* through the dentinal tubules *(direction, arrows).* Note that the cementum *(C)* has already been invaded by the cariogenic microorganisms from the dental biofilm or plaque *(P)* covering the root area. *(From Perry DA, Beemsterboer PL, Taggart EJ: Clinical Periodontology for Dental Hygienists, ed 3, WB Saunders, Philadelphia, 2006.)*

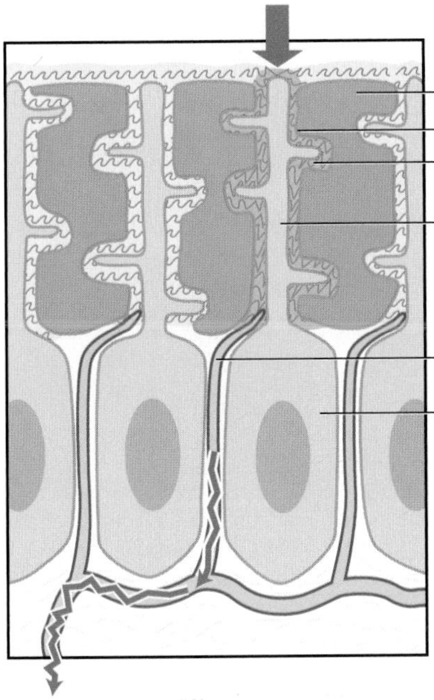

TABLE 13-1	Types of Dentin	
TYPE	**LOCATION/ CHRONOLOGY**	**DESCRIPTION**
Peritubular dentin	Wall of tubules	Highly mineralized
Intertubular dentin	Between the tubules	Highly mineralized
Mantle dentin	Outermost layer	First dentin formed
Circumpulpal dentin	Layer around outer pulpal wall	Dentin formed after mantle dentin
Primary dentin	Formed before completion of apical foramen	Formed more rapidly; more mineralized than secondary
Secondary dentin	Formed after completion of apical foramen	Formed slower; less mineralized than primary
Tertiary dentin	Formed as a result of injury	Irregular pattern of tubules

STIMULATION

- Exposed dentin
- Dentinal tubule
- Change in dentinal fluid
- Odontoblastic process

- Possible nerve location
- Odontoblast cell body in pulp tissue

Pain message sent to brain

FIGURE 13-9 Possible mechanism involved in the hydrodynamic theory of dentinal hypersensitivity. Stimulation of the exposed dentinal tubules (such as with cold water) causes changes in the dentinal fluid, which is then transmitted to the nerves associated with the odontoblast cell bodies in the pulp tissue.

daily 4-μm increment of dentin by the **odontoblasts**, the orientation of the deposited collagen fibers differs slightly. More severe changes occur every fifth day, giving rise at every 20 μm to an imbrication line as noted.

The contour lines of Owen are a number of adjoining parallel imbrication lines that are also present in a stained section of dentin. These specific imbrication lines demonstrate a disturbance in body metabolism that affects the odontoblasts by altering their formation efforts, and they tend to appear together as a series of dark bands. The most pronounced contour line is the **neonatal line** that occurs during the trauma of birth (Figure 13-14). Other contour lines can occur in conjunction with the clinically visible **tetracycline stain** of the teeth, in which the antibiotic taken systemically during tooth development becomes chemically bound to the dentin in varying amounts (see Figure 3-16). Thankfully, most of this intrinsic stain can be lightened with tooth whitening.

Another feature is Tomes' granular layer, which is most often found in the peripheral part of dentin beneath the root's cementum, adjacent to the **DCJ** in a stained section of dentin (Figure 13-15). However, the area only looks granular because of its spotty microscopic appearance; the cause of the visible change in this region of dentin is unknown. It may be due to less mineralized areas of dentin having an increased level of **interglobular dentin** or the presence of branching of the terminal parts of dentinal tubules found near the DCJ, similar to that noted near the DEJ.

AGING AND DENTIN

Assessment of age from dentition constitutes an important step in constructing an identity profile of a decedent. Dentinal translucency is one of the best morphohistological parameters to use for dental age estimation, not only in terms of accuracy but also simplicity, along with use of related software and digital devices.

In addition, with increased age, the diameter of the **dentinal tubule** narrows because of deposition of **peritubular dentin**. This narrowing may be related to the decreased ability of pulp to react to various stimuli with age. With age, the passageways of the tubules to the pulp are not as wide open as when younger; thus the stimuli are not transmitted as rapidly, and in as large amounts, as they were previously (discussed further

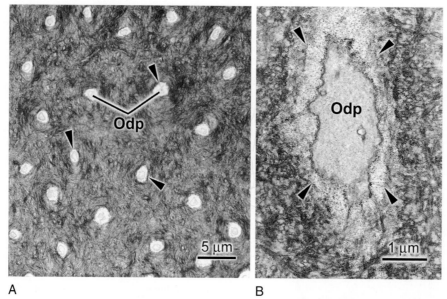

FIGURE 13-10 Cross sections of dentinal tubules composed of peritubular dentin *(arrows)* containing odontoblastic processes *(Odp)* and surrounded by intertubular dentin. **A:** Photomicrograph. **B:** Transmission electromicrograph showing close-up view. *(From Nanci A: Ten Cate's Oral Histology, ed 7, Mosby, St Louis, 2008.)*

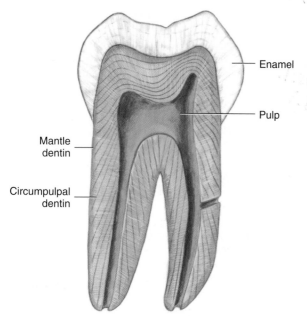

FIGURE 13-11 Main types of dentin and relationship to the enamel and pulp: mantle dentin and circumpulpal dentin.

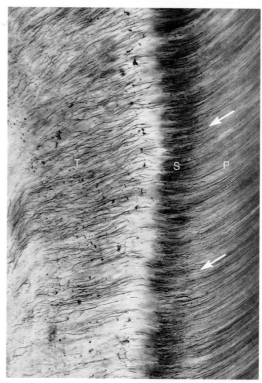

FIGURE 13-12 Microscopic view of various types of dentin showing the relationship to the time of formation (from early to late): primary *(P)*, secondary *(S)*, and tertiary *(T)*, with a dark line between the primary and secondary dentin *(arrows)* caused by an abrupt change in the course of the odontoblasts during apposition. Note also the more irregular course of dentinal tubules in tertiary dentin than in secondary dentin. *(Courtesy of James McIntosh, PhD, Department of Biomedical Sciences, Baylor College of Dentistry, Dallas, TX.)*

in regard to pulp). Studies show the complete obliteration of older tubules with mineralization of the associated odontoblastic processes.

With age, odontoblasts also undergo cytoplasmic changes, including a reduction in organelle content. As discussed previously, dentin becomes more exposed as a result of both attrition and gingival recession, which may or may not lead to **dentinal hypersensitivity** (discussed earlier).

Apart from dentin that is resorbed during the shedding of primary teeth, the dentin formed is mostly stable during the life of the tooth. However, in a few cases it can become resorbed in permanent teeth, but the cause is unknown (idiopathic) and can involve either an internal or external resorption process. It can be noted radiographically, but it is hard to discern between the two processes. In contrast, when

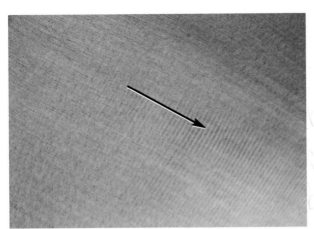

FIGURE 13-13 Imbrication lines of von Ebner that transverse the dentinal tubules in dentin (direction, *arrow*), showing a regular pattern of dentin formation. *(Courtesy of James McIntosh, PhD, Assistant Professor Emeritus, Department of Biomedical Sciences, Baylor College of Dentistry, Dallas, TX.)*

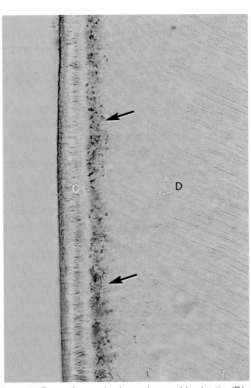

FIGURE 13-15 Tomes' granular layer *(arrows)* in dentin *(D)* near the dentinocemental junction, beneath layers of cementum *(C)*. *(Courtesy of James McIntosh, PhD, Assistant Professor Emeritus, Department of Biomedical Sciences, Baylor College of Dentistry, Dallas, TX.)*

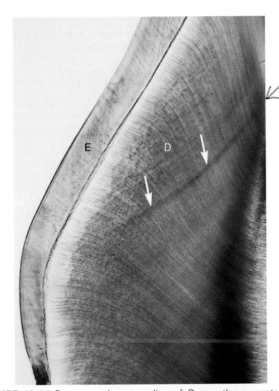

FIGURE 13-14 Pronounced contour line of Owen, the neonatal line *(arrows)*, as well as other parallel adjacent contour lines in dentin *(D)* underlying enamel *(E)*. *(Courtesy of James McIntosh, PhD, Assistant Professor Emeritus, Department of Biomedical Sciences, Baylor College of Dentistry, Dallas, TX.)*

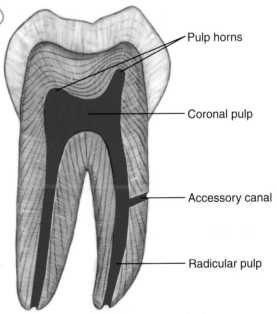

FIGURE 13-16 Anatomy of pulp.

Pulp horns

Coronal pulp

Accessory canal

Radicular pulp

the process begins on the external surface of the root and then penetrates through the cementum into dentin (usually not into the pulp), it can lead to a pinkish crown color noted clinically from the **granulation tissue** seen beneath the translucent enamel.

PULP

The **pulp** is the innermost tissue of the tooth and appears radiolucent (dark) because it is less dense than the radiopaque (or lighter) hard tissues of the tooth. The pulp of a tooth is a **connective tissue** with all

the components of such a tissue (discussed later). Embryologically, the pulp forms from the **central cells of the dental papilla** (see Figure 6-7). Thus, pulp has a background similar to that of dentin, because both are derived from the **dental papilla** of the tooth germ. During odontogenesis, when the dentin forms around the dental papilla, the innermost tissue is considered pulp (see Figures 6-10 and 6-11).

One important consideration that relates to the dentin-pulp complex is that the pulp is involved in the support, maintenance, and continued formation of dentin, because the inner layer of the cell bodies of the **odontoblasts** remain along the outer pulpal wall (discussed later). Another function of the pulp is sensory, because the cell bodies associated with the afferent axons in the dentinal tubules are located among this layer of odontoblasts. When the dentin or pulp is injured, the only sensation perceived by the brain is pain. Therefore, changes in temperature, vibrations, and chemical changes that affect the dentin or pulp are perceived only as painful stimuli. The pulp being a sensory organ mandates that it needs local anesthesia for pain control during most restorative procedures.

Pulp also serves a **nutritional** function for itself as well as dentin, because the dentin contains no blood supply of its own. Dentin depends on the pulp's vascular supply and associated tissue fluids for its nutrition. Nutrition is obtained through the tubules and their connection to the odontoblasts' cell bodies that line the outer pulpal wall.

Finally, the pulp has a protective function because it is involved in the formation of **secondary dentin** or **tertiary dentin**, which increases the coverage of the pulp. In addition, if the pulp suffers any injury that also involves the odontoblasts, its undifferentiated **mesenchyme** contains cells that can differentiate into **fibroblasts**, which then create fibers and intercellular substances, as well as odontoblasts, to create more dentin. The pulp also has white blood cells (**WBCs**) within its vascular system and tissues; these allow triggering of inflammatory and immune responses.

ANATOMY OF PULP

The large mass of pulp is contained within the pulp chamber of the tooth (Figure 13-16). The shape of each pulp chamber corresponds directly to the overall shape of the tooth, and thus is individualized for every tooth (see **Chapters 16 and 17**). The pulp tissue in the pulp chamber has two main divisions: coronal pulp and radicular pulp.

The coronal pulp is located in the **crown** of the tooth. Smaller extensions of coronal pulp into the **cusps** of posterior teeth form the pulp horns. These pulp horns are especially prominent in the **permanent dentition**, under the buccal cusp of **premolars** and the mesiobuccal cusp of **molars** in primary teeth discussed in **Chapter 18**. In contrast, pulp horns are not found on anterior teeth. To prevent exposure of the pulpal tissue, these regions must be taken into consideration during cavity preparation with restorative treatment.

The radicular pulp, or root pulp, is the part of the pulp located in the **root** of the tooth; it is also called the *pulp canal* by patients. The radicular pulp extends from the cervical part of the tooth to each apex of the tooth. This part of the pulp has openings from the pulp through the cementum into the surrounding periodontal ligament. These openings include each apical foramen and possibly accessory canals.

The apical foramen is the opening from the pulp into the surrounding periodontal ligament near each apex of the tooth. If more than one foramen is present on each root, the largest one is designated as the apical foramen and the rest are considered accessory foramina.

This opening is surrounded by layers of cementum and allows arteries, veins, lymphatics, and nerves to enter and exit the pulp from the **periodontal ligament (PDL)** (Tables 13-2 and 13-3). Thus, communication between the pulp and the PDL is possible because of the apical foramen. Each apical foramen is the last part of the tooth to form; it forms after the crown erupts into the oral cavity. In developing teeth, each foramen is large and centrally located. As the tooth matures, each foramen becomes smaller in diameter and is offset in position. Each foramen may be located at each anatomical apex of each of the roots but is usually located slightly more occlusal from each apex.

TABLE 13-2	Arterial Supply to the Teeth and Associated Periodontium
TEETH AND ASSOCIATED PERIODONTIUM	**MAJOR BRANCHES OF MAXILLARY ARTERY**
Posterior maxillary and periodontium	Posterior superior alveolar artery
Anterior maxillary and periodontium	Infraorbital artery
Mandibular and periodontium	Inferior alveolar artery

(From Fehrenbach MJ, Herring SW: *Illustrated Anatomy of the Head and Neck*, ed 3, WB Saunders, Philadelphia, 2007.)

TABLE 13-3	Nerve Supply to the Teeth and Associated Periodontium
TEETH AND ASSOCIATED PERIODONTIUM	**BRANCHES OF TRIGEMINAL NERVE OR FIFTH (V) CRANIAL NERVE**
Maxillary anterior teeth, maxillary anterior facial periodontium	Anterior superior alveolar nerve from maxillary nerve (V$_2$)
Maxillary anterior lingual periodontium	Nasopalatine nerve from maxillary nerve (V$_2$)
Maxillary posterior teeth, maxillary posterior buccal periodontium	Middle superior alveolar and posterior superior alveolar nerve from maxillary nerve (V$_2$)
Maxillary posterior lingual periodontium	Greater palatine nerve from maxillary nerve (V$_2$)
Mandibular teeth and facial periodontium of the mandibular anterior teeth and premolars	Inferior alveolar nerve from mandibular nerve (V$_3$)
Mandibular posterior buccal periodontium	Long buccal nerve from mandibular nerve (V$_2$)
Mandibular lingual periodontium	Lingual nerve from mandibular nerve (V$_2$)

(From Fehrenbach MJ, Herring SW: *Illustrated Anatomy of the Head and Neck*, ed 3, WB Saunders, Philadelphia, 2007.)

Accessory canals may also be associated with the pulp and are extra openings from the pulp to the periodontal ligament (Figure 13-17; see Figure 13-16). Accessory canals are also called *lateral canals,* because they are usually located on the lateral surface of the roots of the teeth. Accessory canals form when **Hertwig's epithelial root sheath** encounters a blood vessel during root formation. Root structure then forms around the vessel, forming the accessory canal.

Teeth have a variable number of these canals, which sometimes poses problems during endodontic therapy or root canal treatment (discussed later). Radiographs do not always indicate the number or position of these canals, unless they are examined with instruments using radiopaque materials during this therapy. Gingival recession may expose the opening of an accessory canal, especially in the furcation area, possibly causing the spread of infection into the pulp from caries or periodontal disease.

Clinical Considerations about Pulp Pathology

Knowing the exact anatomy of a tooth's pulp chamber using radiographs, especially the extension of the pulp horns into the overlying cusps, is important when practicing safe restorative dentistry. However, when the **pulp** is injured by cavity preparation, and even by extensive caries or traumatic injury, it may undergo inflammation, or **pulpitis**. This inflammation initially remains localized within the confines of the dentin. The pressure from this confined pulpitis can result in extreme pain as the inflammatory edema presses on the afferent nerves contained in the pulp.

Pulpitis can later cause a pulpal infection in the form of a periapical abscess or cyst in the surrounding periodontium, spreading through the apical foramen or, possibly, an accessory canal. If the pulp dies from the infection, it must be surgically removed. An inert radiopaque rubbery material (gutta-percha) is then placed within the pulp chamber, including each radicular pulp or root canal during endodontic therapy (or root canal treatment).

When the pulp is removed by this treatment, the tooth is no longer vital, because its nutritional source from the vascular pulp tissue has been removed. Thus, the endodontically treated tooth may darken and become brittle and break during mastication. The darkening is due to degradative products from pulpal necrosis and death being passed along the dentinal tubules. To prolong retention of the tooth, a full-coverage restorative crown is sometimes placed on the natural crown to protect it from breaking and to improve its appearance. Internal or external nonvital whitening may also be necessary to reduce darkening with certain esthetic restorations, or if coverage is deferred. If an abscess or cyst formation develops in the periodontium as a result of pulpitis, further surgery (apicoectomy) must be performed to remove the apical lesion.

Dental professionals must do their utmost to prevent injury to the pulp during preventive and restorative procedures. Such iatrogenic injury to the pulp can result from the heat or vibrations emitted by dental handpiece during cavity preparation, as well as excessive coronal polishing, causing physical damage. The pulp can also be injured by the restorative materials placed in the cavity preparation. Water-cooled handpieces with rapid rotation, which minimize the stress on the tooth, as well as selective polishing techniques, are now used successfully to reduce the incidence of pulpal damage. Liners are also currently placed over dentin when using toxic restorative materials to prevent future pulpal damage. Then cement bases are placed, after the liner, to protect the pulp from restorations that can serve as excellent thermal conductors, such as gold inlays/crowns or silver amalgams.

MICROSCOPIC FEATURES OF PULP

Because pulp is a **connective tissue**, it has all the components of such a tissue: intercellular substance, tissue fluid, certain cells, lymphatics, vascular system, nerves, and fibers (Figure 13-18). As in all forms of connective tissue, the **fibroblasts** are the largest group of cells in the pulp (see Figure 8-5). The **odontoblasts** are the second largest group of cells in the pulp, but only their cell bodies are located in the pulp. The odontoblasts are located only along the outer pulpal wall.

In addition to fibroblasts and odontoblasts, the pulp contains an undifferentiated **mesenchyme** type of stem cells, dental pulp stem cells (DPSCs). These cells are a rich resource for the dentin-pulp complex, because they can transform into fibroblasts and odontoblasts if either cell population is reduced after injury.

The pulp also contains **WBCs** in its tissue and vascular supply, but levels are normally low, unless the cells are ready to be triggered by an inflammatory or immune reaction. The **red blood cells** are located in

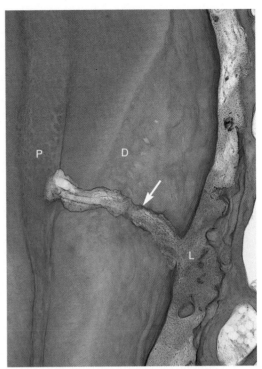

FIGURE 13-17 Accessory canal *(arrow)* located in the root, which is composed of pulp *(P)* and dentin *(D)* covered by cementum. Note that the accessory canal is open to the periodontal ligament *(L)*. *(Courtesy of James McIntosh, PhD, Assistant Professor Emeritus, Department of Biomedical Sciences, Baylor College of Dentistry, Dallas, TX.)*

the extensive vascular supply. The fibers present in the pulp are mainly **collagen fibers** and some **reticular fibers**. The pulp contains no elastic fibers. Also present are an extensive vascular supply and rudimentary **lymphatics**.

Two types of nerves are associated with the pulp, including both myelinated nerves and unmyelinated nerves. The myelinated nerves are the axons of sensory, or afferent, neurons that are located in the dentinal tubules in dentin. The associated nerve cell bodies are located between the odontoblasts' cell bodies in the odontoblastic layer of the pulp. The unmyelinated nerves are associated with the blood vessels.

Pulp stones, or denticles, are sometimes present in the pulp tissue (Figure 13-19). These can be mineralized masses of **dentin** complete with dentinal tubules and odontoblastic processes (true); in other cases, they are amorphous in structure (false). They can be free or unattached to the outer pulpal wall, or they can be attached to the dentin at the dentin-pulp interface. Pulp stones are formed during tooth development, and also later as the pulp ages, and may be due to microtrauma. They are quite common and may fill most of the **pulp chamber**. They are detected as radiopaque masses in radiographs and are only a problem during endodontic therapy.

MICROSCOPIC ZONES IN PULP

Four zones are evident when pulp tissue is viewed microscopically: odontoblastic layer, cell-free zone, cell-rich zone, and pulpal core (Table 13-4; see Figure 13-18). This chapter discusses these zones in order, from the outermost zone closest to the dentin to the center of the pulp.

The first zone of pulp closest to the dentin is the *odontoblastic layer*. This zone lines the outer pulpal wall. It consists of a layer of the cell bodies of odontoblasts, whose odontoblastic processes are located in the dentinal tubules in the adjacent dentin. The odontoblasts are

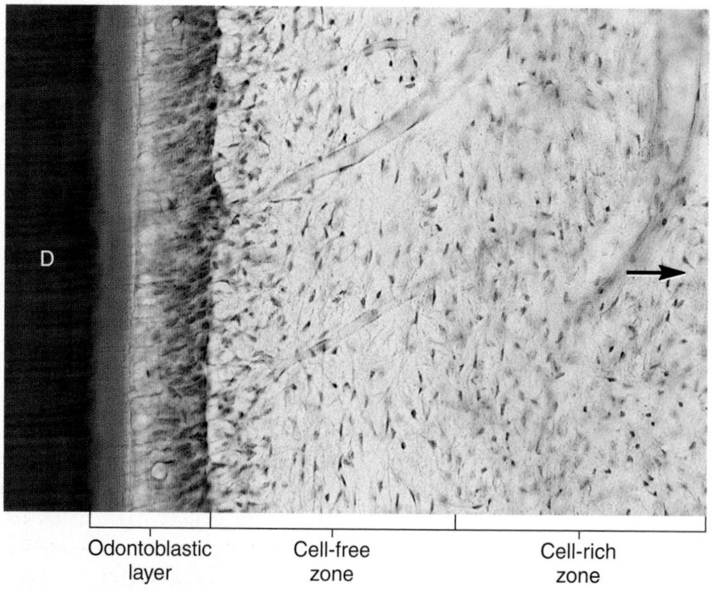

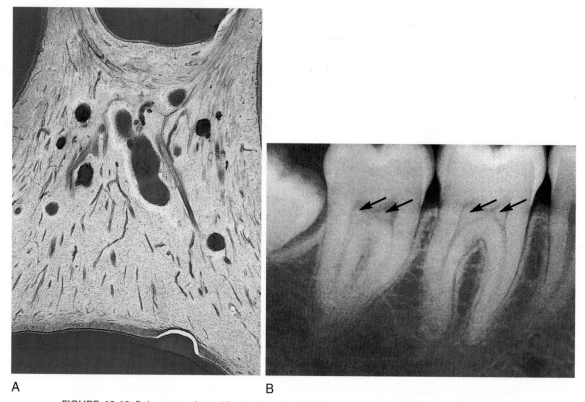

FIGURE 13-18 Pulp tissue zones deep to the dentin *(D)*, from the outer zones to inner zone of the pulpal core (direction, *arrow*). (Courtesy of James McIntosh, PhD, Assistant Professor Emeritus, Department of Biomedical Sciences, Baylor College of Dentistry, Dallas, TX.)

FIGURE 13-19 Pulp stones in multirooted teeth. **A:** Microscopic view. **B:** Radiograph *(arrows).* (**A** *courtesy of James McIntosh, PhD, Assistant Professor Emeritus, Department of Biomedical Sciences, Baylor College of Dentistry, Dallas, TX.)*

capable of forming secondary or tertiary dentin along the outer pulpal wall. If this occurs, the odontoblasts realign on the pulpal side next to this newly formed dentin. In addition, the cell bodies of the afferent axons from the dentinal tubules in dentin are located between the cell bodies of the odontoblasts.

The next zone, nearest to the odontoblastic layer, inward from the dentin is considered the *cell-free zone,* but it is anything but empty.

This zone was so named because it appears to be virtually free of cells, but this is only true when using low-level microscopic powers. In reality, this zone consists of fewer cells in contrast to the odontoblastic layer, but it is not entirely cell free. A nerve and capillary plexus is also located in this zone. No secondary or tertiary dentin is formed here initially, but newly formed dentin may encroach upon this zone.

TABLE 13-4	Microscopic Zones in Pulp
ZONES(FROM OUTER TO INNER ZONES)	**DESCRIPTION**
Odontoblastic layer	Lines outer pulpal wall and consists of cell bodies of odontoblasts, which may form secondary dentin, causing cell bodies to realign themselves; cell bodies of afferent axons from dentinal tubules located between cell bodies of odontoblasts
Cell-free zone	Contains fewer cells than odontoblastic layer; nerve and capillary plexus located here
Cell-rich zone	Contains increased density of cells compared with cell-free zone and more extensive vascular supply
Pulpal core	Located in center of pulp chamber; similar to cell-rich zone with many cells and extensive vascular supply

The next zone after the cell-free zone is the *cell-rich zone,* inward from dentin. The cell-rich zone, as its name implies, has an increased density of cells compared with the cell-free zone but still does not contain as many cells as the odontoblastic layer. This zone also has a more extensive vascular supply than does the cell-free zone.

The final zone of pulp is the *pulpal core,* which is in the center of the pulp chamber. This zone consists of many cells and an extensive vascular supply. Except for its location, it is very similar to the cell-rich zone.

AGING AND PULP

The pulp horns recede with age. Also with increased age, the pulp undergoes a decrease in intercellular substance, water, and cells as it fills with an increased amount of collagen fibers. This decrease in cells is especially evident in the reduced number of undifferentiated mesenchymal cells. Thus, the pulp becomes more fibrotic with increased age, leading to a reduction in the regenerative capacity of the pulp due its loss of these cells. Also, the overall pulp cavity may be smaller by the addition of secondary or tertiary dentin, thus causing pulp recession. The lack of sensitivity associated with older teeth is due to receded pulp horns, pulp fibrosis, addition of dentin, or possibly all these age-related changes; many times restorative treatment can proudly be performed without local anesthesia on older dentitions.

The pulp's apical foramen may also become obliterated with deposits of cementum over time, leading to blockage of blood vessels serving the tissue (see Chapter 14). This can result in vascular congestion and then pulp necrosis and tooth death.

FUTURE CONCERNS WITH DENTIN-PULP COMPLEX

The vitality of the dentin-pulp complex, both during health and after injury, depends on pulp cell activity and the signaling processes that regulate the cell's behavior. This is especially true regarding the DPSCs present. Research has led to a better understanding of the molecular control of cellular behavior. Growth factors play a pivotal role in signaling the events of tissue formation and repair in the dentin-pulp complex. Harnessing these growth factors can provide exciting opportunities for biological approaches to dental tissue repair and the blueprint for replacement tissue engineering of the tooth. These approaches offer significant potential for improved clinical management of dental disease and maintenance of tooth vitality.

In addition, work is continuing directly with the DPSCs, because this particular type of stem cell has the future potential to differentiate into a variety of other cell types that were originally derived from the embryonic mesenchyme, including muscle, bone, cartilage, and fat, as well as dental tissue such as dentin, cementum, PDL, and lamina propria. The DPSCs are most viable in primary teeth; permanent molars, such as thirds, also have the cells, though fewer. Processing has to be quick after removal, and the freezing process is the same as used to store cord blood stem cells. Teeth that merely fall out may have damaged pulp and may not be a useful source, especially if viability standards are not set. The potential for using DPSCs for dental repair, however, remains unclear. Research continues related to using cord blood stem cells to regrow tissue, and possibly to help address diseases like Parkinson's and Alzheimer's, spinal cord injury, stroke, burns, heart disease, diabetes, osteoarthritis, and rheumatoid arthritis.

In addition, identification of the genes controlling odontoblast differentiation might lead to development of methods enabling induction of tertiary dentin formation under carious lesions. Identification of the genes active during dentinogenesis might lead to recognition of regulatory factors, which would cause secondary dentinogenesis to proceed at the rate of primary dentinogenesis, so that present-day restorations would become a thing of the past.

CHAPTER 14

Periodontium: Cementum, Alveolar Bone, and Periodontal Ligament

●●●CHAPTER OUTLINE

Periodontium
Components of the periodontium
  Cementum
    Development of cementum
    Microscopic appearance
    Types of cementum
  Alveolar bone
    Anatomy of the jaws
    Development of the jaws

Periodontal ligament
  Components of the periodontal ligament
  Cells of the periodontal ligament
  Fiber groups of the periodontal ligament

●●●LEARNING OBJECTIVES

- Define and pronounce the key terms in this chapter.
- Discuss the periodontium, and describe the properties of each of its components.
- Describe the development of the periodontium.
- Outline the types of cementum and alveolar bone.
- Label the fiber groups of the periodontal ligament and discuss their functions.
- Indicate and discuss the microscopic features of the periodontium.

- Describe the age-related changes in the periodontium.
- Integrate the knowledge of the histology with the clinical considerations involving the periodontium, especially those changes associated with periodontal pathology in order to promote the health of the periodontium.

●●●NEW KEY TERMS

Alveolar crest (al-**vee**-o-lar), **group**
Alveolar bone proper (al-**vee**-o-lar)
Alveolodental ligament (al-**vee**-o-lo-**dent**-al)
Bone: basal (**bay**-sal), **cortical** (**kor**-ti-kal), **supporting alveolar, trabecular** (trah-**bek**-u-lar)
Canaliculi (kan-ah-**lik**-u-lie)
Cemental caries (see-**men**-tal), **spurs**
Cementicles (see-**men**-ti-kuls)

Cementoenamel junction
Cementum (see-**men**-tum): **acellular, cellular**
Edentulous (e-**den**-tu-lus)
Fibers: principal, Sharpey's (**shar**-peez)
Group: apical, gingival fiber (jin-**ji**-val), **horizontal, interradicular** (in-ter-rah-**dik**-u-lar), **oblique** (o-**bleek**)
Hypercementosis (hi-per-see-men-**toe**-sis)

Interdental septum, ligament (in-ter-**den**-tal)
Interradicular septum (in-ter-rah-**dik**-u-lar)
Lamina dura (**lam**-i-nah **dur**-ah)
Mesial drift (**me**-ze-il)
Periodontal ligament space (pare-ee-o-**don**-tal)
Periodontium (per-e-o-**don**-she-um)

PERIODONTIUM

To understand the pathological changes that occur during the disease states involving the periodontium, dental professionals must first appreciate the histology of the healthy, normal periodontium. Thus, the underlying histological states of these components provide a clue to the clinical features noted visibly with the periodontium, whether in a healthy or diseased state.

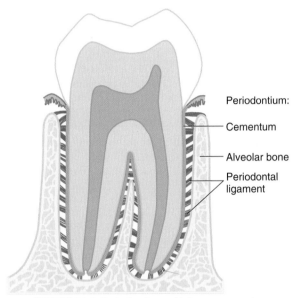

Periodontium:

— Cementum

— Alveolar bone

— Periodontal ligament

FIGURE 14-1 Periodontium with its components.

COMPONENTS OF THE PERIODONTIUM

The periodontium consists of both the supporting soft and hard dental tissue between the tooth and the alveolar bone, as well as parts of the tooth and alveolar bone (Figure 14-1). The periodontium serves to support the tooth in its ongoing relationship to the alveolar bone. Thus, the periodontium includes the cementum, alveolar bone, and periodontal ligament, each one's individual components. Some clinicians may include various types of gingival tissue in the category of the periodontium, but it has only a minor role in the support of the tooth (see Chapter 10).

CEMENTUM

The **cementum** is the part of the periodontium that attaches the teeth to the **alveolar bone** by anchoring the **periodontal ligament** (Figure 14-2). However, in a healthy patient, the cementum is not clinically visible because it usually covers the entire root, overlying **Tomes' granular layer** in dentin, which is not usually exposed in a healthy oral cavity.

Cementum is a hard tissue that is thickest at the tooth's apex or apices and in the interradicular areas of **multirooted** teeth (50 to 200 μm) and thinnest at the cementoenamel junction (CEJ) at the cervix of the tooth (10 to 50 μm). Cementum has no nerve supply and is also avascular, receiving its nutrition through its own imbedded cells from the surrounding vascular periodontal ligament. Like other the dental hard tissue of both dentin and alveolar bone, cementum can form throughout the life of the tooth (see Table 6-2), including after eruption.

Mature cementum is by weight 65% mineralized or inorganic material, 23% organic material, and 12% water. This crystalline formation

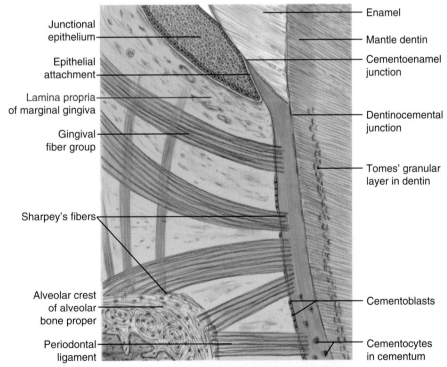

Junctional epithelium —

Epithelial attachment —

Lamina propria of marginal gingiva —

Gingival fiber group —

Sharpey's fibers —

Alveolar crest of alveolar bone proper —

Periodontal ligament —

— Enamel

— Mantle dentin

— Cementoenamel junction

— Dentinocemental junction

— Tomes' granular layer in dentin

— Cementoblasts

— Cementocytes in cementum

FIGURE 14-2 Cementum and its relationship to both the tooth and alveolar bone, with Sharpey's fibers from the periodontal ligament inserting into both tissue types. Note Tomes' granular layer in the underlying dentin.

of mature cementum consists of mainly **calcium hydroxyapatite**, with the chemical formula of $Ca_{10}(PO_4)_6(OH)_2$. The calcium hydroxyapatite found in cementum is similar to that found in higher percentages in both enamel and dentin, but more closely resembles the percentage found in bone tissue such as alveolar bone. Other forms of calcium are also present.

In certain situations, when cementum is initially exposed from **gingival recession,** such as occurs during periodontal disease, it is

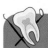
Clinical Considerations about Cemental Pathology

When cementum is exposed through **gingival recession**, it quickly undergoes **abrasion** by mechanical friction because of its low mineral content and thinness. (Figure 14-3; see **Chapter 13**). The exposure of the deeper **dentin** can lead to problems such as extrinsic staining and **dentinal hypersensitivity.**

Studies are showing that such morphology may result in an increased risk of **cemental caries.** The incidence of cemental caries increases in older adults as gingival recession occurs from either trauma or periodontal disease. It is a chronic condition that forms a large, shallow lesion and slowly invades first the root's cementum and then dentin to cause a chronic infection of the pulp (Figure 14-4). Because dental pain is a late finding, many lesions are not detected early, resulting in restorative challenges and increased tooth loss.

Xerostomia (dry mouth), poor manual dexterity for adequate homecare, and poor nutrition in older adults can complicate caries, and all these issues must be addressed during dental treatment of these patients. Increased controversy surrounds treatment of periodontal disease that involves the removal of the outer layers of cementum during scaling of the roots. Dental biofilm and the related hardened calculus are associated with the cemental surface of the root deep inside a diseased **periodontal pocket** (Figures 14-5 and 14-6; see also **Chapter 10**).

In the past, it was believed that bacterial toxins (endotoxins) could be absorbed into the outer part of cementum from the adjacent dental biofilm, and that these outer layers of "toxic" cementum must be removed by manual scaling for the dentogingival tissue to heal and form a more occlusal epithelial attachment. Now it is believed that these toxins are loosely adherent to the cementum and that the cementum does not need to be scaled off to remove them, but, instead, ultrasonic devices can flush these toxins from the cementum without removing any of the hard tissue. More studies in this area are necessary as new treatments of periodontal disease are considered.

a dull pale yellow, lighter than dentin but darker than enamel's whitish shade (discussed later). When instruments are used, cementum feels grainy compared with the harder dentin and the even harder, smoother enamel surfaces. Because of its mineral level, cementum appears more radiolucent (or darker) than either enamel or dentin, but more radiopaque (or lighter) than pulp tissue when viewed radiographically; however, any cemental layer(s) near the CEJ may not be viewable on radiographs due to its thinness.

DEVELOPMENT OF CEMENTUM

Cementum, which develops from the **dental sac**, forms on the root after the disintegration of **Hertwig's epithelial root sheath** (see Figure 6-20). This disintegration allows the undifferentiated cells of the dental sac to come into contact with the newly formed surface of root dentin, inducing these cells to become **cementoblasts**. The cementoblasts then disperse to cover the root dentin area and undergo **cementogenesis**, laying down **cementoid**. Unlike ameloblasts and odontoblasts, which leave no cellular bodies in their secreted products, during the later steps within the stage of apposition, many of the cementoblasts become entrapped by the cementum they produce, becoming **cementocytes** (Figure 14-7). Thus again, cementum is more similar to alveolar bone, with its osteoblasts becoming entrapped osteocytes.

When the cementoid reaches the full thickness needed, the cementoid surrounding the cementocytes becomes mineralized, or matured, and is then considered cementum. Because of the apposition of cementum over the dentin, the **dentinocemental junction (DCJ)** is formed. This interface is not as defined, either clinically or histologically, as that of the dentinoenamel junction, given that cementum and dentin are of common embryological background, unlike that of enamel and dentin.

MICROSCOPIC APPEARANCE OF CEMENTUM

Cementum is composed of a mineralized fibrous matrix and cells (see Figures 14-2 and 14-11). The fibrous matrix consists of both Sharpey's fibers and intrinsic nonperiodontal fibers. Sharpey's fibers are a part of the **collagen fibers** from the **periodontal ligament** that are each partially inserted into the outer part of the cementum at 90 degrees, or at a right angle, to the cemental surface (as well as the alveolar bone on their other end) as they are inserted on the other end, the alveolar bone. These fibers are organized to function as a ligament between the tooth and alveolar bone. The intrinsic nonperiodontal ligament fibers of the cementum are collagen fibers made by the cementoblasts

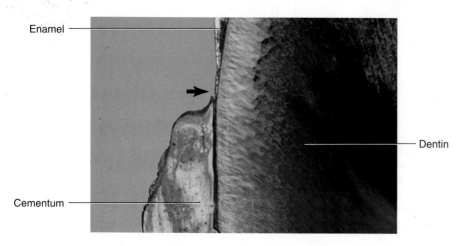

Enamel

Dentin

Cementum

FIGURE 14-3 Phase-contrast image of the cementoenamel junction interface where cementum and enamel do not meet, leaving a gap where dentin is exposed (*arrow*), which may lead to dentinal hypersensitivity. *(Courtesy P. Tambasco de Oliveira. From Nanci A: Ten Cate's Oral Histology, ed 7, Mosby, St Louis, 2008.)*

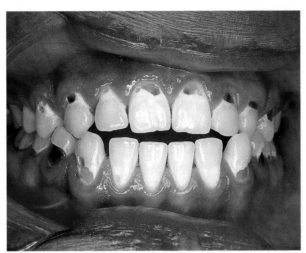

FIGURE 14-4 Cemental caries with some invasion into the adjacent dentin. Pulpal involvement is a late finding due to the initial shallowness of the lesions.

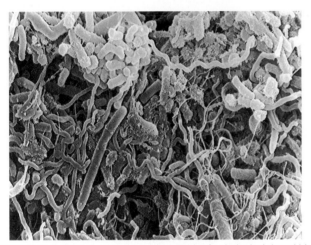

FIGURE 14-5 Scanning electron micrograph of subgingival dental biofilm on the cemental root surface in a deep periodontal pocket. *(Courtesy of Jan Cope, RDH, MS, Associate Professor, Oregon Institute of Technology, Klamath Falls, OR.)*

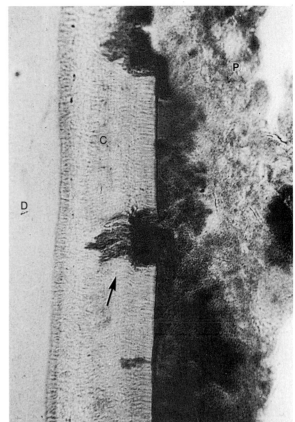

FIGURE 14-6 Calculus *(arrow)* embedded within the cementum *(C)* that overlies the dentin *(D)*. Note that dental biofilm or plaque *(P)* then overlies the rough calculus. Many times the calculus on the root is more mineralized than the cementum or even dentin. *(From Newman MG, Takei HH, Carranza FA: Clinical Periodontology, ed 10, WB Saunders, Philadelphia, 2006.)*

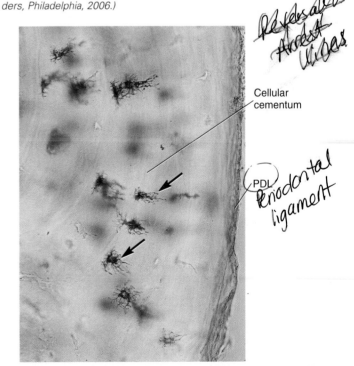

FIGURE 14-7 Microscopic appearance of cellular cementum with its cementocytes within their lacunae *(arrows)*, and the canaliculi oriented toward the periodontal ligament *(PDL)* for nutrition. *(Courtesy of James McIntosh, PhD, Assistant Professor Emeritus, Department of Biomedical Sciences, Baylor College of Dentistry, Dallas, TX.)*

and laid down in a nonorganized pattern, yet all these fibers still run parallel to the DCJ.

The cells of cementum are the entrapped cementoblasts, the cementocytes (see Figure 14-7). Each cementocyte lies in its **lacuna** (plural, **lacunae**), similar to the pattern noted in bone. These lacunae also have **canaliculi** or canals. Unlike those in bone, however, these canals in cementum do not contain nerves, nor do they radiate outward. Instead, the canals are oriented toward the periodontal ligament and contain cementocytic processes that exist to diffuse nutrients from the ligament because it is vascularized.

After the apposition of cementum in layers, the cementoblasts that do not become entrapped in cementum line up along the cemental surface along the length of the outer covering of the periodontal ligament. These cementoblasts can form subsequent layers of cementum if the tooth is injured (discussed later).

Three possible types of transitional interfaces may be present at the **CEJ.** The traditional view was that certain interfaces dominated in certain oral cavities. Studies with the scanning electron microscope indicate that the CEJ may exhibit all of these interfaces in an individual's oral cavity, and there is even considerable variation when one tooth is traced circumferentially (Figure 14-8; see Figure 14-3). In some cases,

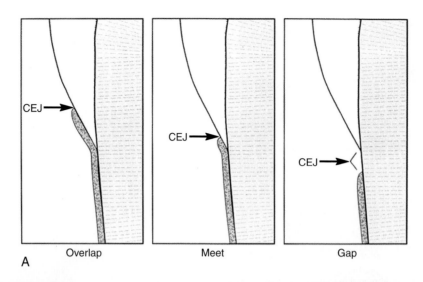

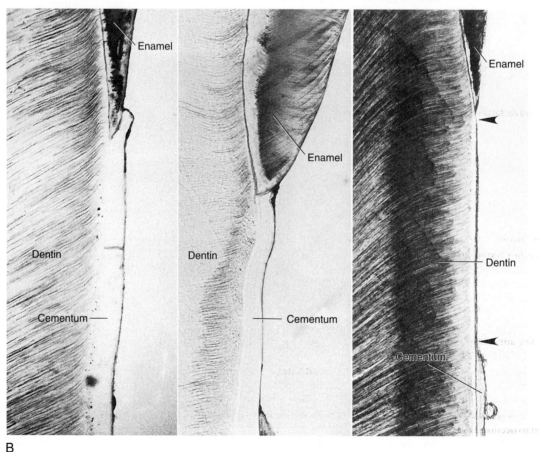

FIGURE 14-8 Three interfaces (*OMG*, or overlap, meet, gap) present at the cementoenamel junction (*CEJ*) throughout an individual's dentition, as well as points along the way *(arrows)*. **A:** Cementum may overlap enamel *(O)*; may meet end-to-end *(M)*; may be a gap between enamel and cementum, leaving dentin exposed *(G)*. **B:** Ground sections of the same three interfaces, with gap exposing dentin highlighted in last section *(arrows)*. *(From Nanci A: Ten Cate's Oral Histology, ed 7, Mosby, St Louis, 2008.)*

the cementum may overlap the enamel at the CEJ (but thankfully fewer times than previously thought) at less than 15%. Novice clinicians may have difficulty discerning the CEJ from calculus deposits around the cervix with this situation. However, compared with the usually spotty placement and roughness of calculus, cementum exhibits a more uniform placement and roughness when using an explorer.

Another possible interface that can occur the CEJ is that the cementum and enamel may meet end to end, presenting no

problems for either the clinician or patient, and it is the most common finding at about 52% of cases. Finally, another possible interface at the CEJ is that a gap may exist between the cementum and enamel, exposing dentin in about 33% of cases (see Figure 14-8). Thus, patients may experience **dentinal hypersensitivity** (see Figure 13-9).

Similar to bone tissue such as alveolar bone, cementum can undergo removal within the tissue as a result of trauma (Figure 14-9).

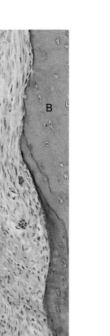

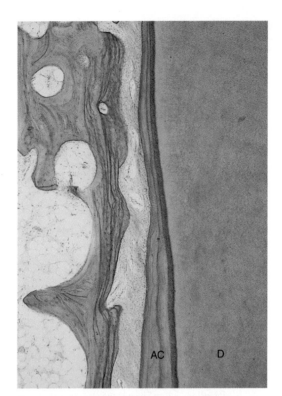

FIGURE 14-9 Reversal lines and arrest lines in cementum with embedded cementocytes (*white arrows*) that has undergone repair due to severe trauma. On the surface of the cementum are the cementoblasts (*dark arrows*) within the surrounding periodontal ligament (*P*). Note that the alveolar bone (*B*) has similar lines noted as a result of bone remodeling. *(Courtesy of James McIntosh, PhD, Assistant Professor Emeritus, Department of Biomedical Sciences, Baylor College of Dentistry, Dallas, TX.)*

This removal involves resorption of cementum by the **odontoclast**, resulting in **reversal lines.** When viewed in a stained section of cementum, these reversal lines appear as scalloped lines, just as in bone. However, cementum is less readily resorbed than bone, an important consideration during orthodontic tooth movement (discussed later).

At the same time, there can be repair of traumatic resorption area by involving the **apposition** of cementum by cementoblasts in the adjacent periodontal ligament. Apposition of this recently formed protective cementum is noted by layers of growth, or **arrest lines,** which, when viewed in a stained section, look like smooth growth rings in a section of a tree similar to what occurs in bone tissue such as alveolar bone. Both reversal and arrest lines are prominent in cementum subjected to **occlusal trauma** or to orthodontic tooth movement, as well as during the shedding of primary teeth and eruption of the permanent tooth. However, unlike bone, cementum does not continually undergo remodeling or repair as part of its makeup, but only when severely traumatized.

TYPES OF CEMENTUM

Two basic types of cementum are formed by cementoblasts: acellular and cellular (Figure 14-10 and Table 14-1). **Acellular cementum** consists of the first layers of cementum deposited at the DCJ, and thus is also considered *primary cementum*. It is formed at a slower rate than other types and contains no embedded cementocytes. At least one layer of acellular cementum covers the entire outer surface of each root with many more layers covering the cervical one third near

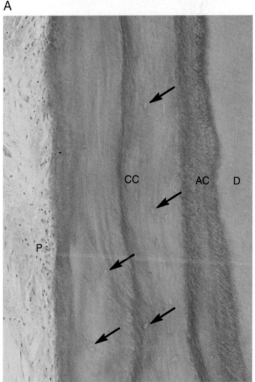

FIGURE 14-10 Two types of cementum on the root surface. **A:** Acellular cementum (*AC*) without cementocytes makes up the first layers deposited at the dentinocemental junction over the dentin (*D*). **B:** Cellular cementum, (*CC*) which contains embedded cementocytes, (*arrows*) are the last layers deposited over the thin layer of acellular cementum (*AC*) adjacent to the dentin (*D*). Cells adjacent to the periodontal ligament (*P*) are cementoblasts. *(Courtesy of James McIntosh, PhD, Assistant Professor Emeritus, Department of Biomedical Sciences, Baylor College of Dentistry, Dallas, TX.)*

TABLE 14-1	Comparison of Two Types of Cementum	
ACELLULAR	**CELLULAR**
First layer(s) deposited	Formed after acellular layer(s)
At least one layer over all of the root, with many layers near cervical one third	Layered over acellular, mainly in apical one third, especially interradicular region
Formed at a slower rate	Formed at a faster rate
No embedded cementocytes	Embedded cementocytes
Width constant over time	Layers sometimes added over time

Clinical Considerations about Cemental Formation

Cementicles are mineralized bodies of cementum found either attached to the cemental root surface or lying free in the periodontal ligament (see Figure 14-11). They form from the apposition of **cementum** around cellular debris in the **periodontal ligament (PDL)**, possibly as a result of microtrauma to **Sharpey's fibers**. They become attached or fused from the continued apposition of cementum, and thus may interfere with periodontal treatment, as well as being noted on radiographs.

Cemental spurs can be found at or near the CEJ. These are symmetrical spheres of cementum attached to the cemental root surface, similar to enamel pearls. Cemental spurs result from irregular deposition of cementum on the root. They can present some clinical problems in differentiation from calculus and may be noted on radiographs; yet, because they are hard dental tissue, they are not easily removed, and thus may also interfere with periodontal treatment.

Hypercementosis is the excessive production of **cellular cementum**, which mainly occurs at the apex or apices of the tooth (Figure 14-12). It may be noted on radiographs as a radiopaque (or lighter) mass at each root apex. This condition can result from **occlusal trauma** caused by occlusal forces and during certain pathological conditions (at a generalized level as noted with Paget's disease), such as chronic periapical inflammation. It may also be a compensatory mechanism in response to attrition to increase occlusal tooth height. However, such deposits form bulbous enlargements on the roots and may interfere with extractions, especially if adjacent teeth become fused (concrescence). It may also result in pulpal necrosis by blocking blood supply via the apical foramen (see **Chapter 13**).

In contrast, an unwanted side effect of orthodontic therapy is root apex resorption, reducing the overall length of the tooth, which is especially noted with permanent maxillary incisors (discussed later). The risk of tooth mobility is also increased. However, with new bioefficient orthodontic therapy being utilized, this effect has been minimized.

the CEJ (see Figure 14-3). The width of acellular cementum never changes.

The other type of cementum is cellular cementum, sometimes called *secondary cementum* because it is deposited later than primary type (Figure 14-11; see Figure 14-6). Cellular cementum consists of the last layers of cementum deposited over the acellular cementum, mainly in the apical one third of each root. It is formed at a faster rate than acellular type, catching the cementoblasts during production, and thus many embedded **cementocytes** are found within it. Lining

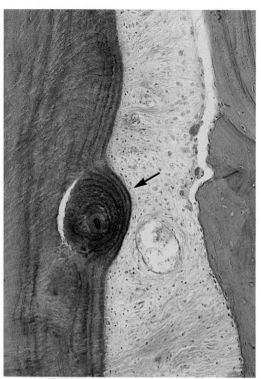

FIGURE 14-11 Cementicle attached to the cemental surface within the periodontal ligament (*arrow*). *(Courtesy of James McIntosh, PhD, Assistant Professor Emeritus, Department of Biomedical Sciences, Baylor College of Dentistry, Dallas, TX.)*

up at its periphery are cementoblasts located in the periodontal ligament, which allow the future production of more cellular cementum, if needed.

Thus, the width of cellular cementum can change during the life of the tooth, especially at the apex or apices of the tooth (discussed next). This type of cementum is especially common in interradicular areas. It is important to note that Sharpey's fibers in acellular cementum are fully mineralized; those in cellular cementum are generally mineralized only partially at their periphery.

ALVEOLAR BONE

The **alveolar bone** is that part of either the **maxilla** or **mandible** that supports and protects the teeth. The alveolar bone is also that part of the periodontium in which the cementum of the tooth is attached to it through the PDL (Figure 14-13). The alveolar bone is a hard, mineralized tissue with all the components of other bone tissue (see Figure 8-9). It is important to note that alveolar bone is more easily remodeled than cementum, thus allowing orthodontic tooth movement (discussed later). When viewing a stained histological section, the remodeled alveolar bone shows **arrest lines** and **reversal lines**, as does all bone tissue.

Like all bone, mature alveolar bone is by weight 60% mineralized or inorganic material, 25% organic material, and 15% water. This crystalline formation consists of mainly **calcium hydroxyapatite** with the chemical formula of $Ca_{10}(PO_4)_6(OH)_2$. This calcium hydroxyapatite is similar to that found in higher percentages in both enamel and dentin, but is most similar to the levels in cementum (see Table 6-2). The minerals of potassium, manganese, magnesium, silica, iron, zinc, selenium, boron, phosphorus, sulfur, chromium, and others are also present but in smaller amounts.

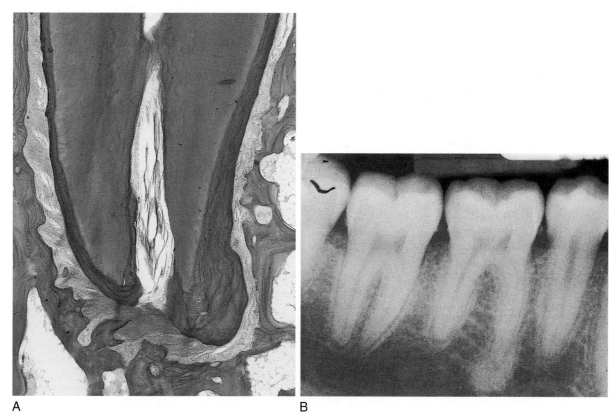

A   B

FIGURE 14-12 Hypercementosis at the root apices due to traumatic occlusal forces on mandibular molar teeth. **A:** Microscopic view with dentin (*D*), cementum (*C*), and radicular pulp tissue (*P*). **B:** Radiograph. (**A** *courtesy of James McIntosh, PhD, Assistant Professor Emeritus, Department of Biomedical Sciences, Baylor College of Dentistry, Dallas, TX.*)

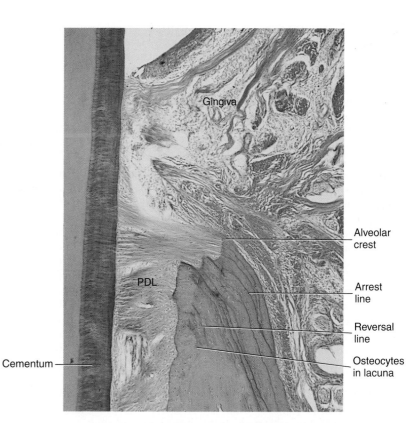

FIGURE 14-13 Alveolar bone with its microscopic components is identified, including arrest and reversal lines. Note that there has been a slight resorption of the alveolar crest showing the beginning of periodontal disease. (*Courtesy of James McIntosh, PhD, Assistant Professor Emeritus, Department of Biomedical Sciences, Baylor College of Dentistry, Dallas, TX.*)

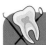

With orthodontic therapy to produce tooth movement for repositioning, bone remodeling is forced (Figure 14-14). The bands, wires, or appliances put pressure on one side of the tooth and adjacent alveolar bone, creating a *compression zone* in the PDL. This compression in the PDL leads to bone resorption. On the opposite side of the tooth and bone, a *tension zone* develops in the PDL and causes the deposition of new bone. Thus, the tooth or teeth are slowly moved along the jaw so as to achieve a dentition that works in harmony (see **Chapter 20**). In this way, the width of the space between the alveoli and the root is kept about the same.

Mesial drift, or physiological drift, is a normal, natural movement phenomenon in which all the teeth move slightly toward the midline of the oral cavity over time (see Figure 20-21). This can cause crowding late in life of a once-perfect dentition. It occurs quite slowly, depending mostly on the degree of wear of the contact points between adjacent teeth and on the number of missing teeth. Overall, amounts may total no more than 1 cm over a lifetime. However, this crowding may lead to poor homecare.

Either occlusal drift or supereruption can also occur, especially with the posterior teeth (see Figures 17-43 and 17-55). The exact mechanism that causes drifting of the dentition is still controversial; it may be an adjustment process to retain balance among the various components of the masticatory apparatus, or may just be related to the wear of the proximal and occlusal tooth surfaces.

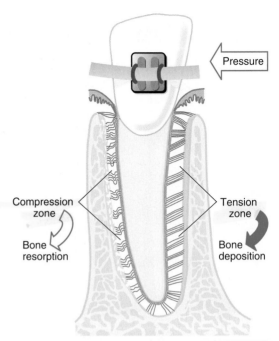

FIGURE 14-14 Process of tooth movement during orthodontic therapy. Appliances put pressure on one side, creating a zone of compression in the periodontal ligament on the opposite side, which leads to bone resorption. On the same side, a zone of tension develops causing deposition of new bone. Thus, the tooth or teeth are slowly moved along the jaw.

ANATOMY OF THE JAWS

Each mature jaw, either the **maxilla** or **mandible**, is composed of two types of bone tissue with differing physiological functioning (discussed later; Figure 14-15). The part that contains the roots of the teeth is the **alveolar bone** (also called the alveolar process or alveolar ridge). The part apical to the roots of the teeth is the basal bone, which then forms the **body of the maxilla** or **body of the mandible**. Both the alveolar bone and basal bone are covered by **periosteum**.

The alveolar bone is divided into the alveolar bone proper and the supporting alveolar bone. Microscopically, both the alveolar bone proper and the supporting alveolar bone have the same components: fibers, cells, intercellular substances, nerves, blood vessels, and lymphatics (see Chapter 8; see Figure 14-13).

The alveolar bone proper is the lining of the tooth socket or **alveolus** (plural, **alveoli**) (see Figure 14-15). Although the alveolar bone proper is composed of **compact bone**, it may be called the *cribriform plate* because it contains numerous holes where **Volkmann's canals** pass from the alveolar bone into the PDL. The alveolar bone proper is also called *bundle bone* because **Sharpey's fibers**, a part of the fibers of the PDL, are inserted here. Similar to those of the cemental surface, Sharpey's fibers in alveolar bone proper are each inserted at 90 degrees, or at a right angle, but are fewer in number, although thicker in diameter than those present in cementum (Figure 14-16). As in cellular cementum, Sharpey's fibers in bone are generally mineralized only partially at their periphery.

The alveolar bone proper consists of plates of **compact bone** that surround the tooth and assume the shape of the tooth. The alveolar bone proper varies in thickness from 0.1 to 0.5 mm. The **lamina propria** of the **attached gingiva** serves as a **mucoperiosteum** for the alveolar bone proper (see Chapter 9). A part of the alveolar bone proper is seen on radiographs as the lamina dura, which is

uniformly radiopaque (or lighter) (Figure 14-17). Integrity of the lamina dura is important when studying radiographs for pathological lesions.

The alveolar crest is the most cervical rim of the alveolar bone proper (Figure 14-18). In a healthy situation, the alveolar crest is slightly apical to the CEJ by approximately 1 to 2 mm. The alveolar crests of neighboring teeth are also uniform in height along the jaw.

A part of the alveolar crest that is between neighboring teeth is seen on radiographs as a radiopaque (or lighter) triangle at the most superior part of the interdental septum or bone (see Figure 14-17). It can be used for educating patients about bone loss levels in periodontal disease; however, it shows only the levels of alveolar bone proper interproximally. In reality, bone loss can occur at any surface of the tooth and in varying amounts around the tooth.

The **supporting alveolar bone** consists of both cortical bone and trabecular bone. The cortical bone, or cortical plates, consists of plates of **compact bone** on the facial and lingual surfaces of the alveolar bone (see Figure 14-15). These cortical plates are usually about 1.5 to 3 mm thick over posterior teeth, but the thickness is highly variable around anterior teeth. The cortical bone is not visible on periapical or bite-wing radiographs but only on occlusal radiographs as a uniformly radiopaque (or lighter) plate, facial and lingual to the teeth (see Figure 14-17).

The trabecular bone consists of **cancellous bone** that is located between the alveolar bone proper and the plates of cortical bone (see Figure 14-15). Only the parts of trabecular bone between the teeth and between the roots are ever seen on any type of radiographs, and this trabecular bone appears less uniformly radiopaque or spongy than the uniformly radiopaque lamina dura of the alveolar bone proper.

The alveolar bone between two neighboring teeth is the interdental septum (or interdental bone) (Figure 14-19). It is easily seen on both periapical and bite-wing radiographs (see Figure 14-17). The interdental septum consists of both the compact bone of the alveolar

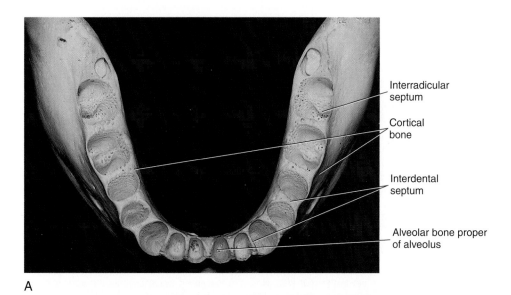

A

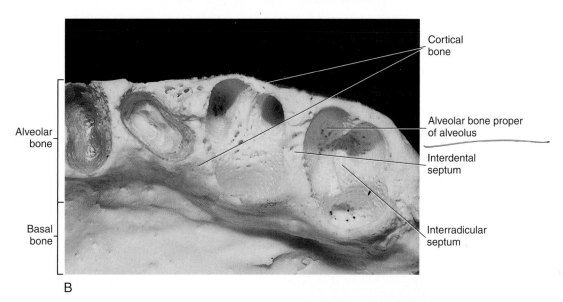

B

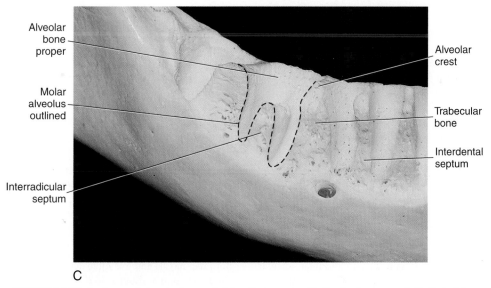

C

FIGURE 14-15 Anatomy of alveolar bone. **A:** Mandibular arch with the teeth removed. **B:** Part of the maxilla with the teeth removed. **C:** Cross section of the mandible with the teeth removed and a molar alveolus highlighted (*dashed lines*).

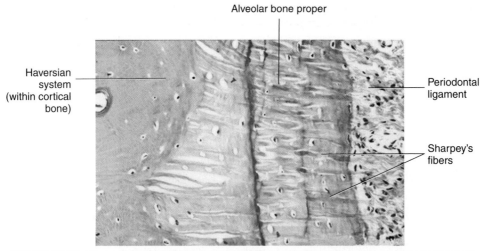

FIGURE 14-16 Microscopic view of the insertion of Sharpey's fibers from the periodontal ligament into the alveolar bone proper in the root area. Note the Haversian system within the cortical bone. *(From Nanci A: Ten Cate's Oral Histology, ed 7, Mosby, St Louis, 2008.)*

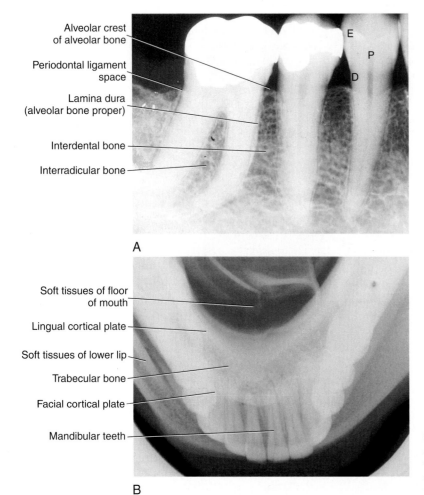

FIGURE 14-17 Radiographs with the anatomy of the alveolar bone of the mandible identified, as well as tooth components for radiographic contrast: enamel *(E)*, dentin *(D)*, and pulp *(P)*. **A:** Periapical radiograph. **B:** Occlusal radiograph.

bone proper and cancellous bone of the trabecular bone. The alveolar bone between the roots of the same tooth is the interradicular septum (or interradicular bone) (Figure 14-20). The interradicular septum consists of both alveolar bone proper and trabecular bone; however, only a part of the interradicular septum is ever seen on periapical or bite-wing radiographs (see Figure 14-17).

DEVELOPMENT OF THE JAWS

Both the maxilla and mandible develop from tissue of the **first branchial arch**, or **mandibular arch**. The maxilla forms within the **maxillary process**, and the mandible forms within the fused mandibular processes of the mandibular arch. Both jaws start as small centers of **intramembranous ossification** located around the **stomodeum**. These centers then increase in diameter, growing into the mature jaws (see Chapter 8.) Both jaws also have several skeletal units during their development, and these are related to the overall morphology, or form, of the bones. Each of these units is influenced in its growth pattern by some adjacent structure that acts on the developing bone.

Development of the Maxilla   The maxilla's primary center of intramembranous ossification for each half of the maxilla appears around the seventh week of prenatal development. It is located at the termination of the infraorbital nerve, just superior to the dental lamina of the primary maxillary canine tooth, in each maxillary process. Secondary ossification centers, the zygomatic, orbitonasal, nasopalatine, and intermaxillary, then appear and fuse rapidly with the primary centers. The two intermaxillary centers generate the alveolar ridge and primary palate region.

The subsequent growth of the maxilla can be subdivided into several skeletal units: the basal body unit, which develops beneath the infraorbital nerve, surrounding it to form the infraorbital canal;

Clinical Considerations with Alveolar Bone Anatomy

After extraction of a tooth, the clot in the alveolus fills in with immature bone, which later is remodeled into mature secondary bone. However, with the loss of teeth, a patient becomes **edentulous,** either partially or completely, and the **alveolar bone** undergoes resorption (Figure 14-21). The underlying **basal bone** of the body of the maxilla or mandible remains less affected, however, because it does not need the presence of teeth to remain viable.

Thus, the alveolar bone depends on the functional stimulation from teeth during mastication and speech for preservation of its structure. Resorption of the alveolar bone can be complicated in postmenopausal women, who experience a shortage of estrogen, which normally helps maintain bone density, and the loss of which may lead to the onset of osteoporosis. The placement of a denture, either partial or full, or a bridge can somewhat mimic the stimulation of the teeth in the alveolar bone. Over time, however, some amounts of bone are lost even with these types of tooth replacements, especially if the prosthesis produces excessive compression of the underlying bone. Loss of bone also accompanies clinical conditions, where blood supply is compromised and hypoxia (reduced oxygen) occurs, such as following inflammation, radiation damage, fracture, and aging.

The loss of alveolar bone, coupled with attrition of the teeth, causes a loss of height of the lower third of the **vertical dimension of the face** when the teeth are in maximum intercuspation (Figure 14-22; see Figures 1-3 and 1-10, **Chapter 20**). The extent of this loss is determined based on clinical judgment using the **Golden Proportions**. This part of the vertical dimension is important in determining the way in which the teeth and jaws function. In addition, a proper amount of height in the lower third of the face reduces the amount of facial wrinkles around the mouth as the skin ages, sags, and loses its resilience. With the loss of vertical dimension in the lower third, older patients can take on a cartoon "Popeye" facial appearance that is aesthetically displeasing and results in poor functioning of the teeth and jaws.

Ideally, an implant placed in an edentulous area preserves the integrity of the bone and serves as a permanent replacement for a lost tooth or teeth, preventing loss of vertical dimension (Figure 14-23). An implant has a core part made of titanium that is surgically implanted in the alveolar bone of either jaw. The high success rate of these current implants has now been demonstrated.

The deeper part of this surgical part of the implant has an open structure, allowing bone to bond to it, undergoing osseointegration of the implant to the surrounding alveolar bone. However, unlike teeth with a fibrous insertion of the PDL into the alveolar bone, an implant has no movement. An implant makes direct contact with the alveolar bone, as well as with the surrounding connective tissue and superficial epithelium, the *periimplant tissue*. Research has shown that a sulcular epithelium that consists of the circular fibers of the PDL surrounds and is also attached to the superior part of the implant by hemidesmosomes in tissue that structurally resembles a junctional epithelium. After osseointegration and healing of the tissue, a prosthetic superstructure of a tooth or denture is then attached to the surgical part of the implant.

Studies have shown that failure to obtain and maintain this cellular junction may lead to apical migration of the epithelium to the bone–implant interface, possible soft tissue encapsulation of the implant, and eventual implant failure resulting from mobility. Thus, special devices are needed for professional and homecare of an implant's superstructure to remove any deposits and prevent periimplant disease, especially because many patients with implants have a history of inadequate homecare.

Now placement of an immediate load implant upon extraction of non-infected tooth or teeth is available. For this placement to be considered successful adequate bone must exist and a sufficiently large implant must be placed; once placed, the implant must be able to resist occlusal forces. The temporary crown must be adjusted so that no forces are placed on it during function. Meeting these criteria allows osseointegration. After a period of 9 weeks, a permanent crown can be placed, shortening treatment time by 4 to 6 months.

During chronic periodontal disease that has affected the periodontium (**periodontitis**), localized bone tissue is also lost (Figure 14-24). This bone loss may be due to the overresponse of the immune system and the activation of certain osteoclast populations; among the bioactive agents implicated are cytokines and prostaglandins. This bone loss is first evident in the **alveolar crest,** which looks moth-eaten microscopically and radiographically (see Figure 14-13). The bone loss slowly continues down the alveolar bone; thus, the tooth becomes increasingly mobile, increasing the possibility of tooth loss. Prevention of further loss of bone, and thus control of the periodontal disease, is paramount in the dental treatment plan for these patients and may include removal of deposits, use of antibiotics, and irrigation.

Bone grafting may be included during periodontal surgery, sourced from either the oral cavity or from other sources, possibly with the use of guided tissue regeneration (GTR) membrane. GTR are surgical procedures that utilize barrier membranes to direct the growth of new bone and soft tissue at sites having insufficient volumes or dimensions for proper function, esthetics, or prosthetic restoration. GTR is based on the long-recognized concept that fibroblasts from the periodontal ligament or undifferentiated **mesenchyme** have the potential to re-create the original periodontal attachment. Using GTR to treat narrow intrabony defects and class II mandibular furcations has been very successful, as well as its use to support new bone growth on an alveolar ridge so as to allow stable placement of dental implant. However, GFR offers limited benefits in the treatment of other types of periodontal defects. Bone repair is also being enhanced by the use of platelet-rich plasma (PRP) in alveoli with bone defects and with implant placement. Treatments similar to those for osteoporosis may be used in the future.

The density of the alveolar bone in a given area also determines the route that dental infection takes with abscess formation, as well as the efficacy of local infiltration during the use of local anesthesia. In addition, the differences in alveolar process density determine the easiest and most convenient areas of bony fracture to be used, if needed during tooth extraction of impacted teeth (see Figure 17-62).

the orbital unit, which responds to the growth of the eyeball; the nasal unit, which depends on nasal septal cartilage for its growth; the alveolar unit, which forms in response to the maxillary teeth; and the pneumatic unit, which reflects maxillary sinus expansion. The primary bone initially formed in the maxilla is soon replaced by secondary bone as the face and oral cavity develop.

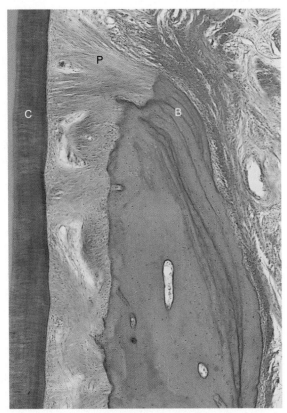

FIGURE 14-18 Photomicrograph of the alveolar crest of the alveolar bone proper (*B*) and its relationship to the root covered by cementum (*C*), with the alveolar crest fibers of the periodontal ligament (*P*) inserting Sharpey's fibers into both tissue types. Note there is some resorption of the alveolar crest showing the beginning of periodontal disease. *(Courtesy of James McIntosh, PhD, Assistant Professor Emeritus, Department of Biomedical Sciences, Baylor College of Dentistry, Dallas, TX.)*

Development of the Mandible   During the sixth week of prenatal development, on each side of the embryo's mandibular arch, a primary ossification center appears in the angle formed by the division of the inferior alveolar nerve and its incisive and mental branches, on the lateral aspect of Meckel's cartilage or the first branchial arch cartilage (see Figures 4-11 and 5-11).

In the seventh week, the first bone tissue in the body of the mandible forms. Bone formation spreads rapidly from the angle anterior to the midline. The anterior bone forms around Meckel's cartilage to produce a trough with medial and lateral plates that unite inferiorly around the incisive nerve. This trough extends to the midline on the embryo, where it comes into close approximation with a similar trough from the other side.

These two separate bilateral centers of ossification of the mandibular arch remain separated at the mandibular symphysis until shortly after birth. The trough turns into the mandibular canal as bone is formed over the incisive nerve joining the lateral and medial plates of initial bone.

Bone formation in the mandibular arch also spreads posteriorly toward the point where the mandibular nerve is divided into its lingual and inferior alveolar branches. This ossification initially forms a gutter, which later evolves into a canal that contains the inferior alveolar nerve.

The mandible subsequently develops as several skeletal units: a condylar unit that forms the articulation with the temporal bone; the body of the mandible, which is the center of all growth of the mandible; the angular unit, which forms in response to the lateral pterygoid and masseter muscles; the coronoid unit, which forms in response to the temporalis muscle development; and the alveolar unit, which forms in response to the mandibular teeth.

Almost all of Meckel's cartilage disappears as the mandible develops. The primary bone formed along Meckel's cartilage is soon replaced by secondary bone. Secondary cartilage appears between the tenth and fourteenth weeks of prenatal development to form the head of the condyle, part of the coronoid process, and the mental protuberance. Separate from Meckel's cartilage, the coronoid cartilage becomes incorporated into the expanding intramembranous bone of the ramus and disappears before birth. In the mental region, a similar situation occurs as the cartilage there disappears when the mandibular processes fuse.

The condylar cartilage appears initially as a cone-shaped structure and is the primordium of the condyle. Chondrocytes differentiate in

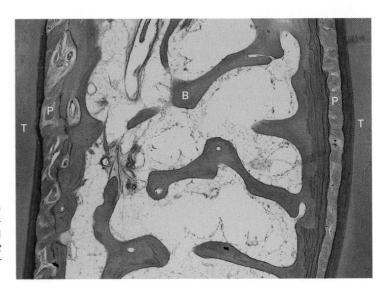

FIGURE 14-19 Microscopic view of interdental septum or bone (*B*) found between the roots of two neighboring teeth (*T*) and surrounded on each side by the horizontal group of the periodontal ligament (*P*). *(Courtesy of James McIntosh, PhD, Assistant Professor Emeritus, Department of Biomedical Sciences, Baylor College of Dentistry, Dallas, TX.)*

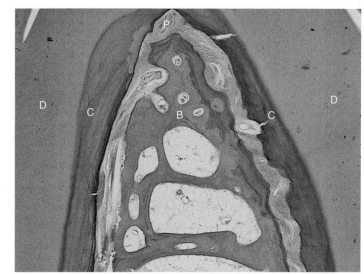

FIGURE 14-20 Microscopic view of interradicular septum or bone between two roots (*B*) of a mandibular molar and surrounded on each side by the interradicular group of the periodontal ligament (*P*). Its roots are composed of dentin (*D*) and cementum (*C*). *(Courtesy of James McIntosh, PhD, Assistant Professor Emeritus, Department of Biomedical Sciences, Baylor College of Dentistry, Dallas, TX.)*

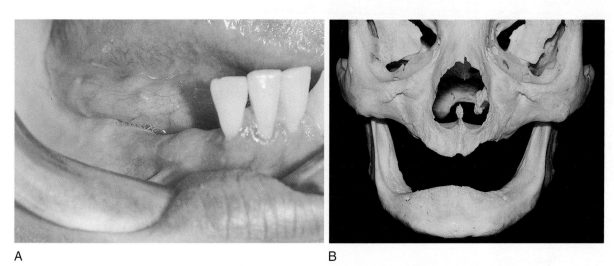

A   B

FIGURE 14-21 Edentulous states with resultant changes in alveolar bone. **A:** Partially edentulous case from the extraction of the posterior teeth, with loss of the alveolar bone of the posterior alveolar ridge of the mandible and only the basal bone remaining. **B:** Complete case from a full mouth extraction of the teeth with the bone loss of both the alveolar ridges and only basal bone remaining.

FIGURE 14-22 Loss of vertical dimension in the inferior third of the face in twenty year increments (age 20, age 40, and age 60) as the alveolar bone is lost. The teeth have also undergone a reduction in height by slight attrition, the mechanical wear of the masticatory surface. Note the increase in wrinkles and lines around the mouth caused by these oral changes. This amount can be dramatically increased with tooth loss, severe periodontal disease, or increased levels of attrition.

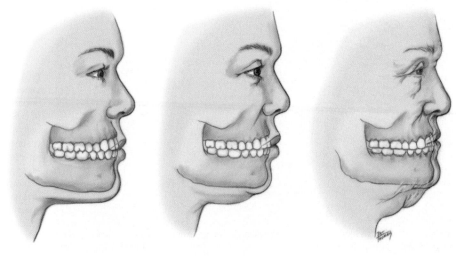

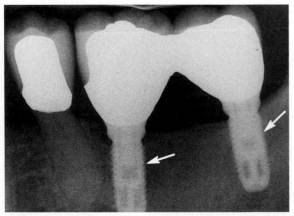

FIGURE 14-23 Radiograph of the implants in the mandible that have successfully undergone osseointegration of the titanium device (*arrows*). *(Courtesy of Dr. William Schmidt, DMD, MSD, Specialist in Prosthodontics and Implants, Seattle, WA.)*

the center and increase by interstitial and appositional growth (see Chapter 8). By the middle of fetal life, most of the condylar cartilage is replaced with bone as a result of endochondral ossification, but its superior end persists into puberty. Thus, the condylar cartilage acts as a growth center for the temporomandibular joint (see Chapter 8 and Figures 8-13 and 19-4).

Developmental Disturbances with Alveolar Bone

The developmental dental anomaly of **anodontia,** in which tooth germs are congenitally absent, may affect the development of the alveolar processes (see Table 6-3, *A*). This occurrence can prevent the **alveolar processes** of either the **maxilla** or the **mandible** from developing. Proper development is impossible because the alveolar unit of each **dental arch** must form in response to the **tooth germs** in the area.

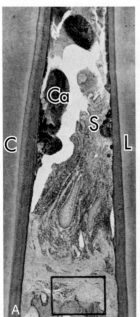

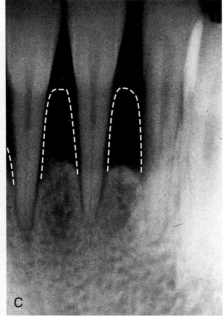

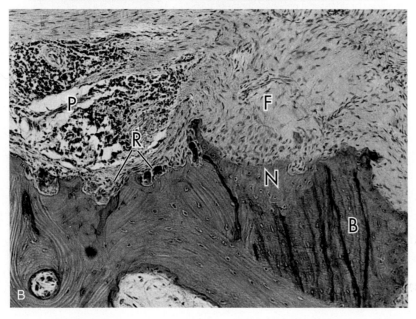

FIGURE 14-24 Bone loss caused by chronic periodontal disease or periodontitis. **A:** Microscopic view of periodontitis between a lateral incisor (*L*) and canine (*C*), showing calculus (*Ca*) and a periodontal pocket with suppuration (*S*). **B:** Close-up view showing bone resorption (*R*) from osteoclast activity beneath the inflammation in the periodontal ligament (*P*); areas of fibrosis (*F*) are also noted in reaction. **C:** Radiograph showing severe bone loss from previously health levels (*outline*). This bone loss initially involved the alveolar crest and moved apically as the periodontal disease progressed. *(**A** and **B** from Newman MG, Takei HH, Carranza FA: Clinical Periodontology, ed 7, WB Saunders, Philadelphia, 2008.)*

PERIODONTAL LIGAMENT

The **PDL** is that part of the **periodontium** that provides for the attachment of the teeth to the surrounding alveolar bone using the **cementum** (see Figure 14-1). The PDL appears on radiographs as the periodontal ligament space, 0.4 to 1.5 mm as a radiolucent area (or darker) located between the denser radiopaque (or lighter) lamina dura of the alveolar bone proper and the similar radiopaque (or lighter) cementum (see Figure 14-17).

The PDL is an organized fibrous connective tissue that also maintains the gingiva in proper relationship to the teeth. In addition, the PDL transmits occlusal forces from the teeth to the bone, allowing for a small amount of movement and acting as a shock absorber for the soft tissue structures around the teeth, such as the nerves and blood vessels (see **Chapter 20**).

Other functions of the PDL are discussed later. These other functions include serving as the periosteum for the cementum and alveolar bone. Cells in the PDL also participate in the formation and resorption of the hard tissue of the periodontium. Additionally, it has blood vessels that provide nutrition for the cells of the ligament and surrounding cells of the cementum and alveolar bone.

Finally, the PDL and its nerve supply provide a most efficient proprioceptive mechanism, allowing us to feel even the most delicate forces applied to the teeth and any displacement of the teeth resulting from these forces (such as metal foil in candy wrappers). Unlike the soft connective tissue of the pulp, the PDL also transmits pain, touch, pressure, and temperature sensations.

Even after patients have endodontic therapy (root canal treatment), and the tooth becomes nonvital, they may feel some level of discomfort when biting down or when the clinician taps the teeth when measuring tooth percussion sensitivity. This discomfort is not due to sensations from the lost pulp tissue, but from sensations within the PDL as it receives pressure from even the slightest intrusive movements of the tooth during mastication. In fact, many times the inflammation associated with **pulpitis** travels through the apical foramen to involve the periodontium, thus causing apical inflammation and destruction. Surgery may have to be performed to remove the apical lesion (apicoectomy).

Similar to the alveolar bone, the PDL develops from the **dental sac** of the tooth germ (see Figure 6-20). Unlike other connective tissue of the periodontium, however, the PDL does not show any overwhelming changes related to aging, although it can undergo drastic changes, such as with the trauma from periodontal disease (discussed later). Guided tissue regeneration (GTR) is being used in the treatment of alveolar bone loss and disorganization of the PDL when caused by periodontal disease. This method to increase bone levels and strengthen the PDL uses a membrane of various materials that allows only osteoblasts and fibroblasts to produce either bone or PDL fibers at the diseased site. GTR is becoming even more successful because the membrane type being used results in less inflammation at the site.

COMPONENTS OF THE PERIODONTAL LIGAMENT

Because the PDL is a connective tissue, it has all the components of a connective tissue, such as intercellular substance, cells, and fibers (Figure 14-25; see **Chapter 8**). The PDL also has a vascular supply, lymphatics, and nerve supply, which enter the apical foramen of the tooth to supply the pulp (see **Chapter 13**). Two types of nerves are found within the PDL. One type is afferent (sensory), which is a myelinated nerve and transmits sensations that occur within the PDL

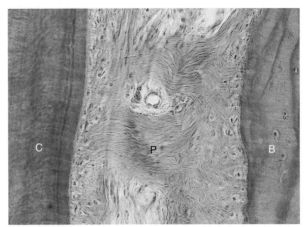

FIGURE 14-25 Microscopic view of the periodontal ligament (*P*), which is located between the alveolar bone (*B*) and cementum (*C*), inserting Sharpey's fibers into both tissue types. *(Courtesy of James McIntosh, PhD, Assistant Professor Emeritus, Department of Biomedical Sciences, Baylor College of Dentistry, Dallas, TX.)*

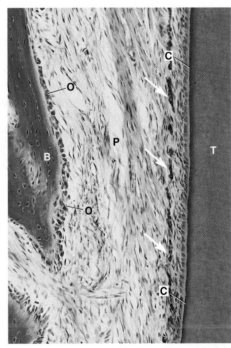

FIGURE 14-26 Microscopic view of the periodontal ligament (*P*) that includes a layer of osteoblasts (*O*) on the periphery of the alveolar bone proper (*B*), with a line of cementoblasts (*C*) on the cemental surface of the tooth (*T*). Note the epithelial rests of Malassez (*white arrows*). *(Courtesy of James McIntosh, PhD, Assistant Professor Emeritus, Department of Biomedical Sciences, Baylor College of Dentistry, Dallas, TX.)*

(as discussed earlier); the other type is an autonomic sympathetic nerve, which regulates the blood vessels.

Cells in the Periodontal Ligament The PDL has all the cells that are in most connective tissue, such as cells of **blood** and **endothelium** (Figure 14-26). However, like all connective tissue, the **fibroblast** is the most common cell in the PDL (see Figure 8-5). The PDL also has cells that are not in other connective tissue, such as a line of **cementoblasts** along the cemental surface. **Osteoblasts** are also present in the PDL at the periphery of the alveolar bone proper. In addition, the PDL has **osteoclasts** as well as **odontoclasts**. Each specific

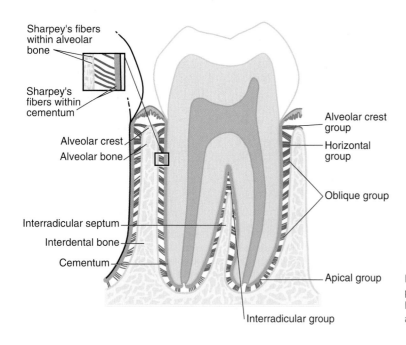

Sharpey's fibers within alveolar bone

Sharpey's fibers within cementum

Alveolar crest
Alveolar bone

Interradicular septum
Interdental bone
Cementum

Alveolar crest group

Horizontal group

Oblique group

Apical group

Interradicular group

FIGURE 14-27 Sagittal section of a multirooted tooth and periodontal ligament. Fiber subgroups of the alveolodental ligament are identified: alveolar crest, horizontal, oblique, and apical, and interradicular group.

cell type can form either cementum or bone, or even resorb the respective tissue, depending on the need of the tissue or the demands of the adjacent environment. Also present are undifferentiated mesenchymal cells, which can differentiate into any of these cells if any of these cell populations are injured. Thus, the PDL serves as a periosteum for the cementum and adjacent alveolar bone.

In addition, the **epithelial rests of Malassez are present** (see Figure 14-26). These groups of epithelial cells become located in the mature PDL after the disintegration of **Hertwig's epithelial root sheath** during the formation of the root (see Figures 6-19, 6-20).

The epithelial rests of Malassez can become cystic, usually forming nondiagnostic, radiolucent apical lesions that can be seen on radiographs. This occurs as a result of chronic periapical inflammation after **pulpitis** occurs. These cysts must be surgically removed and then observed for recurrence on follow-up visits.

FIBER GROUPS OF THE PERIODONTAL LIGAMENT

All the fibers in the PDL are collagen in structure. The PDL is wider near the apex and cervix of the tooth and narrower between the two end points of cementum and bone. Most of the fibers are principal fibers, which are not individual fibers but are organized into groups or bundles according to their orientation to the mature tooth and related function; these bundles resemble spliced ropes. Each is approximately 5 μm in diameter. Histologists refer to these groups by various names, but this text uses the most commonly used names by the dental community. Whether some nonorganized collagen fibers or secondary fibers of the PDL organize to form an indifferent or intermediate plexus remains controversial.

During mastication and speech, certain forces are exerted on a tooth, such as rotational, tilting, extrusive, or intrusive. The principal fibers of the PDL distribute these forces, protecting its soft tissue and allowing some give when they occur similar to a rubber band attached at both ends to two hard objects. The fibers can accomplish this task because the ends of each fiber are anchored within both cementum and the alveolar bone proper, or in cementum alone from adjacent roots or teeth. The ends of the principal fibers that are within either cementum or alveolar bone proper are considered **Sharpey's fibers**

(see Figure 14-16). Sharpey's fibers are each partially inserted into the hard tissue of the periodontium at 90 degrees, or at a right angle. Studies show that the fiber bundles go the length of the periodontal ligament space and then branch along the two end points of cementum and bone, increasing the strength of the ligament.

The main principal fiber group is the alveolodental ligament, which consists of five fiber subgroups: alveolar crest, horizontal, oblique, apical, and interradicular on multirooted teeth (Figure 14-27, Table 14-2). If viewed on sagittal section or from a facial or lingual view of the PDL, the fiber subgroups have different orientations from the cervix to the apex or apices. If the alveolodental ligament is viewed on cross section, the fiber subgroups appear as spokes around the tooth (Figure 14-28). Thus, the overall function of the alveolodental ligament is to resist rotational forces, or twisting of the tooth in its alveolus. Each of the five fiber subgroups also has its own specific function related to its differing orientation to the tooth.

The alveolar crest group of the alveolodental ligament is attached to the cementum just below the CEJ and runs in an inferior and outward direction to insert into the alveolar crest of the alveolar bone proper. Its function is to resist tilting, intrusive, extrusive, and rotational forces.

The horizontal group of the alveolodental ligament is just apical to the alveolar crest subgroup and runs at right angles to the long axis of the tooth from cementum to the alveolar bone proper, just inferior to its alveolar crest. Its function is to resist tilting forces, which work to force the tooth to tip mesially, distally, lingually, or facially, and to resist rotational forces.

The oblique group of the alveolodental ligament is the most numerous of the fiber subgroups and covers the apical two thirds of the root (Figure 14-29). This subgroup runs from the cementum in an oblique direction to insert into the alveolar bone proper more coronally. Its function is to resist intrusive forces, which try to push the tooth inward, as well as rotational forces.

The apical group of the alveolodental ligament radiates from cementum around the apex of the root to the surrounding alveolar bone proper at the base of the alveolus. Its function is to resist extrusive forces, which try to pull the tooth in an outward manner, and rotational forces.

The interradicular group of the alveolodental ligament is found only between the roots of **multirooted** teeth. This subgroup runs

TABLE 14-2	Fiber Subgroups of the Alveolodental Ligament	
FIBER SUBGROUPS	**LOCATION**	**FUNCTION**
Alveolar crest group	Attached to the cementum just below the cementoenamel junction and runs in an inferior and outward direction to insert into the alveolar crest of the alveolar bone proper	To resist tilting, intrusive, extrusive, and rotational forces
Horizontal group	Just apical to the alveolar crest group and runs at right angles to the long axis of the tooth from cementum to the alveolar bone proper, just inferior to its alveolar crest	To resist tilting forces and rotational forces
Oblique group	Runs from the cementum in an oblique direction to insert into the alveolar bone proper more coronally	To resist intrusive forces and rotational forces
Apical group	Radiates from cementum around the apex of the root to the surrounding alveolar bone proper at the base of the alveolus	To resist extrusive forces and rotational forces
Interradicular group (only on multirooted teeth)	Runs from the cementum of one root to the cementum of the other root(s) superficial to the interradicular septum and thus has no bony attachment superficial to the interradicular septum	To resist intrusive, extrusive, tilting, and rotational forces

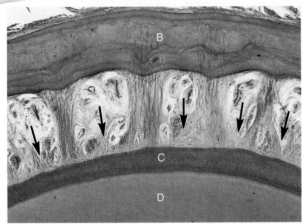

FIGURE 14-28 Microscopic view of the cross section of the tooth composed of cementum (*C*) and dentin (*D*), highlighting the spoke-like arrangement of the fibers subgroups of alveolodental ligament (*arrows*), in most cases running between the cementum and alveolar bone proper (*B*) of the surrounding alveolus. *(Courtesy of James McIntosh, PhD, Assistant Professor Emeritus, Department of Biomedical Sciences, Baylor College of Dentistry, Dallas, TX.)*

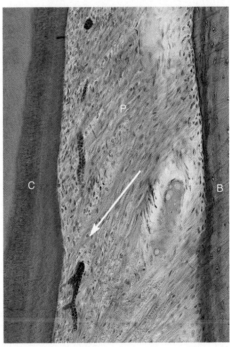

FIGURE 14-29 Photomicrograph of a tooth at the position of the oblique group of the periodontal ligament (*P*), that runs from the cementum (*C*) in an oblique direction (*arrow*) to insert more coronally into alveolar bone proper (*B*). *(Courtesy of James McIntosh, PhD, Assistant Professor Emeritus, Department of Biomedical Sciences, Baylor College of Dentistry, Dallas, TX.)*

from the cementum of one root to the cementum of the other root(s) superficial to the interradicular septum and thus has no bony attachment. This subgroup works together with the alveolar crest and apical subgroups to resist intrusive, extrusive, tilting, and rotational forces.

Another principal fiber other than the alveolodental ligament is the interdental ligament (or transseptal ligament) (Figures 14-30 and 14-31). This principal fiber inserts mesiodistally or interdentally into the cervical cementum of neighboring teeth, at a height superior to the alveolar crest of the alveolar bone proper and inferior to the base of the junctional epithelium. Thus, the fibers travel from cementum to cementum without any bony attachment, connecting all the teeth of the arch. Its function is to resist rotational forces and thus to hold the teeth in interproximal contact.

Some histologists also consider the gingival fiber group to be part of the principal fibers of the PDL (Figure 14-32). These are a separate but adjacent group that is found within the **lamina propria** of the marginal gingiva (see Figures 10-1 and 10-2). These include the fiber subgroups of both the circular and gingival ligament, as well as both the alveologingival and dentoperiosteal ligaments, but other terms may also be used. They do not support the tooth in relationship to the jaw, resisting any forces of mastication or speech; rather, they support only the marginal gingiva to maintain their relationship to the tooth.

The circular ligament encircles the tooth, as shown on a cross section of a tooth, interlacing with the other gingival fiber subgroups. Like the "pulling of the purse strings" of the gingiva, it helps to only maintain gingival integrity.

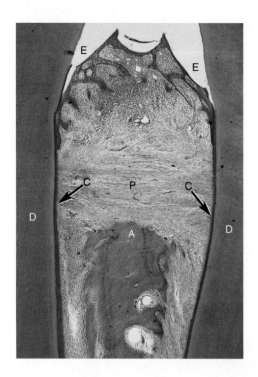

FIGURE 14-30 Microscopic view of interdental ligament of the periodontal ligament (*P*), which is located between the cementum (*C*) of two neighboring teeth with their dentin (*D*) and enamel (space, *E*) and superior to the alveolar crest (*A*). *(Courtesy of James McIntosh, PhD, Assistant Professor Emeritus, Department of Biomedical Sciences, Baylor College of Dentistry, Dallas, TX.)*

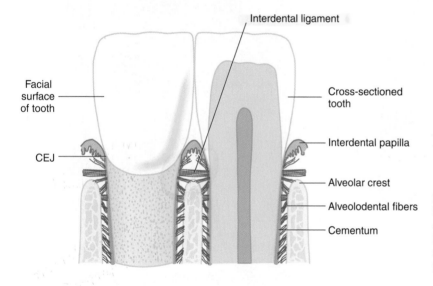

FIGURE 14-31 Diagram of interdental ligament, which inserts mesiodistally or interdentally into the cervical cementum of neighboring teeth superior to the alveolar crest of the alveolar bone proper. Its function is to resist rotational forces and thus hold the teeth in interproximal contact.

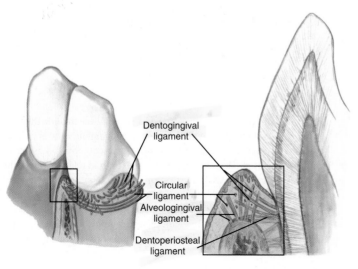

FIGURE 14-32 Fiber subgroups of the gingival fiber group: circular, dentogingival, alveologingival, and dentoperiosteal ligaments. These are located in the lamina propria of the marginal gingiva and support only the gingival tissue in order to maintain its relationship to the tooth.

The dentogingival ligament is the most extensive of the gingival fiber group. It inserts in the cementum on the root, apical to the epithelial attachment, and extends into the lamina propria of the marginal and attached gingiva. Thus, the dentogingival ligament has only one mineralized attachment to the cementum. The dentogingival ligament works with the circular ligament to maintain gingival integrity, mainly of the marginal gingiva.

The alveologingival ligament radiates from the alveolar crest of the alveolar bone proper and extend coronally into the overlying lamina propria of the marginal gingiva. It helps to attach the gingiva to the alveolar bone because of their one mineralized attachment to bone. The dentoperiosteal ligament courses from the cementum, near the CEJ, across the alveolar crest. They anchor the tooth to the bone and protect the deeper PDL.

Clinical Considerations about Periodontal Ligament Changes

It is important to note that occlusal trauma does not cause periodontal disease but can accelerate the progression of existing disease, with certain changes noted in the PDL. When traumatic forces of occlusion are placed on a tooth, the PDL widens to take the extra forces (see **Chapter 20**). Thus, early **occlusal trauma** can be viewed on radiographs as a widening of the radiolucent (or darker) **periodontal ligament space** between the radiopaque (or lighter) lamina dura of the alveolar bone proper and the similar radiopaque (or lighter) cementum (Figure 14-33). Thickening of the **lamina dura** in response is also possible. Clinically, occlusal trauma is noted by the late manifestation of increased mobility of the tooth and possibly the presence of pathological tooth migration (Figure 14-34). This migration is due to the weakened **periodontium**, when even the occlusal forces need not be abnormal if the periodontal support is reduced.

Changes can also be noted histologically in the PDL as a result of occlusal trauma: thrombosis, dilation, and edema of the blood supply; hyalinization of the collagen fibers; the presence of an inflammatory infiltrate; and nuclear changes in the osteoblasts, cementoblasts, and fibroblasts. No histological changes are noted in the gingival collagen fibers or in the adjacent junctional epithelium with occlusal trauma. Histological changes distinct from existing periodontal disease are reversible, if the causes of trauma are eliminated.

The PDL also undergoes drastic changes with chronic periodontal disease that involves the deeper structures of the periodontium (**periodontitis**). The fibers of the PDL become disorganized, and their attachments to either the alveolar bone proper or cementum through Sharpey's fibers are lost because of the resorption of these two hard dental tissue types (see Figures 14-24 and 10-10). The first fibers to be involved in changes caused by periodontal disease is the **alveolar crest group** of the alveolodental ligament, which is located at the most coronal level to the adjacent bone.

The destruction of the PDL with periodontal disease then proceeds in an apical manner, affecting (in order) the horizontal, then oblique, then apical, and then the interradicular subgroups (if present). The teeth involved in advancement of periodontal disease become increasingly mobile, moving in directions that indicate the amount and type of fiber group lost, such as buccal to lingual or with downward pressure, as the periodontal disease progresses inward to the apices of the teeth.

Thus, the principal fiber group that remains the longest in the presence of active periodontal disease, despite the previous destruction of the entire alveolodental ligament, is the **interdental ligament**. The interdental ligament reattaches itself in a more apical manner as the periodontal disease proceeds apically, so that the teeth are at least held in interproximal contact. Thus, when teeth become severely mobile interproximally, mesial to distal (after mobility in other directions is already present), the prognosis is poor because now there is destruction of the interdental ligament. Mobility and its amount and direction per tooth should be charted in the patient record to achieve an overall diagnosis for a dentition with periodontal disease.

To a lesser extent, orthodontic therapy also affects the PDL similar to its response to occlusal trauma or periodontal disease but in a more controlled manner (discussed earlier, see Figure 14-14). On the side under tension, the **periodontal ligament space** will become wider; with the side under pressure, it will become narrower. The interdental ligament is also responsible for the memory of tooth positioning within each dental arch. Therefore, a sufficiently prolonged retention period must be allowed to reattach the interdental ligament fully to its new position and thereby ensure the maintenance of the clinical stability of tooth position established during orthodontic therapy (see earlier discussion). Retainers, removable and permanent, are used to maintain this desirable alignment.

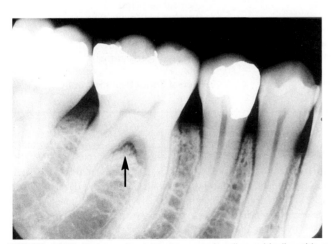

FIGURE 14-33 Early occlusal trauma noted radiographically with a widening of the radiolucent periodontal ligament space between the radiopaque lamina dura of the alveolar bone proper and the similarly radiopaque cementum; thickening of the lamina dura in response is also possible.

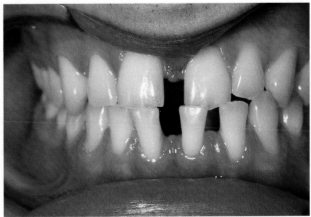

FIGURE 14-34 Pathological tooth migration caused by the weakened periodontium in which the occlusal forces need not be at an abnormal level if the periodontal support is already reduced by periodontal disease.

CHAPTER 15

Overview of the Dentitions

●●●CHAPTER OUTLINE

The dentitions
  Tooth types
  Tooth designation
Dentition periods
  Primary, mixed, and permanent

Dental anatomy terminology
  General dental terms
  Tooth anatomy terms
  Orientational tooth terms
Considerations for tooth study

●●●LEARNING OBJECTIVES

- Define and pronounce the key terms of this chapter when discussing the teeth or portions of a tooth.
- Describe the two dentitions and their relationship to each other.
- Define each dentition period and discuss the important clinical considerations for each dentition period.

- Assign the correct universal designation for a tooth and its correct dentition period when examining a figure or a patient.
- Integrate the knowledge of the dentitions into the dental treatment of patients.

●●●NEW KEY TERMS

Angle: line, point
Anatomical crown, root
Clinical crown, root
Contact area
Cusp (kusp)
D-A-Q-T System
Dental anatomy
Dentition period (den-**tish**-in)
Embrasures (em-**bray**-zhers)
Height of contour

International Standards Organization
  Designation System
Interproximal space (in-ter-
  prok-si-mal)
Occlusion (ah-**kloo**-zhun)
Palmer Notation Method
Quadrants (**kwod**-rints)
Ridges
Root axis line, concavities
Sextants (**sex**-tants)

Surfaces: distal (**dis**-tl),
  incisal (in-**sigh**-zl),
  occlusal (ah-**kloo**-zl),
  masticatory (**mass**-ti-ka-tor-ee),
  mesial (**me**-ze-il),
  palatal (**pal**-ah-tal),
  proximal (**prok**-si-mal)
Thirds
Universal Tooth Designation System

THE DENTITIONS

The term **dentition** is used to describe the natural teeth in the jaws. The dentitions are initially discussed in this beginning of Unit IV. As described in Chapter 6 in relationship to tooth development, a person has two dentitions during a lifetime: primary dentition and permanent dentition.

The first dentition present is the **primary dentition** (Figure 15-1). Child patients and their supervising adults consider the primary teeth to be the *baby teeth*. An older term for the primary dentition is the *deciduous dentition*. This term is derived from the concept that the

primary dentition is exfoliated, or shed (just as deciduous trees shed their leaves), and replaced entirely by the **permanent dentition.** Thus, the permanent dentition is the second dentition to develop (Figure 15-2). The permanent dentition is also sometimes considered the *secondary dentition,* and the permanent teeth are called the *adult teeth.* By recent convention (or convenience), clinicians seem to prefer to mix and match terms when referring to the two dentitions, as in *primary dentition* and *permanent dentition.*

The permanent dentition is also sometimes considered the *succedaneous dentition* because most of these permanent teeth succeed primary predecessors. However, dental professionals must remember

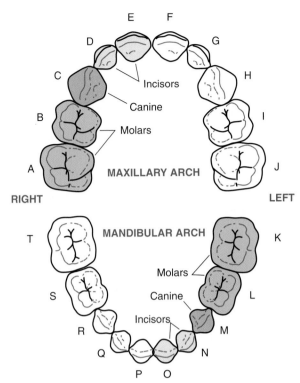

FIGURE 15-1 Occlusal views of the primary dentition during the primary dentition period, with types of teeth identified.

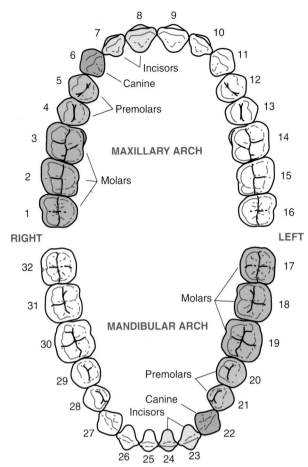

FIGURE 15-2 Occlusal views of the permanent dentition during the permanent period, with types of teeth identified.

that the molars of the permanent dentition are **nonsuccedaneous** because they are without any primary predecessors; only the anteriors and premolars of the permanent dentition are **succedaneous**. Development of the primary dentition, eruption and shedding of the primary teeth, and development of the permanent dentition are discussed further in Chapter 6.

TOOTH TYPES

Teeth comprise around 20% of the surface area of the oral cavity, maxillary more so than mandibular teeth. Tooth types of both arches within the primary dentition include 8 **incisors**, 4 **canines**, and 8 **molars**, for a total of 20 teeth (see Figures 15-1 and 2-4). The anatomy of the primary dentition is discussed further in Chapter 18.

Tooth types of both arches within the permanent dentition include 8 incisors, 4 canines, 8 **premolars**, and 12 molars, for a total of 32 teeth (see Figure 15-2). Note that only the permanent dentition has premolars; in contrast, the primary dentition does not have premolars. The anatomy of the permanent dentition is discussed further in Chapter 16 (anterior teeth) and Chapter 17 (posterior teeth).

Each tooth type has a specific form, no matter which dentition it is in. This tooth form is related to the function during **mastication** for the tooth, as well as to its role in speech and esthetics. The form and function of each tooth type are similar for both the primary and permanent dentitions.

The incisors function as instruments for biting and cutting food during mastication, because of their triangular proximal form. The canines, because of their tapered shape and their prominent cusp, function to pierce or tear food during mastication.

The premolars, which are found only in the permanent dentition, function to assist the molars in grinding food during mastication because of their broad occlusal surface and their prominent cusps.

The premolars also assist the canines in piercing and tearing food with their cusps. Finally, as the teeth with the largest and strongest crowns, the molars function in grinding food during mastication, assisted by the premolars. It is the wide occlusal surfaces of the molars, with their prominent cusps, that help with mastication.

Clinical Considerations for Tooth Type

Variation of teeth within a particular tooth type is a given and is always of interest to clinicians.

The individual tooth form and its related function can be lost as a result of attrition, caries, and trauma. Functional tooth form that has been lost can be approximated by restorative treatment, in many cases, using crowns, bridges, partial or complete dentures, or implants (see Figure 14-23). If not restored, this change in form over time can affect mastication, especially in older patients, who may change to a softer diet that may be poor nutritionally.

Because the specific shape of a tooth varies in each person and possibly within a dentition, a mold of the restored crown is made when integrating artificial crowns (or *caps*) within an individual dentition. The goal is to match as closely as possible the shape of the patient's teeth on the opposite side so the arch appears symmetrical and the crowns fit the space provided. This mold is selected by comparing it with a mold guide of white plastic model crowns provided by various manufacturers.

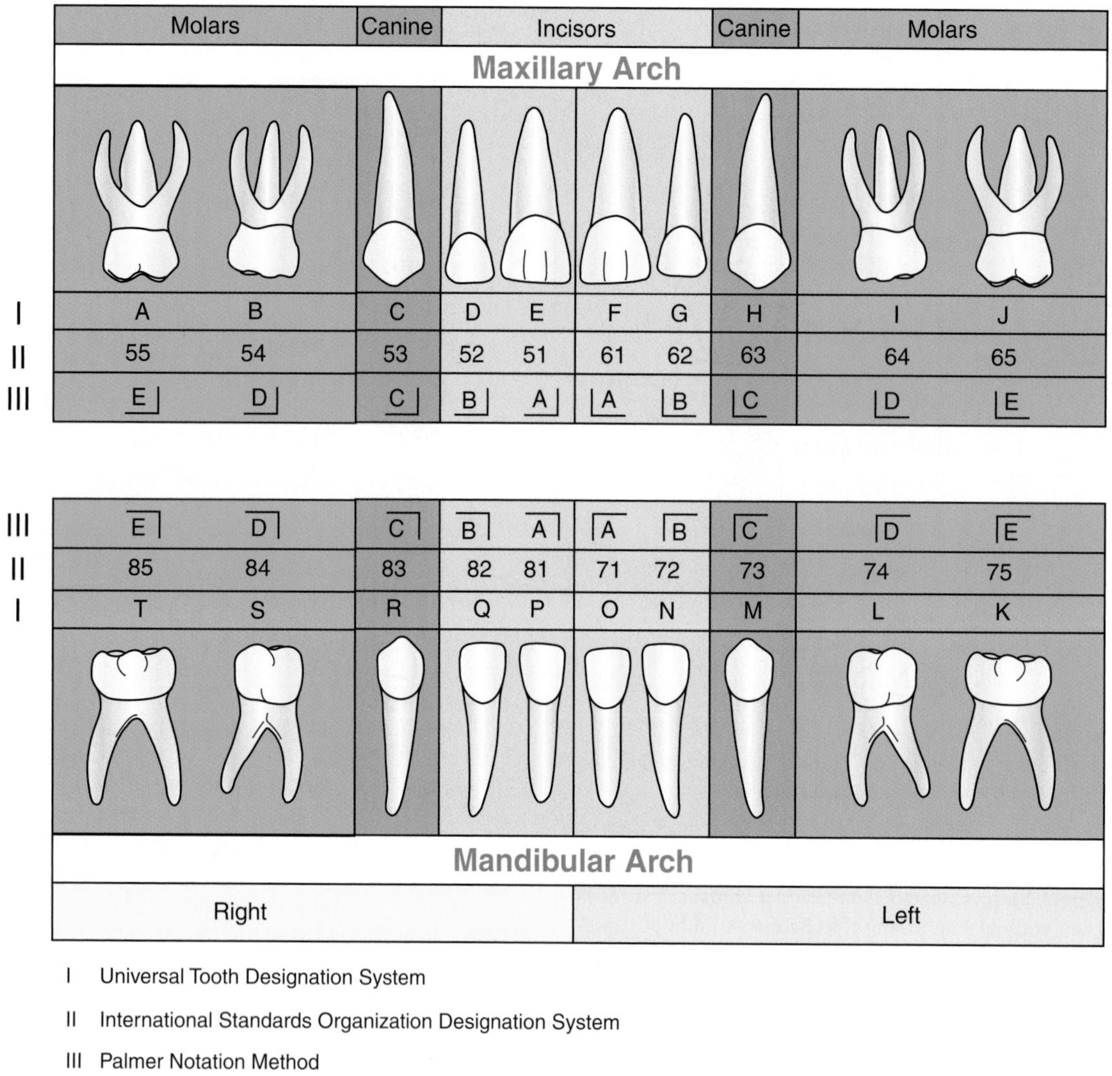

	Molars		Canine	Incisors				Canine	Molars	
	Maxillary Arch									
I	A	B	C	D	E	F	G	H	I	J
II	55	54	53	52	51	61	62	63	64	65
III	E⌋	D⌋	C⌋	B⌋	A⌋	⌊A	⌊B	⌊C	⌊D	⌊E

	Molars		Canine	Incisors				Canine	Molars	
III	E⌉	D⌉	C⌉	B⌉	A⌉	⌈A	⌈B	⌈C	⌈D	⌈E
II	85	84	83	82	81	71	72	73	74	75
I	T	S	R	Q	P	O	N	M	L	K
	Mandibular Arch									
	Right					Left				

I Universal Tooth Designation System

II International Standards Organization Designation System

III Palmer Notation Method

A

FIGURE 15-3 A: Universal Tooth Designation System, International Standards Organization Designation System, and Palmer Notation Method for the primary teeth.

TOOTH DESIGNATION

The primary teeth and the permanent teeth are both designated by the Universal Tooth Designation System (Figure 15-3). This system is the most widely used in United States for the designation of both dentitions because it is adaptable to electronic data transfer; this textbook uses the Universal System. With the Universal Tooth Designation System, the primary teeth are designated in a consecutive arrangement by using capital letters, A through T, starting with the maxillary right second molar, moving clockwise, and ending with the mandibular right second molar (see Figure 15-1).

The permanent teeth are designated by the Universal Tooth Designation System in consecutive arrangement as the patient is observed from in front by using the digits 1 through 32, starting with the maxillary right third molar, moving clockwise, and ending with the mandibular right third molar (see Figure 15-2). The clockwise convention also is also used when charting restorations or periodontal conditions in the oral cavity for a patient.

However, the need for a system that can be used internationally, as well as by electronic data transfer, is recognized; thus the acceptance of the International Standards Organization Designation System (ISO System) by the World Health Organization (see Figure 15-3). With this system, the teeth are designated by using a two-digit code. The first digit of the code indicates the quadrant (see later discussion under general dental terms), and the second indicates the tooth in this quadrant. This is based on the system of the Fédération Dentaire Internationale (FDI).

With the ISO System, the digits 1 through 4 are used for quadrants in a clockwise manner in the permanent dentition, and digits 5 through 8 are used in a clockwise manner for those quadrants of the primary dentition. For the second digit, which indicates the tooth, the digits 1 through 8 are used for the permanent teeth, with this designation using the median line in a distal direction for numbering. The digits 1 through 5 are then used for the primary dentition, with this designation also using the median line in a distal direction for numbering.

Another system that is commonly used in orthodontics is the Palmer Notation Method also known as the *Military Tooth Numbering System* (see Figure 15-3). It is helpful with this dental specialty because it allows immediate discussion of the teeth that require prompt treatment, and it can produce a very graphical

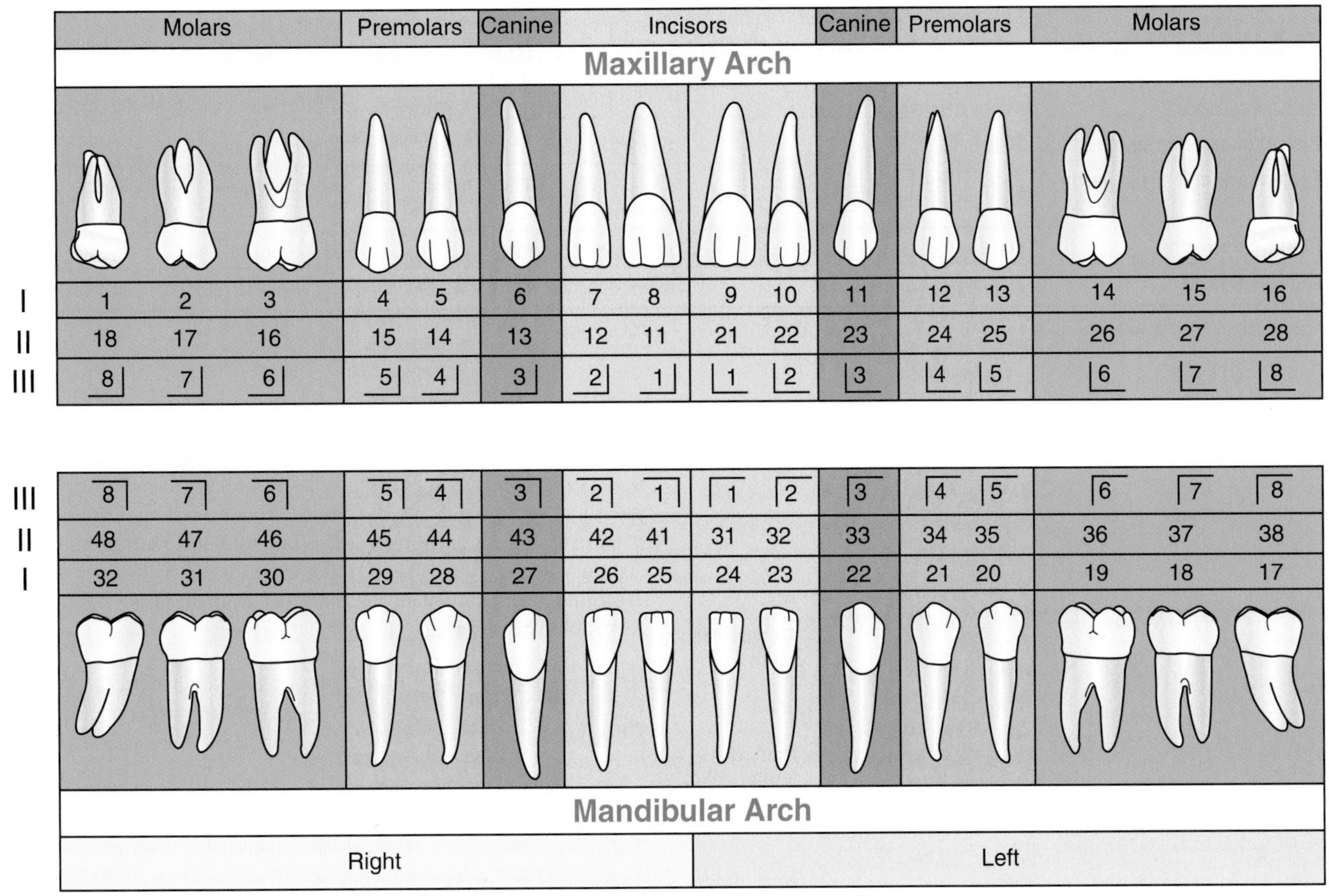

	Molars			Premolars		Canine	Incisors				Canine	Premolars		Molars		

Maxillary Arch

I	1	2	3	4	5	6	7	8	9	10	11	12	13	14	15	16
II	18	17	16	15	14	13	12	11	21	22	23	24	25	26	27	28
III	8⌋	7⌋	6⌋	5⌋	4⌋	3⌋	2⌋	1⌋	⌊1	⌊2	⌊3	⌊4	⌊5	⌊6	⌊7	⌊8

III	8⌉	7⌉	6⌉	5⌉	4⌉	3⌉	2⌉	1⌉	⌈1	⌈2	⌈3	⌈4	⌈5	⌈6	⌈7	⌈8
II	48	47	46	45	44	43	42	41	31	32	33	34	35	36	37	38
I	32	31	30	29	28	27	26	25	24	23	22	21	20	19	18	17

Mandibular Arch

Right	Left

I   Universal Tooth Designation System

II International Standards Organization Designation System

III Palmer Notation Method

B

FIGURE 15-3, cont'd B: Universal Tooth Designation System, International Standards Organization Designation System, and Palmer Notation Method for the permanent teeth.

image, akin to a map of the dentition. In this system, the teeth are designated with a right-angle symbol indicating the quadrants with the tooth number inside, similar in numbering to the ISO System that superseded it.

DENTITION PERIODS

Although there are only two dentitions, there are three dentition periods throughout a person's lifetime, because the time period of the two dentitions overlaps (Table 15-1). Each patient should be assigned a dentition period to allow the most effective dental treatment for that period. This specificity is especially important with the consideration of orthodontic therapy, because growth during certain dentition periods is maximized to allow expansion of the jaws and movement of the teeth.

PRIMARY DENTITION PERIOD

The first dentition period is the *primary dentition period* (see Figure 15-1). This period begins with the eruption of the primary mandibular central incisors. Thus, this period occurs between approximately

6 months and 6 years of age (see Figure 6-22, *A* for chronological order, Table 18-1 for approximate ages, and Figure 20-5 for sequence). Only the primary teeth are present during this time, with their full eruption completed at 30 months, usually when the primary second molars are in occlusion. The jaws are beginning to grow during this period to accommodate the larger permanent teeth. This period usually ends when the first permanent tooth erupts, the permanent mandibular first molar.

MIXED DENTITION PERIOD

The *mixed dentition period* follows the primary dentition period (Figure 15-4, see Chapter 6). This period occurs between approximately 6 and 12 years of age. Both primary and permanent teeth are present during this transitional stage. During this time, both shedding of primary teeth and eruption of permanent teeth begin after their crowns are completed. Thus, this period begins with eruption of the first permanent tooth, a permanent mandibular first molar, which is guided by the distal surface of the primary second molar. This period usually ends with shedding of the last primary tooth, which usually occurs from age 11 to 12.

TABLE 15-1	Dentition Periods and Clinical Considerations		
	PRIMARY DENTITION PERIOD	**MIXED DENTITION PERIOD**	**PERMANENT DENTITION PERIOD**
Approximate time span	~6 months to ~6 years	~6 years to 12 years	After ~12 years
Teeth marking start of period	Eruption of primary mandibular central incisor	Eruption of permanent mandibular first molar	Shedding of the last primary tooth
Dentition present	Primary	Primary and permanent	Usually permanent
Growth of jaws	Beginning	Fastest and most noticeable	Slowest and least noticeable

Adapted from Nelson S: *Wheeler's Dental Anatomy, Physiology and Occlusions*, ed 9, WB Saunders, Philadelphia, 2009.

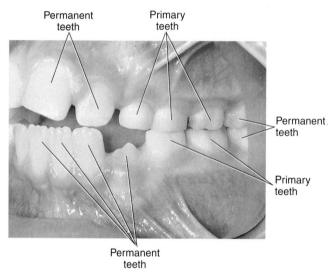

FIGURE 15-4 Example of the oral cavity during the mixed dentition period, with the primary and permanent teeth identified.

The color differences between the primary and permanent teeth become apparent during this middle phase, as any supervising adult has noticed in the child and routinely points it out to the dental professionals. The primary crowns are lighter in color than the darker permanent crowns owing to the fact that the permanent teeth having less opaque enamel, and thus the underlying yellow dentin is more visible. Also more evident is the difference in the crown size and root length between the smaller and shorter primary teeth and the larger and longer permanent teeth.

The jaws undergo their fastest and most noticeable growth during this period, consistent with the onset of puberty, to accommodate the larger teeth of the adult. Females shed their primary teeth and receive their permanent teeth slightly earlier than males, possibly reflecting the earlier overall physical maturation achieved.

PERMANENT DENTITION PERIOD

The final dentition period is the *permanent dentition period* (see Figure 15-2). This period begins with shedding of the last primary tooth. Thus, this dentition period begins just approximately after 12 years of age. Included is the eruption of all the permanent teeth, except for teeth that are congenitally missing or impacted and cannot erupt, usually involving the third molars (see Figure 6-22, *B* for chronological order, Table 15-2 and **Appendix D** for approximate ages, and Figure 20-6 for sequence).

The permanent teeth are usually the only teeth present during this period. Growth of the jaws is not noticeable as it slows and then eventually stops. Thus, little growth of the jaws occurs overall during this period, given that puberty has passed. Tooth types tend to erupt in pairs so that, if any asymmetry exists in a patient, a radiograph of the area may be required. When a child patient is unusually early or late regarding the usual sequential eruption of teeth, the family dental history should be reviewed.

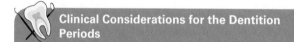

Clinical Considerations for the Dentition Periods

The clinical considerations associated with the primary and permanent dentition periods are discussed later in each appropriate chapter. However, the *mixed dentition period* also has characteristic physiological and psychological effects. This dentition period is sometimes considered an *ugly duckling stage*, because of the different tooth colors, disproportionately sized teeth, and various clinical crown heights. The patient's smile shows temporary edentulous areas and crowding. Additionally, in many cases, the surrounding gingiva responds to all these changes, as well as hormonal fluctuations, by becoming inflamed.

Homecare may be difficult for patients during the mixed dentition period because these changes, such as crowding, may promote dental biofilm retention. Child patients and supervising adults must be reminded to be especially diligent about oral hygiene care and be reassured that this stage is only temporary. Early interceptive orthodontic therapy may also be initiated during this dentition period; panoramic radiograph is important for monitoring tooth development (see Figure 6-27, *A* and **Chapter 20**).

If in the primary and/or mixed dentition, gingival inflammation is only slight, with little dental biofilm formation, but bone loss around the newly erupted permanent first molars and lower anteriors is severe, early aggressive periodontitis (previously referred to as *juvenile periodontitis*) may be suspected. Early intervention in this serious periodontal disease can prevent further bone loss.

DENTAL ANATOMY TERMINOLOGY

Dental professionals must be able to understand and use dental anatomy terminology. **Dental anatomy** is the area of the dental sciences dealing with the morphology, or form, of the teeth, both crown and root. Restorative dentistry uses many specific dental anatomy terms when discussing treatment. Periodontal treatment of the teeth also necessitates using many of these detailed terms, such as line angles, when performing procedures such as probe readings.

GENERAL DENTAL TERMS

As noted earlier, each tooth is surrounded and supported by the bone of the tooth socket, or **alveolus** (plural, **alveoli**) (Figure 15-5). Each alveolus is located in the **alveolar process,** or tooth-bearing part of each jaw. Each alveolar process of the jaws is also considered a **dental arch**, either the **maxillary arch** or **mandibular arch**.

TABLE 15-2	Approximate Eruption and Root Completion Ages for Permanent Teeth (in Years)	
MAXILLARY TEETH	**ERUPTION**	**ROOT COMPLETION**
Central incisor	7–8	10
Lateral incisor	8–9	11
Canine	11–12	13–15
First premolar	10–11	12–13
Second premolar	10–12	12–14
First molar	6–7	9–10
Second molar	12–13	14–16
Third molar	17–21	18–25
MANDIBULAR TEETH	**ERUPTION**	**ROOT COMPLETION**
Central incisor	6–7	9
Lateral incisor	7–8	10
Canine	9–10	12–14
First premolar	10–12	12–13
Second premolar	11–12	13–14
First molar	6–7	9–10
Second molar	11–13	14–15
Third molar	17–21	18–25

Adapted from Nelson S: *Wheeler's Dental Anatomy, Physiology and Occlusions,* ed 9, WB Saunders, Philadelphia, 2009.

The teeth in the **maxilla** are the **maxillary teeth;** the teeth in the **mandible** are the **mandibular teeth** (see Figure 15-5). **Occlusion** is the method by which the teeth of the mandibular arch come into contact with those of the maxillary arch. The term occlusion is also used to describe the anatomical alignment of the teeth and their relationship to the rest of the masticatory system (see Chapter 20).

Each dental arch has a midline, an imaginary vertical plane that divides the arch into two approximately equal halves, a right and a left (Figure 15-6). The midline is similar to the median, or midsagittal, plane of the body. The midline is an important consideration in the evaluation of a patient's smile. Thus, each dental arch can be further divided into two quadrants, with four quadrants in the entire oral cavity. Thus, teeth are described as being located in one of the four quadrants: maxillary right quadrant, maxillary left quadrant, mandibular right quadrant, and mandibular left quadrant. This designation

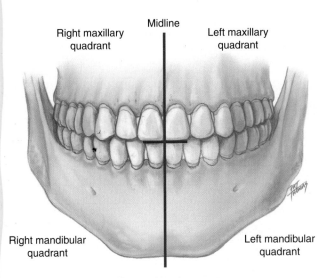

Anterior teeth - shown white
Posterior teeth - shown yellow

FIGURE 15-6 Oral cavity with the permanent teeth, with the midline, quadrants, and anterior and posterior teeth identified.

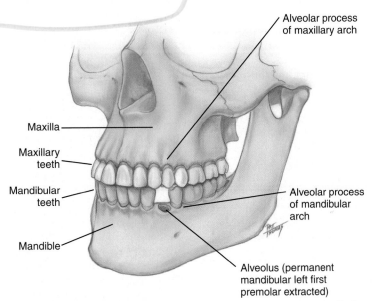

FIGURE 15-5 Oral cavity with the permanent teeth, with the maxillary and mandibular arches and other structures identified.

is useful when planning a course of dental treatment for a patient, because it allows the treatment of only one or more oral regions at a time.

Thus, the correct sequence of words when describing a tooth is based on a **D-A-Q-T System**: **D** for dentition, **A** for arch, **Q** for quadrant, and **T** for tooth type. An example would be the permanent (*D*) mandibular (*A*) left (*Q*) first premolar (*T*).

Teeth can also be described according to their position in each dental arch and in relationship to the midline (see Figure 15-6). The incisors and canines are considered **anterior teeth** because they are closer to the midline. In contrast, the molars (and premolars, if present) are considered **posterior teeth** because they are farther from the midline.

Some dental treatment plans also include the use of sextants, which further divide each dental arch into three portions according to the relationship to the midline: right posterior sextant, anterior sextant, and left posterior sextant. Thus, the permanent maxillary right central incisor is in the maxillary anterior sextant. This division follows the mapping of oral nerve pathways, especially in the maxillary arch; so, the use of sextants can be useful in treatment plans, such as those that use local anesthesia for patient pain control.

TABLE 15-3	ISO System for Designation of Areas of Oral Cavity
Whole oral cavity	00
Maxillary area	01
Mandibular area	02
Upper right quadrant	10
Upper left quadrant	20
Lower left quadrant	30
Lower right quadrant	40
Upper right sextant	03
Upper anterior sextant	04
Upper left sextant	05
Lower left sextant	06
Lower anterior sextant	07
Lower right sextant	08

To prevent miscommunication internationally, the ISO System also includes the designation of areas in the oral cavity (used also in their tooth designation system). These areas are designated by a two-digit number, and at least one of the two digits is zero (Table 15-3). An example of this system is that *00* designates the whole of the oral cavity, and *01* designates the maxillary area only.

TOOTH ANATOMY TERMS

Each tooth consists of a **crown** and one or more **roots** (Figure 15-7, see Figure 2-5). The crown has **dentin** covered by **enamel**, and each root has dentin covered by cementum. The inner part of the dentin of both crown and root also covers the pulp cavity of the tooth. The **pulp cavity** has a **pulp chamber**, **pulp canal** (or canals) with an **apical foramen** (or foramina), and possibly **pulp horn** (or horns).

In this textbook, the illustrations of the head and neck, as well as any structures related to them, are oriented according to the patient's head being in anatomical position unless otherwise noted (see Appendix A). This is the same as if the patient were being viewed straight on while sitting upright in the dental chair. Thus, maxillary teeth show the root superior to the crown; mandibular teeth show the root inferior to the crown (see Figure 15-3).

Orientation of the dental chart is traditionally from the dental professional's view, that is, the patient's right corresponds to the notation chart's left. The designations "left" and "right" on the chart, however, nonetheless correspond to the patient's left and right, respectively. Other dental charts may show each of the teeth "unfolded" so that the facial, occlusal or incisal, and lingual surfaces of the teeth can be shown.

The enamel of the crown and cementum of the root usually meet close to the **cementoenamel junction (CEJ)**, an external line at the neck or cervix of the tooth (see Figure 14-8). There are three possible interfaces at the CEJ. At the CEJ, the cementum over the neck of each tooth may overlap the enamel, the enamel may meet the cementum edge to edge, or a small area of underlying dentin may be exposed because there is a gap between the enamel and cementum. The CEJ usually feels smooth or evenly grainy or has a slight groove when explored.

Parts of the crown and root of a tooth can also be designated using more specific terms in order to assist the clinician during patient dental charting (Figure 15-8). The anatomical crown is the part covered by enamel. It remains mostly constant throughout the life of the tooth, except for attrition and other physical wear. The clinical crown is that

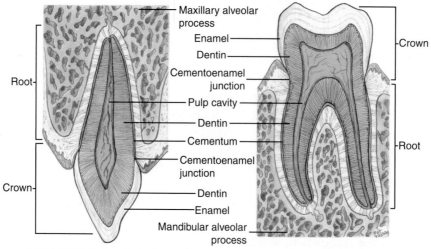

FIGURE 15-7 Anterior and posterior tooth showing the involved dental tissues.

Labels (left tooth): Root, Crown. Center labels: Maxillary alveolar process, Enamel, Dentin, Cementoenamel junction, Pulp cavity, Dentin, Cementum, Cementoenamel junction, Dentin, Enamel, Mandibular alveolar process. Right tooth labels: Crown, Root.

part of the anatomical crown that is visible and not covered by the **gingiva**. Its height is determined by the location of the **marginal gingiva**. The clinical crown of a tooth can change over time, especially with **gingival recession** as the marginal gingiva recedes toward the root (see Figure 13-1). This textbook, when discussing the crown of a tooth, refers to the anatomical crown unless designated otherwise.

Similarly, the anatomical root is that part of the root covered by **cementum**. The clinical root of a tooth is that part of the anatomical root that is visible, subject to variability over time, again related to **gingival recession** (see Figure 13-1). This textbook, when discussing the root of a tooth, refers to the anatomical root of a healthy tooth unless designated otherwise.

Some clinicians describe features of a tooth related to the root axis line (RAL), which is an imaginary line representing the long axis of a tooth, drawn in a way to bisect the root and the crown in the cervical area (see Figure 20-9). However, it is important to note that the tooth's crown and root are never strictly vertically placed within the alveolar bone but have some degree of angulation.

Teeth may have one or more roots, but all the roots of both dentitions have common traits. All roots are widest at the CEJ and taper toward the apex of the tooth. Roots have more bulk on the facial surface than on the lingual surface. The root tapers more dramatically on the lingual surface. Many surfaces of the roots have indentations, or root concavities. These commonly occur on the proximal root surfaces of anteriors and posteriors, and the buccal and lingual surfaces of molars. These can become exposed to the oral environment due to periodontal disease but still hidden to the clinician under a **periodontal pocket**, presenting complications during instrumentation and homecare (see Figure 10-10).

Historically in dental education, the importance of clinical crown anatomy was emphasized, with limited emphasis on clinical root anatomy. Subsequently, dental professionals have seen an increased educational emphasis placed on detailed knowledge of root anatomy. This change in emphasis is due to a new recognition of the importance of precise periodontal root instrumentation to achieve oral health in cases of disease, as well as preserving of the crown of the teeth by restorations. Initially, pocket analysis using periodontal probes yields the situational root morphology and deposit level in a patient with periodontal disease. Once **root morphology** is understood and the

patient's periodontal needs ascertained, the dental professional can also choose the most effective treatment plan, including instrumentation. In addition, the awareness of root morphology will prevent the destruction of the root by overinstrumentation by hand.

Root concavities should be carefully explored during instrumentation appointments and charted in the patient's record. Treatment failures have been linked to any deposits remaining either after therapy or with continued poor homecare because these deposits contribute to the continuation of the disease process. However, a significantly greater attachment loss for root surfaces with proximal root grooves occurs as compared with those that lack proximal root grooves. Whereas these concavities can act as predisposing factors in the periodontal disease process, the depressions also increase the attachment area, producing a root shape more resistant to damaging occlusal forces. Thus, root contours present both harmful and protective effects that must be considered individually in the patient's periodontal prognosis.

Until recently, clinicians were not able to visualize the root surface unless access to periodontal surgery was performed to remove the

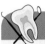

Clinical Considerations with Tooth Anatomy

Certain restorations may cover the entire **anatomical crown** area; these are full restorative crowns (or *caps*, as called by patients). Pins may be placed within the crown and root to help with the buildup of restorative materials to support an individual crown restoration.

A full crown should ideally cover the entire prepared anatomical crown, but enlarged gingival tissue or loss of anatomical crown structure may require a surgical periodontal procedure, called *crown lengthening,* to increase the amount of the **clinical crown** and reduce the surrounding **gingival tissue** by removal. However, many clinicians feel that a restored crown, instead, should be partial if possible, avoiding the CEJ region that is in contact with the gingival tissue in order to preserve tissue health. In a case with poorer prognosis, a root (or roots) may be retained without the crown(s) if there is enough structure and gingival attachment, so as to support a removable prosthesis, such as an overdenture.

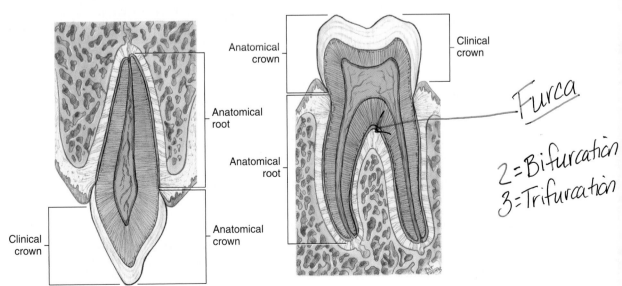

FIGURE 15-8 Anterior and posterior tooth showing the anatomical crown and root, as well as the clinical crown. The clinical root is not shown because this is a healthy periodontal situation without recession, which would expose a clinical root.

overlying oral mucosa and had to rely only on tactile sense and resultant mental picture to understand the subgingival topography. However, with the recent development of endoscopic technology, with its small camera that can fit within a deepened sulcus, clinicians today are able to see the root surface in real time. When incorporated into more clinical practice settings in the future, such devices may change the way many dental procedures are performed.

ORIENTATIONAL TOOTH TERMS

Each tooth has five surfaces: facial, lingual, masticatory, mesial, and distal surfaces. Thus, each tooth is like a box with sides. Some of the surfaces of the tooth are identified by their orientational relationship to other orofacial structures, similar to the designation of the soft tissue of the oral cavity (Figure 15-9, see Figure 2-1). Tooth surfaces closest to the surface of the face are considered facial surfaces. Those facial tooth surfaces closest to the lips are termed the labial surfaces. Those facial tooth surfaces closest to the inner cheek are considered the buccal surfaces. Therefore, the anterior teeth have a labial surface, and posterior teeth have a buccal surface.

Those tooth surfaces closest to the tongue are termed the lingual surfaces. Those lingual surfaces closest to the palate on the maxillary arch are sometimes also termed the palatal surfaces. The masticatory surface is the chewing surface on the most superior surface of the crown. This is the incisal surface for anterior teeth and the occlusal surface for posterior teeth.

The **masticatory surfaces** of both anterior and posterior teeth have linear elevations, or ridges, which are named according to location. The masticatory surfaces of both canines and posterior teeth also have at least one major elevation, the cusp; cusps contribute to a significant portion of the tooth's surface. Maxillary and mandibular canines have one cusp, and maxillary premolars and the mandibular first premolars usually have two cusps. Mandibular second premolars frequently have three cusps: one buccal and two lingual. Maxillary molars have two buccal cusps and two lingual cusps; a fifth cusp that may form on these teeth is known as the **cusp of Carabelli**. In contrast, mandibular molars may have five or four cusps.

Surfaces of both the crown and the root are also defined by their relationship to the midline (see Figure 15-9). The surface closest to the midline is considered the mesial surface; the surface farthest away from the midline is considered the distal surface.

Together, both the mesial and the distal surfaces between adjacent teeth are considered the proximal surface. In other words, either surface of a tooth that is next to an adjacent tooth is referred to as a proximal surface, which may therefore be either the mesial or the distal surface. The area between adjacent tooth surfaces is the interproximal space.

The area where the crowns of adjacent teeth in the same arch physically touch each proximal surface is the contact area (see Figure 15-9), or, as referred to by clinicians, the *contact*. Its presence is checked when dental floss is passed between two teeth and some resistance is felt.

The contact areas on the mesial and distal are usually also considered the location of the height of contour on the proximal surfaces. The height of contour, or crest of curvature, is the greatest elevation of the tooth either incisocervically or occlusocervically on a specific surface of the crown (Figure 15-10). The facial and lingual surfaces of a tooth also have a height of contour that is easily seen when viewing the tooth's profile from the proximal.

It is noted when viewing teeth overall that the proximal **CEJ** curvature is greatest on the anterior and the least on the posterior teeth.

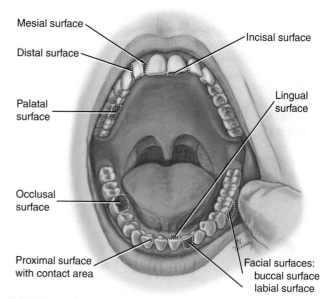

FIGURE 15-9 Surfaces of the teeth, with the orientational relationship to other oral cavity structures, to the midline, and to other teeth.

However, this curvature is approximately similar on mesial and distal surfaces of the two teeth that face each other. In addition, on any given tooth, the height of the CEJ curvature is greater on the mesial aspect of that tooth than it is on the distal.

When two teeth in the same arch come into contact, their curvatures next to the contact areas form spaces considered embrasures (Figure 15-11). These consist of triangular-shaped spaces between two teeth, created by the sloping away of the mesial and distal surfaces, and may diverge facially, lingually, occlusally, or apically with loss of tissue. The embrasures are continuous with the interproximal spaces between the teeth, and there is an increasing angle of the occlusal embrasures anteroposteriorly. They form spillways between teeth to direct food away from the gingiva. Also, they provide a mechanism for teeth to be more self-cleansing. Lastly, they protect the gingiva from undue frictional trauma but also provide the proper degree of stimulation to the tissues.

All these tooth contours, such as contact areas, heights of contour, and embrasures, are important in the function and health of the masticatory system (see Chapter 20). These specific forms and alignments of the teeth serve to shelter the vulnerable gingivosulcular area from damage.

Each tooth can also be divided by imaginary lines to designate specific crown areas. A line angle is formed by the lines created at the junction of two crown surfaces, and the name is derived by combining the names of those two surfaces (Figure 15-12). When combining terms such as *mesial* and *labial*, the *al* from the end of the first surface is dropped and an *o* is added and combined with the second surface, thus creating *mesiolabial*. If the first letter of the second word will result in doubling a vowel, such as *mesio-occlusal*, a hyphen is placed between the words, such as *mesio-occlusal*. An example of line angle would be the mesiolabial line angle, which is the junction of the mesial and labial surfaces.

Posterior teeth have eight line angles per tooth: mesiobuccal, distobuccal, mesiolingual, distolingual, mesio-occlusal, disto-occlusal, bucco-occlusal, and linguo-occlusal. Anterior teeth have only six line angles per tooth: mesiolabial, distolabial, mesiolingual, distolingual, labioincisal, and linguoincisal. Anteriors have fewer line angles than posteriors because the mesial and distal incisal line angles are

ANTERIOR   POSTERIOR

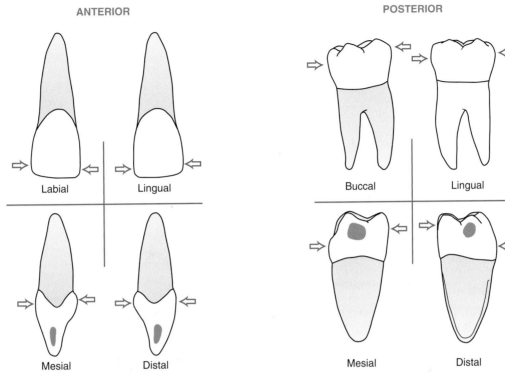

FIGURE 15-10 Anterior and posterior tooth, with the height of contour for each surface noted and contact areas highlighted.

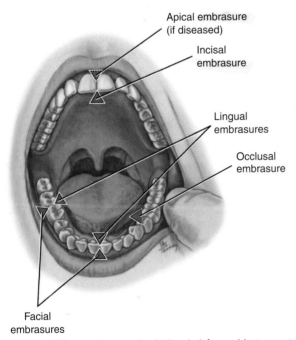

FIGURE 15-11 The embrasures (*red triangles*) formed between two teeth created by the sloping away of the mesial and distal surfaces, which may diverge facially, lingually, incisally/occlusally, or apically with loss of tissue.

rounded; thus, the mesioincisal and distoincisal line angles are practically nonexistent.

A **point angle** is another way to determine a specific area of the crown (Figure 15-13). The junction of three surfaces of the crown, the point angle, takes its name from those three surfaces. Each tooth has

four point angles. Examples of point angles are mesiolabioincisal for an anterior tooth or mesiolabio-occlusal for a posterior tooth.

Finally, a crown surface can be divided both horizontally and vertically into three portions, or **thirds,** to designate specific tooth areas (Figure 15-14). An example is the middle third of the labial surface of a crown. The root can be divided into thirds only horizontally. An example is the cervical third of the buccal surface of a root. The root is also divided vertically into halves by the root axis line, such that the halves are either labial-buccal-lingual or mesial-distal.

Note that in reference to line angles, point angles, thirds, or even a direction, there is an accepted sequencing of combined names of the involved surfaces. The accepted sequence allows that the one term *mesial* precedes *distal,* and also that both *mesial* and *distal* precede all other terms. The terms *labial, buccal,* and *lingual* follow *mesial* or *distal* but precede *incisal* or *occlusal* in any combination.

 Clinical Considerations for Tooth Surfaces

The tooth's angles, height of contour, and spaces define the front or *face* of a tooth when the design of a patient's smile is considered, because these features are what people see first when contemplating someone's smile. Altering placement and shape of these features changes the face of a tooth and its perceived size and the appearance of the smile. Note that ideally the mesial part of the face and silhouette of a tooth is more angled vertically than the distal part of the face of a tooth.

After studying the surfaces of a tooth, dental professionals must be careful to note that access to proximal surfaces and interproximal space is more difficult than access to facial and lingual surfaces (although line angles can also present problems). This access problem occurs for the patient during oral care, as well as for the clinician during instrumentation and restoration procedures.

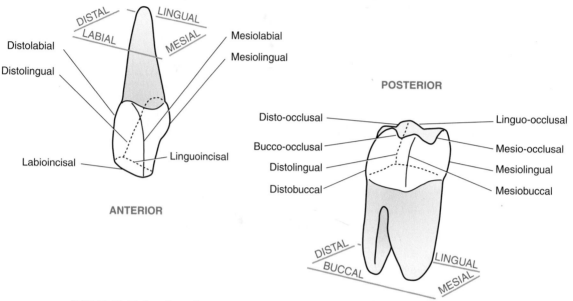

FIGURE 15-12 Anterior and posterior tooth, with the designation of line angles of the crown.

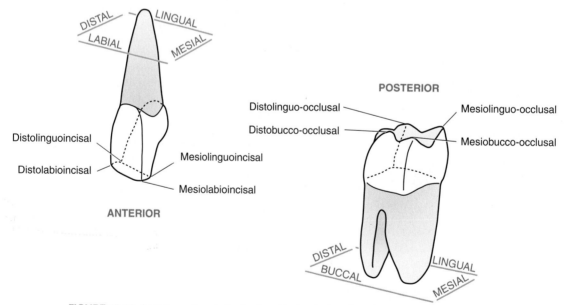

FIGURE 15-13 Anterior and posterior tooth, with the designation of point angles of the crown.

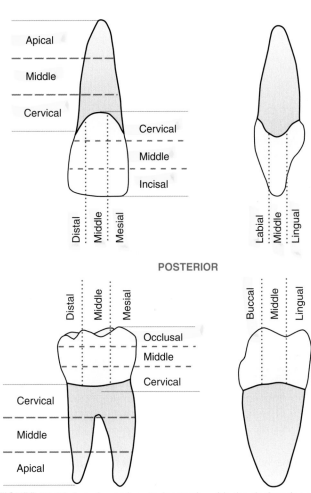

FIGURE 15-14 Anterior and posterior tooth, with the designation of crown and root thirds.

CONSIDERATIONS FOR TOOTH STUDY

Appendix C in this textbook includes charts of the measurements of the permanent dentition. Dental professionals should note that the values are mean values of ideal teeth; real teeth vary in size among patients and do not always directly reflect jaw size. Dental professionals should also note that most of the descriptions in this textbook are also of ideal teeth. Even though the drawn figures are larger than life-size, size relationships among teeth are retained (similar to those to be drawn and also shown in the flashcards from the *Workbook for Illustrated Dental Embryology, Histology, and Anatomy*).

These ideal teeth also have no wear or pathology, similar to plastic model teeth. The features on most extracted specimens are sometimes harder to see because they show signs of wear on both the crown and even the root apex, and the teeth may also show the trauma related to caries and restorative treatment.

However, many of the specific distinguishing features of a tooth can be seen only when the tooth is an extracted specimen. Extraction allows both the **anatomical crown** and the **anatomical root** to be viewed. Fewer features can be seen clinically when portions of the CEJ and root are covered by **gingival tissue** and only the **clinical crown** is visible. However, clinical views of the teeth are still important for observation of overall tooth arrangements and relationships.

Thus, extracted teeth provide a more realistic form of dental anatomy than plastic model teeth, because they have more clearly formed cusps, ridges, fossae, and pits; variations of the ideal tooth form can thus be seen. Extracted teeth can also provide an opportunity to view relatively rare, as well as more common, dental anomalies. However, infection control procedures must be followed when handling extracted teeth (see the *Workbook for Illustrated Dental Embryology, Histology, and Anatomy* for detailed procedures).

CHAPTER 16

Permanent Anterior Teeth

●●● LEARNING OBJECTIVES

- Use the correct names and universal designation numbers of each permanent anterior tooth when examining a diagram and a patient.
- Demonstrate the correct location of each permanent anterior tooth on a diagram and a patient.
- Use and pronounce the key terms when discussing the permanent anterior teeth.
- Describe the general and specific features of permanent anterior teeth and of each permanent anterior tooth type.

- Discuss the important clinical considerations and developmental disturbances based on the anatomy of the permanent anterior teeth.
- Integrate the knowledge of dental anatomy of the permanent anterior teeth into the dental treatment of patients to preserve them.

●●● NEW KEY TERMS

Avulsion (ah-**vul**-shin)
Cingulum (**sin**-gu-lum)
Cusp slope (kusp), **tip**
Cuspid (**kus**-pidz)
Developmental depressions, groove, pits
Diastema (di-ah-**ste**-mah)

Fossa (**fos**-ah) (plural, **fossae, fos**-ay)
Hutchinson's incisors (**hutch**-in-suns in-**sigh**-zers)
Impacted (im-**pak**-ted)
Incisal angle (in-**sign**-sl), **edge, ridge**
Mamelons (**mam**-ah-lons)

Mesiodens (**me**-ze-oh-denz)
Peg lateral
Ridge: labial (**lay**-be-al), **lingual, marginal**
Supplemental groove

PERMANENT ANTERIOR TEETH

Permanent **anterior teeth** include the **incisors** and **canines** (Figure 16-1, see Figure 2-4, 15-1). All anterior teeth are composed of four developmental lobes: three labial lobes named *mesiolabial, middle labial,* and *distolabial,* and one lingual lobe (Figure 16-2). Two vertical labial developmental depressions outline the separations among the labial developmental lobes, the *mesiolabial* and *distolabial developmental depressions.* All permanent anterior teeth are **succedaneous,** which means that each one replaces the primary tooth of the same type. The development of the permanent dentition is discussed in Chapter 6.

The long **crown** of an anterior tooth has an incisal surface, which is its **masticatory surface** (Figure 16-3). From the labial and lingual, the crown outline is trapezoidal, or four-sided, with only two parallel sides. The longer of the two parallel sides is toward the incisal.

The crown outline is triangular when viewed from the proximal, with the base of the triangle at the cervical and the apex at the incisal edge (Figure 16-4). These teeth are wider mesiodistally than labiolingually when compared with posteriors. For anteriors, the **height of contour,** or crest of curvature, for both the crown's labial and lingual surfaces is in the cervical third. Each **contact area** of anteriors is usually centered labiolingually on their **proximal surfaces** and has a smaller area than the contacts of posterior teeth (see Figure 15-10).

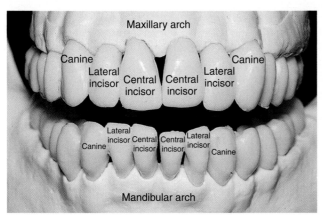

FIGURE 16-1 Permanent anterior teeth identified, which include the incisors and canines.

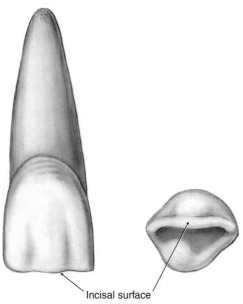

FIGURE 16-3 Example of an incisal surface on a permanent anterior tooth.

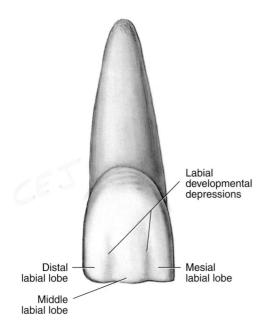

Labial View

FIGURE 16-2 Example of lobe development in a permanent anterior tooth.

On each proximal surface, the **cementoenamel junction (CEJ)** curvature of all anteriors is greater than that of the posteriors.

The **lingual surfaces** of all anteriors have a cingulum (Figure 16-5). The cingulum is a raised, rounded area on the cervical third of the lingual surface in varying degrees of prominence or development on anteriors. The cingulum corresponds to the lingual developmental lobe. **Ridges** may also be present on the lingual surface. The lingual surface on anteriors is bordered mesially and distally on each side by a rounded raised border, the marginal ridge.

Some anteriors have a more complex lingual surface with a fossa or even fossae, which are shallow, wide depressions (Figure 16-6). Some may also have developmental pits, which are located in the deepest part of each fossa. Other anteriors may have on their lingual surface a developmental groove, or primary groove, a sharp, deep, V-shaped linear depression that marks the junction among the developmental lobes.

In addition, a supplemental groove, or secondary groove, may also be present on the lingual surface of anteriors (Figure 16-6).

Clinical Considerations for Anterior Teeth

Patients may have difficulty in maintaining homecare of anteriors because their **dental arch** position naturally may allow the lips to overhang the teeth. Thus, patients may clean only the incisal two-thirds of the crowns of anteriors with their toothbrushes, missing the associated cervical area and facial gingival tissue. This overhanging of the lips may also make instrumentation difficult.

Instrumentation may also be compromised in the area where the greater curvature of the **CEJ** is present interproximally on anteriors, where accessibility is limited and the teeth are in close proximity. The **grooves** on the lingual surface of anteriors may present areas for dental biofilm retention if they extend to the root and are near the adjacent gingival tissue; for this reason, the grooves may be reduced with a dental bur during a minor odontoplasty.

When the anterior teeth are restored, the **Golden Proportions** can be useful guidelines to balance the size of the teeth with one another. These guidelines designate that the ideal width of the maxillary lateral incisor as a factor of 1.0×, the width of the central incisors as 1.618×, and the width of the canines as 0.168× when observed in two dimensions from the facial aspect. Other formulas state that the maxillary central should be 60% wider than the lateral, and the lateral should be 60% wider than the canine from its midline to its mesial aspect. In addition, each incisor should also ideally have an 8:10 width-to-length ratio.

In addition, consideration of smile design may involve the drawing of a line following the ideal outline formed by the **incisal edges** of the maxillary anterior teeth; this line should be 1 to 3 mm parallel or equidistant to the lower lip line. Some variation will occur with aging. Older patients lose elasticity in the lips, which results in sagging, prominence of the mandibular teeth, and diminution of the maxillary teeth. Straight smiles are perceived as more masculine and feminine smiles as more curved. In addition, if the upper lip line appears to be convex instead of concave compared with the lower lip line, the smile will be perceived as more youthful (see Figure 14-22).

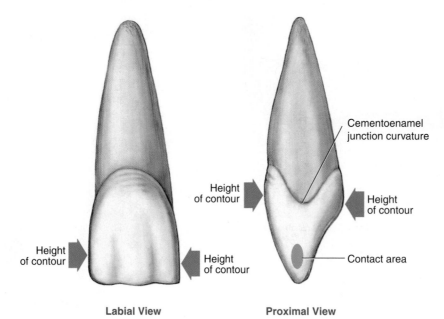

FIGURE 16-4 Example of a permanent anterior tooth, with the contact area and height of contour identified.

This is a shallower, more irregular linear depression. Supplemental grooves branch from the developmental grooves but are not always present in the same pattern on each different tooth type. In general, the more anterior the tooth is located in the arch, the fewer supplemental grooves are present and the smoother the lingual surface.

Anteriors usually have a single **root**, with some exceptions. Each root of the maxillary anterior teeth has great lingual and slight distal inclination (see Figure 20-9). Each root of the mandibular anterior teeth varies in angulation from nearly vertical to great lingual inclination, with the canines possibly having a slight distal root inclination.

PERMANENT INCISORS

GENERAL FEATURES

Permanent incisors are the eight most anterior teeth of the permanent dentition, with four in each dental arch (Table 16-1). The two types are the **central incisors** and the **lateral incisors**. The centrals are closest to the midline, and the laterals are the second teeth from the midline. One of each type is present in each quadrant of each dental arch. Both types are mesial to the permanent canines when the permanent dentition is fully erupted. The permanent incisors are **succedaneous** and replace the primary incisors of the same type. On occasion, the permanent incisors seem to spread out across the arch as a result of spacing during initial eruption and with the eruption of the permanent canines, these spaces often close. When newly erupted, each incisor also has three mamelons, or rounded enamel extensions on the incisal ridge from the labial or lingual views (Figures 16-7 and 16-8, *B*). The mamelons are extensions from the three labial developmental lobes.

The incisors are also the only permanent teeth with two incisal angles formed from the incisal ridge or *incisal edge* (discussed later) and each proximal surface. Incisors of both types are the only permanent teeth with a nearly straight incisal ridge, which is a linear elevation on the masticatory or incisal surface when newly erupted—thus the name incisors.

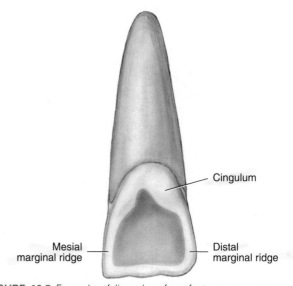

FIGURE 16-5 Example of lingual surface features on a permanent anterior tooth.

The lingual surface has a **cingulum** that corresponds to the lingual developmental lobe, although its prominence or development differs for each type of incisor. These teeth also have a **lingual fossa** and **marginal ridges** on the lingual surface, again in differing developmental levels for each type of incisor. The **height of contour** for both labial and lingual surfaces of all incisors is at the cervical third, as is the case for all anteriors.

PERMANENT MAXILLARY INCISORS

GENERAL FEATURES

Permanent maxillary incisors are the four most anteriorly placed teeth of the maxillary arch. Each has a crown that is larger in all dimensions, especially mesiodistally, compared with a mandibular incisor. In addition, the labial surfaces are rounder from the incisal aspect, with the tooth tapering toward the lingual.

Clinical Considerations for Incisors

Incisors function as instruments for biting and cutting food during mastication, because of their incisal ridge, triangular proximal form, and arch position. They also support the lips and face, as well as maintain **vertical dimension of the face**. Additionally, they contribute to overall normal arch appearance. Finally, they are involved during the articulation of speech and assist in guiding jaw closure as the teeth come together.

Because of the anterior position of the incisors, esthetic concerns are important during restorative procedures. However, restorative replacement of only a part of the **incisal edge** of this tooth after traumatic fracture may also be difficult to maintain owing to this tooth's function in biting and cutting food.

The mamelons on the incisal ridge of incisors usually undergo **attrition**, the wearing away of a tooth surface caused by tooth-to-tooth contact, shortly after eruption as the tooth moves into occlusion (Figures 16-8, *A* and 16-9, *C*, see Figure 16-17 and **Chapter 20**). The incisal ridge, thus, now appears flattened from its labial, lingual, or incisal views and becomes the **incisal edge**. Thus, **mamelons** are usually most noticeable immediately after eruption, becoming undetectable as the tooth undergoes attrition over time. With attrition, the maxillary incisors' incisal edges show lingual inclination and the mandibular incisors have a labial inclination to their incisal edges. Thus, with this arrangement, the incisal edges of the maxillary and mandibular incisors are now usually parallel to one another and mesh correctly during mastication. Excessive attrition can sometimes create a bow-shaped wear pattern on the incisal edge when viewed from the incisal.

If mamelons are still present on the incisal ridge in an adult, it is because these teeth are not in occlusion, whereby they undergo normal attrition, such as with an anterior **open bite** relationship (Figure 16-8, *B*, see Figure 20-22). Thus mamelons occasionally do not wear down, especially when malalignment of the teeth and loss of tooth-to-tooth contact with occlusion exist. Many young adults do not like the appearance of mamelons and sometimes request to have them polished off; some patients even request placement of restorative materials to achieve a straight-appearing incisal edge. Part of the reason that the mamelons are so noticeable, if present long after eruption, is that these extensions are made of enamel, with no dentin layer underneath.

This factor and their thinness contribute overall to their translucent appearance, as opposed to the rest of the clinical crown, which is usually more opaque than the mamelons. Given this translucent quality, mamelons often appear to be a different shade than the rest of the tooth, sometimes making them much more distinct. With the addition of tooth whitening (bleaching), this incisal translucency may become even more noticeable.

All lingual surface features, including the marginal ridges, lingual fossa, and cingulum, are more prominent on the maxillary incisors than on the mandibular incisors. Finally, the incisal edge is just labial to the long axis of the root from either proximal view.

Each root is short compared with those of other maxillary teeth and usually is without root concavities. Bulbous and pronounced crowns may also create deep mesial and distal concavities at the CEJ.

The central and lateral incisors of the maxillary arch resemble each other more than they resemble the similar type of incisors of the opposing arch. Generally, a maxillary central incisor is larger than a maxillary lateral incisor, but overall they have a similar form. Both types of maxillary incisors are wider mesiodistally than labiolingually.

Developmental Disturbances of Incisors

The crown of a permanent incisor can be affected with **dens in dente** (see Table 6-3, *D*). This disturbance leaves the tooth with a deep lingual pit resulting from invagination of the **enamel organ** into the **dental papilla**. This pit may lead to pulpal exposure and pathology. Dens in dente may be hereditary and is more common with a maxillary lateral incisor.

The crowns of permanent incisors, similar to molars, can be affected in children with congenital syphilis. A pregnant woman infected with **syphilis** transmits the spirochete *Treponema pallidum*, a sexually transmitted microorganism, to her **fetus** via the **placenta**. This microorganism may cause localized enamel hypoplasia, which can result in **Hutchinson's incisors**, occurring during tooth development (see Figure 3-16).

A Hutchinson's incisor has a crown with a screwdriver shape from the labial view and is wider cervically and narrow incisally, with a notched incisal edge. Children may also have other developmental anomalies, such as blindness, deafness, and paralysis from congenital syphilis. Treatment of these teeth with restorative materials may improve their appearance.

A sharp, small, extra cusp, or *talon cusp* (claw), occasionally appears as a projection from the cingulum of incisor teeth and can happen in both dentitions. These types of cusps can interfere with occlusion; however, grinding them down is a hazardous endeavor. They often contain a prominent pulp horn, which is at an increased risk of exposure during restorative procedures.

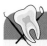

Clinical Considerations for Maxillary Incisors

If a maxillary incisor has increased prominence of the lingual **marginal ridges** and a deeper **lingual fossa**, it may be considered a shovel-shaped incisor (Figure 16-9, *A*). It can also have an accentuated **cingulum** (Figure 16-9, *B*), with deepened **grooves**, and show incisal edge **attrition** (Figure 16-9, *C*).

Another lingual feature, if present on the maxillary incisors, a lingual pit, is at increased risk of caries development due to both increased dental biofilm retention and the weakness of the enamel forming the walls of the pit (Figure 16-10, *A* to *C*, see **Chapter 12**). If the lingual pit is deep, a developmental disturbance of **dens in dente** must be considered, and needed changes made in the patient's treatment plan (discussed earlier). Also present may be a vertically placed linguogingival groove (Figure 16-10, *D*), which originates in the lingual pit and extends cervically and slightly distally onto the cingulum, and is also more common on maxillary laterals, possibly resulting in caries.

Clinicians need to be aware of these lingual **pit and groove patterns** on maxillary incisors when they examine a dentition in order to determine the patient's caries risk level. All pits and grooves must be checked for decay with an explorer and mirror. Light-induced devices that measure changes in laser fluorescence of hard tissue allow dental professionals to better diagnose early lesions in pits and grooves. Maxillary incisors with deep pit and groove patterns but without incipient decay should have enamel sealants placed as soon as they erupt.

In addition, supragingival tooth deposits such as dental biofilm and stain can collect in the prominent lingual surface concavities of maxillary incisors (see Figure 16-9, *D*). During instrumentation, the proximal surfaces of these teeth are more accessible from the lingual than the facial approach because of the increased tapering of the tooth to the lingual. Dental professionals must be careful to check for deposits in any mesial and distal **root concavities** at the CEJ if this area is exposed as a result of recession.

Finally, many dental professionals believe that competency of the lips to maintain a lip seal, when at a **resting posture,** can affect the position of the maxillary incisors (see **Chapter 20**). Competent lips allow these

Continued

tooth tips to lie below the lower lip border, helping to maintain normal inclination. Incompetent lips that fail to provide a lip seal do not control this inclination and may even allow the maxillary incisors to lie in front of the lower lip, exaggerating already buccally-inclined teeth and possibly become lingually inclined. A **tongue thrust** is a complicating factor that may be associated with this problem (see **Chapter 20**).

PERMANENT MAXILLARY CENTRAL INCISORS #8 AND #9

Specific Overall Features (Figure 16-11) Permanent maxillary central incisors erupt between 7 to 8 years of age (root completion at age 10). Thus, these teeth usually erupt after the mandibular central incisors. Many child patients want these two teeth to come in fast to fill their wide arch space when they shed their four primary maxillary incisors, as in the old song, *All I Want for Christmas Is My Two Front Teeth*.

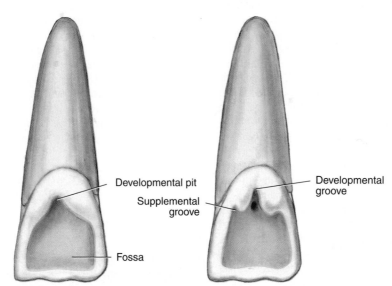

Developmental pit
Supplemental groove
Fossa
Developmental groove

FIGURE 16-6 Additional examples of lingual surface features on a permanent anterior tooth.

TABLE 16-1	Anatomical Information on Permanent Incisors			
	MAXILLARY CENTRAL INCISOR	**MAXILLARY LATERAL INCISOR**	**MANDIBULAR CENTRAL INCISOR**	**MANDIBULAR LATERAL INCISOR**
Universal number	#8 and #9	#7 and #10	#24 and #25	#23 and #26
General crown features	Incisal edge and incisal angles			
Specific crown features	Widest crown MD, greatest CEJ curve, and height of contour; distal offset cingulum, shallow lingual fossa, marginal ridges	Greatest crown variation, like a smaller maxillary central, prominent lingual surface; centered cingulum, pronounced marginal ridges	Smallest and simplest tooth, bilaterally symmetrical; small centered cingulum, subtle lingual fossa, and equal subtle marginal ridges	Like a larger mandibular central, not bilaterally symmetrical; appears twisted distally; small, distally placed cingulum; lingual fossa and moderate mesial marginal ridge longer than distal
Height of contour	Cervical third			
Mesial contact	Incisal third			
Distal contact	Junction of incisal and middle thirds	Middle third or junction with incisal third	Incisal third	Incisal third
Distinguishing right from left	Sharper MI angle, rounder DI angle, more pronounced mesial CEJ curvature			
General root features	Single-rooted			
Specific root features	Overall conical shape; no proximal root concavities		Bow shaped on cross section; root is longer than the crown; proximal root concavities give double-rooted appearance	
	Rounded apex; triangular in cross section		Root curves distally, with sharp apex; oval in cross section; same or longer than central but thinner	

CEJ, Cementoenamel junction; DI, distoincisal; MD, mesiodistally; MI, mesioincisal.

The maxillary central incisors are the most prominent teeth in the permanent dentition because of both their large size and their anterior arch position. In consideration of a patient's smile design, the central incisors should be dominant with perspective in such a way that each tooth posteriorly appears to get smaller. In addition, they are the largest of all the incisors, and the two usually share a mesial contact area. The outline of the crown from the labial or lingual view is trapezoidal (four-sided with two parallel sides); it has the widest crown mesiodistally of any permanent anterior tooth.

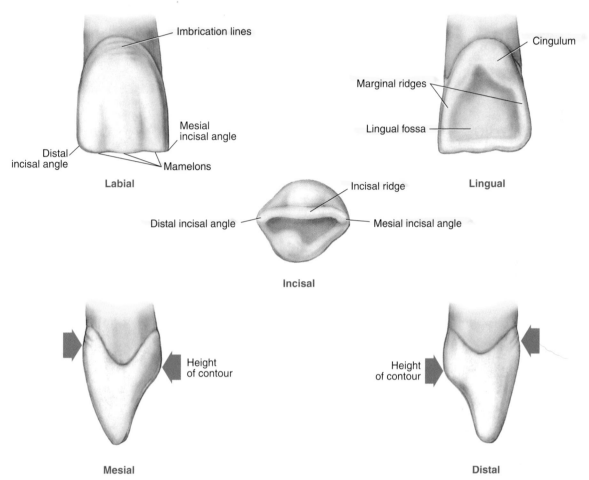

FIGURE 16-7 Views of a newly erupted permanent incisor, with the features noted.

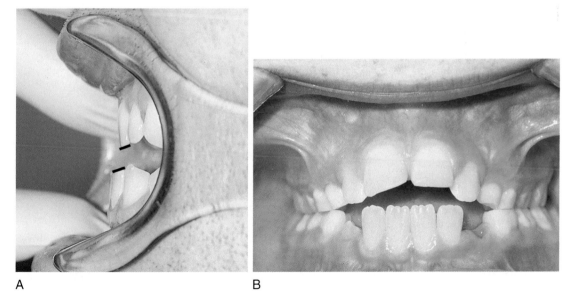

FIGURE 16-8 Examples of the incisal edges on permanent incisors. A: Lateral view of permanent incisors altered by attrition on the incisal surfaces (see the *dark lines* on incisal edges). B: Mamelons present on the incisal edges of permanent incisors in a mixed dentition, resulting from an open bite.

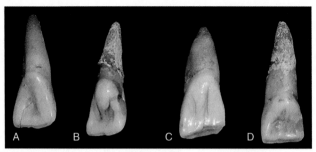

FIGURE 16-9 Lingual views of permanent maxillary incisors. **A:** Shovel shape. **B:** Accentuated cingulum, with deepened grooves. **C:** Attrition on incisal surface and showing lingual inclination. **D:** Stain in the lingual fossa.

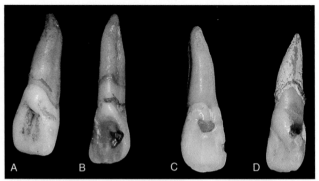

FIGURE 16-10 Lingual views of permanent maxillary incisors. **A:** Lingual pit. **B:** Lingual pit with caries. **C:** Lingual pit caries repaired. **D:** Linguogingival groove, resulting in caries.

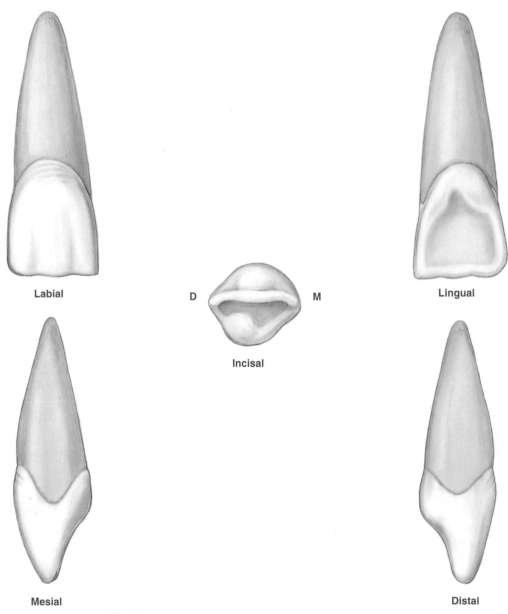

Labial

D ⏜ M

Incisal

Lingual

Mesial

Distal

FIGURE 16-11 Views of a permanent maxillary right central incisor.

The maxillary central incisor has a single conical root, smooth and slightly straight, usually with a rounded apex. Thus, the root is thick in the cervical third and narrows through the middle to the blunt apex and is one and one half times the length of the crown. The root is also about the same length, or shorter, but wider than the lateral of the same arch. Bulbous crowns may create deep mesial and distal concavities at CEJ. The pulp cavity mirrors the shape of the tooth; there is only one root canal, which is rather large (Figure 16-12).

The pulp chamber of the maxillary central incisor has three sharp elongations, the mesial, distal, and central pulp horns. These pulp horns correspond to the three labial developmental lobes of the tooth. The central pulp horn is usually shorter than the other two and more rounded. The root is oval in cervical cross section, being slightly wider on the labial surface and narrower at the lingual.

Labial View Features The crown of a maxillary central incisor is narrowest at the cervical third and becomes wider toward the incisal edge on the labial surface (see Figure 16-11). The incisal ridge is nearly straight. Two labial developmental depressions may extend the length of the crown from the cervical to the incisal, showing the division of the surface into three labial developmental lobes. The crown usually has **imbrication lines,** or slight ridges, that run mesiodistally

in the cervical third, and between them are the grooved **perikymata.** The CEJ on the labial surface has more curvature to the distal.

From the labial view, both incisal angles can be seen on the maxillary central incisor. The overall mesial outline is slightly rounded, with a sharp mesioincisal angle. The overall distal outline is even rounder, with a definite rounded distoincisal angle. The difference in sharpness of the central's mesioincisal and distoincisal angle *helps to distinguish the right maxillary central incisor from the left.*

The mesial contact with the other maxillary central is in the incisal third (see Figure 16-7). The distal contact with the maxillary lateral is at the junction of the incisal and middle third, located farther cervically than the mesial contact.

Lingual View Features The lingual surface of the crown of a maxillary central incisor is narrower overall than the labial surface (Figure 16-13). The CEJ usually has more curvature to the distal. The single cingulum is wide and well developed in size, as well as being located slightly off center toward the distal.

From the lingual view, the mesial marginal ridge is longer than the distal marginal ridge. The single lingual fossa is wide yet shallow and is located immediately incisal to the cingulum. The lingual fossa varies in depth and diameter. Outlining the incisal border of the lingual fossa, the raised linguoincisal edge is on the same level as the bordering marginal ridges.

On the lingual surface, a horizontally placed lingual groove may be present (although it is more common on maxillary laterals), separating the cingulum from the lingual fossa. The lingual groove may make the cingulum appear scalloped.

A lingual pit may also be present at the incisal border of the cingulum in the lingual groove. Also present may be a vertically placed linguogingival groove, which originates in the lingual pit and extends cervically and slightly distally onto the cingulum.

Proximal View Features The CEJ curvature on the mesial surface is deep incisally and has the greatest depth of curvature of any tooth surface in the permanent dentition, which *helps to distinguish the right maxillary central incisor from the left* (see Figure 16-11). The height of contour for both the labial and lingual surfaces is also greater on this tooth than on any tooth in the permanent dentition and is located at the cervical third, as in all incisors.

The incisal edge is located slightly labial to the long axis of the tooth. The incisal outline is also sloped toward the lingual from its longest

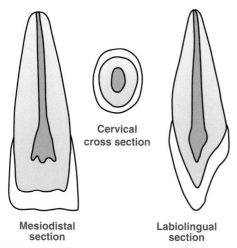

Cervical cross section

Mesiodistal section **Labiolingual section**

FIGURE 16-12 Pulp cavity of a permanent maxillary right central incisor.

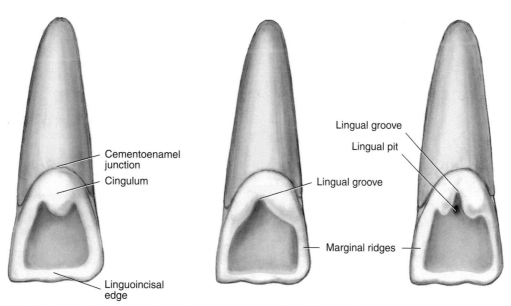

Cementoenamel junction

Cingulum

Lingual groove

Lingual groove

Lingual pit

Lingual groove

Marginal ridges

Linguoincisal edge

FIGURE 16-13 Variations of the lingual surface of the permanent maxillary right central incisor, with the lingual fossae highlighted.

and, also, most labial part. The distal view is similar to the mesial, although the curvature of the CEJ is less on the distal than on the mesial surface.

Incisal View Features   Overall, the shape of the crown of a maxillary central incisor from the incisal view is triangular, with the labial outline broadly rounded. This is a useful view for observing the slight distal placement of the cingulum. On the lingual surface of the incisal view, the mesial marginal ridge again appears longer than the distal marginal ridge. Note that the incisal edge lies just labial to the long axis of the root.

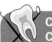

Clinical Considerations with Maxillary Central Incisors

The incisal edge, or even the entire maxillary central incisor, is especially at risk for traumatic fracture or tooth displacement because of the tooth's most anterior and labial position (especially its incisal edge) and its early eruption into the oral cavity. Because of these two factors and without full root completion, the entire tooth in a child may undergo **avulsion**, which is complete displacement of the tooth from the socket, resulting from extensive trauma to the area. Even if the tooth only undergoes fracture, pulpal pathology may occur in the tooth and result in the need for endodontic therapy or loss of tooth vitality as the pulp dies.

An open contact, or **diastema**, can also exist between the maxillary central incisors, which can be a wide, and to some patients, an unattractive space (see Table 6-3*H*). Both the cause and treatment of this type of diastema are controversial. Treatment may involve surgery to reduce the impact of a tight maxillary **labial frenum**, with or without additional orthodontic therapy. Incisors may appear *winged* looking when looking at the patient's smile, but they are not a disturbance of development but, rather, a case of tooth rotation, usually bilateral rotation to the mesial.

Developmental Disturbances of Maxillary Central Incisors

One common location for a supernumerary tooth is between the two maxillary central incisors or **mesiodens** (see Table 6-3, *B*). It is due to the presence of an extra **tooth germ** resulting from an abnormal **initiation stage** during tooth development, a **supernumerary tooth**. The presence of this extra tooth may affect spacing in the maxillary arch, whether it is erupted or not. The tooth may also have a dwarfed root, which results in a lack of periodontal support for the tooth and may negatively affect the prognosis of the tooth if it is involved in periodontal disease.

PERMANENT MAXILLARY LATERAL INCISORS #7 AND #10

Specific Overall Features (Figure 16-14)   Permanent maxillary lateral incisors erupt between 8 to 9 years of age (root completion at age 11). Thus, these teeth usually erupt after the maxillary central incisors.

The crown of a maxillary lateral incisor has the greatest degree of variation in form of any permanent tooth, except for the third molars. A maxillary lateral usually resembles a maxillary central incisor in all views of the tooth but has a smaller and slightly rounder crown.

A maxillary lateral incisor has a single conical root that is relatively smooth and straight but may curve slightly to the distal. Its crown is one to one and one half times shorter than the length of the root. The root is also about the same length as or longer than the central, but it is thinner, particularly mesiodistally, as well as being wider labiolingually. This tooth is frequently confused with a small permanent mandibular canine, but the root usually has no depressions on the proximal surface, as is common on a mandibular canine. A linguogingival groove may be present on the root (and possibly on the crown). The apex of the root is not rounded like the central but is sharp.

The pulp cavity of the maxillary lateral incisor is simple in form, with a single pulp canal and a pulp chamber (Figure 16-15). The pulp chamber does not have three sharp pulp horns as it does in a maxillary central incisor; instead, it usually has one rounded form or two less-sharp pulp horns, a mesial and distal pulp horn. The shape of the root on cross section is oval.

Labial View Features   The labial developmental depressions and imbrication lines on the labial surface are less common on a maxillary lateral than on a central incisor (see Figure 16-14). The crown is smaller than that of a central incisor and less symmetrical.

Generally, it resembles a central in its mesial outline, with the mesial contact with the maxillary central at the incisal third or at the junction of the incisal and the middle third, farther cervically than the central. The distal outline is always rounder than the central and has a more cervical distal contact area with the maxillary canine, at the middle third or at the junction of the incisal and the middle third.

From the labial view, both incisal angles are rounder on a maxillary lateral than on a central incisor. Although similar to a central incisor, a maxillary lateral has different incisal angles from the labial. The lateral's mesioincisal angle is sharper than the distoincisal angle, which *helps to distinguish the right maxillary lateral incisor from the left*.

Lingual View Features   The lingual surface of the crown of a maxillary lateral incisor is narrower than the labial surface, as is the case with a central (Figure 16-16). It has a prominent, yet centered and narrower cingulum than does a central incisor, with a deeper lingual fossa. The marginal ridges are pronounced: The longer mesial marginal ridge is nearly straight, and the shorter distal marginal ridge is quite straight. The linguoincisal ridge is also noticeably well developed in size.

On the lingual surface, a horizontal lingual groove that separates the cingulum from the lingual fossa is more common on a maxillary lateral and better developed than on a central. A lingual pit is more common on a lateral than on a central and is located on the incisal surface of the cingulum, along the lingual groove.

Additionally present on the lingual surface may be a vertical linguogingival groove that originates in the lingual pit and extends cervically and slightly distally onto the cingulum. The linguogingival groove may extend onto the root surface. The linguogingival groove is also more common on this tooth than on a maxillary central. Rarely, the root has a deep distolingual marginal groove, a developmental groove that starts on the distal marginal ridge on the lingual surface and extends onto the root.

Proximal View Features   The crown of a maxillary lateral incisor is triangular on a mesial view, as are all anterior teeth (see Figure 16-14). The CEJ curvature is similar to that of a central, although it is not as deeply curved on a lateral. Also similar to a central, a lateral's CEJ is more curved on the mesial surface than the distal of this tooth, which *helps to distinguish the right maxillary lateral incisor from the left*. The incisal edge is usually labial to the long axis of the tooth. The distal view is similar to that of the mesial, although the CEJ is not as deeply curved.

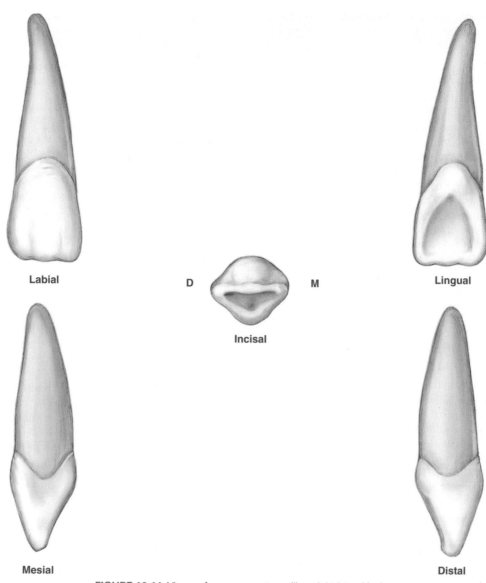

Labial

D   **Incisal**   M

Lingual

Mesial

Distal

FIGURE 16-14 Views of a permanent maxillary right lateral incisor.

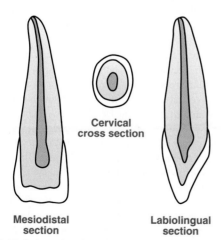

Mesiodistal section   **Cervical cross section**   **Labiolingual section**

FIGURE 16-15 Pulp cavity of a permanent maxillary right lateral incisor.

Clinical Considerations with Maxillary Lateral Incisors

Because of the variations in form and the possibility of developmental disturbances (see the next section), maxillary lateral incisors present challenges during preventive, restorative, and orthodontic procedures. Open contacts that seem unattractive to patients may be easily visible in this region of the dental arch due to these variations in form, as well as asymmetrical in both tooth size and position across the maxillary arch.

The linguogingival groove can be considered a clinically adverse factor because deposits can accumulate in the nichelike groove. This condition can track apically the periodontal destruction as the groove advances, resulting in the formation of a deeply localized periodontal lesion. A deeper mean probing pocket depth and a greater degree of severe **gingivitis** is usually present in an involved **groove** region. Careful, repeated pocket depth probing with associated root exploration is essential to monitor these high-risk areas for periodontal complications in a patient.

Developmental Disturbances of Maxillary Lateral Incisors

A maxillary lateral incisor is one of the most common teeth of the permanent dentition to exhibit partial **microdontia** (see Table 6-3, C). This disturbance leads to a smaller lateral incisor crown, or **peg lateral**, present either unilaterally or bilaterally. This disturbance occurs in the process of **proliferation** during tooth development. It may be hereditary or may result from other factors. Treatment to improve appearance may include restorative materials that increase the size of the tooth.

The maxillary laterals are also more commonly involved in partial **anodontia** (hypodontia) and thus may be congenitally missing. This disturbance results from an absence of the appropriate individual **tooth germ** (or germs) in the area, unilaterally or bilaterally at around 1% to 2%, from a failure in the initiation process during tooth development. Partial anodontia may present esthetic problems for patients and can result in problems in occlusion; thus, these missing teeth may require a prosthetic replacement or an implant.

Finally, a maxillary lateral may have one or more **tubercles**, or accessory **cusps**, on the **cingulum**. The **dilaceration** of the crown or root, showing angular distortion, may occur, making extraction and endodontic treatment difficult.

Incisal View Features The outline of the crown of a maxillary lateral incisor is round or oval from the incisal view, not triangular, as is a central. The crown's mesiodistal measurement is somewhat wider than the labiolingual measurement. Thus, the labial surface of the lateral is rounder than that of a central.

PERMANENT MANDIBULAR INCISORS
GENERAL FEATURES

Permanent mandibular incisors are the smallest teeth of the permanent dentition and the most symmetrical. More uniformity in form is seen among these teeth than among any other of the permanent dentition. The lateral and central incisors of the mandibular arch resemble each other more than do the similar types of incisors of the maxillary arch.

Generally, a mandibular lateral is slightly larger than a central, exactly the opposite of the situation in the maxillary arch. The **incisal ridge** usually also wears from attrition mainly on the labial surface to become the **incisal edge**. The incisal edge is just lingual to the long axis of the root. Each mandibular incisor has a crown that is wider labiolingually than mesiodistally, this being unlike the maxillary incisors. Both mandibular incisors also have smoother and less complex **lingual surface** features than the maxillary incisors, including a cingulum, lingual fossa, and marginal ridges.

Proximal **root concavities** are also present on both types of mandibular incisors and, if deep enough, give the teeth a double-rooted appearance. The root of a mandibular incisor is elliptical, an elongated oval on cervical cross section. Thus, the root is extremely narrow on the labial and lingual surfaces and wide on both proximal surfaces. The root is longer than the crown for both incisors (see Figures 16-18 and 16-20).

PERMANENT MANDIBULAR CENTRAL INCISORS #24 AND #25

Specific Overall Features (Figure 16-18) Permanent mandibular central incisors erupt between 6 to 7 years of age (root completion at age 9). Thus, these teeth usually erupt before the maxillary

Clinical Considerations with Mandibular Incisors

Although the concavity of the **lingual surface** of all mandibular incisors is smoother than that of maxillary incisors, supragingival tooth deposits, such as dental biofilm, calculus, and stain, tend to collect in the concavity. This buildup of deposits is aided by the mandibular incisors' position in the oral cavity near the **duct** openings of the **submandibular salivary gland** and **sublingual salivary glands** in the **floor of the mouth**. **Saliva**, with its mineral content, is released from these glands, causing the dental biofilm to mineralize quickly into calculus.

With **attrition**, the wearing away of a tooth surface caused by tooth-to-tooth contact, the incisal edge can change on the mandibular incisors (see **Chapter 20**). Thus, these incisors may lose their symmetrical form, exposing the inner **dentin** (Figure 16-17). With severe attrition, the incisal edge also becomes a concavity lined with exposed dentin; this porous dentin becomes intrinsically stained and unattractive or can be affected by **dentinal hypersensitivity** (see Figure 13-9).

Instrumentation may be more difficult in this area because many patients have overlapping mandibular incisors owing to inadequate mandibular arch size and other occlusal factors. This crowding increases with age because of normal physiological **mesial drift** (see Figure 20-21). If the incisors tip incisally back toward the tongue, instrumentation is also extremely difficult, and use of a mouth mirror for indirect vision is essential.

Prolonged hand instrumentation can narrow even further the already narrow labial and lingual root surfaces of the mandibular incisors. The crowns of the teeth can thus be placed in jeopardy during mastication because of unsupported cervical enamel. Finally, the proximal surface of the roots is difficult to explore with instruments because of the limited interproximal space and the oval root shape, and the presence of proximal root concavities may also increase the difficulty.

central incisors. They are the smallest and simplest teeth of the permanent dentition; thus, they are smaller than the lateral incisors of the same arch. Due to its smallness, the tooth has only one antagonist in the maxillary arch. This tooth and the maxillary third molar are the only teeth that have one antagonist; all others have two. However, equally different is that the two mandibular centrals usually share a mesial contact area.

This tooth has a simple root, which is widest labiolingually and then mesiodistally. The root has pronounced proximal root concavities, which vary in both length and depth, and a shallow depression extends longitudinally along the midportion of root. Dental professionals must remember that root proximation with a contralateral tooth may cause access difficulty.

The pulp cavity of the mandibular central is quite simple, because it has a single pulp canal and three pulp horns (Figure 16-19). The root is a narrow oval in cross section.

Labial View Features The crown of a mandibular central incisor is quite symmetrical from the labial view, having a fan shape (see Figure 16-18). The imbrication lines and developmental depressions usually are not present or are extremely faint. The mesial contact with the other mandibular central is at the incisal third. The distal contact with the lateral incisor is also at the incisal third.

From the labial view, both the incisal angles, mesioincisal angle and distoincisal angle, are sharp or only slightly rounded; the mesioincisal angle is slightly sharper than the distoincisal angle, which *helps to distinguish the right mandibular central incisor from the left*. Nevertheless, distinguishing between the right and left central incisors is often

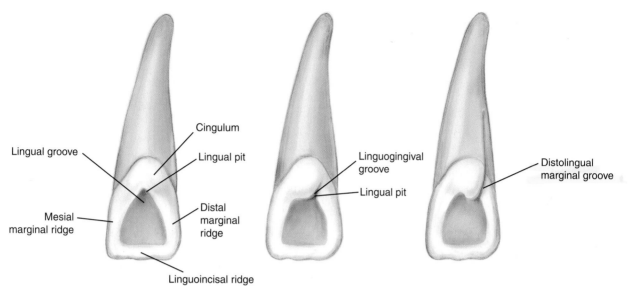

FIGURE 16-16 Variations of the lingual surface of the permanent maxillary right lateral incisor, with the lingual fossae highlighted.

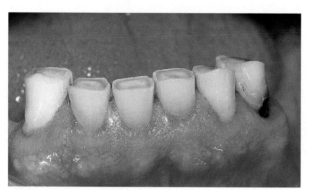

FIGURE 16-17 Attrition noted on the incisal surface of the permanent mandibular incisors, as well as canines.

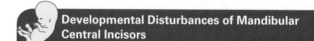

Developmental Disturbances of Mandibular Central Incisors

Developmental disturbances are rarely noted in the mandibular central incisors. One rare exception is that the teeth may have an **accessory root** or **bifurcated** root, with the two branches having labial and lingual orientations.

PERMANENT MANDIBULAR LATERAL INCISORS #23 AND #26

Specific Overall Features (Figure 16-20) Permanent mandibular lateral incisors erupt between 7 to 8 years of age (root completion at age 10). Thus, these teeth usually erupt after the mandibular central incisors. It is slightly larger overall than a central; there is also more variation in form. The crown is also slightly larger than that of a central, but it resembles a central in most other ways. From both the labial and lingual views, the crown appears tilted or twisted distally in comparison with the long axis of the tooth; this gives the impression that the tooth has been bent at the CEJ.

The single root of a mandibular lateral is usually straight, slightly longer, and wider than that of a central. The root, like that of a mandibular central, has pronounced proximal root concavities, especially on the distal surface. These vary in both length and depth. The pulp cavity for this tooth is quite simple, because it has a single pulp canal and three pulp horns (Figure 16-21).

Labial View Features The crown of a mandibular lateral incisor is not as symmetrical as that of a central and appears tilted or twisted distally on the root from the labial view (see Figure 16-20). The tooth is not symmetrical because the distal outline is slightly rounder and shorter compared with the slightly flatter and longer mesial outline. The incisal angles are different: The mesioincisal angle of the incisal edge is sharper than the distoincisal angle, which *helps to distinguish the right mandibular lateral incisor from the left.* The labial developmental depressions are deeper than on the central incisors.

From the labial view, the mesial contact with a mandibular central incisor is in the incisal third. The distal contact with a mandibular canine is in the incisal third but is located more cervically than the mesial contact.

difficult. The mesial and distal outlines are nearly straight from the CEJ to the relatively straight incisal edge.

Lingual View Features The crown of a mandibular central incisor is narrower on the lingual surface than the labial, with its outline that is the reverse of the labial view. However, its outline of the crown is the most symmetrical of all incisors, either maxillary or mandibular. Overall, the lingual surface is smooth and has a small, centered cingulum.

On the lingual surface, the single lingual fossa is barely noticeable; therefore, the mesial marginal ridge and distal marginal ridge are barely noticeable as well. Because the cingulum is centered, the faint mesial and distal marginal ridges have the same length.

Proximal View Features The CEJ curvature is higher incisally on the mesial than on the distal surface, which *helps to distinguish the right mandibular central incisor from the left.* The incisal edge is usually straight but can be rounded and is lingual to the long axis of the root. The distal view is similar to the mesial view of the tooth, except that the CEJ curves less incisally on the distal than on the mesial surface.

Incisal View Features The mandibular central incisor has a nearly symmetrical crown outline on the incisal view. The incisal edge is usually at a right angle, or perpendicular, to the labiolingual axis of the crown of the tooth and overall is just lingual to the long axis of the root. The labiolingual measurement is also wider than the mesiodistal measurement on incisal view. Again, on the lingual surface, the faint mesial marginal ridge and distal marginal ridge are the same length.

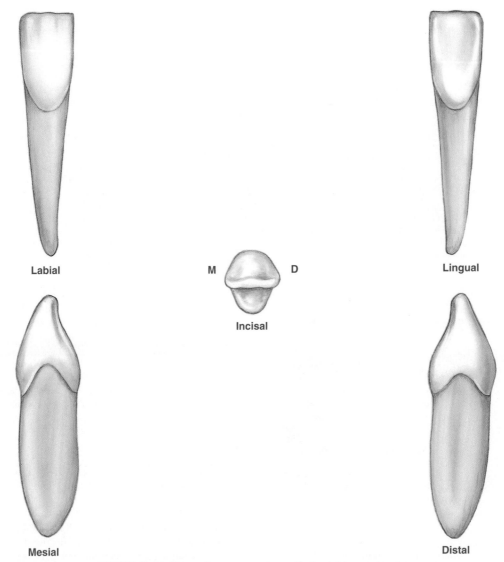

Labial

M D

Incisal

Lingual

Mesial

Distal

FIGURE 16-18 Views of a permanent mandibular right central incisor.

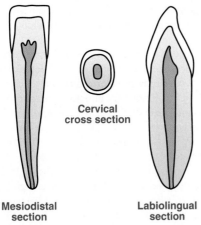

**Cervical
cross section**

**Mesiodistal
section**

**Labiolingual
section**

FIGURE 16-19 Pulp cavity of a permanent mandibular right central incisor.

The small single cingulum lies just distal to the long axis of the root.

On the lingual surface, both the mesial marginal ridge and distal marginal ridge are more developed than on a central, although the mesial marginal ridge is longer than the distal marginal ridge. A single lingual fossa is also present, but a lingual pit is rarely present on a lateral, although more often than on a central.

Proximal View Features The greater height of the CEJ curvature on the mesial than the distal surface *helps to distinguish the right mandibular lateral incisor from the left.* Also, from the mesial view, more of the lingual surface is visible because of the distal tilt or twist of the incisal edge. The distal view is similar to the mesial view of the tooth, but the CEJ is curved less on the distal than the mesial surface.

Incisal View Features A rounder appearance is noted both labially and lingually from the incisal view of a mandibular lateral incisor as compared with that of a central. The entire incisal edge is not straight mesiodistally, as it is in a central; instead, the incisal edge curves toward the lingual in its distal part. Additionally the incisal angles are different: The distoincisal angle is visibly at a distinctly lingual location compared to the mesioincisal angle, and the cingulum appears displaced toward the distal. Again, on the lingual surface, the mesial marginal ridge is longer than the distal marginal ridge.

Lingual View Features The crown of a mandibular lateral incisor lacks bilateral symmetry and appears tilted or twisted distally on the root from the lingual view, with its outline the reverse of the labial view. Overall, the lingual surface has more prominent features as compared to the lingual surface of a central incisor.

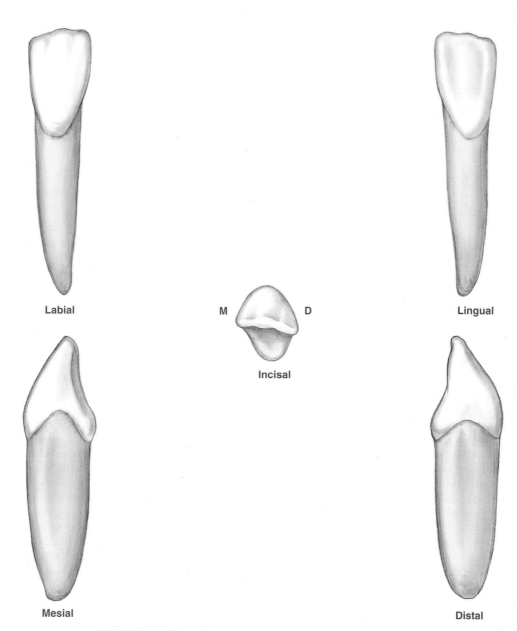

Labial

M   D

Incisal

Lingual

Mesial

Distal

FIGURE 16-20 Views of a permanent mandibular right lateral incisor.

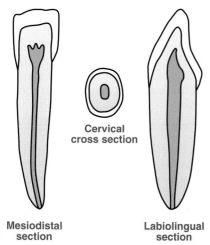

Mesiodistal
section

Cervical
cross section

Labiolingual
section

FIGURE 16-21 Pulp cavity of a permanent mandibular right lateral incisor.

**Developmental Disturbances of Mandibular
Lateral Incisors**

Developmental disturbances are rare in a mandibular lateral incisor, as is the case with a central. One rare exception is that the tooth may have an **accessory root** or **bifurcated** root, with the two branches having labial and lingual orientation.

PERMANENT CANINES

GENERAL FEATURES

Permanent **canines** are the four anterior teeth located at the corners of each quadrant for each dental arch (Table 16-2). Thus, it is the third tooth from the midline in each quadrant, distal to the incisors and

TABLE 16-2	Anatomical Information on Permanent Canines	
	MAXILLARY CANINE	**MANDIBULAR CANINE**
Universal number	#6 and #11	#22 and #27
General crown features	Single cusp, with tip and slopes, labial ridge, marginal ridges and lingual ridge, cingulum, and lingual fossae; longest tooth in each arch or dentition	
Specific crown features	Prominent lingual anatomy, sharp cusp tip	Smoother lingual anatomy, less sharp cusp tip
Height of contour	Labial: cervical third	
	Lingual: middle third	
Mesial contact	Junction of incisal third and middle thirds	Incisal third
Distal contact	Middle third	Junction of incisal and middle thirds
Distinguishing right from left	Shorter mesial cusp slope, more cervical contact on distal, more pronounced mesial CEJ curvature	
	Shorter distal outline on labial view with depression between the distal contact and CEJ	Shorter and rounder distal outline on labial view, with a shorter mesial slope than distal
General root features	Long, thick single root; ovoid on cross section; proximal root concavities	
Specific root features	Blunt root apex	Developmental depressions on mesial and distal giving tooth double-rooted appearance; pointed apex

CEJ, Cementoenamel junction.

mesial to the posteriors. The permanent canines are **succedaneous** and replace the primary canines of the same type.

Patients commonly call the canines the *eye teeth;* an older term was cuspids, because they were the only teeth in the permanent dentition with one cusp. The more commonly used name of *canines* comes from the Latin word for dog, because they resemble dogs' teeth. Patients often complain of the slightly deeper yellow color of their permanent canines compared with their incisors, a normal color tone in the dentition that is actually placed in dentures to mimic a natural look.

Both the maxillary and mandibular canines resemble one another. The crown of each is about the same size and, when viewed from the proximal, appears triangular, like all anterior teeth. When viewed from the labial or lingual, however, its crown outline appears pentagonal, with five sides, similar to the premolars. Canines are also wider labiolingually than the incisors, even wider than maxillary central incisors.

Similar to the other anteriors, each of the canines has an **incisal edge** (Figure 16-22). Different from the incisors is the cusp tip, which is in line with the long axis of the root for both maxillary and mandibular canines when first erupted. Because of the presence of the cusp tip, the incisal edge is divided into two cusp slopes or ridges, rather than being nearly straight across like the incisors.

The mesial cusp slope is usually shorter than the distal cusp slope for both the maxillary and mandibular canines when they first erupt. The mesial cusp slope of a maxillary canine occludes with the distal cusp slope of a mandibular canine. The length of these cusp slopes and position of the cusp tip can change with **attrition** (discussed later).

The canines are the only teeth in the permanent dentition with a vertical and centrally placed labial ridge. This labial ridge is a result of greater development of the middle labial developmental lobe in comparison with the mesial and distal labial developmental lobes. Mamelons are not normally present on the incisal edge as they are on incisors, but a small notch may be seen on either cusp slope. The height of contour on labial and lingual surfaces is in the cervical third for the canines, similar to all anteriors.

Each canine also has a **cingulum** and **marginal ridges** on its **lingual surface**, like the incisors (Figure 16-23). The cingulum corresponds to the lingual developmental lobe, as in the incisors, but is

larger than on any incisor. As with the incisors, however, its crown is narrower on the lingual surface than on the labial surface, with the crown tapering lingually.

In addition, canines have a vertical, centrally placed lingual ridge that extends from the cusp tip to the cingulum. The lingual ridge creates two separate and shallow lingual **fossae** between it and the bordering **marginal ridges**; these lingual fossae are more pronounced on the maxillary canines than on the mandibular.

The permanent canines are the longest teeth in the dentition. Each has a particularly long, thick root, and the root is usually one and one half times the length of the crown. The long and large root is externally manifested by the vertically oriented and labially placed bony ridge called the **canine eminence** of the alveolar bone, which is especially noted on the maxilla. Proximal **root concavities** are located on both proximal root surfaces. The root is ovoid or egg shaped on cervical cross section (see Figures 16-26 and 16-29).

Clinical Considerations with Canines

Because of their tapered shape and prominent cusp, the canines function to pierce or tear food during mastication—and because of their arch position, serve as a major support of facial muscles and keep the overall **vertical dimension of the face** intact. Without their presence, normal facial contours cannot be maintained, and a loss of height occurs in the lower third of vertical dimension. Anatomists consider the canines the cornerstones of the **dental arch** because of their arch position, tooth form, and function.

The canines also support the incisors and premolars in their functions during mastication and speech. During occlusal movement, they act as guideposts (see Figure 20-13). In this respect, they serve as a protective functional device for a type of mandibular movement that is termed *lateral deviation.* Finally, they can help relieve any excessive horizontal forces imposed on posteriors.

The canines are the most stable teeth in the dentition, one reason being their long root length, which offers an increased amount of periodontal tissue support. In addition, the proximal root concavities help to provide an increased periodontal anchorage for these teeth. Thus, these teeth have a significantly reduced risk of loss as a result of periodontal disease or traumatic injury, usually making them the last teeth lost in a failing dentition. The canines (or many times only the roots) often serve as the stabilizing anchors for replacements of lost teeth in prosthetic procedures, such as the placement of partial dentures or permanent bridges. These teeth are also important esthetically because each one holds the commissure out, reducing the appearance of any lip lines or wrinkles present.

Caries usually does not occur with canines, another factor that makes them an extremely stable tooth in the dentition. This is because the crown part usually has a form that promotes self-cleansing and does not easily retain dental biofilm or other deposits.

However, changes can occur in the length of each canine **cusp slope** and in the movement of the position of the usually centered **cusp tip**. In older patients, the lengths of the cusp slopes are often altered by **attrition**, the wearing away of a tooth surface caused by tooth-to-tooth contact (Figure 16-24). With wear, each cusp tip of the maxillary canines is moved to the distal of center, with mesial displacement of the cusp tip for the mandibular canine. This wear also lengthens the mesial cusp slope, shortens the distal slope for the maxillary canines, and shortens the mesial cusp slope and lengthens the distal slope for the mandibular canines. The wear pattern on a canine from the incisal view can appear either diamond shaped or triangular.

It is also noted that proximal surfaces of the canines are more accessible from the lingual than the facial approach during instrumentation. This is because of the convergence of the proximal surfaces toward the lingual.

PERMANENT MAXILLARY CANINES #6 AND #11
SPECIFIC OVERALL FEATURES

Permanent maxillary canines erupt between 11 to 12 years of age (root completion between ages 13 to 15) (Figure 16-25). Thus, these teeth usually erupt after the mandibular canines, after the maxillary incisors, and possibly after the maxillary premolars.

The crown of a maxillary canine is similar in length, or even shorter, than that of a maxillary central incisor. Labiolingually, the crown is considerably wider than that of a central incisor, but a canine crown is noticeably narrower mesiodistally. The cingulum on the lingual surface is more developed and larger than that of a central incisor of the same arch, making the tooth stronger during mastication.

A maxillary canine does somewhat resemble a mandibular canine. However, the cusp is more developed and larger, and the cusp tip is sharper on a maxillary tooth. In addition, the entire lingual surface features of the maxillary canine are more prominent, including the lingual ridge and marginal ridges.

Finally, an entire maxillary canine is as long as a mandibular canine, but the crown is as long as, or slightly shorter, than that of a mandibular canine. The long root is single and has a blunt apex; it is the longest root in the maxillary arch. Developmental depressions are evident on both proximal surfaces of the root but are especially pronounced on the distal surface owing to the distal prominence of crown at CEJ. Moderate to deep proximal concavities are also possible. The pulp cavity consists of a single pulp canal and a large pulp chamber (Figure 16-26). The pulp chamber usually has only one pulp horn.

LABIAL VIEW FEATURES

The mesial half of the crown of a maxillary canine resembles a part of an incisor, and the distal half resembles a part of a premolar, showing the transition from the incisors to the premolars in the maxillary arch (see Figure 16-25). Normally, both imbrication lines and perikymata are present in the cervical third of the surface, especially in newly erupted teeth.

Two faint and vertical mesial and distal labial developmental depressions extend from the cervical to the incisal and separate the three labial developmental lobes. These depressions are located on either side of the vertical, centrally placed labial ridge, and this ridge is most noticeable in the incisal part of the labial surface.

The mesial outline of the labial surface of the maxillary canine is usually rounded from the mesial contact area to the CEJ, but overall it is straighter than the distal outline. The distal outline is shorter than the mesial outline and usually has a depression between the distal contact area and the CEJ, which *helps to distinguish the right maxillary canine from the left*. From the labial view, the mesial and distal contacts are on two different levels of the tooth, which *helps to distinguish the right maxillary canine from the left*. The mesial contact with the lateral incisor is at the junction of the incisal and middle thirds. The distal contact with the first premolar is more cervical because it is at the middle third.

As previously discussed, the single cusp is round, and the mesial cusp slope of a maxillary canine is shorter than the distal cusp slope when first erupted, which *helps to distinguish the right maxillary canine from the left*. The cementoenamel junction or CEJ on the labial surface is evenly curved toward the root.

LINGUAL VIEW FEATURES

The mesial, distal, and incisal lingual outlines of a maxillary canine are similar to those on the labial view of the tooth (Figure 16-27). The overall dimension of the lingual surface is less than that of the labial surface, however, because the mesial and distal surfaces converge slightly toward the lingual. The cingulum is large and usually smooth and is centered mesiodistally on the lingual surface.

The lingual surface also has a prominent mesial marginal ridge and distal marginal ridge. A vertical, centrally placed lingual ridge is also present from the cingulum to the cusp tip, separating two lingual fossae, the shallow but visible mesiolingual fossa and distolingual fossa. Each of the major features of this tooth are "variations on a theme": The cingulum and incisal half of the lingual surface are sometimes separated by a shallow lingual groove, and this groove may contain a lingual pit near its center, or the pit may also be present without the lingual groove.

PROXIMAL VIEW FEATURES

The mesial and distal aspects present a triangular outline. They resemble the maxillary incisors but are more robust, especially in the cingulum region. The CEJ curves higher incisally on the mesial than on the distal surface, which *helps to distinguish the right maxillary canine from the left* (see Figure 16-26). The cusp tip is toward the labial. The distal view of the tooth is similar to the mesial view, but the CEJ curvature is less on the distal than on the mesial surface.

INCISAL VIEW FEATURES

Again, the labiolingual width of a maxillary canine is large in comparison with that of any other anterior tooth, making it an extremely strong tooth during mastication. Additionally, the crown outline is asymmetrical; the

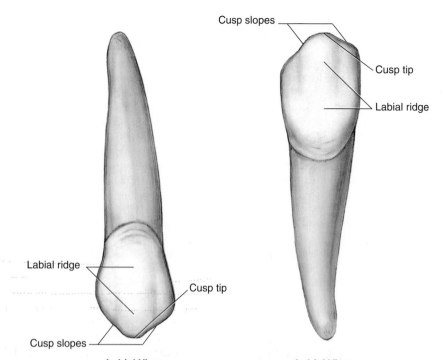

Labial View
Permanent Maxillary Right Canine

Labial View
Permanent Mandibular Right Canine

FIGURE 16-22 Labial views of newly erupted permanent canines, with features noted.

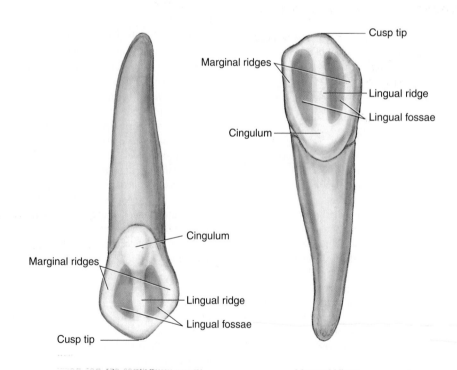

Lingual View
Permanent Maxillary Right Canine

Lingual View
Permanent Mandibular Right Canine

FIGURE 16-23 Lingual views of permanent canines and their features, with lingual fossae highlighted.

mesial part of the crown has greater labiolingual bulk. The distal part of the crown appears thinner than the mesial and gives the impression of being stretched to make contact with the first premolar.

More specifically, the mesial half of the labial outline is quite rounded, and the distal half is frequently concave. The distal half of

the lingual outline is also frequently concave, because the distal fossa is deeper and thus more pronounced. The mesial marginal ridge is longer than the distal marginal ridge. The cusp slopes seem to form a nearly straight line; the tip of the cusp is displaced labially and mesial to the central long axis.

Clinical Considerations with Maxillary Canines

Because the maxillary canines erupt after the maxillary incisors and possibly the maxillary premolars, their **dental arch** space often is partially closed, and they may erupt labially or lingually to the surrounding teeth. The maxillary canines may also fail to erupt fully, remaining **impacted** within the alveolar bone. An impacted tooth is an unerupted or partially erupted tooth that is positioned against another tooth, bone, or even soft tissue in a way that makes complete eruption unlikely. As a result, surgical exposure and follow-up orthodontic therapy may be needed, which may be prevented by careful evaluation of mixed dentition, and institution of any needed interceptive orthodontic therapy. In addition, the distal prominence of the crown is at the CEJ, which may cause instrumentation difficulties on the distal root surface.

Developmental Disturbances of Maxillary Canines

The cingulums on the maxillary canines may exhibit **tubercles**, or extra **cusps** that are located near the most incisal level of the **cingulum** (see Table 6-3*G*). A lingual pit is often associated with the presence of tubercles.

In a separate developmental disturbance, the **root** of maxillary canines may undergo distorted angulations or **dilaceration**, and there may be several curvatures along its length. With root curvature in the apical third, the root is usually curved distally. Finally, developmental cyst formation may occur within the dental tissue of an impacted crown of a maxillary canine (see earlier discussion), resulting in a **dentigerous cyst**.

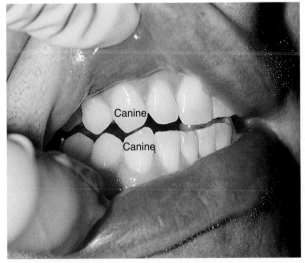

FIGURE 16-24 Lateral view of permanent canines altered on the incisal surfaces by attrition. The cusp tip of maxillary canines is moved to the distal of center, with mesial displacement of the cusp tip for the mandibular canine. This also lengthens the mesial cusp slope, as well as shortening the distal one for the maxillary canines, and shortens the mesial cusp slope and lengthens the distal one for the mandibular canines.

PERMANENT MANDIBULAR CANINES #22 AND #27
SPECIFIC OVERALL FEATURES

Permanent mandibular canines erupt between 9 to 10 years of age (root completion between ages 12 to 14) (Figure 16-28). Thus, these teeth usually erupt before the maxillary canines and after most of the incisors have erupted.

A mandibular canine closely resembles a maxillary canine. Although the entire tooth is usually as long, a mandibular canine is narrower labiolingually and mesiodistally than a maxillary canine. The crown of this tooth can be equal to in length, or even longer than that of a maxillary canine.

The single cusp is not as well developed in size, and the two cusp ridges are thinner labiolingually than those of a maxillary canine. The single cusp tip usually is not as sharp. In addition, the cusp tip is on a line with the long axis of the root, but it is sometimes positioned lingually, similar to the mandibular incisors.

The lingual surface of the crown of a mandibular canine is smoother than that of a maxillary canine and has a less developed cingulum and two marginal ridges. Thus, the lingual surface of this crown more closely resembles the form of the lingual surface of the adjacent mandibular lateral incisors, despite the added feature of a lingual ridge.

The single root of a mandibular canine may be as long as that of a maxillary canine but is usually somewhat shorter, although it still has the longest mandibular root. The root has a slight mesial inclination. The mesial developmental depression on the root is more pronounced and often deeper compared with that of a maxillary canine. A distal developmental depression similar to the mesial one is also apparent. These proximal concavities may extend the full length of the root. These depressions may be extremely pronounced, to the point of creating a facial and lingual component in the apical third and giving the tooth a double-rooted appearance. The root apex is also more pointed on this tooth than on a maxillary canine.

The pulp cavity of a mandibular canine resembles that of a maxillary canine in that they both usually have a single pulp canal and a large pulp chamber (Figure 16-29). There is also only one pulp horn. The major difference is that a mandibular canine may have two separate pulp canals. If the tooth has two canals, one is placed labially and the other lingually; the canals may join at the apex or have separate apical foramina.

LABIAL VIEW FEATURES

The labial surface on a mandibular canine is not as rounded as that on a maxillary canine, especially in the incisal two thirds of the tooth (see Figure 16-29). In contrast, however, a mandibular canine is generally rounder than a mandibular incisor.

Imbrication lines are not normally present on the labial surface, unlike a maxillary canine. Two faint and vertically placed mesial and distal labial developmental depressions separate the three labial lobes, similar to the maxillary canine and incisors. These depressions are located on either side of the vertical, centrally placed labial ridge, which is not as prominent as that of a maxillary canine.

From the labial view, the mesial outline is almost a straight line from the mesial contact to the CEJ, straighter than on a maxillary canine. The distal outline is shorter and rounder than the mesial outline, similar to a maxillary canine, which *helps to distinguish the right mandibular canine from the left*.

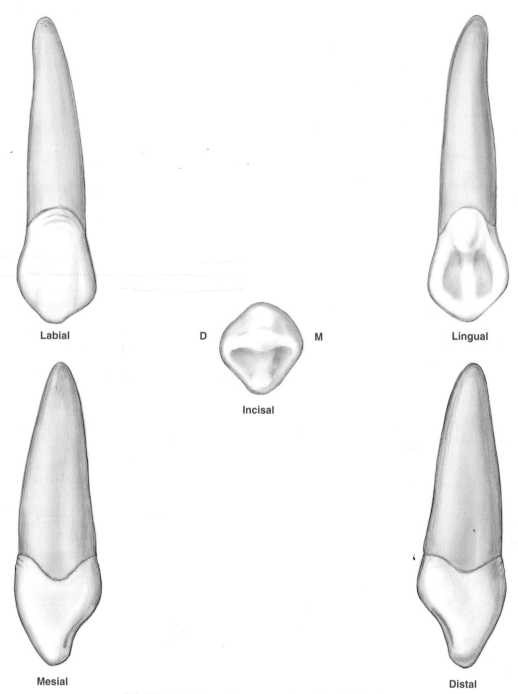

Labial

D   M

Incisal

Lingual

Mesial

Distal

FIGURE 16-25 Views of a permanent maxillary right canine.

From the labial view, similar to a maxillary canine, the mesial and distal contacts are on different levels of the tooth, which *helps to distinguish the right mandibular canine from the left*. The mesial contact with the lateral incisor is in the incisal third. The distal contact with the first premolar is at the junction of the incisal and middle thirds, at a more cervically placed location than that on the mesial side.

As discussed before, the cusp slopes are different: The mesial cusp slope of a mandibular canine is shorter than the distal cusp slope when first erupted from the labial view, which *helps to distinguish the right mandibular canine from the left*. With attrition, the central cusp tip moves to the mesial, shortening the already short mesial cusp

slope and further lengthening the distal cusp slope. The CEJ is evenly curved toward the root.

LINGUAL VIEW FEATURES

The lingual surface is relatively smooth, except for the faintly demarcated features of a lingual ridge, mesial marginal ridge, distal marginal ridge, and two lingual fossae, the distolingual fossa and mesiolingual fossa. The less developed cingulum on a mandibular canine is not centered as on a maxillary canine but lies distal to the long axis of the root. In addition, the cingulum also does not extend as far incisally as it does in the maxillary canines. Rarely are there any lingual pits or lingual grooves on this surface.

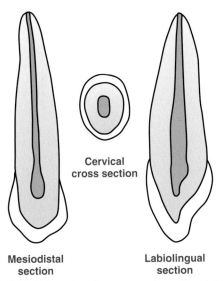

Mesiodistal section   **Cervical cross section**   **Labiolingual section**

FIGURE 16-26 Pulp cavity of a permanent maxillary right canine.

PROXIMAL VIEW FEATURES

A mandibular canine is, again, similar to a maxillary canine from a mesial view, with a similar triangular shape and pointed cusp on the crown. Again, the less-developed cingulum and thinner marginal ridges are seen. The cusp tip is more lingually inclined without incisal wear, unlike the labially placed cusp tip on a maxillary canine.

The CEJ curvature on the mesial surface is more toward the incisal when compared to the same surface of a maxillary canine. Additionally, the CEJ curve is more toward the incisal on the mesial surface than the distal on this same tooth, which *helps to distinguish the right mandibular canine from the left.* The distal view is similar to the mesial aspect. The one exception is that the CEJ is curved less on the distal than on the mesial surface.

INCISAL VIEW FEATURES

A mandibular canine from this view is similar to a maxillary canine, but it is slightly more symmetrical compared with the maxillary tooth. Additionally, the crown is wider labiolingually than mesiodistally and is offset toward the mesial. The less developed cingulum is offset toward the distal. This placement still gives the tooth only a slight asymmetrical appearance from this view, less than a maxillary canine.

The mesial marginal ridge is longer than the distal marginal ridge. The labial outline is also rounder mesiodistally than that of the mandibular incisors because of the pronounced labial ridge.

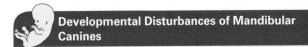

Developmental Disturbances of Mandibular Canines

The **dilaceration** of the **root** can also occur with a mandibular canine, similar to a maxillary canine (see **Chapter 6**). Another developmental disturbance is an **accessory root** or **bifurcated** root in the apical third, with labial and lingual branches. This tooth is the anterior tooth most likely to have a bifurcated root, although this still is rare.

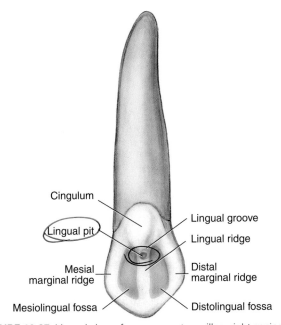

Cingulum

Lingual pit

Lingual groove

Lingual ridge

Mesial marginal ridge

Distal marginal ridge

Mesiolingual fossa

Distolingual fossa

FIGURE 16-27 Lingual view of a permanent maxillary right canine and features, with lingual fossae highlighted.

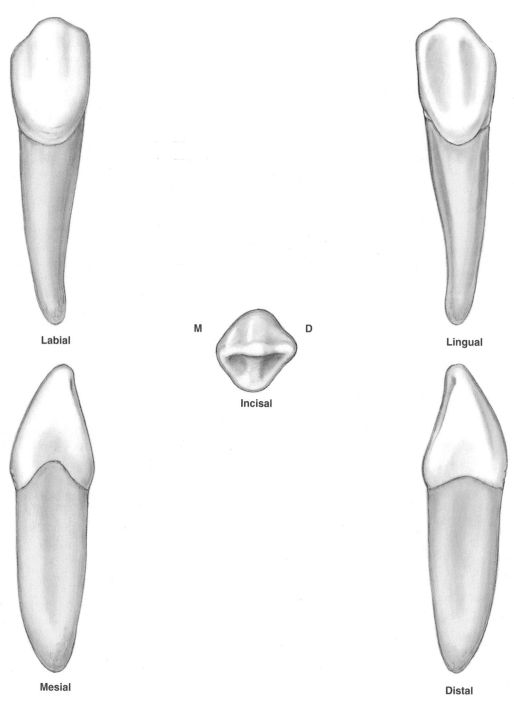

Labial

Lingual

M   D

Incisal

Mesial

Distal

FIGURE 16-28 Views of a permanent mandibular right canine.

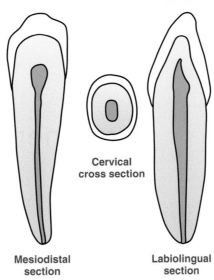

Cervical
cross section

Mesiodistal
section

Labiolingual
section

FIGURE 16-29 Pulp cavity of a permanent mandibular right canine.

Permanent Posterior Teeth

●●● CHAPTER OUTLINE

●●● LEARNING OBJECTIVES

- Use the correct names and universal designation numbers of each permanent posterior tooth when examining a diagram and a patient.
- Demonstrate the correct location of each permanent posterior tooth on a diagram and a patient.
- Define and pronounce the key terms when discussing the permanent posterior teeth.
- Describe the general and specific features of posterior teeth and each posterior tooth type of the permanent dentition.

- Discuss the important clinical considerations and developmental disturbances based on the anatomy of the permanent posterior teeth.
- Integrate the knowledge of dental anatomy of the permanent posterior teeth into the dental treatment of patients in order to preserve them.

●●● NEW KEY TERMS

Bicuspid (bi-**kus**-pid)
Bifurcated (bi-fer-**kay**-ted)
Cusp planes (kusp), **ridges**
Cusp of Carabelli (kusp kare-ah-**bell**-ee), **groove**
Dilaceration (di-las-er-**ay**-shun)

Fluting
Fossa (**fos**-ah) (plural, **fossae, fos**-ay): **central, triangular**
Furcation (fer-**kay**-shin), **crotches**
Groove: central, marginal, triangular
Inclined cuspal planes (**kusp**-al)
Molars (**mo**-lers): **mulberry** (**mull**-bare-ee), **peg**

Occlusal (ah-**kloo**-zl) **developmental pits, table**
Ridge: oblique (o**bleek**), **transverse** (trans-**vers**), **triangular**
Root fusion
Trifurcated (try-fer-**kay**-ted)

PERMANENT POSTERIOR TEETH

The permanent **posterior teeth** include the **premolars** and **molars** (Figure 17-1, see Figures 2-4, 15-2). The **crown** of each has an occlusal surface as its **masticatory surface**, bordered by the raised **marginal ridges** that are located on both the **distal surface** and **mesial surface** (Figure 17-2). The **occlusal surface** also has two or more **cusps**. Some anatomists liken a cusp to a *gothic pyramid*, with four cusp ridges descending from each cusp tip. Between these cusp ridges are sloping areas, or four inclined cuspal planes. These planes are named by

combining the names of the two cusp ridges that are between them. Some inclined planes are functional and thus involved in the **occlusion** of the teeth (see **Chapter 20**).

The occlusal surface of permanent posteriors creates an inner occlusal table bordered by the marginal ridges (Figure 17-3). There are also triangular ridges, which are cusp ridges that descend from the cusp tips toward the central part of the occlusal table (Figure 17-4). They are so named because the slopes of each side of the ridge are inclined in a way that resembles two sides of a triangle. Thus, the triangular ridges are specifically named for the cusps to which they

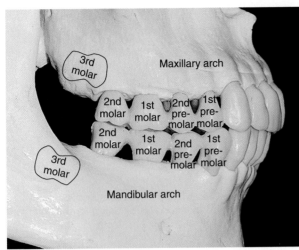

FIGURE 17-1 Permanent posterior teeth identified, which include the premolars and molars. Note that the third molars, or *wisdom teeth*, have not erupted yet.

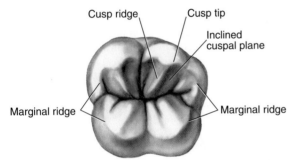

FIGURE 17-2 Example of the occlusal surface on a permanent posterior tooth, with its features noted.

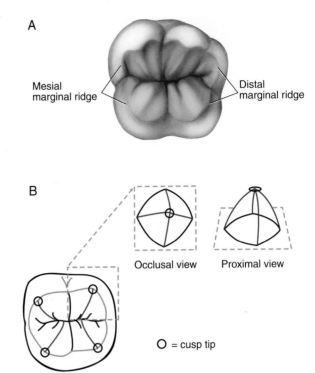

FIGURE 17-3 Occlusal views of a permanent posterior tooth. **A:** Occlusal table highlighted. **B:** Triangular ridges highlighted, with a close-up of the *gothic pyramid* shape of the cusp that many anatomists refer to when discussing these features.

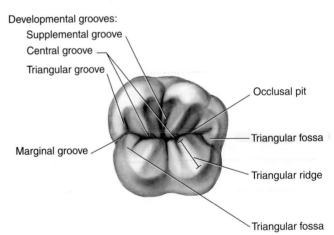

FIGURE 17-4 Example of the other features of the occlusal table on a permanent posterior tooth, including the central groove.

belong. Additionally present on many posteriors is a transverse ridge, a collective term given to the joining of two triangular ridges crossing the occlusal table transversely, or from the labial to the lingual outline.

Each shallow and wide depression on the occlusal table is a **fossa,** (plural, **fossae**). One type of fossa on posteriors, the central fossa, is located at the convergence of the cusp ridges in a central point, where the grooves meet. Another type of fossa is the triangular fossa, which appears to have a triangular shape at the convergence of the cusp ridges, and is associated with the termination of the triangular grooves (discussed next). Sometimes located in the deepest parts of the fossae are occlusal developmental pits; each pit is a sharp pinpoint depression where two or more grooves meet.

Developmental grooves, or primary grooves, are also found on the occlusal table. The developmental grooves on each different posterior tooth type are located in the same place and mark the junction between the developmental lobes. The grooves are sharp, deep, V-shaped linear depressions. The most prominent developmental groove on posteriors is the central groove, which generally travels mesiodistally and separates the occlusal table buccolingually.

Other developmental grooves are marginal grooves, which cross the marginal ridges and serve as a spillway, allowing food to escape during mastication. Finally, there are triangular grooves that separate a marginal ridge from the triangular ridge of a cusp, and at their terminations form the triangular fossae.

In contrast, **supplemental grooves**, or secondary grooves, appear as shallower, more irregular linear depressions (Figure 17-5). Supplemental grooves branch from the developmental grooves, but these

grooves are not always present in the same pattern on the occlusal table of each different tooth type. In general, the more posterior a tooth is located in the dental arch, the more supplemental grooves are present, such that the occlusal table appears more wrinkled.

When examined from the buccal and lingual views, the crown outline of the posteriors is trapezoidal, or four-sided with only two parallel sides (not including the occlusal surface cusp form of posteriors). Thus, the longer of the two parallel sides is toward the occlusal aspect. This arrangement is quite important in the functioning of the teeth.

For posteriors, the **height of contour**, or crest of curvature, for the crown's buccal surface is in the cervical third, and the lingual surface is in the middle or occlusal third (Figure 17-6). When compared with

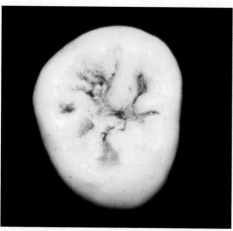

FIGURE 17-5 Example of supplemental grooves on the occlusal surface of a permanent posterior tooth.

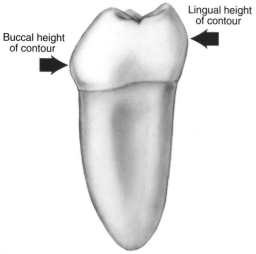

Lingual height of contour

Buccal height of contour

FIGURE 17-6 Height of contour on a permanent posterior tooth.

Clinical Considerations for Posterior Teeth

The complex **pit and groove patterns** on the occlusal surface of posteriors can put them at an increased risk of caries (Figure 17-7). This susceptibility is due to increased dental biofilm retention and the weakness of enamel forming the walls of the pits and grooves (see Figure 12-4, *A*). All pits and grooves must be checked for decay with an explorer and mirror. Clinicians need to be aware of these pit and groove patterns on posteriors when they examine dentitions to assess the patient's caries risk level. All pits and grooves must be checked for decay with an explorer and mirror. Light-induced devices that measure changes in laser fluorescence of hard tissue allow dental professionals to better diagnose early lesions in pits and grooves. Posteriors with deep pit and groove patterns, but without incipient decay, should have enamel sealants applied as soon as they erupt.

anteriors, the posteriors are wider labiolingually than mesiodistally, except for the mandibular molars.

In another comparison with anteriors, the **contact areas** of each of the posteriors is wider, usually located to the buccal of center, and is nearer the same level on each **proximal surface** (see Figure 15-10). In addition, on each proximal surface is a **cementoenamel junction**

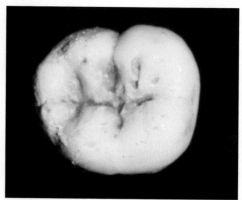

FIGURE 17-7 Example of a complex pit and groove pattern on the occlusal surface of a permanent posterior tooth.

(CEJ) curvature that is less pronounced on the posteriors than on the anteriors. In fact, the CEJ is often quite straight for posteriors.

Like anterior teeth, **multirooted** premolars and molars originate as a single root on the base of the crown. This part on these posterior teeth is considered the **root trunk.** The cervical cross section of the root trunk initially follows the form of the crown. However, the root of a posterior tooth divides from the root trunk into the correct number of root branches for its tooth type, either two (**bifurcated**) or three (**trifurcated**) (see Figure 6-21).

PERMANENT PREMOLARS

GENERAL FEATURES

Permanent premolars are the most anteriorly placed posteriors in the permanent dentition (Figure 17-8, Table 17-1). Each dental arch has four premolars, two to each quadrant.

There are two types of premolars: **first premolar** and **second premolar**. One of each type is present in each quadrant of each dental arch. The first is closer to the midline at the fourth position from it. The second is next to the first premolar and is in the fifth position from the midline. Both types are distal to the permanent canine and mesial to the permanent first molar when full eruption of the permanent dentition has occurred. Permanent premolars are **succedaneous,** because they replace the primary first and second molars.

As posterior teeth, premolars have a shorter crown than anterior teeth. The buccal surface is rounded and has a prominent vertical buccal ridge in the center of the crown (Figure 17-9). Two buccal developmental depressions are noted on each side of the buccal ridge. The **buccal ridge** of premolars is similar to the labial ridge of the canines and may be related to the increased development of the middle buccal lobe. The height of contour, or crest of curvature, of the crown buccally is in the cervical third, as in anterior teeth. Lingually, the height of contour for premolars is in the middle third.

An older term for a premolar was bicuspid, because of the usual presence of two cusps on the occlusal surface, one more cusp than in the canines. However, the mandibular second premolar frequently has three cusps. Thus, the name *premolar* is more widely used because these teeth are located anterior to the molars.

Finally, in addition to the cusps, the occlusal surface of a premolar, similar to all posteriors, has marginal ridges, triangular ridges, developmental grooves, and occlusal developmental pits. The boundaries of the occlusal surface, the marginal ridges and cusp ridges, form an inner occlusal table.

Clinical Considerations for Premolars

Premolars function to assist the molars in grinding food during **mastication,** because of their broad occlusal surface and their prominent cusps. Premolars also assist the canines in piercing and tearing food with those cusps. These teeth, along with the canines, also help maintain the height of the lower third of the **vertical dimension of the face** and support the facial muscles, especially those muscles in the corners of the mouth. Thus, the premolars are involved in esthetics and speech, less so than the anteriors but more so than the molars.

Single, permanent premolars can be extracted in each quadrant during orthodontic therapy to improve dental arch spacing. If a premolar has been extracted, the distinctive pit and groove patterns on the occlusal surface will help in identifying the remaining premolars when the arch space from the extraction is lost if the remaining molars are not restored. However, orthodontic therapy tends instead to include expansion of the jaw, if needed, instead of removing premolars to retain a more natural rounded curved shape to the arches. If extraction is unavoidable, first premolars are usually extracted more often than second premolars. Additionally, they present difficulties in instrumentation of the root because they have proximal **root concavities**, especially on the mesial of the maxillary first premolar.

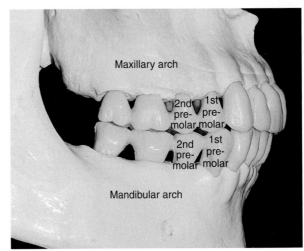

FIGURE 17-8 Permanent premolars identified.

TABLE 17-1	**Anatomical Information on Permanent Premolars**			
	MAXILLARY FIRST PREMOLAR	**MAXILLARY SECOND PREMOLAR**	**MANDIBULAR FIRST PREMOLAR**	**MANDIBULAR SECOND PREMOLAR**
Universal number	#5 and #12	#4 and #13	#21 and #28	#20 and #29
General crown features	Occlusal table with marginal ridges and cusps, with tips, ridges, inclined planes, grooves, fossae, pits; buccal ridge			
Specific crown features	Larger than second, with buccal cusp longer of two, long central groove	Smaller than first, two cusps same length, short central groove, no mesial surface features like first, increased supplemental grooves	Smaller than second, smaller lingual cusp of two, mesial surface features	Larger than first, usually three cusps: Y groove pattern or two cusps: H or U groove pattern, increased supplemental grooves
Mesial and distal contact	Just cervical to the junction of occlusal and middle thirds			
Distinguishing right from left	Longer mesial cusp slope, mesial features: marginal groove, developmental depression, deeper CEJ curvature	Lingual cusp offset to the mesial	Shorter mesial cusp slope, mesiolingual groove, deeper mesial CEJ curvature	Distal marginal ridge more cervically located, thus more occlusal surface visible from distal view
General root features	Proximal root concavities			
Specific root features	Bifurcated with root trunk; elliptical on cross section	Single-rooted; elliptical on cross section	Single-rooted; ovoid or elliptical on cross section	

CEJ, Cementoenamel junction.

In addition, most premolars usually have one root, except for the permanent maxillary first premolar, which has two roots. Whether one or two roots are present, they have proximal **root concavities**.

PERMANENT MAXILLARY PREMOLARS

GENERAL FEATURES

Both types of maxillary premolars resemble each other more than do the mandibular premolars. A maxillary first premolar is larger than a maxillary second premolar, but, in contrast, a mandibular first premolar is smaller than a mandibular second premolar. Both maxillary premolars erupt earlier than the mandibular premolars.

The crown of a maxillary premolar is shorter occlusocervically than that of a maxillary canine, but is slightly longer than that of a molar. The crown outline from the proximal aspect is trapezoidal, or four-sided with only two parallel sides, similar to all maxillary posterior teeth.

The crown is also centered over the root and shows no lingual inclination, which is unlike the mandibular premolars or other mandibular posteriors. They also have a greater buccolingual width than mesiodistal width compared with the mandibular premolars or other mandibular posterior teeth when viewed from the occlusal. The outline for both maxillary premolars is somewhat hexagonal, with six sides, and almost oval compared with the rounder mandibular premolars.

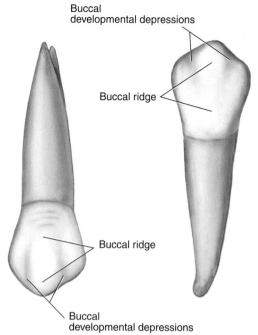

Buccal
developmental depressions

Buccal ridge

Buccal ridge

Buccal
developmental depressions

FIGURE 17-9 Buccal features of permanent premolars.

Both maxillary premolars have two cusps of almost equal size. In contrast, the mandibular premolars can have more than two cusps, but any lingual cusps are always smaller. The cusps of all premolars are centered over the long axis of the tooth from either proximal view. The maxillary premolars are composed of four developmental lobes: three buccal and one lingual.

Additionally, the roots of the maxillary premolars are shorter than the maxillary canine's roots, but the root length is the same as that of the molars. The roots show slight lingual and distal inclination. The roots on cervical cross section are elliptical, or an elongated oval, which may be slightly altered by proximal root concavities.

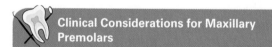

Clinical Considerations for Maxillary Premolars

The roots of maxillary premolars may penetrate the anterior part of the **maxillary sinus** as a result of accidental trauma or during tooth extraction because of the close relation of these roots to the sinus walls (see Figure 11-21). In addition, the discomfort of **sinusitis** can be mistakenly interpreted as tooth-related (stemming from the maxillary premolar), and vice versa. Thus, radiographic study of the tooth or maxillary sinus and other diagnostic tests are necessary to determine the true cause of the discomfort.

PERMANENT MAXILLARY FIRST PREMOLARS #5 AND #12

Specific Overall Features (Figure 17-10) Permanent maxillary first premolars erupt between 10 and 11 years of age (root completion between ages 12 to 13). These teeth erupt distal to the primary maxillary canines or their arch space, and thus are the succedaneous replacements for the primary maxillary first molars.

The crown of a maxillary first premolar has an angular shape with sharp outlines compared with a maxillary second premolar's more rounded shape. The tooth's two cusps are also sharply defined, with the buccal cusp usually about 1 mm higher than the lingual cusp. The tooth appears bent mesially when viewed from the occlusal compared with the second premolar of the same arch. The central groove on the occlusal surface is also longer on the maxillary first premolar than on the second.

Most maxillary first premolars are bifurcated, having two root branches in the apical third, with a buccal root and a lingual (palatal) root. This is unlike the other premolars, which are single-rooted. Maxillary first premolars originate as a single root on the base of the crown, as do other premolars and anteriors; this part is considered the root trunk.

A cervical cross section of the root trunk follows the form of the crown. The root trunk usually makes up half the length of the entire root, and the root branches make up the other half. The roots are rounded overall and taper to sharp apices. The buccal root of this tooth is larger but not longer than the lingual root. A distinct mesial root concavity is present on the root trunk of the maxillary first premolar, extending from the contact area to the bifurcation. The mesial surface groove on the root puts this tooth possibly at an increased risk for periodontal disease because it allows an increased deposit level. The distal surface has a groove that is reduced in depth, creating a convex or flat surface.

This trunk can also have a root fusion, with little of the root bifurcated. If a single root is present, which occurs in 20% of the population, it is wider buccolingually than mesiodistally, the buccal and lingual surfaces are rounded, and the root is tapered to a blunt apex. In cross section, the root becomes kidney shaped. A single root also has a deep and wide mesial surface root concavity, which ranges from relatively shallow to deep enough to almost bifurcate the root. Three-rooted, or trifurcated teeth have been noted, with two buccal roots and a single lingual root.

The pulp cavity for a two-rooted tooth usually shows two pulp horns (one for each cusp) and two pulp canals (one for each root) (Figure 17-11). Even if there is only one undivided root, as for the maxillary second premolar, two pulp canals are usually found, although they often combine to form one apical foramen.

Buccal View Features The crown of a maxillary first premolar is the widest mesiodistally of all the premolars (Figure 17-12). This tooth's crown is wide at the level of the contact areas, becoming narrower at the CEJ, similar to the maxillary canine. The mesial contact with the maxillary canine is just cervical to the junction of the occlusal and middle thirds. The distal contact with the maxillary second premolar is the same, just cervical to the junction of the occlusal and middle thirds.

The mesial and distal outlines of the crown of the maxillary first premolar are almost straight from the contact areas to the CEJ, but the mesial outline is more rounded. Both these outlines converge more toward the cervical than they do on the maxillary second premolars. Imbrication lines and perikymata are found on the buccal surface, and these extend mesiodistally in the cervical third. The CEJ curvature of the tooth is evenly rounded toward the apex of the tooth and has less depth than on anterior teeth.

The buccal cusp of a maxillary first premolar is high and sharp, located slightly distal to the long axis of the tooth because the two cusp slopes of the buccal cusp are not equal in height. This tooth is the only tooth in the permanent dentition that has a buccal cusp with the mesial cusp slope longer than the distal cusp slope, which *helps to distinguish the right maxillary first premolar from the left*. This relationship of the cusp slopes normally exists upon eruption; attrition may change it. A bulge may be found occasionally on the buccal cusp of this tooth.

Lingual View Features The lingual surface of the maxillary first premolar is rounded in all directions but is smaller than the buccal surface. The shorter lingual cusp is sharp but not as sharp as the

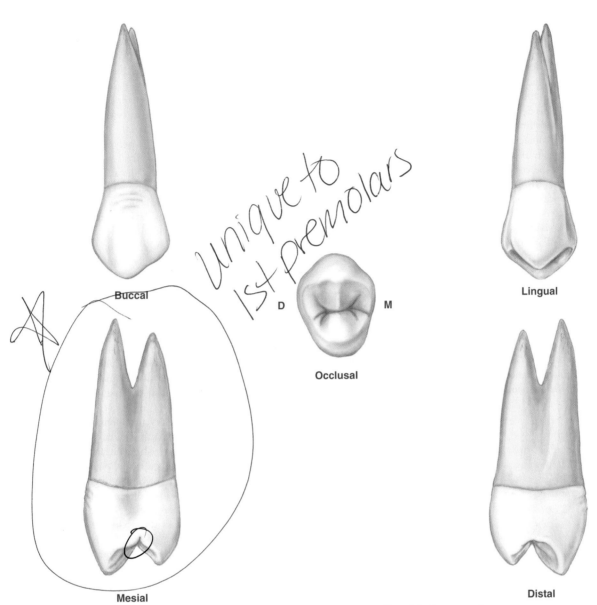

Unique to 1st premolars

Buccal

Lingual

Occlusal

D   M

Mesial

Distal

FIGURE 17-10 Views of the permanent maxillary right first premolar.

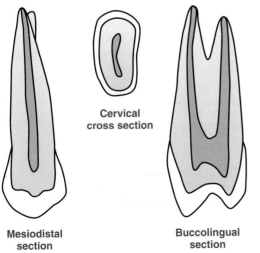

Cervical
cross section

Mesiodistal
section

Buccolingual
section

FIGURE 17-11 Pulp cavity of the permanent maxillary right first premolar.

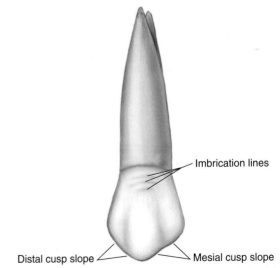

Imbrication lines

Distal cusp slope

Mesial cusp slope

FIGURE 17-12 Buccal features of the permanent maxillary right first premolar.

buccal cusp and is offset toward the mesial. Thus, the cusp slopes of the lingual cusp are again not equal in length. From the lingual aspect, however, the mesial cusp slope is shorter than the distal cusp slope.

Proximal View Features On the mesial surface of the crown of a maxillary first premolar, the mesial marginal ridge is present on the concave occlusal margin. A mesial marginal groove is also sometimes present (Figure 17-13). This developmental groove crosses the mesial marginal ridge and extends from the occlusal to the middle third of the crown, lingual to the contact area.

The mesial surface usually also has a mesial developmental depression located cervical to the contact area, across the CEJ, normally extending onto the root. On the root, the depression joins a deep developmental root concavity between the roots. The CEJ curvature is more occlusally located on the mesial than on the distal surface. All these prominent mesial features from the proximal view *help to distinguish the right maxillary first premolar from the left.*

The distal surface is similar to the mesial, except that it does not have a depression, and more of the occlusal surface shows because the distal marginal ridge is more cervically located than is the mesial marginal ridge. A distal marginal groove is sometimes located across the distal marginal ridge, but this distal groove is shallower than the groove on the mesial surface. Additionally, the CEJ curvature on the distal surface is not as deep cervically as the mesial.

Occlusal View Features The outline of the occlusal surface of a maxillary first premolar is somewhat hexagonal, or six-sided, but is wider buccolingually than mesiodistally (Figure 17-14). The buccal

ridge (or buccal cusp ridge of the buccal cusp, as discussed later) is prominent on the buccal margin, and the lingual margin of the occlusal outline is almost a semicircle. The mesial and distal margins are straight as they converge toward the lingual. Thus, the lingual part of the tooth is narrower mesiodistally than the buccal part. When the mesial marginal groove is prominent, it may create a dip in the mesial outline.

Occlusal Table Components The buccal cusp of a maxillary first premolar is sharper and higher than the lingual cusp. The occlusal function of the buccal cusp involves only its lingual surface. Four buccal cusp ridges descend from the buccal cusp tip, each named for its location: buccal, lingual, mesial, and distal. Because this is the first occlusal table of a posterior tooth under discussion, this text provides specific details on each of the occlusal table features; this information can then be related to the occlusal tables of other posterior teeth.

The buccal cusp ridge of the buccal cusp extends cervically from the cusp tip on the buccal surface and corresponds to the buccal ridge. The lingual cusp ridge extends lingually from the buccal cusp tip to the central groove (also called the *buccal triangular ridge* or *buccal part of the transverse ridge,* as discussed later). The mesial cusp ridge of the buccal cusp extends mesially from the cusp tip to the mesiobucco-occlusal point angle. The distal cusp ridge extends distally from the buccal cusp tip to the distobucco-occlusal point angle.

Between the cusp ridges are four buccal-inclined cuspal planes, named for the two cusp ridges between which they lie: mesiobuccal, mesiolingual, distobuccal, and distolingual. However, only the mesiolingual- and distolingual-inclined cuspal planes function during occlusion.

The lingual cusp of the maxillary first premolar is rounder, less sharp, and shorter than the buccal cusp. This cusp is also located well to the lingual and offset to the mesial. Again, there are four lingual cusp ridges and four lingual-inclined cuspal planes similar to those associated with the buccal cusp, but all the lingual inclined cuspal planes are functional. This is because the entire lingual cusp functions during occlusion, unlike the buccal cusp.

Extending mesiodistally, across the occlusal table of the maxillary first premolar, is a long central groove, evenly dividing the tooth buccolingually. The central groove is a developmental groove that is sharply defined; it is deep and V-shaped. A few supplemental grooves appear irregular in shape and shallower, and they branch from the central groove. Thus, the occlusal surface is relatively smooth compared with the adjacent maxillary second premolar.

The lingual cusp ridge, which runs from the buccal cusp tip to the central groove, is also termed the buccal triangular ridge (Figure 17-15). The buccal cusp ridge of the lingual cusp is also termed the lingual triangular ridge, because it runs from the lingual cusp tip to the central groove. Perpendicular to the central groove is a transverse ridge, the collective term given to the joining of the buccal triangular ridge and the lingual triangular ridge.

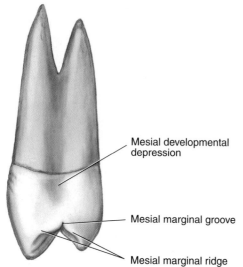

Mesial developmental depression

Mesial marginal groove

Mesial marginal ridge

FIGURE 17-13 Mesial features of the permanent maxillary right first premolar.

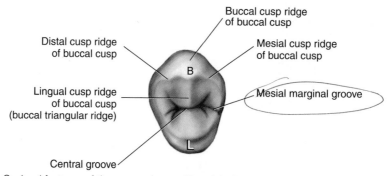

Buccal cusp ridge of buccal cusp

Distal cusp ridge of buccal cusp

Mesial cusp ridge of buccal cusp

Lingual cusp ridge of buccal cusp (buccal triangular ridge)

Mesial marginal groove

Central groove

FIGURE 17-14 Occlusal features of the permanent maxillary right first premolar, with occlusal table highlighted.

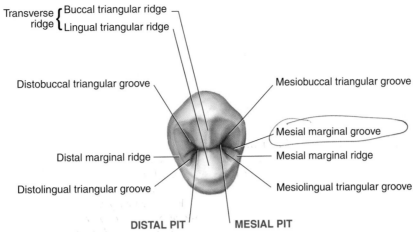

FIGURE 17-15 Additional occlusal features of the permanent maxillary right first premolar, with fossae highlighted.

The central groove of the maxillary first premolar also crosses to the mesial marginal ridge, which is shorter than the distal marginal ridge. Extending from the central groove, another developmental groove, the mesial marginal groove, crosses the mesial marginal ridge and travels onto the mesial surface of the tooth.

Descending down the slope of the buccal cusp, and just inside the distal and mesial marginal ridges, are two developmental grooves, the mesiobuccal triangular groove and the distobuccal triangular groove. Across the occlusal table, the lingual cusp also has two developmental grooves, the mesiolingual triangular groove, and the distolingual triangular groove.

Each of these triangular grooves ends in a triangular depression called a *triangular fossa*. These fossae are the deeper mesial triangular fossa, which surrounds the mesiobuccal triangular groove, and the shallower distal triangular fossa, which surrounds the distobuccal triangular groove.

The boundaries of the mesial triangular fossa are the mesial marginal ridge, the transverse ridge, and the mesial cusp ridges of the two cusps. The distal triangular fossa has boundaries similar to those of the mesial fossa in a mirror-image fashion. The deepest parts of these fossae are the occlusal developmental pits. These are termed the mesial pit and distal pit, respectively, and they are connected by the central groove.

PERMANENT MAXILLARY SECOND PREMOLARS #4 AND #13

Specific Overall Features (Figure 17-16) Permanent maxillary second premolars erupt between 10 to 12 years of age (root completion between ages 12 to 14). These teeth erupt distal to the permanent maxillary first premolars, and thus are the succedaneous replacements for the primary maxillary second molars.

A maxillary second premolar resembles a first premolar, except that its crown is less angular and more rounded. Additionally, more crown variations, especially in its occlusal surface anatomy, are noted in this tooth as compared with maxillary first premolars.

Unlike a maxillary first premolar, a maxillary second premolar usually has only a single root, but it may occasionally have two roots. The dimensions between the maxillary second and the first premolars are usually about the same overall, except for greater root length of the second. The mesial concavity is not as pronounced as in a first

premolar. The pulp cavity of this tooth has two pulp horns and one single pulp canal (Figure 17-17).

Buccal View Features The buccal cusp of a maxillary second premolar is neither as long nor as sharp as that of a maxillary first premolar (see Figure 17-16). All other features of the buccal surface of a maxillary second are similar to those of the first. Again, the mesial contact with a maxillary first premolar is just cervical to the junction of the occlusal and middle thirds on the buccal surface. The distal contact with a maxillary first molar is the same, just cervical to the junction of the occlusal and middle thirds.

Lingual View Features All lingual surface features of a maxillary second premolar are similar to those of a maxillary first premolar. One noteworthy exception is that the lingual cusp is larger, almost the same height as the buccal cusp on a maxillary second premolar. In addition, the lingual cusp is slightly displaced to the mesial, which *helps to distinguish the right maxillary second premolar from the left*. In addition, less of the occlusal surface is seen from this view because the crown is longer on the lingual.

Proximal View Features The mesial surface of a maxillary second premolar is similar to that of a maxillary first premolar, except that the cusps are closer to being the same size, and no mesial developmental depression is present on the crown and root. Instead, this area cervical to the contact area is rounder.

In addition, this tooth has no mesial marginal groove. Both the contact areas and mesial marginal ridge are more cervically located than those on a maxillary first premolar. The distal surface is the same as the mesial surface without any distal marginal groove, but the contact area is larger.

Occlusal View Features The outline of the occlusal surface of a maxillary second premolar is more rounded and larger overall than that of a maxillary first premolar from the occlusal view. Thus, the hexagonal outline of the crown from the occlusal is more difficult to see.

Occlusal Table Components The central groove is shorter on a maxillary second premolar than on a maxillary first premolar (Figure 17-18). This groove ends in a mesial pit and distal pit, which are closer together and thus more to the middle of the occlusal table.

A maxillary second premolar has numerous supplemental grooves radiating from the central groove. This gives the tooth a more wrinkled appearance compared with a maxillary first premolar. Other features and the overall anatomy of this tooth's occlusal surface are similar to those of a maxillary first premolar.

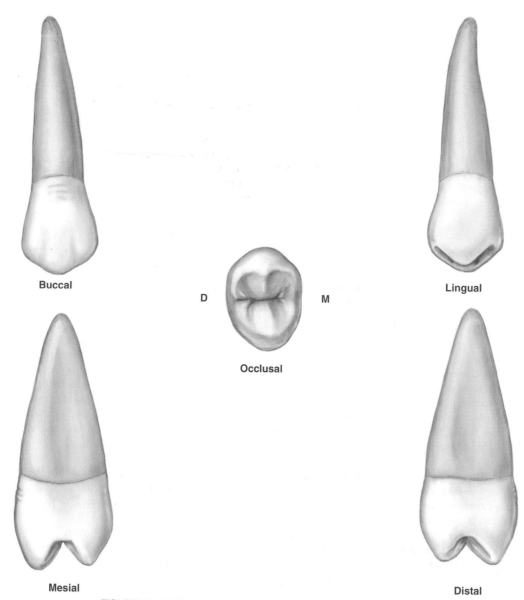

Buccal

Lingual

D   M

Occlusal

Mesial

Distal

FIGURE 17-16 Views of the permanent maxillary right second premolar.

Clinical Considerations for Maxillary Second Premolars

With premature loss of a primary maxillary second molar, the developing permanent maxillary first molar inclines and drifts mesially. The developing permanent maxillary second premolar is prevented from normal eruption because its arch **leeway space** is nearly closed (see Figure 20-3). This situation can allow the maxillary second premolar to become **impacted** against the first molar. An impacted tooth is an unerupted or partially erupted tooth that is positioned against another tooth, bone, or even soft tissue, making complete eruption unlikely. Additionally, the leeway space can be compromised if the permanent maxillary second molar erupts before the maxillary second premolars, the arch perimeter is significantly shortened, and occlusal disharmony is likely to occur, as is with **malocclusion**. These problems may be prevented by careful evaluation of patients with mixed dentition and use of interceptive orthodontic therapy, such as space maintainers (see Figure 20-4).

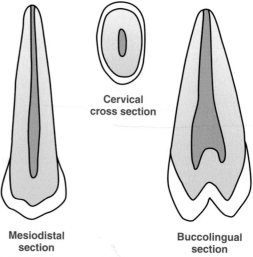

Cervical cross section

Mesiodistal section

Buccolingual section

FIGURE 17-17 Pulp cavity of the permanent maxillary right second premolar.

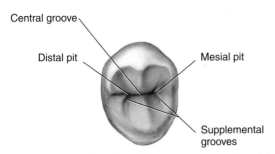

Central groove

Distal pit

Mesial pit

Supplemental grooves

FIGURE 17-18 Occlusal features of the permanent maxillary right second premolar, with occlusal table highlighted.

PERMANENT MANDIBULAR PREMOLARS

GENERAL FEATURES

Mandibular premolars do not resemble each other as much as do the maxillary premolars. In addition, a mandibular first premolar is smaller than a mandibular second premolar; in contrast, a maxillary first premolar is larger overall than the second premolar. Generally, both mandibular premolars erupt into the oral cavity later than do the maxillary premolars.

Quite distinct from maxillary premolars, the buccal outline of the crown of all mandibular premolars shows a strong lingual inclination when viewed from the proximal, similar to all mandibular posterior teeth. The permanent mandibular premolars also have an equal buccolingual and mesiodistal width when viewed from the occlusal, making the outline almost round. In addition, both types of premolars have a similar buccal outline of both the crown and root.

The mesial and distal contact areas of mandibular premolars are on nearly the same level. Similar CEJ curvatures are also found on both premolars. From each proximal view, both the crown outlines of mandibular premolars are rhomboidal, with four sides, having the opposite sides parallel, like all mandibular posteriors. The crowns thus incline lingually on their root bases, bringing the cusps into proper occlusion with their maxillary antagonists and the distribution of forces along their long axes.

Unlike the maxillary premolars, both of which have two cusps of almost equal size, the mandibular premolars can have more than two cusps; however, any lingual cusps are always smaller than the buccal cusp.

These teeth usually have a single root; the angulation of the roots of mandibular premolars may show slight distal inclination. The root on cervical cross section is either ovoid (egg-shaped) or elliptical (an elongated oval), shapes that may be slightly altered by the presence of proximal root concavities. These proximal **root concavities** are most frequently found on the mesial surface of the root.

Clinical Considerations for Mandibular Premolars

Both types of mandibular premolars can present difficulties during instrumentation due to narrow lingual surfaces combined with the lingual inclination of the crown, especially with subgingival placement. In addition, patients may have problems performing adequate homecare because of the lingual inclination of the crown, which causes some patients to miss the associated lingual gingival tissue and clean only the occlusal surface with a toothbrush. The nearby tongue also makes homecare and instrumentation more difficult on the lingual surface.

PERMANENT MANDIBULAR FIRST PREMOLARS #21 AND #28

Specific Overall Features (Figure 17-19) Permanent mandibular first premolars erupt between 10 to 12 years of age (root completion between ages 12 to 13). These teeth erupt distal to the permanent mandibular canines, and thus are the succedaneous replacements for the primary mandibular first molars.

A mandibular first premolar resembles a mandibular canine in many more ways than it does a mandibular second premolar. This is true despite the fact that a premolar is smaller overall than a canine. However, the buccolingual width of this tooth is similar to that of a mandibular canine. Thus, a mandibular first premolar shows a transition in the dental arch from the canine to the molar-like second premolar.

A mandibular first premolar has a buccal cusp that is long and sharp and is the only functional cusp during occlusion, similar to a mandibular canine. The lingual cusp of a mandibular first premolar is usually small and nonfunctioning. The lingual cusp, then, is similar in appearance to the cingulum found on some maxillary canines, but it can vary considerably. Finally, the occlusal surface of the mandibular first premolar has a similar outline and slopes sharply to the lingual, and the mesiobuccal cusp ridge is shorter than the distobuccal cusp ridge, features similar to the mandibular canine.

A mandibular first premolar has a smaller and shorter root than does a mandibular second premolar, although it is closer to the length of a second premolar than to that of a mandibular canine. The buccal aspect of the root is more conical, but the lingual aspect is tapered. A deep groove may be found on the distal root surface. The tooth occasionally has a bifurcated root, with the root divided into buccal and lingual parts.

The pulp cavity of this tooth consists of two pulp horns and a single pulp canal (Figure 17-20). Each pulp horn is located within a cusp. The buccal pulp horn is more pronounced, and the lingual pulp horn is smaller and less significant.

Buccal View Features The outline of the crown of a mandibular first premolar from the buccal is nearly symmetrical (see Figure 17-19). The middle developmental lobe is visibly well developed, resulting in a prominent buccal ridge and a large, pointed buccal cusp. In contrast, the buccal ridge is not as prominent as on a maxillary first premolar. Two buccal developmental depressions are often seen among the three buccal lobes. Imbrication lines are not usually found on the buccal surface.

The buccal cusp is also located slightly to the mesial of the center of the crown, again similar to a mandibular canine. Thus, the two cusp slopes of the premolar are not equal in length. The mesial cusp slope of the buccal cusp is shorter than the distal cusp slope, which *helps to distinguish the right mandibular first premolar from the left.*

The mesial outline of the mandibular first premolar is slightly concave from the mesial contact to the CEJ. The distal outline is rounder and shorter. Again, the mesial contact with the maxillary first premolar is just cervical to the junction of the occlusal and middle thirds. The distal contact with the maxillary first molar is the same, just cervical to the junction of the occlusal and middle thirds.

Lingual View Features The lingual surface is much narrower than the buccal on a mandibular first premolar, with the crown tapering to the lingual (Figure 17-21). Most of the mesial and distal surfaces, therefore, can be seen from the lingual. The lingual cusp is small and nonfunctional during occlusion, and the lingual cusp tip is often pointed.

Because the lingual cusp is small, most of the occlusal surface can be seen from this view. The lingual cusp tip lines up with the buccal triangular ridge. The mesial fossa and distal fossa are on each side of

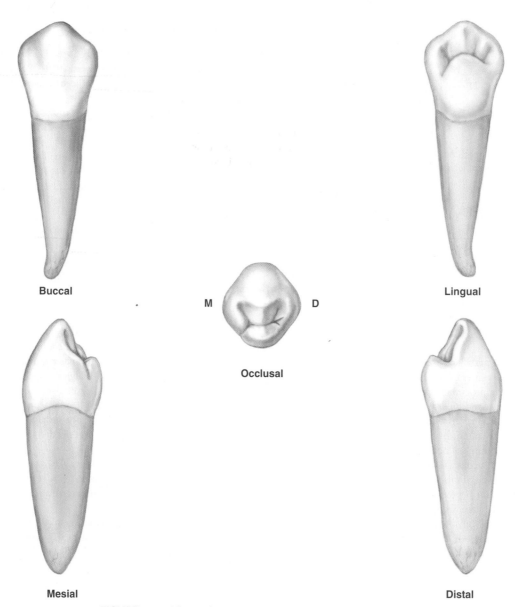

Buccal

M   D

Lingual

Occlusal

Mesial

Distal

FIGURE 17-19 Views of the permanent mandibular right first premolar.

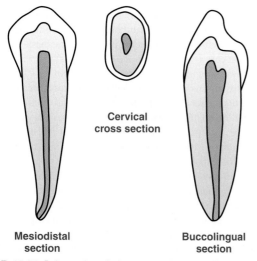

Cervical
cross section

Mesiodistal
section

Buccolingual
section

FIGURE 17-20 Pulp cavity of the permanent mandibular right first premolar.

this ridge. A developmental groove, the mesiolingual groove, usually separates the mesial marginal ridge from the mesial cusp slope of the small lingual cusp.

Proximal View Features From the mesial, the crown of a mandibular first premolar tilts noticeably toward the lingual at the cervix, as do all mandibular posteriors (see Figure 17-19). Thus, the buccal outline is longer than the lingual outline. This lingual inclination of the crown also places the buccal cusp tip almost over the root axis line. Thus, the lingual cusp tip is usually in line vertically with the lingual surface of the cervical part of the root. The transverse ridge slopes at a 45-degree angle from the buccal cusp tip to the occlusal surface and then nearly flattens out to the lingual cusp tip.

The mesial marginal ridge is nearly parallel to the angulation of the transverse ridge at a more cervical level. The slope of the mesial marginal ridge is similar to that of anteriors. The mesiolingual groove, again, can be seen near the lingual margin. The CEJ curvature is also more occlusal on the mesial surface. Both these mesial surface features *help to distinguish the right mandibular first premolar from the left.*

The distal view of the mandibular first premolar is similar to the mesial, except for the absence of a groove near the lingual margin. The distal marginal ridge is much more developed than that of the mesial, and its continuity is unbroken by any deep developmental grooves. Additionally, the distal marginal ridge does not show quite as steep a slope toward the lingual, as is present on the mesial.

Occlusal View Features   The crown outline of the mandibular first premolar is diamond shaped from the occlusal, with a notch in the mesial outline at the mesiolingual groove (Figure 17-22). The prominent buccal ridge is located on the buccal margin. The lingual margin is much shorter than the buccal outline. The mesial margin is slightly rounded to nearly straight, except in the area near the mesiolingual groove. The distal margin is even more rounded than the mesial margin.

Occlusal Table Components   Both the cusps and transverse ridge of the mandibular first premolar are offset to the mesial, leaving the distal part of the tooth larger than the mesial part. The larger and functioning buccal cusp has four buccal cusp ridges and four functioning buccal inclined cuspal planes, all of which are named for their location. The lingual cusp ridge of the buccal cusp is also the buccal triangular ridge.

The lingual cusp is quite small, usually no more than half the height of the buccal cusp. It also has four lingual cusp ridges and four lingual inclined cuspal planes. The buccal cusp ridge of the buccal cusp is also the lingual triangular ridge.

The transverse ridge is composed of the joining of the buccal triangular ridge of the lingual cusp and the lingual triangular ridge of the buccal cusp. The buccal triangular ridge is longer than the lingual, thus making up a greater part of the transverse ridge. The transverse ridge is perpendicular to the central groove. This groove, which slightly separates the two triangular ridges, is sometimes rather indistinct, and thus the two triangular ridges appear to be continuous.

The mesial marginal ridge closely resembles the angulation of the marginal ridges of anterior teeth, especially the canine. This is because it slopes from the buccal to the lingual at a 45-degree angle (Figure 17-23). The mesial marginal ridge is less prominent and shorter than the distal marginal ridge. The distal marginal ridge also does not have quite as steep a slope toward the lingual.

The mesial fossa and distal fossa, and associated mesial pit and distal pit, are also found on the occlusal table. The mesial fossa is shallower than the distal. Although both are circular, the mesial fossa is slightly more linear. The mesial pit is the junction of the central groove, mesiolingual groove (previously described on the lingual and mesial aspects), and mesiobuccal triangular groove (similar in location to that of the maxillary premolars). The distal pit is the junction of the central groove, distal marginal groove, distolingual triangular groove, and distobuccal triangular groove.

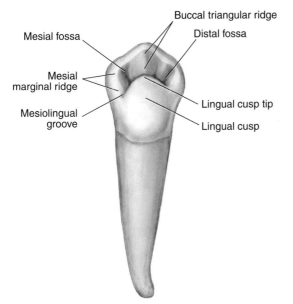

FIGURE 17-21 Lingual features of the permanent mandibular right first premolar, with occlusal table highlighted.

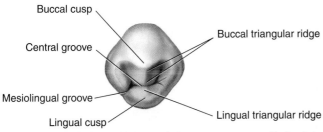

FIGURE 17-22 Occlusal features of the permanent mandibular right first premolar, with occlusal table highlighted.

Clinical Considerations for Mandibular First Premolars

When mandibular first premolars have Class I metallic restorations in their mesial and distal **fossae,** these restorations are sometimes nicknamed *snake eyes* because of the roundness of the two fossae (Figure 17-24). This type of restoration can also be noted on the occlusal surface of mandibular second premolars. Tooth-colored restorative materials are now more commonly placed on the occlusal surface of these smaller posterior teeth to achieve a more esthetic appearance.

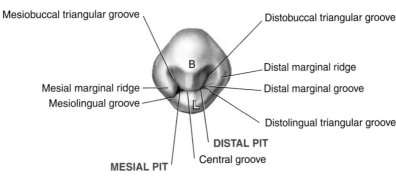

FIGURE 17-23 Additional occlusal features of the permanent mandibular right first premolar, with fossae highlighted.

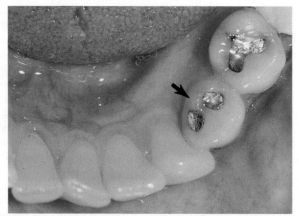

FIGURE 17-24 Restorations on the permanent mandibular first premolar, which are considered as *snake eyes* (*arrow*).

PERMANENT MANDIBULAR SECOND PREMOLARS #20 AND #29

Specific Overall Features (Figure 17-25) The permanent mandibular second premolars erupt between 11 to 12 years of age (root completion between ages 13 to 14). These teeth erupt distal to the mandibular first premolars, and thus are the succedaneous replacements for the primary mandibular second molars.

There are two forms of the mandibular second premolars: three-cusp type (tricuspidate form) and two-cusp type (or bicuspidate form; Figure 17-26). Unlike mandibular first premolars, the more common (55% frequency) three-cusp type has three cusps: one large buccal cusp composed of the three buccal lobes and two smaller lingual cusps composed of the two lingual lobes. Thus, the three-cusp type is composed of five developmental lobes: three buccal and two lingual.

Similar to mandibular first premolars, the less common (45% frequency) two-cusp type has a larger buccal cusp and a single smaller lingual cusp. The two-cusp type is thus composed of four developmental lobes: three buccal and one lingual.

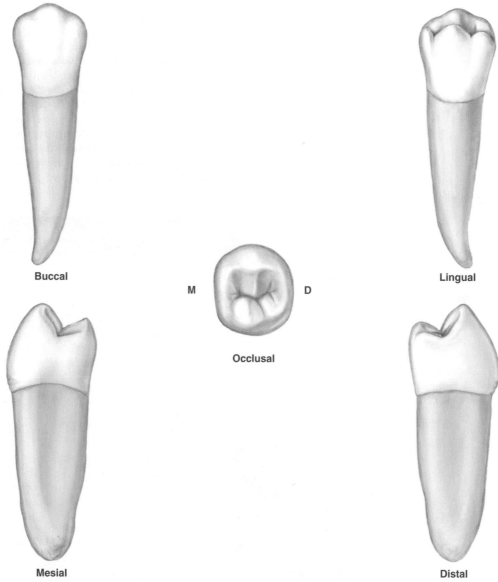

Buccal

M   D

Occlusal

Lingual

Mesial

Distal

FIGURE 17-25 Views of the permanent mandibular right second premolar of the three-cusp type.

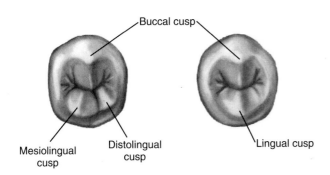

FIGURE 17-26 Occlusal view of the two types of permanent mandibular right second premolars: three-cusp type and two-cusp type, with occlusal table highlighted.

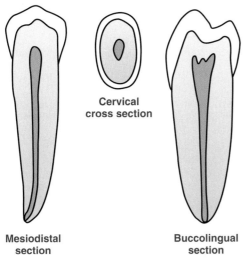

FIGURE 17-27 Pulp cavity of the permanent mandibular right second premolar of the three-cusp type.

Both types of mandibular second premolars have more supplemental grooves than the first premolar of the same arch. The two types of this tooth differ mainly in their occlusal features, but other surface features are similar. The three-cusp type also appears more angular from the occlusal view, and the two-cusp type appears more rounded.

Although a mandibular first premolar resembles a mandibular canine, the more common three-cusp type of mandibular second premolar resembles a small molar because its lingual cusps are well developed, which places both marginal ridges horizontal and superior on the occlusal table. A more efficient occlusion thus results, with the premolars in the opposite arch, similar to the molars. A mandibular second premolar thus represents a transition from a canine-like first premolar to the molars.

The single root of a mandibular second premolar is larger and longer than that of a first premolar but shorter than the maxillary premolars. Proximal root concavities are pronounced. In addition, the apex of this tooth is blunter than that of a first molar or of the maxillary premolars. The pulp cavity of the three-cusp type shows three pointed pulp horns (Figure 17-27). Two pulp horns are present with the two-cusp type. No matter the number of pulp horns, all pulp horns are more pointed in the mandibular second premolar than the first.

Buccal View Features A mandibular second premolar has a shorter buccal cusp than does a mandibular first premolar (see Figure 17-25). The cusp slopes of the buccal cusp are also more rounded. The

mesial contact and distal contact are wide and at the same location, just cervical to the junction of the occlusal and middle thirds.

Lingual View Features From the lingual, a mandibular second premolar shows considerable differences from a first premolar (Figure 17-28). The lingual cusp or cusps, depending on the type, are longer. Thus, less of the occlusal surface can be seen from this view. Because the lingual cusp is still smaller than the buccal cusp, however, part of the buccal part of the occlusal surface may be seen.

And the differences between its two types can also be noted. In the three-cusp type, the mesiolingual cusp is wider and longer than the distolingual cusp. A developmental groove, the lingual groove, is located between the cusps, extending a short distance on the lingual surface and usually distal to the center of the crown because the mesiolingual cusp is wider.

With the two-cusp type of the mandibular second premolar, the single lingual cusp development is at an equal height with the mesiolingual cusp of the three-cusp type but is higher than that of a first premolar. The two-cusp type has no groove noted lingually but does show a distolingual developmental depression where the lingual cusp ridge joins the distal marginal ridge.

Proximal View Features From the mesial, a mandibular second premolar has a shorter buccal cusp and is located more to the buccal than a first premolar (see Figure 17-25). Therefore, the distance between the cusp tips of this tooth is shorter than for the first. In addition, the crown is wider buccolingually, and the lingual cusp or cusps are larger. The mesial marginal ridge is at almost a right angle, or 90 degrees, to the long axis of the tooth. There is no mesiolingual groove.

The distal view is similar, although more of the occlusal surface can be seen from this view because the distal marginal ridge is more cervically located than the mesial marginal ridge, which *helps to distinguish the right mandibular second premolar from the left.*

Occlusal View Features The general shape of the crown outline of a mandibular second premolar is more nearly square, especially in the three-cusp type, than a mandibular first premolar (see Figure 17-25). The convergence of the mesial and distal margins toward the lingual is equally severe.

Occlusal Table Components In both the three-cusp and two-cusp types of mandibular second premolar, the buccal cusp is similar. Thus, the two types are the same in that part of the occlusal table, which is buccal to the mesiobuccal and distobuccal cusp ridges. Each of the cusps has buccal ridges, triangular ridges, and cuspal inclined planes, named for their location and orientation.

On the three-cusp type, the cusps are separated by two developmental grooves, a V-shaped central groove, and a linear lingual groove (Figure 17-29). The lingual groove extends lingually between the two lingual cusps and ends on the lingual surface of the crown just below the meeting of the lingual cusp ridges. These two grooves together form a distinctive Y-shaped groove pattern on the occlusal table.

On the three-cusp type, a deep central pit is located at the junction of the central groove and the lingual groove, toward the lingual. The central pit is also more to the distal between the mesial marginal ridge and distal marginal ridge because the mesiolingual cusp is wider than the distolingual cusp. Some anatomists prefer to separate the central groove on this tooth into two grooves, a mesial groove, and a distal groove.

On the three-cusp type of a second mandibular premolar, the mesial part of the central groove travels in a mesiobuccal direction and ends in a mesial pit surrounded by a mesial triangular fossa just distal to the mesial marginal ridge, which is often crossed by a mesial marginal groove (Figure 17-30). The distal part of the central groove travels in a distobuccal direction, is slightly shorter than the mesial groove, and ends in a distal pit surrounded by a distal triangular fossa mesial to the distal marginal ridge.

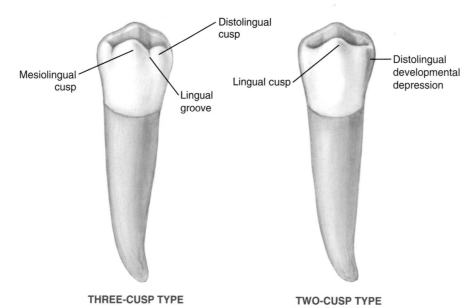

THREE-CUSP TYPE   TWO-CUSP TYPE

FIGURE 17-28 Lingual view of both types of permanent mandibular right second premolars, with occlusal table highlighted.

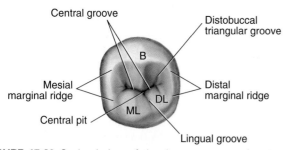

FIGURE 17-29 Occlusal view of the three-cusp type of permanent mandibular right second premolar showing the Y-shaped groove pattern, with occlusal table highlighted.

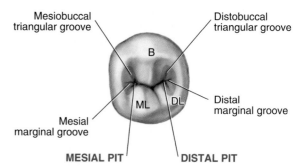

FIGURE 17-30 Additional occlusal features of the three-cusp type of permanent mandibular right second premolar, with fossae highlighted.

These triangular fossae are shallow, irregularly shaped, but overall more linear in form than the triangular fossae of the maxillary premolars. In addition, a mesiobuccal triangular groove, which extends into the mesial pit, is on the occlusal table. The distobuccal triangular groove, distolingual triangular groove, and possibly a distal marginal groove also extend into the distal pit.

In contrast, the two-cusp type is rounder lingual to the buccal cusp ridges (Figure 17-31). The mesial and distal margins converge slightly, making the lingual part narrower than the buccal, but never to the degree of a mandibular first premolar. The larger and longer buccal cusp is seen directly opposite the smaller and shorter lingual cusp. On the two-cusp type, a central groove on the occlusal table travels in a mesiodistal direction.

The central groove is most often crescent shaped, forming an U-shaped groove pattern on the occlusal table. Less often, the central groove may be straight, forming an H-shaped groove pattern on the occlusal table. The lingual cusp of the type with the H-shaped groove pattern is larger and sharper than the one with the U-shaped groove pattern, and is often offset to the mesial. The buccal cusp for both occlusal groove patterns of the two-cusp type has four functional inclined planes, and the lingual cusp has two.

The central groove of the two-cusp type has its terminal ends centered in the mesial fossa and distal fossa, which are circular depressions having supplemental grooves radiating from them. Some of

2-cusp type have a mesial pit and distal pit centered in mesial and distal fossae, instead of an unbroken central groove; most have a distolingual developmental depression crossing the distolingual cusp ridge. None of the 2-cusp types have a lingual groove or central pit.

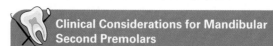

Clinical Considerations for Mandibular Second Premolars

With premature loss of a primary mandibular second molar, the developing permanent mandibular first molar inclines and drifts mesially. The developing permanent mandibular second premolar is prevented from normal eruption because its arch **leeway space** is nearly closed (see **Chapter 20**). This situation can allow the mandibular second premolar to become **impacted** against the first molar. An impacted tooth is an unerupted or partially erupted tooth that is positioned against another tooth, bone, or even soft tissue, making complete eruption unlikely. Additionally, the leeway space can be compromised if the permanent mandibular second molars erupt before the mandibular second premolars, the arch perimeter is significantly shortened, and occlusal disharmony is likely to occur, as is **malocclusion**. These problems may be prevented by careful evaluation of patients with mixed dentition and use of interceptive orthodontic therapy, such as space maintainers.

Permanent mandibular second premolars are commonly involved in partial **anodontia** (hypodontia) and thus are congenitally missing (see Table 6-3, *A*). With this disturbance, the appropriate individual tooth germ (or germs) in the area is absent because of failure of the initiation process during tooth development; this condition can be bilateral or unilateral. This extremely important information must be obtained by careful patient evaluation when primary mandibular second molars are retained in a mixed or mature dentition, which would include radiographs. Missing permanent teeth may require prosthetic replacement or an implant and can result in problems in spacing and occlusion.

Dental professionals should note that these retained primary molars, without the presence of their underlying **succedaneous** permanent teeth, may not be shed (or exfoliated) for many years. Thus, these primary teeth can serve as functioning replacements for the permanent premolar teeth and should not be extracted unless they are involved in root pathology or are uncomfortably **mobile.**

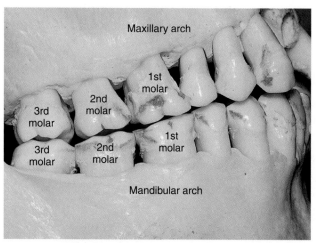

FIGURE 17-32 Permanent molars identified per arch.

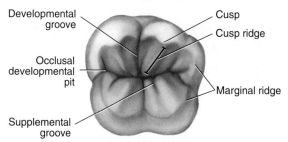

FIGURE 17-33 Occlusal view of a permanent molar, with occlusal table highlighted.

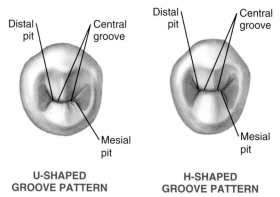

FIGURE 17-31 Occlusal view of the two-cusp type of permanent mandibular right second premolar, showing the U-shaped and H-shaped groove patterns, with fossae highlighted.

PERMANENT MOLARS

GENERAL FEATURES

Permanent **molars** are the most posteriorly placed **posterior teeth** of the **permanent dentition**, distal to the premolars (Figure 17-32). Molars are also the largest teeth in the dentition. Each dental arch usually has six molars, three in each quadrant, if all have erupted. The name *molar* comes from the Latin word for *grinder*, one of the functions of the molar teeth.

There are three types of molars: **first molars**, **second molars**, and **third molars** (see Figure 17-32). The first molars and second molars are called the 6-year molars and 12-year molars, respectively, because of their eruption times.

The third molars, also known as the *wisdom teeth*, are extremely variable in their eruption time, as well as in their anatomical size and form. They were given this unusual nickname in ancient times when it was thought that only educated men had this important type of molar. Many dental professionals jokingly argue against the wisdom sometimes shown in young adults, given that these teeth erupt between 17 to 21 years of age.

Eruption of the third molars usually marks the end of the growth of the jaws. The first molar usually is overall the largest, and the second and third are each progressively smaller. Only the permanent dentition has three types of molars; the primary dentition only has two types. One of each type of molar is present in each quadrant of each dental arch. The first molars are closer to the midline, at the sixth position from it, and at the same time, they are distal to the permanent second premolars when full eruption of the permanent dentition has occurred. The second molars are distal to the first molars and are in the seventh position from the midline. Finally, the third molars are distal to the second molars and are in the eighth position from the midline.

All three types of molars erupt in order distal to the primary second molars, long after all the primary teeth have erupted and are functioning. Thus, all the permanent molars are **nonsuccedaneous** because they do not replace any primary teeth. Because of the continued elongation of the facial bones during development, these teeth usually have enough space as they progressively erupt (except in some cases for third molars, discussed later).

Each molar has an extremely large crown compared with the rest of the permanent dentition, but the crown is shorter occlusocervically in contrast to the teeth anterior to it. Each buccal surface of a molar has a prominent **cervical ridge** running mesiodistally in the cervical one third.

Like all posterior teeth, molars have an **occlusal surface** with usually three or more **cusps**, of which at least two are buccal cusps (Figure 17-33). Unlike anterior teeth and premolars, molars do not exhibit buccal developmental depressions. Evidence of developmental lobe separation is in the developmental grooves on the occlusal table. In addition to cusps, the **occlusal table** of the molar is bordered by **cusp ridges** and **marginal ridges**. The occlusal table of molars is even more complex than that of premolars, because it has more developmental grooves,

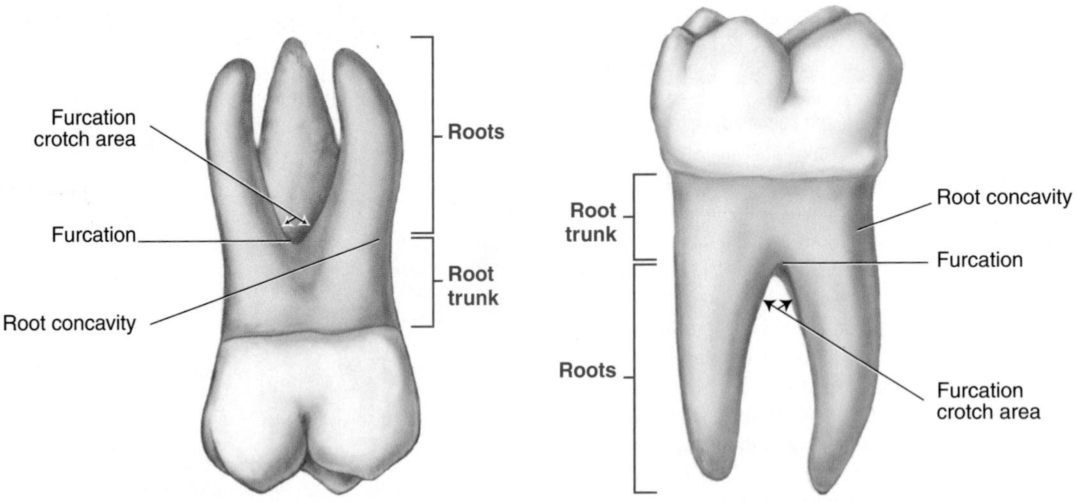

FIGURE 17-34 Buccal root features of a permanent maxillary and mandibular molar.

Clinical Considerations for Molars

As the largest and strongest crowns of the permanent dentition, the molars, assisted by the premolars, function in grinding food during **mastication**. This grinding function is possible because molars have wide occlusal surfaces with prominent cusps. These teeth also support the soft tissue of the cheek, especially the facial muscles. They maintain the height of the lower third of the **vertical dimension of the face** and arch continuity. Thus, they are involved in esthetics and speech, but less so than the premolars, due to their posterior position.

Multiple roots give molars increased periodontal tissue support. However, with the loss of periodontal tissue support caused by advanced periodontal disease (**periodontitis**), the **furcations**, **furcation crotches**, and **root concavities** of the molars can lose their bony coverage in varying degrees. The horizontal component of a furcation invasion can be located by using a Nabor's probe within a **periodontal pocket**; if **gingival recession** has occurred, they can become clinically exposed. Dental biofilm and other deposits can be retained in the exposed furcation crotches and root concavities, leading to further periodontal tissue disease. Molars are lost to periodontal disease more than single rooted teeth partially due to the presence of furcations.

Therefore, furcation crotches and root concavities on these molars present a challenge during both instrumentation and performance of homecare in the area, due to lack of access. Approximately half of molar furcations are too narrow for access by instruments, decreasing the prognosis if periodontally involved. To allow better access, the furcations of a tooth may

be reduced by a dental bur with a minor odontoplasty, and any occluding gingival tissue is removed during surgical intervention. In addition, when roots are extremely close to each other, access to interproximals may be even more difficult. The cervical ridge on molars also presents challenges during instrumentation around the cervical area.

In addition, awareness of root trunk dimensions and their relationship to the furcations is critical to the periodontal prognosis of a molar. Short root trunks are most commonly found buccally on both maxillary and mandibular molars, whereas long root trunks are more commonly found mesially in both maxillary molars. Additionally, short root length is associated with longer root trunks, and these long root trunks are more commonly found on the second molar than on the first molars. There is also a strong correlation between length of the root trunk and furcation invasion by periodontal disease.

Surgical removal of third molars is a controversial procedure, with around 25% of patients designated to have their third molars removed before age 25. Often, patients are not even aware of the troubled nature of their third molars. More than 40% of adult patients who never had their third molars removed during adolescence develop infection, caries, cyst formation, or periodontal disease (discussed later) by age 45, thus requiring extraction; the risk of surgical complications in adults is increased by approximately 30% compared with adolescents. However, surgeons now refrain from automatically removing functioning third molars that are not causing any problems. Thus, an evaluation of the third molars by age 25 is generally recommended.

supplemental grooves, and occlusal developmental pits. The grooves and pits are located on the occlusal and lingual surfaces of maxillary molars and on the occlusal and buccal surfaces of mandibular molars.

In addition, molars usually are **multirooted**. Maxillary molars usually have three root branches (**trifurcated**), and mandibular molars have two (**bifurcated**) (Figure 17-34). Molars, as do other teeth, originate as a single root on the base of the crown, which is considered the **root trunk**. The cervical cross section of root trunk follows the form of the crown, but the root then divides from the root trunk into the number of root branches for its type (see Figure 6-21).

Between two or more of these root branches, before they divide from the root trunk, is an area called the furcation (Figures 17-34 and 17-35). The spaces between the roots at the furcation are called furcation crotches. Teeth with two roots, such as mandibular molars, have

two furcation crotches; teeth with three roots can have three furcation crotches. Such crotches can be either facial and lingual or mesial and distal, depending on tooth type, each with a slightly different individual configuration. The furcation crotches may be close to the CEJ or far from it. **Root concavities** are also found on many of the root branches of molar teeth, as well as on the furcal surfaces. In a molar, the root canals join the pulp chamber apical to the CEJ.

PERMANENT MAXILLARY MOLARS
GENERAL FEATURES

Permanent maxillary molars erupt between 6 months to 1 year after the corresponding permanent mandibular molars (Table 17-2). They are usually the first permanent teeth to erupt into the maxillary arch.

Developmental Disturbances of Molars

Permanent molar teeth may have one or more tubercles, or accessory cusps, on the occlusal surface (see Table 6-3, G). In addition, similar to incisors, the molars may be affected in children with congenital **syphilis**. The spirochete *Treponema pallidum*, a sexually transmitted microorganism, is passed from an infected pregnant woman to her **fetus** via the **placenta**. This microorganism may cause localized **enamel hypoplasia** and result in mulberry molars, a disturbance that occurs during tooth development (see Figure 3-16). This tooth has a crown with an abnormally shaped occlusal surface characterized by berry-like nodules or **tubercles** of enamel instead of cusps. Children with this condition may also have other developmental anomalies, such as blindness, deafness, and paralysis caused by congenital syphilis. Treatment using full-coverage crowns may be performed to improve the appearance of these teeth.

Another disturbance associated with molars is the **enamel pearl** (or enamel projection) (see Table 6-3, J). Mainly found on the buccal surfaces of second molars, these deposits of enamel apical to the level on the CEJ have a tapered form and extend into root **furcation** areas. They are present on over 28% of maxillary and 17% of mandibular molars, and on most mandibular molars with isolated furcation involvement. Teeth were also found to have deeper **root concavities** compared with teeth that lacked cervical enamel projections. Unlike calculus, which it resembles radiographically, the enamel pearl cannot be removed by instrumentation. Instead, it must be ground away to restore the normal contour of the tooth.

Finally, dilaceration of the root(s) can also occur, making extraction and endodontic treatment difficult (Figure 17-36, see **Chapter 6**). Another disturbance is **root fusion**, which creates deep developmental grooves when the molar roots fuse. These can function as pathways to accumulate deposits that are not easily accessible to professional periodontal therapy or homecare. The highest prevalence of permanent molars with root fusion occurs in maxillary second molars, followed by mandibular second molars, maxillary first molars, and finally, mandibular first molars; females present a higher incidence overall of root fusion than males.

Clinical Considerations for Maxillary Molars

The roots of maxillary molars may penetrate the middle and posterior parts of the **maxillary sinus** as a result of accidental trauma, or during tooth extraction because of the close relation of these roots to the sinus walls (see Figure 11-21). In addition, the discomfort of **sinusitis** can be mistakenly interpreted as tooth-related (stemming from the maxillary molars), and vice versa. Thus, radiographic study of the tooth or maxillary sinus and other diagnostic tests become necessary to determine the true cause of the discomfort in this area.

Because of the arch position of maxillary molars, with the natural overhang of the cheek, instrumentation and homecare of the buccal surface may be difficult. Instrumentation and homecare of the proximal furcation crotch areas of the maxillary molars have the easiest access from the lingual because the furcations are located closer to the lingual surface. However, the furcation entrances diameters can be 0.75 mm or less, making instrumentation access limited.

A possible lingual pit on the lingual surface of maxillary molars is at an increased risk of caries (Figure 17-38). This is due to both increased dental biofilm retention and the thinness of enamel forming the walls of the pit (see **Chapter 12**). An enamel sealant should be placed on each lingual surface of the erupting teeth. However, because of the histology of enamel in the area, enamel sealants do not bond as easily on the lingual surface as on the occlusal surface.

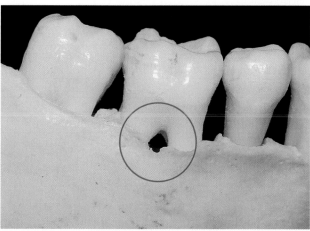

FIGURE 17-35 Example of exposed root surface on permanent molars on a skull due to periodontal disease, exposing the furcation area and crotch on the mandibular first molar (circled).

In addition, maxillary molars are overall the largest and strongest teeth of the maxillary arch. They are usually shorter occlusocervically than are the crowns of teeth anterior to them, but they are larger in all other measurements than other maxillary teeth.

All maxillary molars are wider buccolingually than mesiodistally; in comparison, the mandibular molars are wider mesiodistally.

From the occlusal, the outline of the crown of maxillary molars is rhomboidal, or four-sided with opposite sides parallel. Like all maxillary posteriors, the crown outline is also trapezoidal from each proximal view—again four-sided but with only two parallel sides. In addition, the crown is also centered over the root and shows no lingual inclination, similar to maxillary molars, but unlike mandibular molars.

Each maxillary molar usually has four major cusps, with two cusps on the buccal part of the occlusal table and two on the lingual (Figure 17-37). An oblique ridge is a unique feature is present on the occlusal table of most except the third molar. This type of transverse ridge crosses the occlusal table obliquely, forming by the union of the triangular ridge of the distobuccal cusp and distal cusp ridge of the mesiolingual cusp. In contrast, an oblique ridge is never present on mandibular molars.

Maxillary molars usually have three root branches, or are **trifurcated**, unlike mandibular molars, which usually have only two root branches (bifurcated) (see Figure 17-34). These roots are the mesiobuccal, distobuccal, and lingual (or palatal). The lingual root is usually the largest and longest. The farther distal a molar is in the maxillary arch, the shorter and more varied in size, shape, and curvature are the roots. The roots also become less divided (or divergent) on the teeth located farther distally. Thus, a first molar has longer, more divergent roots than a third molar and has more consistency in the root's size, shape, and curvature. Roots of maxillary molars show great lingual and moderate distal inclination within the alveolar bone.

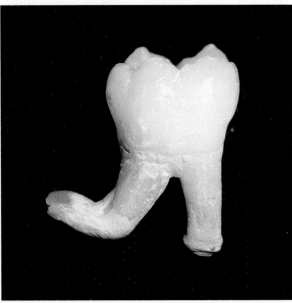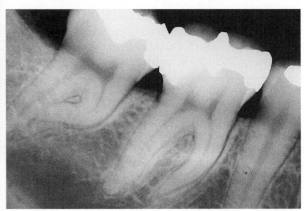

FIGURE 17-36 Dilaceration of mandibular first and second molars, respectively *(From Ibsen OAC, Phelan JA:* Oral Pathology for Dental Hygienists, *ed 5, WB Saunders, Philadelphia, 2009.)*

TABLE 17-2	Anatomical Information on Permanent Maxillary Molars		
	MAXILLARY FIRST MOLAR	**MAXILLARY SECOND MOLAR**	**MAXILLARY THIRD MOLAR**
Universal number	#3 and #14	#2 and #15	#1 and #16
General crown features	Occlusal table with marginal ridges, cusps with tips, inclined planes, ridges, grooves, fossae, and pits; buccal cervical ridge		
Specific crown features	Largest tooth in arch, largest crown in dentition; four major cusps, with buccal cusps almost equal in height; fifth minor cusp of Carabelli associated with mesiolingual cusp and prominent oblique ridge	Smaller crown than first, heart-shaped or rhomboidal crown outline, thus three or four cusps; oblique ridge less prominent, with mesiobuccal cusp longer than distobuccal cusp and no fifth cusp; distolingual cusp smaller than on first or absent	Smaller crown than second, variable in form, heart-shaped or rhomboidal crown outline, thus three or four cusps
Mesial contact	Junction of occlusal and middle thirds	Middle third	Middle third
Distal contact	Middle third	Middle third	None
Distinguishing right from left	Mesiolingual cusp outline longer and larger but not as sharp as distolingual cusp	Mesiolingual cusp outline longer and larger but not as sharp as distolingual cusp	Distobuccal cusp shorter than mesiobuccal cusp, and roots curved distally
Root features	Trifurcated roots, with furcations, root trunks, and root concavities		Usually fused roots, curving distally
	Divergent roots; furcations well removed from the CEJ	Less divergent roots	

CEJ, Cementoenamel junction.

Because maxillary molars are trifurcated, the three furcations are usually located on the mesial, buccal, and distal surfaces. All **furcations** on maxillary teeth usually begin near the junction of the cervical and middle thirds of the root. The buccal furcation is located midway between the mesial and distal surfaces. The mesial and distal furcations are located more to the lingual than the buccal surface. **Root concavities** are found on the mesial surface of the mesiobuccal root, the lingual surface of the lingual root, and all three furcal surfaces.

PERMANENT MAXILLARY FIRST MOLARS #3 AND #14

Specific Overall Features (Figure 17-39) Permanent maxillary first molars erupt between 6 to 7 years of age (root completion between ages 9 to 10). Thus, these teeth are the first permanent teeth

to erupt into the maxillary arch. They erupt distal to the primary maxillary second molars and thus are nonsuccedaneous, not having primary predecessors.

The maxillary first molar is the largest tooth in the maxillary arch, as well as having the largest crown in the permanent dentition. It has a much more complex crown form than do the nearby maxillary premolars. Of all the maxillary permanent molars, the first is the least variable in form.

This tooth is composed of five developmental lobes: two buccal and three lingual. These are named in the same manner as their associated cusps: mesiobuccal, distobuccal, mesiolingual, distolingual, and an additional minor cusp on the lingual (discussed later). Evidence of lobe separation can be found in the developmental grooves on the occlusal surface.

The roots of maxillary first molars are larger and more divergent than those of the second molars, and are more complex in form than

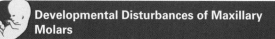

Developmental Disturbances of Maxillary Molars

Maxillary molars are some of the most common teeth of the permanent dentition to be involved in **concrescence** (see Table 6-3, *I*). Concrescence is the union of the root structure of two or more teeth through the **cementum** only. The teeth involved are initially separate but join because of excessive cementum deposition in one or more teeth following eruption. It occurs as a result of traumatic injury or crowding of the teeth in the area during the stages of **apposition** and **maturation** of tooth development. This disturbance may present problems during extraction and endodontic treatment; thus, preoperative radiographs are important.

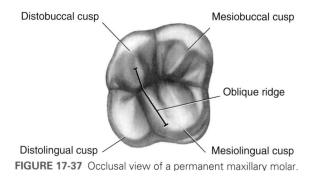

Distobuccal cusp   Mesiobuccal cusp

Oblique ridge

Distolingual cusp   Mesiolingual cusp

FIGURE 17-37 Occlusal view of a permanent maxillary molar.

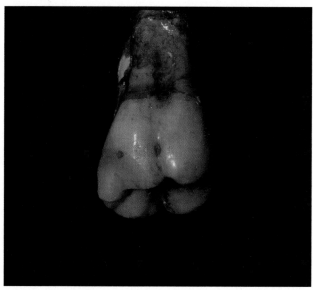

FIGURE 17-38 Example of lingual surface anatomy of a lingual pit on the crown of the permanent maxillary molar, with view of palatal root.

those of the maxillary premolars. The roots are twice as long as the crown. Thus, the furcations are well removed from the cervical area of the tooth, and the distal furcation crotch is wider than the mesial crotch.

The lingual, or palatal, root is the largest and longest, inclines lingually, and extends beyond the crown outline. It has a banana-like curvature toward the buccal. A vertical depression may be present on the palatal surface of the root that is more pronounced at the cervical third.

Both the mesiobuccal and distobuccal roots have an extreme curvature that, together, makes them look like the handles on a set of pliers. The mesiobuccal root is the second largest and longest, is inclined mesially and buccally, and has its apical third curving distally. The distobuccal root is the smallest, shortest, and thus the weakest of the three. This root inclines distally and buccally, and its apical one third curves mesially, with its buccal furcation about 4 mm apical to the CEJ.

The maxillary first molar's furcation concavity depths are only 0.1 mm to 0.7 mm, limiting deposit removal during instrumentation. The mesial furcation is 3 mm from the CEJ and not centered. Its entrance is dictated by the size of mesiobuccal root and located two thirds of the buccolingual width of the root trunk from the buccal and one third of the buccolingual width of the root trunk from the lingual, and it is wider buccolingually than mesiodistally. The distal furcation is 5 mm from the CEJ and is predisposed to develop periodontal disease owing to the proximity of the divergent distobuccal root to the adjacent second molar, limiting access to its already narrow furcation entrance.

The pulp cavity of a maxillary first molar usually has one pulp horn for each major cusp (Figure 17-40). Thus, the four pulp horns are mesiobuccal, distobuccal, mesiolingual, and distolingual. Three main pulp canals are usually present, one for each of the three roots. The lingual pulp canal is the largest, the distobuccal the smallest, and the mesiobuccal between these two in size. It sometimes has four pulp canals, with two pulp canals in the mesiobuccal root.

Buccal View Features The general shape of a maxillary first molar from this view is trapezoidal, with the longer parallel side toward the occlusal (see Figure 17-39). The entire buccal surface is larger than that of the adjacent premolar. Despite this fact, the occlusocervical measurement is slightly smaller.

Parts of all four major and functioning cusps are seen from this view: mesiobuccal cusp, distobuccal cusp, mesiolingual cusp, and distolingual cusp. This is because the two lingual cusps are slightly offset to the distal relative to the buccal cusps. The occlusal outline of the mesiobuccal cusp is wider, but the distobuccal cusp tip is sharper. However, the two buccal cusps are nearly the same height, and the mesiolingual cusp tip is seen between them.

The occlusal outline of a maxillary first molar is divided symmetrically by the buccal groove. This developmental groove extends between the two buccal cusps, runs apically about halfway to the CEJ, and is parallel with the long axis of the tooth. There it can fade out, but it may end in a buccal pit. In addition, the buccal groove may end in two short, slanting grooves, with or without a buccal pit.

The mesial outline is flat from the CEJ occlusally to the mesial contact. The mesial contact is at the junction of the occlusal and middle thirds. The mesial contact is initially with a primary maxillary second molar, until that tooth is exfoliated, or shed; later the tooth's contact is with the permanent second premolar after it erupts. As noted occlusally from the mesial contact, the mesial outline is rounded.

Instead of being flat like the mesial, the distal outline of the maxillary first molar is rounded or convex from the CEJ to the occlusal surface. The distal contact is in the middle third. However, no distal contact occurs until the permanent maxillary second molars erupt. The CEJ is slightly but irregularly curved apically but with less curvature than that on teeth anterior to it. A sharp dip or point may be observed just occlusal to the furcation area.

Lingual View Features The lingual surface of the maxillary first molar is almost as wide mesiodistally as the buccal surface, as well as trapezoidal. However, the lingual surface is more rounded or convex than the buccal. Both the mesial and distal outline and CEJ curvature are about the same, except that the distal outline is shorter because the distolingual cusp is smaller than the distobuccal cusp.

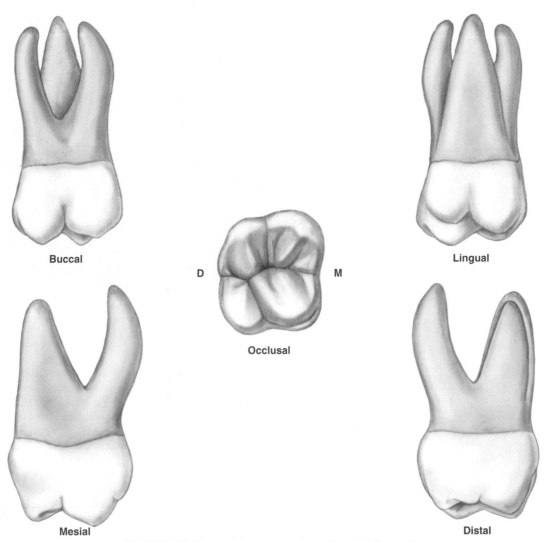

Buccal

D   M

Lingual

Occlusal

Mesial

Distal

FIGURE 17-39 Views of the permanent maxillary right first molar.

Similar to the buccal surface, the lingual surface has a distolingual groove that divides the occlusal outline into two asymmetrical parts. Dissimilar to the buccal surface, only the two lingual cusps can be seen from this view. The distolingual groove usually ends in a lingual pit in the middle of the lingual surface, but it may fade out. Being the largest cusp on the occlusal surface, the mesiolingual cusp outline is much longer and larger, but the cusp is not as sharp as the distolingual cusp, which *helps to distinguish the right maxillary first molar from the left*. The distolingual groove usually ends in a lingual pit in the middle of the lingual surface, but it may fade out.

Commonly arising from the lingual surface of the mesiolingual cusp of the maxillary first molar is a fifth nonfunctioning cusp, the cusp of Carabelli, named for its discoverer. This minor cusp is set apart from the rest of the mesiolingual cusp by its associated cusp of Carabelli groove. Its presence can be variable; it is not present in all dentitions. If present, this small cusp, and its equally small groove, varies in prominence from tooth to tooth.

Proximal View Features   The only two cusps of the maxillary first molar that are seen from the mesial are the mesiobuccal cusp and mesiolingual cusp. A mesial marginal groove usually notches the mesial marginal ridge about midway along its length. The contact area on the mesial is situated slightly to the buccal.

The distal view is the same as the mesial, the exception being that the mesial cusp tips are seen projecting beyond the outline of the distobuccal cusp and distolingual cusp from proximal. The distal marginal ridge is less prominent and dips farther cervically than on the mesial, with a distal marginal groove halfway along its length. On both proximal views, the CEJ usually curves slightly toward the occlusal, and may even be a straight line on some teeth on the distal.

Occlusal View Features   The overall rhomboidal outline of the occlusal surface of a maxillary first molar is seen from the occlusal view (Figure 17-41) because it is four-sided with opposite sides parallel. The buccal outline is divided unequally into two parts by the buccal groove, and the mesial part is longer than the distal part. The lingual outline is also divided unequally into two parts by the distolingual groove, with the mesial part longer and less rounded than the distal part.

The mesial marginal ridge is longer and more prominent than the distal marginal ridge. Both marginal ridges are crossed by a mesial marginal ridge groove and distal marginal ridge groove, respectively. Because this is the first molar a student will study, a detailed discussion of the occlusal table follows, and this information can be applied to the other molars, especially the maxillary molars.

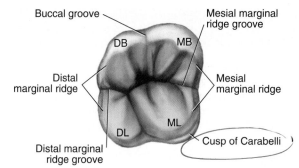

FIGURE 17-41 Occlusal features of the permanent maxillary right first molar, with occlusal table highlighted.

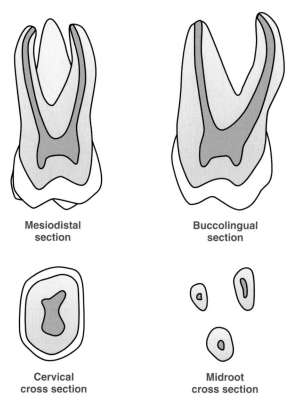

FIGURE 17-40 Pulp cavity of the permanent maxillary right first molar.

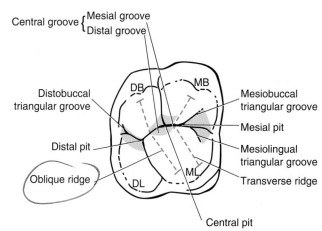

FIGURE 17-42 Additional occlusal features of the permanent maxillary right first molar, with fossae highlighted.

Occlusal Table Components The two marginal ridges and the mesial and distal cusp ridges of the four major cusps on the buccal and lingual border the occlusal table of the maxillary first molar (Figure 17-42). Each major cusp has a triangular ridge and three other cusp ridges. Also present are four inclined cuspal planes with each major cusp.

The mesiobuccal cusp has a sharp cusp tip and is the second largest cusp. It has a mesial cusp ridge that extends from the cusp tip to the mesiobuccal occlusal point angle. The mesiobuccal cusp on the first maxillary first molar is important in classifying the permanent dentition using **Angle's classification of malocclusion** in relation to the mandibular arch (see Table 20-1).

The distal cusp ridge runs from the cusp tip to the buccal groove. The buccal cusp ridge passes from the cusp tip to the CEJ on the buccal surface. Finally, the lingual cusp ridge runs from the cusp tip to the central groove and is the triangular ridge of the mesiobuccal cusp. The mesiobuccal cusp has four inclined planes, with all the lingual parts functional.

The distobuccal cusp has the sharpest cusp tip and is the third largest cusp. Its triangular ridge, cusp ridges, and inclined planes are named similarly to those of the mesiobuccal cusp.

The mesiolingual cusp is the largest cusp, with a rounded cusp tip. Its cusp ridges are similar to those of the other cusps, except that the distal triangular ridge extends from the mesiolingual cusp tip in an oblique distobuccal direction. There the distal triangular ridge meets the lingual triangular ridge of the distobuccal cusp to form a prominent oblique ridge. The mesiolingual cusp also has four inclined planes, all of which are functional. A typical transverse ridge is also present and is formed by the buccal triangular ridge of the mesiolingual cusp and the lingual triangular ridge of the mesiobuccal cusp.

The smallest cusp, when present on the maxillary first molar, is the minor and nonfunctional cusp, the cusp of Carabelli, with its cusp of Carabelli groove.

The distolingual cusp is the smallest of the major cusps and is the most variable of this group. The triangular ridge, cusp ridges, and inclined planes are similar to those of other cusps, except that all the inclined planes are functional.

Four fossae are also present, along with associated developmental grooves and occlusal pits: central, mesial triangular, distal triangular, and distal. The central fossa is mesial to the oblique ridge and has a central pit in its most central, deepest part. The central pit divides the central groove into two parts, a mesial groove and a distal groove. Thus, the central pit is at the junction of three developmental grooves: buccal, mesial, and distal. Along with the central groove and other developmental grooves, supplemental grooves can be present.

Three triangular grooves are present: mesiobuccal triangular groove, mesiolingual triangular groove, and distobuccal triangular groove. The buccal groove extends onto the buccal surface. The mesial groove, as part of the central groove, extends from the central pit to the mesial pit. The mesial pit is in the mesial triangular fossa, distal to the mesial marginal ridge. Thus, the mesial pit is at the junction of four developmental grooves: mesial, mesiobuccal triangular, mesiolingual triangular, and mesial marginal.

As part of the central groove, the distal groove usually extends from the central pit across the oblique ridge to the distal pit. Thus, it is sometimes referred to as the transverse groove of the oblique ridge. The distal pit is in the distal triangular fossa, mesial to the distal marginal ridge, making the distal pit located at the junction of five

Clinical Considerations for Maxillary First Molars

Because of their arch position, and because the permanent maxillary first molars are the first permanent teeth to erupt in the maxillary arch, they are considered important in the development of **occlusion** (see Table 20-1). The importance of this role in occlusion is shown if this tooth is lost (Figure 17-43). Loss of this tooth now commonly results from periodontal disease, whereas, in the past, it resulted from caries.

Loss of the tooth is followed by mesial inclination and drift of the maxillary second molar into the open arch space, and the mandibular first molar, if present, also supererupts. Occlusion and then mastication are disabled, causing an increased risk of further periodontal disease around the irregularly spaced teeth. Prosthetic replacement may prevent these situations.

The distobuccal surfaces of the permanent first molars may have increased supragingival tooth deposits. This is mainly due to the maxillary first molars' position in the oral cavity, opposite the duct openings of the **parotid salivary glands** on the inner cheek at the **parotid papilla**. **Saliva**, with its mineral content, is released from these glands, causing the dental biofilm to mineralize quickly into supragingival calculus.

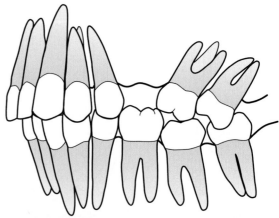

FIGURE 17-43 Changes that can occur in the permanent dentition when the maxillary first molar is lost. Arch undergoes mesial inclination and drift of the maxillary second molar into the adjacent open space, with supereruption of the mandibular first molar into opposing space.

developmental grooves: distal, distolingual, distobuccal triangular, distal marginal, and distal lingual triangular. The last fossa is the distal fossa, a linear rather than circular depression that is distal and parallel to the oblique ridge and thus is in the distolingual groove.

PERMANENT MAXILLARY SECOND MOLARS #2 AND #15

Specific Overall Features (Figure 17-44)   Permanent maxillary second molars erupt between 12 to 13 years of age (root completion between ages 14 to 16). These teeth erupt distal to the permanent maxillary first molars and thus are nonsuccedaneous.

Much variation in the form of the maxillary second molars is observed, especially in the size of the distolingual cusp. The crown usually has four cusps similar to the four major cusps of the first molar, but it can have three cusps. This tooth is composed of four developmental lobes, all named in the same manner as their associated cusps. Evidence of lobe separation can be found in the developmental grooves on the occlusal surface.

The three roots on maxillary second molars are smaller than the first molars. They are also less divergent, as well as placed at a more parallel position than on the first molars. The lingual root is still the largest and longest and extends beyond the crown outline, but it is usually straighter and not as curved toward the buccal as the lingual root of the first molars. The furcation notches are also narrower than those in the first molars, and all depressions are shallower. Thus, the chance of fusion, especially of the buccal roots or even of all three roots, is greater for the second than for the first molars.

The pulp cavity of a maxillary second molar consists of a pulp chamber and three main pulp canals, one for each of the three roots (Figure 17-45). Each major cusp usually has one pulp horn, giving it four pulp horns: mesiobuccal, distobuccal, mesiolingual, and distolingual.

Buccal View Features   Maxillary second molar is shorter occlusocervically and narrower mesiodistally than a first molar (see Figure 17-44). The buccal groove is located farther distally on the buccal surface of the second than the first. The mesiobuccal cusp is longer and has a less sharp cusp tip than the distobuccal cusp. Both the mesial contact and distal contact are in the middle third.

Lingual View Features   The distolingual cusp of the maxillary second molar is smaller and shorter than on the first molar and is sometimes not present. Thus, the outline of the largest cusp of the occlusal surface, the mesiolingual cusp, is much longer and larger, but the cusp is not as sharp as the distolingual cusp, which *helps to distinguish the right maxillary second molar from the left*. In addition, a fifth cusp (or cusp of Carabelli) usually does not exist. From this view, the cusp tips of the distobuccal cusp and the mesiobuccal cusp can be seen.

A lingual pit is usually present at the end of the distolingual groove, which does not extend as far mesially or cervically as the groove on the first molar. Thus, the distolingual groove ends at a point that is occlusal and distal to the center of the lingual surface.

Proximal View Features   From the mesial, the mesial contact area of a maxillary second molar is larger, and the cervical flattening or concavity is never as pronounced as in a first molar. From the distal, the distobuccal cusp and distolingual cusp are smaller on a second than a first molar, thus showing more of the occlusal surface. Note that no distal contact area is present until the third molar possibly erupts and moves into occlusion.

Occlusal View Features   The outline of the crown of a maxillary second molar is narrower mesiodistally than that of a maxillary first molar but is about the same width buccolingually. Two types of crown outlines are possible on this tooth when viewed from the occlusal: rhomboidal and heart-shaped (Figure 17-46). The more common rhomboidal type has four sides with opposite sides parallel; this type is similar to that of the first molar but with an even more accentuated outline. The heart-shaped type is the less common and is similar to the typical maxillary third molar.

Occlusal Table Components   With the rhomboidal type on a maxillary second molar, the cusps present are similar to the major cusps of a maxillary first molar. With the heart-shaped type, the distolingual cusp is quite small, with the other three cusps completely overshadowing it. The distolingual cusp is sometimes absent in the heart-shaped type, and the distolingual groove is confined to the occlusal table.

The cusp ridges, triangular ridges, transverse ridge, oblique ridge, developmental grooves, fossae, and occlusal pits for both types of a second molar are similar to those of the first molar of the same arch. However, the oblique ridge is less prominent on the second than on the first molar. Instead, an increased number of supplemental grooves are usually present on the occlusal table of the second.

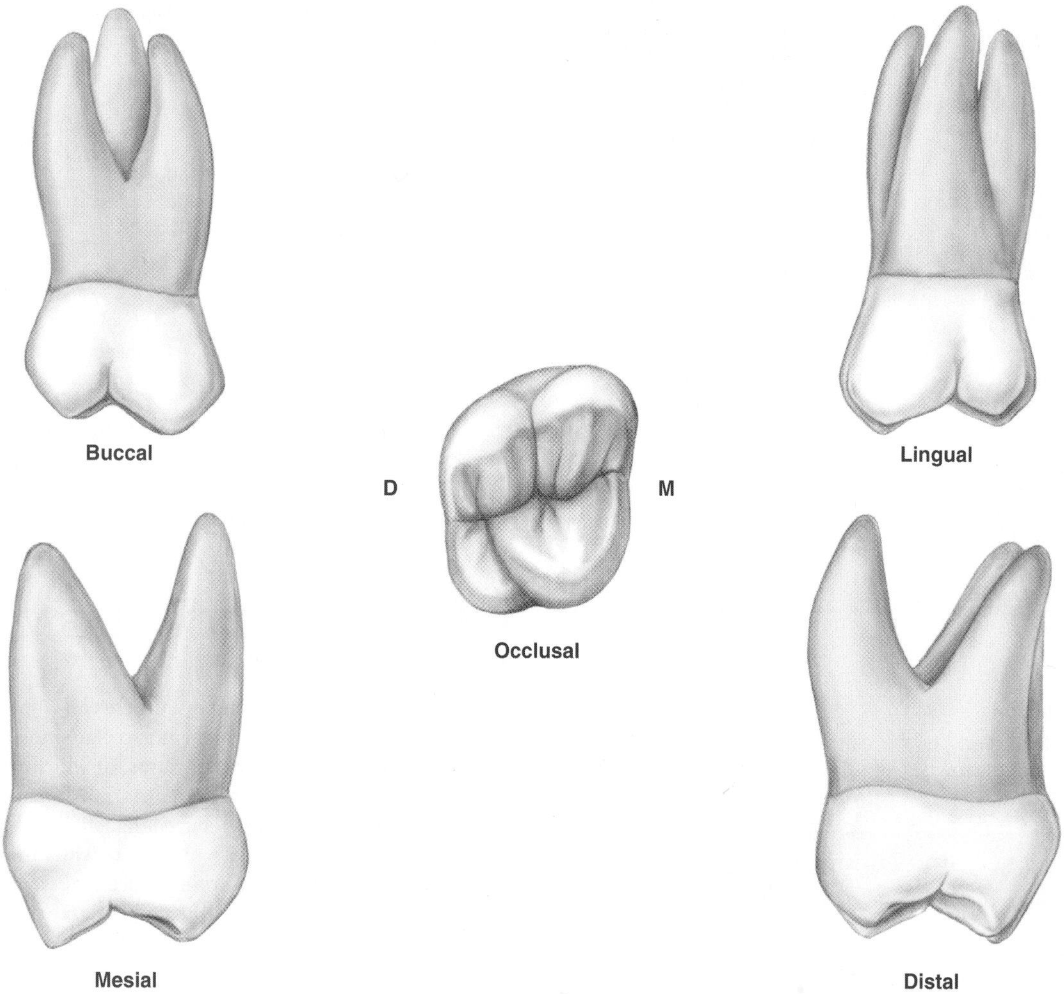

FIGURE 17-44 Views of the permanent maxillary right second molar that has the rhomboidal crown outline.

PERMANENT MAXILLARY THIRD MOLARS #1 AND #16

Specific Overall Features (Figure 17-47) Permanent maxillary third molars may erupt between 17 to 21 years of age (root completion is between ages 18 to 25). If they erupt (see the later section on clinical considerations), they erupt distal to the permanent maxillary second molars and thus are nonsuccedaneous. The tooth's mesial contact is in the middle third, but it does not have a distal tooth contact because it may be the last tooth in both maxillary arches. In addition, because of its very distal arch position, the tooth has only one antagonist in the mandibular arch. This tooth and the very small mandibular central incisor are the only teeth that have one antagonist; all others have two.

This tooth is the smallest molar and most variable tooth in shape in the permanent dentition. Without any standard form observed for this tooth, describing a typical maxillary third molar is therefore difficult. Generally, it is smaller in all dimensions than a second maxillary molar, and its crown is poorly developed when compared with the other maxillary molars. The tooth is composed of four developmental lobes.

Two types of crown outlines are possible for a maxillary third molar when viewed from the occlusal (Figure 17-48). The most common type is heart shaped, similar to a maxillary second molar but with more supplemental grooves on the occlusal table. Generally, with the heart-shaped type, the tooth has only three cusps: mesiobuccal, distobuccal, and mesiolingual, but not any distolingual cusp.

If a fourth cusp is present, it is a rhomboidal type, with a small and nonfunctioning distolingual cusp, and there is not any oblique ridge present. For both types of occlusal forms, the distobuccal cusp is much shorter than the mesiobuccal cusp, which *helps to distinguish the right maxillary third molar from the left.*

Like other maxillary molars, the maxillary third molars are trifurcated. However, the roots are sometimes so close together that they are fused, either partially or fully, and thus may give the appearance of a single root. All roots of the third are also poorly developed, like the crown, and shorter than that of a second molar. The distobuccal root usually is the smallest and often is found tucked under the crown. The roots are curved distally, which *helps to distinguish the right maxillary third molar from the left.*

The pulp cavity of a maxillary third molar may have a pulp chamber and three pulp canals (Figure 17-49). The tooth may sometimes have one large pulp canal, if the root is fused, to as many as four pulp canals, if there are four roots. The number of pulp horns varies and depends on the number of cusps; if there are three cusps, there are three pulp horns.

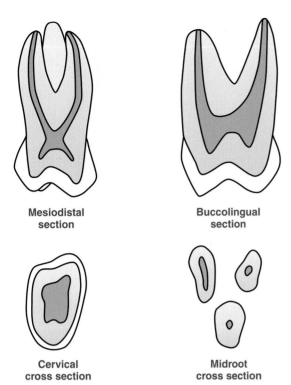

Mesiodistal section   **Buccolingual section**

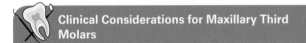

Cervical cross section   **Midroot cross section**

FIGURE 17-45 Pulp cavity of the permanent maxillary right second molar, with rhomboidal crown.

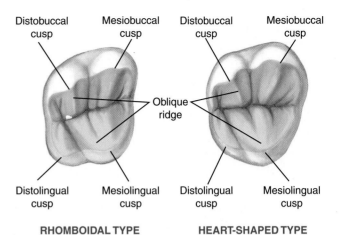

| Distobuccal cusp | Mesiobuccal cusp | Distobuccal cusp | Mesiobuccal cusp |

Oblique ridge

| Distolingual cusp | Mesiolingual cusp | Distolingual cusp | Mesiolingual cusp |

RHOMBOIDAL TYPE   **HEART-SHAPED TYPE**

FIGURE 17-46 Occlusal view of the two types of crowns of the permanent maxillary right second molars: rhomboidal and heart-shaped, with occlusal tables highlighted.

> ### Clinical Considerations for Maxillary Third Molars
>
> Permanent maxillary third molars may also fail to erupt and remain **impacted** within the alveolar bone. An impacted tooth is an unerupted or partially erupted tooth that is positioned against another tooth, bone, or even soft tissue in such a way that only partial eruption is likely, if at all. This impaction usually occurs because the maxilla is underdeveloped, and space or arch length is insufficient to accommodate these teeth because they are the last to erupt in the maxillary arch; thus, surgical removal may be necessary (see earlier discussion). Any homecare procedures or instrumentation may also be difficult when these teeth are erupted because of their extreme posterior arch position.

> ### Developmental Disturbances of Maxillary Third Molars
>
> Permanent maxillary third molars, along with the mandibular third molars, commonly exhibit partial **anodontia** (hypodontia) and thus are congenitally missing (see **Chapter 6**). With this disturbance, the appropriate individual **tooth germ** in the area is missing owing to failure of the **initiation stage** during tooth development. This situation usually has no harmful consequences, however.
>
> This tooth also commonly exhibits partial microdontia, which leads to a smaller molar crown with one cusp, or **peg molar,** either unilaterally or bilaterally, owing to failure in the **proliferation** process during tooth development (Figure 17-50, see Table 6-3, *C*). This tooth may also have **accessory roots** that complicate extraction procedures. Finally, developmental cyst formation may occur within the dental tissue of an **impacted** crown, resulting in a **dentigerous cyst** (see earlier discussion).

PERMANENT MANDIBULAR MOLARS
GENERAL FEATURES

Permanent mandibular molars erupt between 6 months to 1 year before the corresponding permanent maxillary molars (Table 17-3). The crown has four or five major cusps, of which there are always two lingual cusps of about the same width. All mandibular molars are wider mesiodistally than buccolingually, similar to anterior teeth. In comparison, maxillary molars are wider buccolingually, as are all posterior teeth. Thus, from an occlusal view, the outline of the crown is also rectangular, with four sides, or pentagonal, with five sides.

Quite distinct from maxillary molars, the buccal crown outline of all mandibular molars also shows a strong lingual inclination when viewed from the proximal, like the nearby premolars. Thus, from each proximal view, the crown outline is rhomboidal, or four-sided with opposite sides parallel, like all mandibular posterior teeth. The crown is thus inclined lingually on the root base, bringing the cusps into proper occlusion with their maxillary antagonists and distributing the forces along the long axis.

Mandibular molars are usually **bifurcated**, having two roots, a mesial root and distal root (see Figure 17-34). Both these roots show great to moderate distal root inclination. Because these teeth are bifurcated, the two **furcations** are located on the buccal and lingual surfaces midway between the proximal surfaces. These furcations are at a level of one fourth the root length from the CEJ. **Root concavities** are also found on the mesial surface of the mesial root and on furcal surfaces of both the mesial and distal roots. The root concavities on the mesial root are especially prominent, if this root also has two root canals.

PERMANENT MANDIBULAR FIRST MOLARS #19 AND #30

Specific Overall Features (Figure 17-51) The permanent mandibular first molars erupt between 6 to 7 years of age (root completion between ages 9 to 10). These teeth are usually the first permanent teeth to erupt in the oral cavity. They erupt distal to the primary mandibular second molars and thus are nonsuccedaneous.

The crown of a mandibular first molar usually has five cusps: three buccal and two lingual. Thus, these teeth are usually composed of five

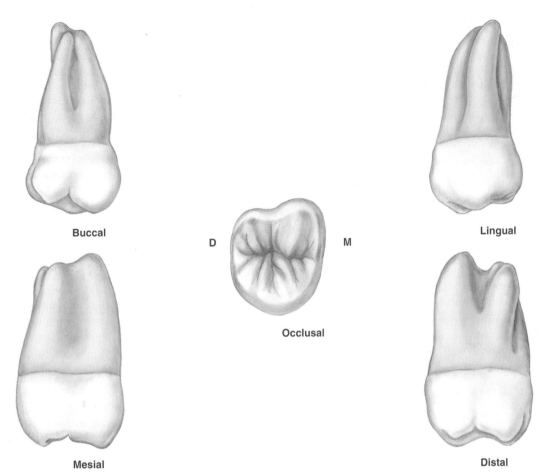

Buccal

D   **Occlusal**   M

Lingual

Mesial

Distal

FIGURE 17-47 Views of the permanent maxillary right third molars with heart-shaped occlusal outline.

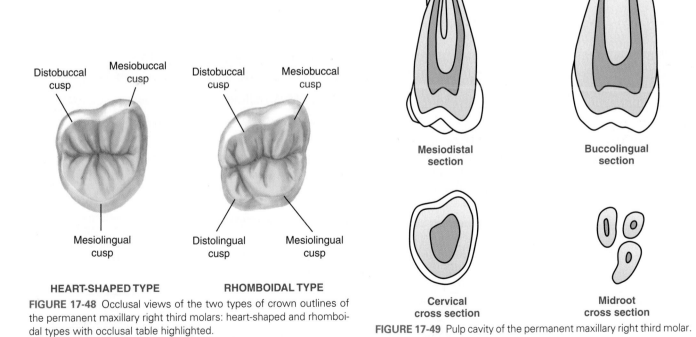

Distobuccal cusp   Mesiobuccal cusp

Distobuccal cusp   Mesiobuccal cusp

Mesiolingual cusp

Distolingual cusp   Mesiolingual cusp

HEART-SHAPED TYPE   **RHOMBOIDAL TYPE**

FIGURE 17-48 Occlusal views of the two types of crown outlines of the permanent maxillary right third molars: heart-shaped and rhomboidal types with occlusal table highlighted.

Mesiodistal section   **Buccolingual section**

Cervical cross section   **Midroot cross section**

FIGURE 17-49 Pulp cavity of the permanent maxillary right third molar.

developmental lobes, like the maxillary first molars but unlike the other mandibular molars, which have four. The lobes are named for their associated cusps. Evidence of lobe separation is also found in the developmental grooves on the occlusal surface. Occasionally, the distal cusp is missing and, more rarely, in large molars the distal cusp is joined by a sixth cusp.

Clinical Considerations for Mandibular Molars

All three types of mandibular molars can present difficulties in instrumentation because of their narrow lingual surfaces combined with the lingual inclination of the crown; therefore, instrument placement subgingivally can be difficult.

In addition, patients may have difficulty in performing homecare because of the lingual inclination of the crown. They may miss the associated interface with the lingual gingival tissue and clean only the occlusal surface with a toothbrush. The proximity of the tongue also makes homecare and instrumentation more difficult on the lingual surface.

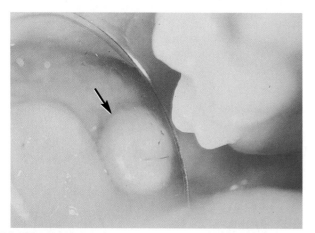

FIGURE 17-50 Peg third molar of the permanent maxillary arch (*arrow*).

The two roots, mesial and distal, of a mandibular first molar are larger and more divergent than the second, leaving the roots widely separated buccally. The root trunk of the first is also shorter than that of the second. Both roots are usually the same length, but if one is longer, it is the mesial root. The mesial root is also the wider and stronger of the two. If this molar has three roots, it is because the mesial root has both buccal and lingual branches.

Fluting, an elongated developmental depression, is noted on many surfaces of the root branches, especially on the mesial surface of the mesial root, but none is observed on the distal surface of the distal root. Furcations are well removed from the CEJ but the entrance diameter is small at only around 1 mm or less, making access to instrumentation limited. The buccal furcation entrance diameter is even smaller than that of the lingual furcation and is 3 mm from the CEJ; the lingual furcation is 4 mm from the CEJ.

The pulp cavity of a mandibular first molar is more likely to have three root canals: distal, mesiobuccal, and mesiolingual, and five pulp horns (Figure 17-52). The distal pulp canal is much larger than the other two canals and is usually the only canal in the distal root. The mesial root usually has two pulp canals: mesiobuccal and mesiolingual. Rarely, these two mesial canals join into one single apical foramen, or only one pulp canal is found in the mesial root. Again, rarely, two canals are present in the distal root, just as with the mesial root.

Buccal View Features The crown of a mandibular first molar is larger mesiodistally than occlusocervically (see Figure 17-51). It is the widest tooth mesiodistally of any permanent tooth because it has a fifth major cusp. From this view, at least some part of all five cusps is visible.

The mesiobuccal cusp is the largest, widest, and highest cusp on the buccal part. The distobuccal cusp is slightly smaller, shorter, and sharper than the mesiobuccal cusp. The distal cusp, despite its name, is considered a buccal cusp; it is the lowest cusp and slightly sharper than the other two. The occlusal outline is divided into three sections by the two grooves, as they pass into the buccal surface: the mesiobuccal and distobuccal grooves. These sections of the crown surface decrease in size distally. The mesiobuccal groove on a first mandibular molar is important in classifying the permanent dentition using

TABLE 17-3	Anatomical Information on Mandibular Molars		
	MANDIBULAR FIRST MOLAR	**MANDIBULAR SECOND MOLAR**	**MANDIBULAR THIRD MOLAR**
Universal number	#19 and #30	#18 and #31	#17 and #32
General crown features	Occlusal table with marginal ridges, cusps with tips, inclined planes, ridges, grooves, fossae, and pits		
Specific crown features	First permanent tooth to erupt, with widest crown mesiodistally of dentition; five cusps, with Y-shaped groove pattern and with buccal groove possibly ending in buccal pit	Smaller crown than first; four cusps with cross-shaped groove pattern	Smaller crown than second
Mesial and distal contact	Junction of occlusal and middle thirds	Middle third	Mesial: middle third distal: none
Distinguishing right from left	Distal cusp smallest, with a sharp cusp	Difference in height of contour for buccal and lingual from each proximal surface; wider on the mesial than distal	Wider buccolingually on mesial than on distal
General root features	Bifurcated roots, with root trunks, furcation, and root concavities		Fused root, irregularly curved, with sharp apices
Specific root features	Divergent roots, with furcations well removed from the CEJ	Less divergent roots, with furcations closer to CEJ	

CEJ, Cementoenamel junction.

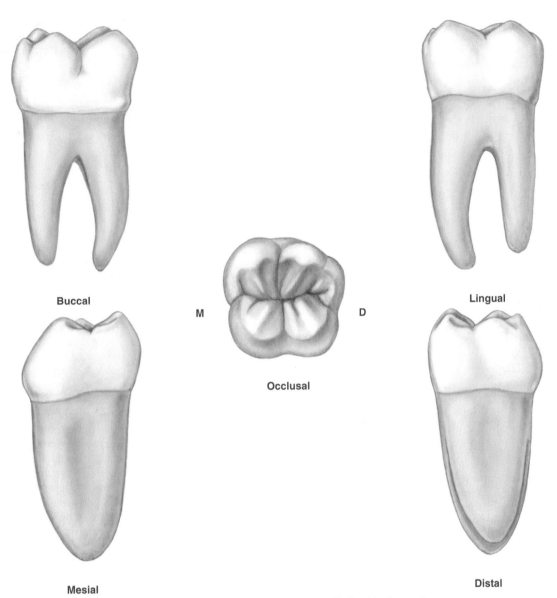

Buccal

M   D

Occlusal

Lingual

Mesial

Distal

FIGURE 17-51 Views of the permanent mandibular right first molar.

Angle's classification of malocclusion in relation to the maxillary arch (see Table 20-1).

The mesiobuccal groove extends straight cervically to a point about midway occlusocervically, but slightly mesial to the center mesiodistally, and usually ends in the buccal pit. Additionally, it may end in two short, slanting grooves or may fade out after a short distance. The distobuccal groove extends cervically, similarly to the mesiobuccal groove, but is slightly distal to the center mesiodistally, and usually ends in a distobuccal pit but sometimes just fades out.

A buccal cervical ridge, which has a mesiodistally-oriented roundness in the cervical third of the buccal surface, is apparent. It is usually more prominent in its mesial part. In addition, a shallow concavity may extend mesiodistally in the middle third.

The mesial outline on a mandibular first molar is slightly concave from the contact area cervically and is rounded occlusal to the contact. The distal outline is more rounded than the mesial. Both the mesial contact and distal contact are at the junction of the occlusal and middle thirds.

Lingual View Features The lingual surface of a mandibular first molar is smaller than the buccal surface. The mesial and distal outlines of the lingual are similar to the buccal. The occlusal outline is divided by the lingual groove between the mesiolingual cusp and the distolingual cusp.

Proximal View Features The crown of a mandibular first molar is smaller buccolingually than mesiodistally and cervico-occlusally. The crown is also inclined toward the lingual, as are the other mandibular posterior teeth. Additionally, the crown outline is rhomboidal, 4-sided with opposite sides parallel, because the surface is wider at the cervical than the occlusal.

The buccal margin on the mesial surface is usually rounded, especially at the buccal cervical ridge. The buccal cervical ridge is in the cervical third, where the height of contour is also located. The lingual margin on the mesial is either straight or slightly rounded from the CEJ to the height of contour in the middle third. It is then rounded from the height of contour to the occlusal. The CEJ is either straight or slightly curved occlusally, but always is located at a more occlusal level on the lingual part of the mesial surface.

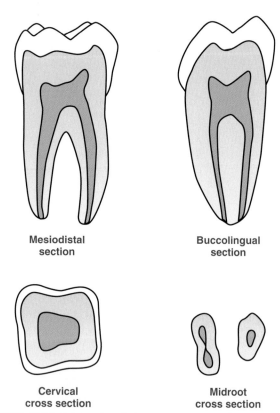

FIGURE 17-52 Pulp cavity of the permanent mandibular right first molar.

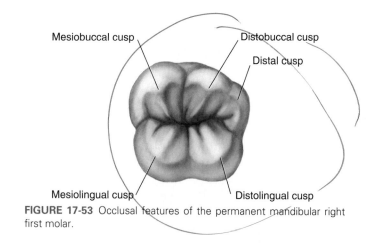

FIGURE 17-53 Occlusal features of the permanent mandibular right first molar.

The mesial marginal groove notches the mesial marginal ridge on a mandibular first molar. It has a flattened or slightly concave area centrally located in the gingival third, comparable to the mesial concavity of a maxillary first premolar.

The distal surface is similar to the mesial but smaller, especially in the buccolingual dimension. The distal marginal ridge is notched by the distal marginal groove and is located more cervically than the mesial marginal ridge.

Occlusal View Features The crown outline of the mandibular first molar is roughly pentagonal, with the fifth side created by the distal cusp. The distal part of the buccal outline converges toward the distal to create the fifth side of the outline. The buccal outline has rounded line angles, which is divided into three parts by the two buccal grooves, the mesiobuccal groove and the distobuccal groove. The length of each of the buccal cusps decreases distally, as noted from the buccal view.

The lingual outline is divided into two parts by the lingual groove. The mesial outline is divided into two parts by the mesial marginal groove. The distal outline, the shortest of the five sides, is divided by the distal marginal groove.

Occlusal Table Components The mandibular first molar usually has five functional cusps (listed from largest to smallest): mesiobuccal, mesiolingual, distolingual, distobuccal, and distal (Figure 17-53). The cusps from highest to lowest: mesiolingual, distolingual, mesiobuccal, distobuccal, and distal cusp. Each cusp has four cusp ridges, a triangular ridge, and four inclined cuspal planes.

The mesiobuccal cusp is the bulkiest cusp, although it has a blunt tip. Except for the distal cusp, the distobuccal cusp is the smallest of the cusps and has a rounded tip. The mesiolingual cusp is second in size to the mesiobuccal cusp and has the sharpest tip. The distolingual cusp is also quite sharp but is slightly smaller than the

Clinical Considerations with Mandibular First Molars

Because of their arch position, and because the permanent mandibular first molars are the first permanent teeth to erupt in the mandibular arch, they are considered important in regard to the development of occlusion (see Table 20-1).

The importance of the role of this tooth in **occlusion** is shown when the tooth is lost (Figure 17-55). This loss might more easily occur because this tooth is the first permanent tooth to erupt into the oral cavity. It has a greater chance of being affected by caries because child patients are just beginning to master homecare and diet restrictions. In addition, early dental restorative intervention of the caries may be neglected.

With the loss of the tooth, the mandibular second molar, and possibly the third molar, incline and drift mesially into the newly opened arch space, allowing the maxillary first molar to supererupt into the space. Occlusion and then mastication are disabled, and the risk of further caries, and possibly periodontal disease around the irregularly spaced teeth, is greatly increased. Interceptive orthodontic therapy is important to prevent these situations after tooth loss.

Buccal pits that may occur on the buccal surface of mandibular first molars are at increased risk of caries, because of both increased dental biofilm retention and the thinness of enamel forming the walls of the pit (Figure 17-56, see **Chapter 12**). An enamel sealant should be placed on each buccal surface as the tooth begins to erupt. Sealants on the buccal surface do not bond as easily as on the occlusal surface, however, because of the histology of the area. If caries does occur, tooth-colored restorative materials can be used to achieve a more esthetic appearance, and thus the presence of the buccal pit may not now be easy to discern clinically.

---

mesiolingual cusp. The distal cusp is the smallest and has a sharp cusp, which *helps to distinguish the right mandibular first molar from the left.*

The mandibular first molar has the most complex developmental groove pattern of all the permanent mandibular molars (Figure 17-54). The Y-shaped groove pattern is formed on the occlusal table around the cusps by the mesiobuccal groove, distobuccal groove, and lingual groove. Two marginal ridges border the occlusal table, the mesial marginal ridge and the distal marginal ridge. No transverse ridges are found on the occlusal, unlike a maxillary first molar and a mandibular second molar.

The occlusal table also has three fossae: large central fossa, smaller mesial triangular fossa, and distal triangular fossa. Three pits are

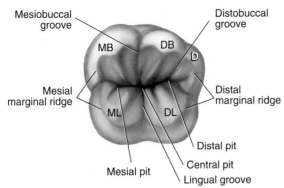

FIGURE 17-54 Additional occlusal features of the permanent mandibular right first molar, with occlusal table highlighted.

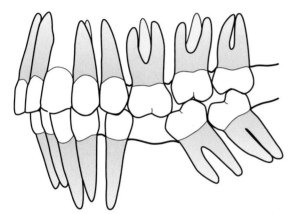

FIGURE 17-55 Changes that can occur in the permanent dentition with the loss of the mandibular first molar. Teeth become inclined, and there is mesial drift of the mandibular second molar and possibly third molar, with supereruption of the maxillary first molar into the opposing open space.

associated with the fossae: mesial pit, central pit, and distal pit. The central pit is the also the deepest pit and divides the central groove into two grooves, the mesial groove and distal groove.

The central pit is the junction of three grooves: mesiobuccal, distobuccal, and lingual. The mesial pit is the junction of four grooves: mesial, mesiobuccal triangular, mesiolingual triangular, and mesial marginal. The distal pit is the junction of three grooves: the distal, the distolingual, and distal marginal.

PERMANENT MANDIBULAR SECOND MOLARS #18 AND #31

Specific Overall Features (Figure 17-57) The permanent mandibular second molars erupt between 11 to 12 years of age (root completion between ages 14 to 15). These teeth erupt distal to the permanent mandibular first molars and thus are nonsuccedaneous.

The crown measurements of a mandibular second molar are generally smaller when compared to a first molar. The four cusps of a second are nearly equal in size compared with the five cusps of differing sizes of a first molar. Like the mandibular third molars, the mandibular second molars are usually composed of four developmental lobes, unlike the mandibular first molars, which have five lobes. The lobes are named for the associated cusps, and the developmental grooves on the occlusal surface show lobe division.

The two roots of a second molar are smaller, shorter, and less divergent in placement than those of a first molar. The lack of separation

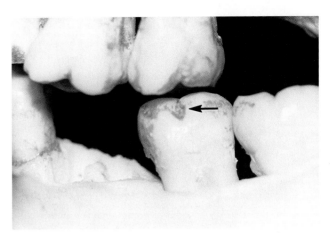

FIGURE 17-56 Example on a skull of a buccal pit (*arrow*) on the permanent mandibular first molar.

making detection and deposit removal difficult if exposed. The root trunk of a second is also longer than that of a first. The mesial root of the second is not as broad as that of a first, but the furcation is farther from the CEJ. All root depressions are shallower. Overall, root variability is greater than in the first molar.

The pulp cavity of a mandibular second molar can have two pulp canals (one for each root). However, it is more likely to have three pulp canals, similar to a mandibular first molar: distal, mesiobuccal, and mesiolingual canals (the latter two being together in the mesial root) (Figure 17-58). The tooth usually has only four pulp horns, which correspond to the four cusps.

Buccal View Features The buccal groove divides the same-size mesiobuccal cusp and distobuccal cusp of a mandibular second molar (see Figure 17-57). The mesial contact is at the junction of the occlusal and middle third. The distal contact is slightly cervical, but still at the junction of the occlusal and middle third.

Lingual View Features The mesiolingual cusp and distolingual cusp have the same size and shape as the buccal cusps, although they have sharper cusp tips. Because the crown converges lingually, a part of the mesial and distal surfaces can be seen from this view.

Proximal View Features The buccal height of contour is in the cervical third, and the lingual height of contour is in the middle third for the mandibular second molar. The crown also tapers distally when viewed from the mesial aspect. That is because the molar is also wider buccolingually on the mesial surface than on the distal. Both these mesial surface features *help to distinguish the right mandibular second molar from the left*. The buccal cervical ridge is less pronounced on the second molar than on the first or the proximal.

The CEJ curvature on both proximal surfaces of a second is less pronounced than that of a first. Neither the mesial, nor distal marginal ridge is divided by a marginal groove.

Occlusal View Features The outline of the crown of a mandibular second molar is rectangular (Figure 17-59). The tooth has four cusps, two buccal and two lingual cusps: mesiobuccal, distobuccal, mesiolingual, and distolingual. With this view, the occlusal surface of a second is considerably different from that of a first because there is no distal cusp, and all cusps are of equal size.

Occlusal Table Components A cross-shaped groove pattern is formed where the well-defined central groove is crossed by the buccal groove and lingual groove, dividing the occlusal table into four parts that are nearly equal. There are three occlusal pits present: central, mesial, and distal. Cusp slopes on a second are less smooth than on a first because second molars have an increased number of supplemental grooves.

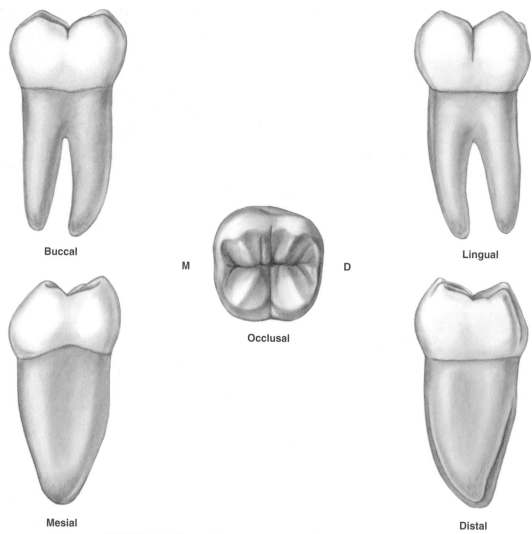

Buccal

M

Occlusal

D

Lingual

Mesial

Distal

FIGURE 17-57 Views of the permanent mandibular right second molar.

Unlike a mandibular first molar, this tooth has two transverse ridges. The triangular ridges of the mesiobuccal and mesiolingual cusps meet to form a transverse ridge, as do the distobuccal and distolingual cusps.

PERMANENT MANDIBULAR THIRD MOLARS #17 AND #32

Specific Overall Features (Figure 17-60) The mandibular third molars may erupt between 17 to 21 years of age (root completion between ages 18 to 25). If they erupt (see later discussion), they erupt distal to the permanent mandibular second molars.

Similar to maxillary thirds, the mandibular thirds are variable in shape, having no standard form. Thus, a typical mandibular third molar is difficult to describe. This molar usually is smaller in all dimensions than the second molar, and it sometimes is the same size as the first molar.

Like the mandibular second molars, the mandibular third molars are usually composed of four developmental lobes, unlike the mandibular first molars, which have five lobes. The lobes are named for

the associated cusps, and the developmental grooves on the occlusal surface show lobe division.

The crown of a mandibular third molar tapers distally when viewed from the mesial aspect. That is because the molar is also wider buccolingually on the mesial surface than on the distal surface, which *helps to distinguish the right mandibular third molar from the left,* like all mandibular molars. The crown is usually smaller in all dimensions than that of a second molar.

The occlusal outline of the crown is more oval than rectangular, although the crown usually resembles that of a second molar. The two mesial cusps are larger than the two distal cusps. The occlusal surface appears quite wrinkled, with an irregular groove pattern, numerous supplemental grooves, and occlusal pits; if an excess of these features exists, the occlusal surface is described as *crenulated.*

A mandibular third molar usually has two roots that are fused, irregularly curved, and shorter than a mandibular second molar. Additionally, the roots are usually smaller in proportion to the crown and have sharp apices. The pulp cavity is usually similar to that of the second molars, with four pulp horns and two or three pulp canals (Figure 17-61).

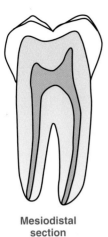
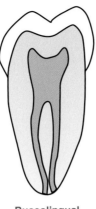

Mesiodistal
section

Buccolingual
section

Cervical
cross section

Midroot
cross section

FIGURE 17-58 Pulp cavity of the permanent mandibular right second molar.

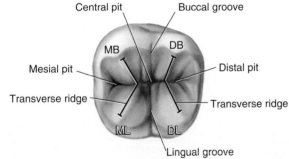

Central pit   Buccal groove

MB   DB

Mesial pit   Distal pit

Transverse ridge

Transverse ridge

ML   DL

Lingual groove

FIGURE 17-59 Occlusal features of the permanent mandibular right second molar, with occlusal table highlighted.

Developmental Disturbances of Mandibular Third Molars

Permanent mandibular third molars, along with the maxillary third molars, are permanent teeth commonly involved in partial **anodontia** (hypodontia), being congenitally missing either unilaterally or bilaterally (see **Chapter 6**). With this disturbance, the appropriate individual **tooth germ** in the area is missing because of a failure in the **initiation stage** during tooth development. However, anodontia of this tooth or teeth usually has no harmful consequences.

These teeth may also have **accessory roots**, which complicate extraction procedures. Finally, developmental cyst formation may occur within the dental tissue of an impacted crown, resulting in a **dentigerous cyst** (see earlier discussion, Figure 6-30).

Clinical Considerations for Mandibular Third Molars

Permanent mandibular third molars may also fail to erupt and remain **impacted** within the surrounding alveolar bone (Figure 17-62), which occurs more frequently than with the maxillary counterparts. An impacted tooth is an unerupted or partially erupted tooth that is positioned against another tooth, bone, or even soft tissue, making complete eruption unlikely, and surgical removal may be necessary (see earlier discussion). This impaction usually occurs because the mandible is underdeveloped, and space or arch length is insufficient to accommodate these teeth, which are the last to erupt in the mandibular arch. They may also be partially erupted, causing the surrounding gingival tissue (which may even cover the occlusal surface) to have an increased risk of periodontal infections (pericoronitis) from poor homecare of the area. Due its arch position, this infection can become serious (Ludwig's angina) and impact breathing.

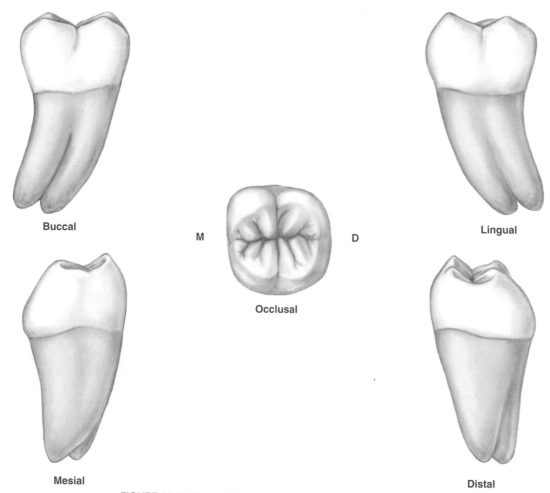

Buccal

M   D

Lingual

Occlusal

Mesial

Distal

FIGURE 17-60 Views of the permanent mandibular right third molar.

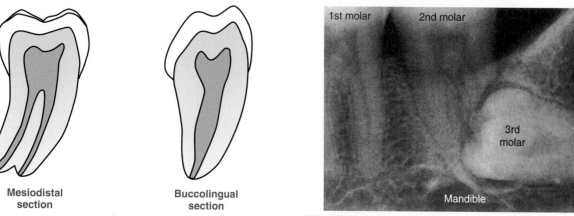

Mesiodistal
section

Buccolingual
section

1st molar   2nd molar

3rd
molar

Mandible

FIGURE 17-62 Radiograph of an impacted permanent mandibular third molar.

Cervical
cross section

Midroot
cross section

FIGURE 17-61 Pulp cavity of the permanent mandibular right third molar.

Primary Dentition

●●●LEARNING OBJECTIVES

- Use the correct name and universal designation letter for each primary tooth when examining a diagram and a patient.
- Demonstrate the correct location of each primary tooth on a diagram and a patient.
- Define and pronounce the key terms when discussing the primary teeth.
- Describe the general features of primary teeth and of each primary tooth type.

- Describe the specific features of each primary tooth.
- Discuss the important clinical considerations and developmental disturbances based on the anatomy of the primary teeth.
- Integrate the knowledge of dental anatomy of the primary teeth into the dental treatment of patients in order to maintain them.

●●●NEW KEY TERMS

Early childhood caries
Primate spaces

PRIMARY TEETH

The first set of teeth is the **primary dentition** (Figure 18-1). The primary dentition is exfoliated, or shed, and replaced by the **permanent dentition**. There are 20 total primary teeth when the primary dentition period is completed, 10 per **dental arch**. These include the tooth types of **incisors, canines**, and **molars** (see Figure 15-1). These are designated in the **Universal Tooth Designation System** by the capital letters *A* through *T*. There are no premolars in the primary dentition as there are in the permanent dentition.

Mineralization of the primary teeth begins in utero at 13 to 16 weeks. By 18 to 20 weeks during **prenatal development**, all the primary teeth have started to mineralize. There are usually no primary teeth visible in the oral cavity at birth. The first eruption of a primary tooth, a primary mandibular central incisor, occurs at an average age of 6 to 10 months, with the further eruption of the rest of the primary dentition following (Table 18-1).

The primary dentition takes between 2 to 3 years to be completed, beginning with the initial mineralization of the primary mandibular central incisors, and later being completed with root formation in the primary maxillary second molar (see Figure 6-22, *A*). A 6-month delay, or acceleration, is considered normal for an individual child. If a child patient is unusually early or late in getting their teeth, it is important to inquire about the family's dental history concerning this issue.

The actual dates are not as important as the eruption sequence because, even though there can be a great deal of variation in the actual dates of eruption noted in various texts. However, the sequence tends to be uniform (see Figure 20-5). In addition, the specific tooth types tend to erupt in pairs so that if there is any asymmetry noted within the primary dentition, a radiograph of the area may be required. Young girls tend to both shed their primary teeth and have their permanent teeth slightly earlier than young boys, possibly reflecting the earlier overall physical maturation achieved.

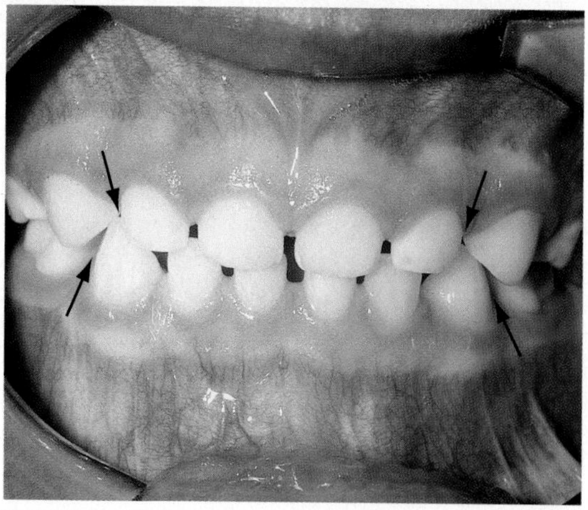

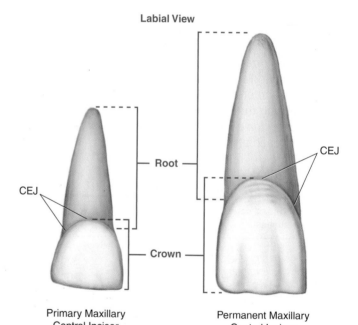

FIGURE 18-1 Labial view of the primary dentition with the possible primate spaces of the primary dentition indicated *(arrows)*. Note the attrition of the masticatory surfaces, which may normally be present, and a tendency for an end-to-end bite. *(From Bird DL, Robinson DS: Modern Dental Assisting, ed 9, WB Saunders, Philadelphia, 2008.)*

Also, certain **interproximal spaces** between the primary teeth are considered normal in most child patients, because space is necessary for the proper alignment of the future permanent dentition. These spaces still may concern the supervising adults, and they may need reassurance. These spaces are considered primate spaces, mainly involving spaces between the primary maxillary lateral incisor and canine, and also between the primary mandibular canine and first molar (see Figure 18-1, Chapter 20).

COMPARISON OF PRIMARY TO PERMANENT TEETH

Primary teeth are smaller overall than permanent teeth. However, the primary teeth should not be considered just *mini-me* permanent teeth, because there are important differences that occur in the structure of primary teeth compared with that of permanent teeth (Figures 18-2 to 18-4).

The **crown** of any primary tooth is short in relation to its total length. The crowns are also more constricted, or narrower, at the **cemento-enamel junction (CEJ)**, making them appear bulbous in comparison to the thinness of the tooth neck. A prominent **cervical ridge** is present on both the labial and lingual surfaces of **anterior teeth** and on buccal surfaces of the molars, even more so than any similar structure on the even larger permanent molars (see Figure 18-4).

Roots of primary teeth are also narrower and longer than the crown length (see Figures 18-2 to 18-4). Each crown to root ratio of primary teeth are smaller than those ratios of their permanent dentition counterparts. Roots may also show partial resorption as the teeth begin to be shed, which can be noted radiographically (see Figure 6-27, *A*).

The **pulp cavity** on primary teeth shows that **pulp chambers** and **pulp horns** are relatively large in proportion to those of the permanent teeth, especially the mesial pulp horns of the molars (Figure 18-5). Overall, the dentin of the primary dentition is thinner than that of the permanent counterparts. However, the dentin thickness between the pulp chambers and the enamel is increased, especially in the primary mandibular second molar. The enamel is also relatively thin in comparison to permanent counterparts, but has consistent thickness overlying the dentin of the crown. However, primary teeth also have whiter enamel on their crowns than the permanent teeth, because of

TABLE 18-1	Approximate Eruption and Shedding Ages for Primary Teeth	
MAXILLARY TEETH	**ERUPTION, MEAN (RANGE)**	**SHEDDING, RANGE**
Central incisor	10 (8-12 months)	6-7 years
Lateral incisor	11 (9-13 months)	7-8 years
Canine	19 (16-22 months)	10-12 years
First molar	16 (13-19 months, males and 14-19 months, females)	9-11 years
Second molar	29 (25-33 months)	10-12 years
MANDIBULAR TEETH	**ERUPTION**	**SHEDDING**
Central incisor	8 (6-10 months)	6-7 years
Lateral incisor	13 (10-16 months)	7-8 years
Canine	20 (17-23 months)	9-12 years
First molar	16 (14-18 months)	9-11 years
Second molar	27 (23-31 months, males and 24-30 months, females)	10-12 years

Adapted from Nelson S: *Wheeler's Dental Anatomy, Physiology and Occlusion*, ed 9, WB Saunders, Philadelphia, 2009.

Labial View

FIGURE 18-2 Differences between the crowns of the primary and permanent teeth. Note, especially, the different crown/root ratios, as well as the differences at the cementoenamel junction (CEJ).

the increased opacity of the enamel, which covers the underlying yellow dentin.

PRIMARY INCISORS
GENERAL FEATURES

Each dental arch has four primary **incisors**. As in the permanent dentition, each quadrant has two incisor types: **central incisor** and **lateral incisor**. Both primary incisors resemble their permanent successor,

Clinical Considerations for the Primary Dentition

Child patients and supervising adults sometimes discount the importance of the teeth of the primary dentition, because they believe they are temporary and soon replaced. It is true that a 70-year-old person will have spent 91% of his or her time chewing on permanent teeth but only 6% with the primary dentition. Thus, the primary dentition generally functions in esthetics, mastication, and speech for a child for only 5 to 12 years. However, these teeth also serve the important function of holding open the eruption space for the succedaneous permanent teeth, which will replace the primary teeth. Individually, each primary tooth also functions in the same way as its permanent counterpart, when present.

In the past, many carious primary teeth were extracted instead of repaired, resulting in crowding and potential occlusal complications in the permanent dentition (see **Chapter 20**). Worse still, many carious primary teeth were ignored, resulting in serious oral infections and discomfort for the child patient.

The value of primary teeth is now more realistically appreciated, and more are saved from caries because of early dental care. Still, the value of these teeth must be imparted to child patients and supervising adults. Supervision of oral hygiene must begin early, as soon as the first primary teeth erupt into the oral cavity, to prevent premature loss of the primary teeth. Because the enamel and dentin are thinner, the risk of endodontic complications is greater for the primary dentition. In addition, because the **pulp chamber** and **pulp horns** are also larger, there is increased risk of pulpal exposure during cavity preparation. Bulging of the **cervical ridge** of primary teeth must also be taken into account when these teeth are involved in any restorative procedure.

These factors can be coupled with the increased possibility of poor homecare in the child patient, especially if lacking direction by supervising adults. Prolonged nighttime use of a baby bottle with a cavity-causing beverage or sugar on a pacifier must also be considered as an etiological factor in a child patient with extensive acute caries of the primary teeth.

This is diagnosed as **early childhood caries (ECC)**, which is more commonly called *baby bottle tooth decay* (Figure 18-6).

A child's first dental appointment should occur within 6 months of the eruption of the first primary tooth and no later than 12 months of age. The intent of this recommendation is to provide information to the child's supervising adults, which will help to establish positive preventive behaviors, prevent serious dental problems, and allay concerns. This early initial visit affords the dental professional the opportunity to provide basic, timely information, and to do this in 6-month increments.

Early dental care is important not only for keeping the primary dentition healthy but also for assessing for any appropriate, needed interceptive orthodontic therapy. This may include the use of space maintainers, retainers, and removal of any extraneous bulbous proximal crown width. Also, removal of retained primary teeth (or retained roots), as needed, may allow the correct eruption sequence and alignment of the permanent teeth later (see Figure 20-4).

Extraction procedures of primary teeth should always be performed with caution and with radiographic confirmation of a permanent replacement, especially with primary molars. If the permanent teeth are missing (**anodontia**), which can occur with second premolars, the extraction of the primary tooth (primary molar) must be avoided because retention is preferred and may cover many years of use (see Table 6-3, *A*). Extensive extrinsic staining of the primary teeth may be attributed to **Nasmyth's membrane** (see Figure 6-29).

In addition, if severe periodontal inflammation and destruction in the primary and/or mixed dentition are found with evidence of little dental biofilm, either locally or generally, early aggressive periodontitis must be suspected (considered *juvenile periodontitis* in the past). Early intervention with this severe yet uncommon periodontal disease can prevent further periodontal destruction. Thus, a periodontal probe should always be present on the dental tray with child patients.

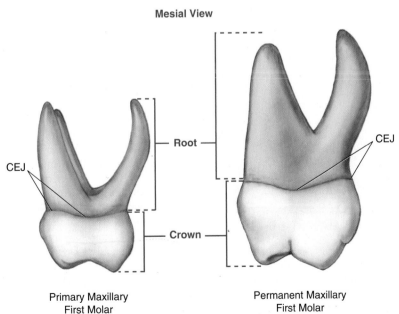

Mesial View

CEJ · Root · Crown · CEJ

Primary Maxillary
First Molar

Permanent Maxillary
First Molar

FIGURE 18-3 Differences between the crowns and roots of the primary and permanent teeth, especially the differences at the cementoenamel junction (CEJ).

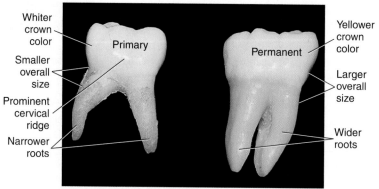

FIGURE 18-4 Extracted teeth showing the differences between the primary and permanent teeth.

Mesiodistal Section

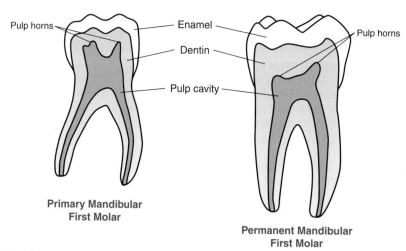

FIGURE 18-5 Differences between the relatively large pulp chambers and pulp horns of the primary teeth and those of permanent teeth, which are relatively smaller.

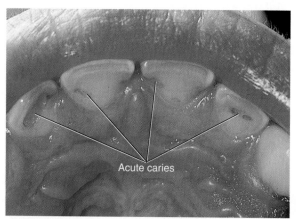

FIGURE 18-6 Acute caries on the primary maxillary anterior teeth caused by *baby bottle tooth decay* or early childhood caries.

with some exceptions such as a more prominent **cervical ridge** present on both the labial and lingual surfaces. Also, both have the same arch position, function, and general shape as the permanent counterpart, and they function as such for about 5 years.

Dental professionals sometimes note extensive wear or **attrition** of the **incisal edges** of the primary incisors from **bruxism** (grinding),

and the possible formation of an end-to-end bite between the arches. The significance of this finding and its possible relevance to later adult **parafunctional habits** are unknown (see Figures 18-1, 20-22).

PRIMARY MAXILLARY CENTRAL INCISOR *E* AND *F*

Specific Features (Figure 18-7) From the labial aspect, the crown of the primary maxillary central incisor appears wider mesiodistally than incisocervically, the opposite of its permanent successor. In fact, it is the only anterior tooth of either dentition with this crown dimension. Additionally, its mesial and distal outlines are more rounded than the permanent central incisor as a result of the cervical constriction. The incisal outline is relatively straight from this view, but it slopes toward the distal with attrition.

Unlike their permanent successors, the primary maxillary central incisors have no mamelons, leaving the labial surface smooth. In addition, these teeth rarely have developmental depressions or imbrication lines, and no pits are evident on the lingual surface. However, the cingulum and marginal ridges on the lingual surface all are more prominent than on the permanent successor, and the lingual fossa is deeper.

Both proximal surfaces of the maxillary central incisor appear similar. Because of the short crown and its wide labiolingual

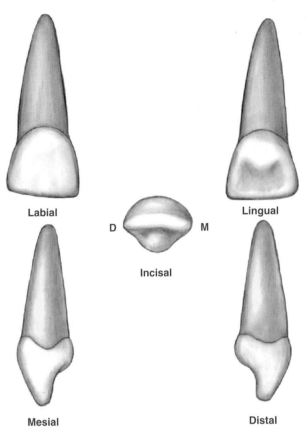

FIGURE 18-7 Views of the primary maxillary right central incisor.

measurement, the crown appears thick, even at the incisal third. The CEJ curves distinctly toward the incisal but not as much as on its permanent successor. This curvature is less distal than mesial, as in the permanent successor. From the incisal surface, the crown appears wider mesiodistally than labiolingually, and the incisal edge appears nearly straight. The single root is generally round and tapers evenly to the apex, but it is longer, relative to crown length, than the permanent central incisor.

PRIMARY MAXILLARY LATERAL INCISOR *D* AND *G*

Specific Features (Figure 18-8) The crown of the primary maxillary lateral incisor is similar to the central incisor but is much smaller than the central in all dimensions. The lateral is also longer incisocervically than mesiodistally, exactly the opposite of the central. The incisal angles are also more rounded than the central. The root is also similar to that of the central, but the lateral's root is longer in proportion to its crown compared with the same proportions of the central, and its apex is sharper.

PRIMARY MANDIBULAR CENTRAL INCISOR *O* AND *P*

Specific Features (Figure 18-9) The crown of the primary mandibular central incisor looks more like the primary mandibular lateral incisor than its permanent successor or any other primary maxillary incisor. This tooth is also quite symmetrical, however, similar to its permanent successor. It is also not as constricted at the CEJ as the primary maxillary central incisor. From the labial aspect, the crown appears wide compared with its permanent successor.

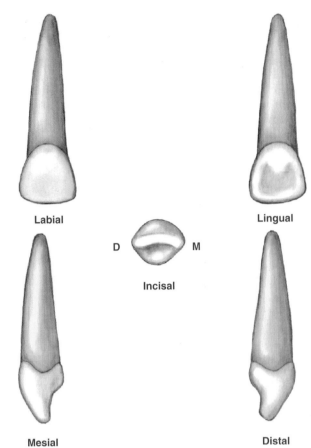

FIGURE 18-8 Views of the primary maxillary right lateral incisor.

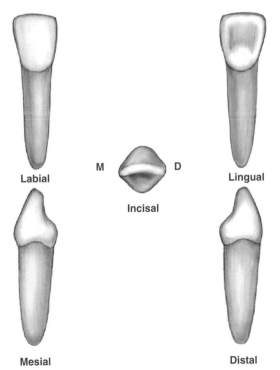

FIGURE 18-9 Views of the primary mandibular right central incisor.

Its mesial and distal outlines from the labial aspect also show that the crown tapers evenly from the contact areas.

The lingual surface of the primary mandibular central incisor appears smooth and tapers toward the prominent cingulum. The marginal ridges are less pronounced than those of the primary maxillary incisor are; however, the lingual fossa is also shallow. Again, the CEJ curvature on the mesial side is greater than on the distal. From the mesial aspect, this tooth is much wider labiolingually than its permanent successor.

The incisal edge is centered over the root from the proximal and incisal views and divides the labial and lingual into equal halves.

The root is single, long, and slender. The labial and lingual surfaces of the root are rounded, but the proximal surfaces are slightly flattened.

PRIMARY MANDIBULAR LATERAL INCISOR Q AND N

Specific Features (Figure 18-10) The crown of the primary mandibular lateral incisor is similar in form to the central incisor of the same arch, but the crown is wider and longer than that of the central. The cingulum is also more developed, and the lingual fossa is slightly deeper than that of the central incisor.

The incisal edge slopes distally, and its distoincisal angle is more rounded, as is the distal margin. From the incisal aspect, the crown is not as symmetrical as is the central, because the cingulum is offset toward the distal, which is the same cingulum position as its permanent successor. The root may have a distal curvature in its apical third, and it usually has a distal longitudinal groove.

PRIMARY CANINES
GENERAL FEATURES

There are four primary **canines**, two in each dental arch. These primary canines mainly resemble the outline of their permanent successors, with some exceptions, such as a more prominent **cervical ridge** present on both the labial and lingual surfaces.

PRIMARY MAXILLARY CANINE C AND H

Specific Features (Figure 18-11) The crown of the primary maxillary canine has a relatively longer and sharper cusp than that of its permanent successor, when first erupted. The mesial and distal outlines of the primary maxillary canine are rounder, however, and greatly overhang the cervical line. The mesial cusp slope is longer than the distal cusp slope on this tooth, just the opposite of the primary mandibular canine and, also, the opposite of the permanent counterpart.

On the lingual surface, the cingulum is well developed, as are the lingual ridge and marginal ridges. The lingual ridge extends from the cingulum to the cusp tip and divides the lingual surface into a shallow mesiolingual fossa and distolingual fossa. A **tubercle** is often present on the **cingulum**, extending from the cusp tip to the cingulum.

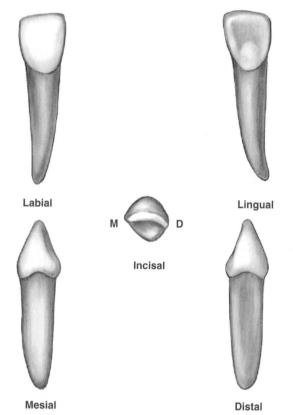

Labial

Lingual

M D

Incisal

Mesial

Distal

FIGURE 18-10 Views of the primary mandibular right lateral incisor.

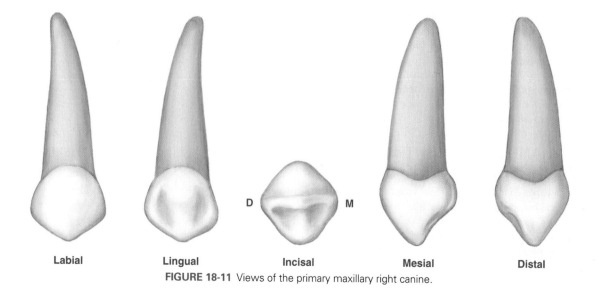

Labial   Lingual   Incisal   Mesial   Distal

D   M

FIGURE 18-11 Views of the primary maxillary right canine.

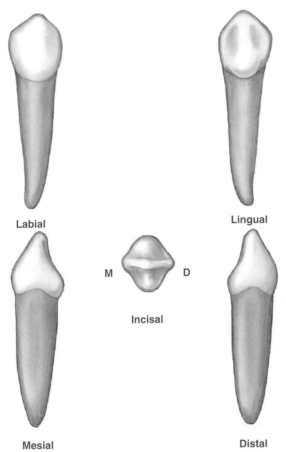

Labial

Lingual

M D

Incisal

Mesial

Distal

FIGURE 18-12 Views of the primary mandibular right canine.

From the incisal aspect, the crown is diamond-shaped and the cusp tip is slightly offset to the distal. The root is twice as long as the crown and more slender than that of its permanent successor, and it is inclined distally.

PRIMARY MANDIBULAR CANINE M AND R

Specific Features (Figure 18-12) The crown of the primary mandibular canine resembles that of the primary maxillary canine, although some dimensions are different. This tooth is much smaller labiolingually. The distal cusp slope is much longer than the mesial cusp slope, as is the case on its permanent counterpart.

The lingual surface is smoother than the primary maxillary canine and is marked by a shallow lingual fossa. The incisal edge of the primary mandibular canine is straight and is centered over the crown labiolingually. The root is long, narrow, and almost twice the length of the crown, although shorter and more tapered than that of a primary maxillary canine.

PRIMARY MOLARS
GENERAL FEATURES

There are eight primary molars, with two types, a **first molar** and **second molar**. One of each type is located in each quadrant of both dental arches. Both have the similar arch position, function, and general shape as the permanent counterpart, and they function as such for approximately 9 years. Primary molars are replaced when shed by the permanent premolars. However, none of the primary first molars resembles any other tooth in either dentition, but, instead, the crown

of each primary second molar in both arches resembles the **first molars** of the **permanent dentition** that will erupt **distal** to them. Each molar crown is shorter occlusocervically than mesiodistally. A prominent **cervical ridge** is present on the buccal surfaces.

The **occlusal table** of a primary molar is more constricted buccolingually than with a permanent molar, rather like a rope around a corral (Figure 18-13). This constriction is due to the buccal and lingual surfaces of a primary molar being flatter occlusal to the CEJ curvatures, thus narrowing the occlusal table. The occlusal anatomy of the **cusps** is also not as pronounced as on the permanent successors.

The **roots** of the molars are flared beyond the crown outlines, widely separating the roots (see Figure 18-13). Additional space is thus created between the roots for the developing permanent premolar crowns. The primary molars have a short **root trunk**, as with permanent posterior teeth; the roots branch a short distance from the base of the crown. Again, this arrangement creates more space for the developing permanent premolar crowns.

PRIMARY MAXILLARY FIRST MOLAR B AND I

Specific Features (see Figure 18-13) The crown of the maxillary first molar does not resemble any other crown of either dentition. From the buccal aspect, the mesial and distal outlines are rounded and constricted at the CEJ. The CEJ on the mesial half of the buccal surface curves around an extremely prominent buccal cervical ridge. The height of contour on the buccal is at the cervical one third and for the lingual at the middle one third.

The occlusal table of the maxillary first molar can have four cusps: mesiobuccal, mesiolingual, distobuccal, and distolingual, with the two mesial cusps being the largest and the two distal cusps being quite small. It can also have only three cusps because the distolingual cusp may be absent. The occlusal table also has an extremely prominent transverse ridge. Additionally, an oblique ridge extends between the mesiolingual cusp and the distobuccal cusp; however, it is not as prominent as the one on its permanent counterpart.

The tooth also has an H-shaped groove pattern and three fossae: central, mesial triangular, and distal triangular. The central groove connects the central pit with the mesial pit and distal pit, at each end of the occlusal table.

The buccal groove originates in the central pit and extends buccally, separating the mesiobuccal and distobuccal cusps. The distal triangular fossa contains the disto-occlusal groove, which extends obliquely and is parallel to the oblique ridge just distal to it. Both the buccal and disto-occlusal grooves remain on the occlusal table, unlike its permanent counterpart.

Primary maxillary first molars do have the same number and position of the roots of the primary first molars as the permanent maxillary molars. The three root branches are thinner and have greater flare than on the permanent molar, and the root trunk is short. The mesiobuccal root is wider buccolingually than the distobuccal root and the lingual root is the longest and most divergent.

PRIMARY MAXILLARY SECOND MOLAR A AND J

Specific Features (Figure 18-14) The primary maxillary second molar is larger than the primary maxillary first molar. This tooth most closely resembles the form of the permanent maxillary first molar but is smaller in all dimensions. Thus, it usually has a **cusp of Carabelli**, the minor fifth cusp, as does its permanent counterpart.

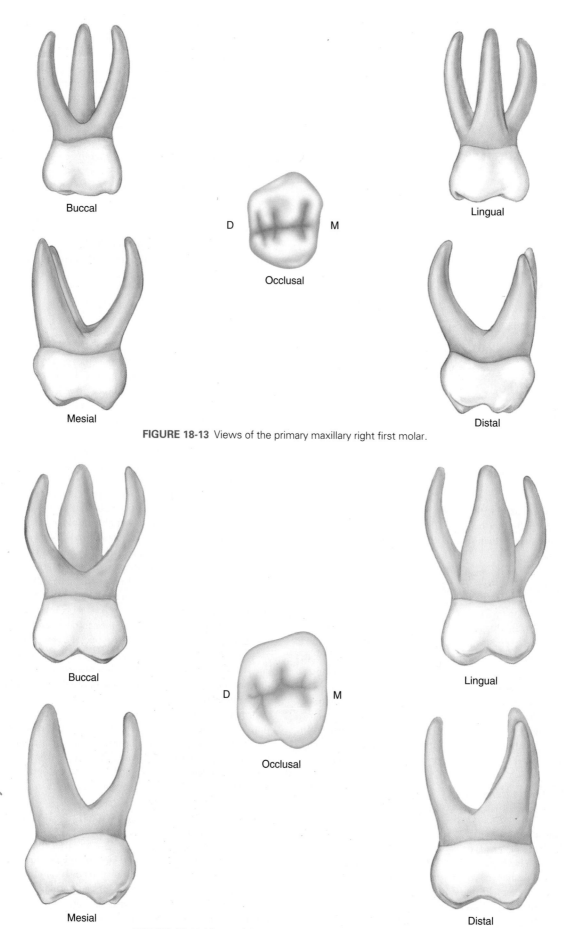

Buccal

Lingual

D M

Occlusal

Mesial

Distal

FIGURE 18-13 Views of the primary maxillary right first molar.

Buccal

Lingual

D M

Occlusal

Mesial

Distal

FIGURE 18-14 Views of the primary maxillary right second molar.

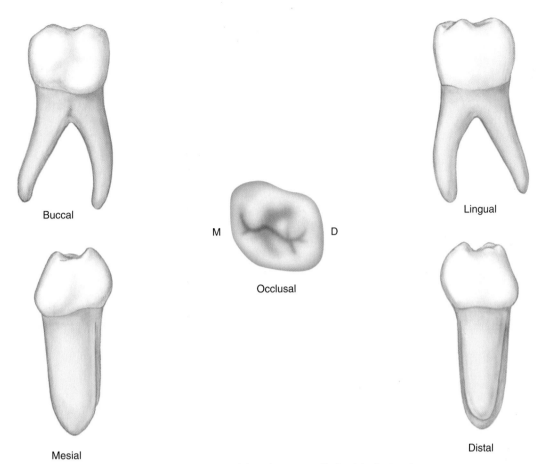

Buccal

Lingual

M D

Occlusal

Mesial

Distal

FIGURE 18-15 Views of the primary mandibular right first molar.

PRIMARY MANDIBULAR FIRST MOLAR *L* AND *S*

Specific Features (Figure 18-15) The primary mandibular first molar has a crown unlike any other tooth of either dentition. The tooth does have a prominent buccal cervical ridge, also on the mesial half of the buccal surface, similar to other primary molars. The height of contour on the buccal is at the cervical one third and for the lingual is in the middle one third. The mesiolingual line angle of the crown is rounder than any other line angles.

The tooth has four cusps, with the mesial cusps larger. The mesiolingual cusp is long, pointed, and angled in on the occlusal table. A transverse ridge passes between the mesiobuccal and mesiolingual cusps. The tooth does have two roots, which are positioned similarly to those of other primary and permanent mandibular molars.

PRIMARY MANDIBULAR SECOND MOLAR *K* AND *T*

Specific Features (Figure 18-16) The primary mandibular second molar is larger than the primary mandibular first molar. The tooth most closely resembles the form of the permanent mandibular first molar that erupts distal to it because it has five cusps. The three

buccal cusps are nearly equal in size, however, and the primary mandibular second molar has an overall oval occlusal shape.

Clinical Considerations with Primary Molars

Child patients within the mixed dentition period and their supervising adults may not notice the presence of the newly erupted permanent first molar of either arch because, when it erupts, it appears just like a larger primary second molar that is adjacent to it (Figure 18-17). These child patients and their supervising adults must be reminded that, to last a lifetime, these new posterior permanent teeth require careful homecare and possibly enamel sealants applied to the occlusal surface.

The greater root spread of primary molars, along with their narrow shape and lack of root trunk, make primary molars susceptible to fracture during extraction procedures. Dental professionals should also remember that shedding of primary teeth is an intermittent process, with resorption of the dental tissues being followed by apposition. A loose primary tooth may tighten and thus may not be as ready as thought for extraction, a procedure which should always be considered with caution in these young patients (see earlier discussion, **Chapter 6**).

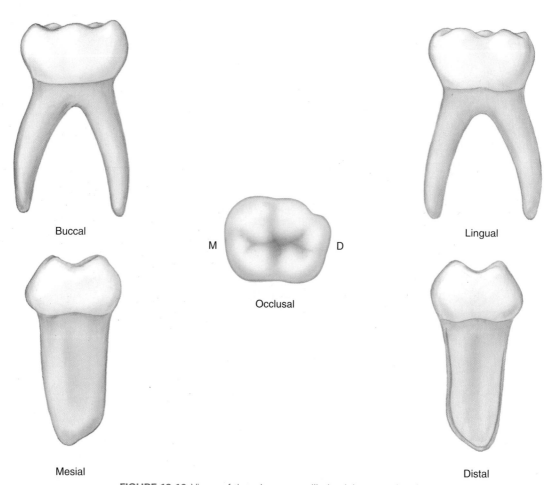

Buccal

Lingual

M   D

Occlusal

Mesial

Distal

FIGURE 18-16 Views of the primary mandibular right second molar.

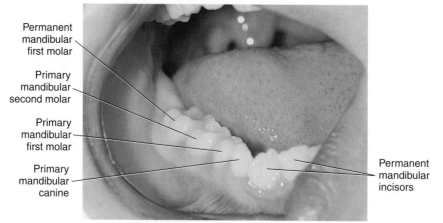

Permanent mandibular first molar

Primary mandibular second molar

Primary mandibular first molar

Primary mandibular canine

Permanent mandibular incisors

FIGURE 18-17 The mixed dentition with the eruption of the permanent mandibular first molar distal to the primary mandibular second molar. Note that the eruption of the permanent molar is difficult to discern because it appears similar to the adjacent primary molar.

Temporomandibular Joint

●●● CHAPTER OUTLINE

●●● LEARNING OBJECTIVES

- Define and pronounce the key terms in this chapter.
- Locate and identify the specific anatomical landmarks of the temporomandibular joint on a diagram, a skull, and a patient.
- Describe the histology of each component of the temporomandibular joint and how it relates to its clinical features.

- Outline the movements of the temporomandibular joint as well as demonstrating them.
- Discuss the disorders of the temporomandibular joint.
- Integrate the knowledge of the anatomy and histology of the temporomandibular joint into the dental treatment of the patient in order to promote its health.

●●● NEW KEY TERMS

Articular eminence (ar-**tik**-you-ler), **fossa**
Depression of the mandible (de-**presh**-in)
Disc of the joint
Elevation of the mandible (el-eh-**vay**-shun)
Joint capsule

Lateral deviation of the mandible (de-vee-**ay**-shun)
Muscles of mastication (mass-ti-**kay**-shin)
Postglenoid process (post-**glen**-oid)
Protrusion of the mandible (pro-**troo**-zhin)

Retraction of the mandible (re-**trak**- shun)
Subluxation (sub-luk-**say**-shun)
Synovial (sy-no-**vee**-al) **fluid, cavities, membrane**
Temporomandibular disorder (tem-poh-ro-man-**dib**-you-lar)

TEMPOROMANDIBULAR JOINT

The **temporomandibular joint (TMJ)** is a joint on each side of the head that allows for movement of the mandible for mastication, speech, and respiratory movements; it is the most complex set of joints in the body. The TMJ can be palpated just anterior to each ear (see Figure 1-3).

Patients may have a disorder associated with the TMJ (discussed later). Thus, dental professionals must understand the anatomy, histology, and normal movements of the TMJ before being able to understand any possible disorders associated with the joint.

The TMJ develops in the eleventh to twelfth week of prenatal development, during the proliferation of the associated ligaments, muscles, and bones of the joint, as well as the joint spaces and articular disc.

BONES OF THE JOINT

The TMJ is the articulation of the temporal bone and the mandible on each side of the head (Figure 19-1). Knowing the basic anatomy of the bones is necessary, as well as the histology and actions of the TMJ.

TEMPORAL BONE

The articulating area on the temporal bone of the TMJ is located on the bone's inferior aspect (Figure 19-2). This articulating area includes the bone's articular eminence and the articular fossa. The articular eminence is positioned anterior to the articular fossa, and consists of a smooth, rounded protuberance on the inferior aspect of the zygomatic process.

The **articular fossa**, or mandibular fossa, is posterior to the articular eminence, and consists of a depression on the inferior aspect of the temporal bone, posterior and medial to the **zygomatic arch** (see Figure 1-3). Posterior to the articular fossa is a sharper ridge, the **postglenoid process**.

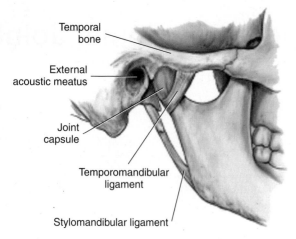

FIGURE 19-1 Temporomandibular joint and its associated bony components. *(From Fehrenbach MJ, Herring SW: Illustrated Anatomy of the Head and Neck, ed 3, WB Saunders, Philadelphia, 2007.)*

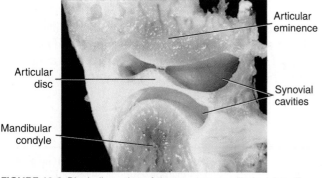

FIGURE 19-2 Block dissection of the temporomandibular joint. *(From Nanci A: Ten Cate's Oral Histology, ed 7, Mosby, St Louis, 2008.)*

The temporal bone consists of **compact bone** overlying **cancellous bone** (Figure 19-3; see Chapter 8). The outermost surface of compact bone is covered by **periosteum**. Like all bones, the innermost part of the bone consists of **endosteum** and the medullary cavity with its **bone marrow**. The articulating bony surface of the joint is covered by **fibrocartilage** immediately overlying the periosteum.

MANDIBLE

The mandible articulates with each temporal bone at the heads of the **mandibular condyle**, with their **articulating surface of the condyle**, which has histology similar to the articulating surface of the temporal bone. In a mature adult, each condyle consists of compact bone overlying cancellous bone (see Figure 19-2). Periosteum overlies the compact bone of the condyle, and the endosteum and bone marrow are located on the innermost part of the bone. Fibrocartilage then overlies the periosteum.

However, in contrast to the articulating surface of the temporal bone, a growth center is located in the head of each mandibular condyle before an individual reaches maturity (Figure 19-4). This growth center consists of **hyaline cartilage** underneath the periosteum on the articulating surface of the condyle. This is the last growth center of bone in the body and is multidirectional in its growth capacity, unlike a typical long bone.

This area of cartilage within the bone grows in length by appositional growth as the individual grows to maturity. Over time, the cartilage is replaced by bone, using **endochondral ossification** (see Figure 8-13). This mandibular growth center in the condyle allows the increased length of the mandible needed for the larger permanent teeth, as well as for the larger brain capacity of the adult. This growth of the mandible also influences the overall shape of the face, and thus is charted and referred to during orthodontic therapy (see Chapter 20). When an individual reaches full maturity, the growth center of bone within the condyle has disappeared.

JOINT CAPSULE

A **joint capsule** completely encloses the TMJ (see Figures 19-3 and 19-5). The capsule wraps around the margin of the temporal bone's articular eminence and articular fossa superiorly. Inferiorly, the capsule wraps around the circumference of the mandibular condyle, at the level of the condyle's neck.

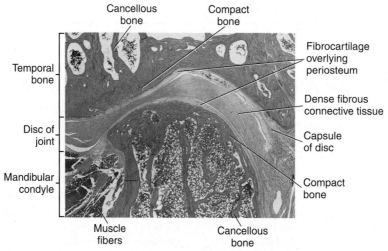

FIGURE 19-3 Sagittal section of the temporomandibular joint, including the articulating area of the temporal bone, articulating surface of the condyle, and disc and capsule of the joint.

The joint capsule has two layers. The outer layer is a firm, fibrous **connective tissue** supported by the surrounding ligaments associated with the joint. The inner layer is a synovial membrane, which consists of a thin connective tissue that contains nerves and blood vessels. The blood vessels in the synovial membrane produce synovial fluid. Synovial fluid is a thick substance that fills the joint, lubricates it, and provides nutrition to the avascular parts of the disc (discussed next).

JOINT DISC

A joint disc is located on each side between the temporal bone and mandibular condyle (Figure 19-6, see Figures 19-2 and 19-3). On section, each disc appears caplike on the mandibular condyle, with its superior aspect concavoconvex from anterior to posterior and its inferior aspect concave. As is shown, this shape of the disc conforms to the shape of the adjacent articulating bones of the TMJ and is related to normal joint movements.

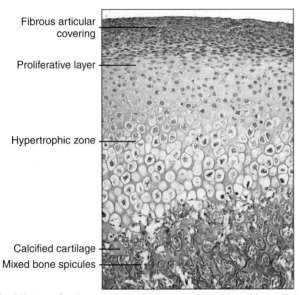

Fibrous articular covering

Proliferative layer

Hypertrophic zone

Calcified cartilage

Mixed bone spicules

FIGURE 19-4 Section taken through growth center of mandibular condyle, with endochondral transformation into bone using interstitial growth. *(From Nanci A: Ten Cate's Oral Histology, ed 7, Mosby, St Louis, 2008.)*

The disc completely divides the TMJ into two compartments. These two compartments are synovial cavities, which consists of an upper and a lower synovial cavity. The **synovial membrane** lining the joint capsule produces the **synovial fluid** that fills these cavities.

The disc is attached to the lateral and medial poles of the mandibular condyle. The disc is not attached to the temporal bone anteriorly, except indirectly through the capsule. Posteriorly, the disc is divided into two areas that attach to the disc. The upper division of the posterior part is attached to the temporal bone's **postglenoid process**, and the lower division attaches to the neck of the **mandibular condyle**. The disc blends with the capsule at these two points. This posterior area of attachment of the disc to the capsule is one of the regions where nerves and blood vessels enter the joint.

The disc consists of **dense connective tissue** (Figure 19-7). The central area of the disc is avascular and lacks innervation, and, in contrast, the peripheral region has both blood vessels and nerves. Few cells are present, but **fibroblasts** and **white blood cells** are among these. The central area is also thinner but of denser consistency than the peripheral region, which is thicker but has a more cushioned consistency. The **synovial fluid** in the **synovial cavities** provides the nutrition for the avascular central area of the disc. With age, the entire disc thins and may undergo addition of cartilage in the central part, changes that may lead to impaired movement of the joint (discussed later).

MOVEMENTS OF THE JOINT

Two basic types of movement of the mandible are performed by the joint and its associated muscles of mastication: a gliding movement and a rotational movement (Figures 19-8 and 19-9, see Tables 19-1 and 19-2). These muscles are involved in **mastication** using these two movements.

The *gliding movement* of the TMJ occurs mainly between the disc and the articular eminence of the temporal bone in the upper synovial cavity, with the disc plus the mandibular condyle moving forward or backward, down and up the articular eminence. The gliding movement allows the lower jaw to move forward or backward. Bringing the lower jaw forward involves protrusion of the mandible (see Figure 20-15). Bringing the lower jaw backward involves retraction of the mandible.

The *rotational movement* of the TMJ occurs mainly between the disc and the mandibular condyle in the lower synovial cavity. The axis of rotation of the disc plus the mandibular condyle is transverse, and the movements accomplished are depression or elevation of the mandible.

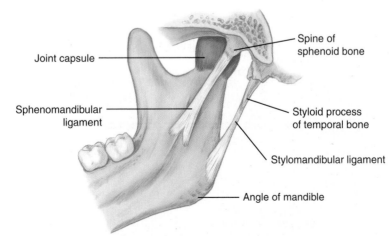

Joint capsule

Sphenomandibular ligament

Spine of sphenoid bone

Styloid process of temporal bone

Stylomandibular ligament

Angle of mandible

FIGURE 19-5 Joint capsule of the temporomandibular joint. *(From Fehrenbach MJ, Herring SW: Illustrated Anatomy of the Head and Neck, ed 3, WB Saunders, Philadelphia, 2007.)*

The **depression of the mandible** is the lowering of the lower jaw. The **elevation of the mandible** is the raising of the mandible.

With these two types of movements, gliding and rotation, and with the right and left TMJs working together, the finer movements of the jaw can be accomplished. These include opening and closing the jaws and shifting the lower jaw to one side.

Opening the jaws, which occurs during mastication, speech, and respiratory movements, involves both depression and protrusion of the mandible. When the jaws close, both elevation and retraction of the mandible occur. Thus, the natural opening and closing of the jaws involve a combination of gliding and rotational movements of the TMJs in their respective joint cavities. The disc plus the condyle glides on the articular fossa in the upper synovial cavity, moving forward or backward on the articular eminence. At approximately the same time, the mandibular condyle rotates on the disc in the lower synovial cavity.

Lateral deviation of the mandible, or lateral excursion, which involves shifting the lower jaw to one side, occurs during mastication (see Figure 20-13). Thus, lateral deviation involves both gliding and rotational movements of opposite TMJs in their respective joint cavities. During lateral deviation, one disc plus the mandibular condyle glides forward and medially on the articular eminence in the upper synovial cavity, while the other condyle and disc remain relatively stable in position in the articular fossa. These actions produce rotation around the more stable condyle.

During mastication, the power stroke (when the teeth crunch the food) involves a movement from a laterally deviated position back to the midline. If the food is on the right side of the mouth, the mandible is deviated to the right. The power stroke returns the mandible to the center, and thus the movement is to the left and involves retraction of the left side; the reverse situation occurs if the food is on the left.

DISORDERS OF THE JOINT

Patients may have a chronic disorder associated with one or both of their TMJs, or a **temporomandibular disorder (TMD)** (or dysfunction). Patients may experience chronic joint tenderness, swelling, and painful muscle spasms. They may also have difficulties in moving the joint, such as a limited or deviated mandibular opening. In a healthy joint, the surfaces in contact with one another (bone and cartilage) do not have any receptors to transmit the feeling of pain. The pain therefore originates from one of the surrounding soft tissues. When receptors from one of these areas are triggered, the pain causes a reflex to limit the mandible's movement. Furthermore, inflammation of the joints can cause constant pain, even without movement of the jaw.

Recognition of TMD includes palpation of the joint as the patient performs all the movements of the joint, as well as the associated muscles of mastication. All signs and symptoms related to the TMD, such as the amount of mandibular opening and facial pain, should be noted in the patient record, as should any **parafunctional habits** and related systemic diseases. To aid in diagnosis, a traditional skull radiograph is taken, or magnetic resonance imaging (MRI) of the joint may be requested in more severe cases because this noninvasive procedure for imaging soft tissue uses no ionizing radiation (Figure 19-10).

Many controversies are associated with the etiology of these disorders. TMD is a heterogeneous, complex disorder involving many factors, such as behavioral stressors and **parafunctional habits** (**clenching** and/or **bruxism** [grinding]) (see **Chapter 20**). Trauma to the jaw may cause TMD, with the disc having adhesions to the bony surfaces; however, this is not the most common etiological factor as are stressors and habits. Jaw thrusting (causing unusual speech and chewing habits) and excessive gum chewing or nail biting, as well as the size of food eaten, are other factors to be considered. Poor posture can also be an important factor in TMJ symptoms. For example, holding the head forward, while looking at a computer all day, strains the muscles of the face and neck.

Systemic diseases such as osteoarthritis may involve parts of the TMJ and contribute to TMD. Aging of the disc, which causes wear and hardening, may also be a factor in TMD; however, TMD does not usually become worse with age.

Not all patients with TMD have abnormalities in the joint disc or the joint itself; most symptoms seem to originate from the

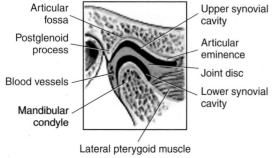

Articular fossa
Postglenoid process
Blood vessels
Mandibular condyle
Upper synovial cavity
Articular eminence
Joint disc
Lower synovial cavity
Lateral pterygoid muscle

FIGURE 19-6 Disc of the temporomandibular joint and its synovial cavities. *(From Fehrenbach MJ, Herring SW: Illustrated Anatomy of the Head and Neck, ed 3, WB Saunders, Philadelphia, 2007.)*

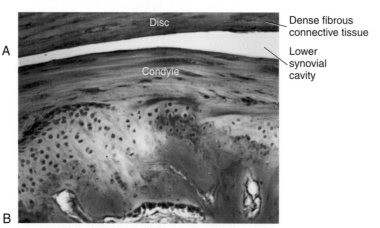

Disc
Dense fibrous connective tissue
Condyle
Lower synovial cavity
A
B

FIGURE 19-7 Microscopic appearance of the temporomandibular joint from **(A)** an inferior section of the disc of the joint and **(B)** mandibular condyle.

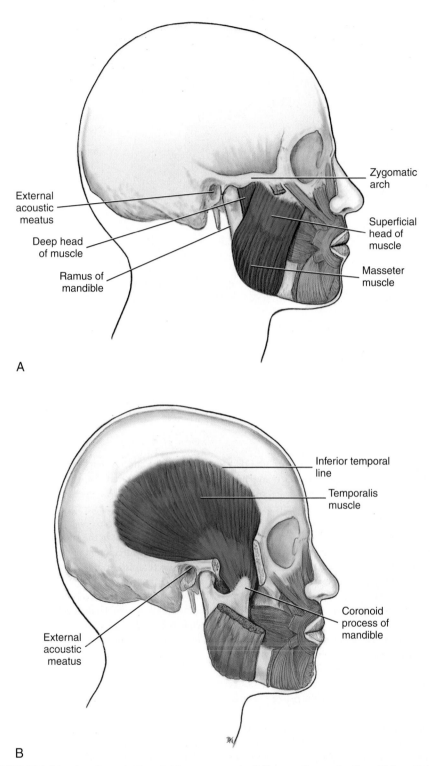

FIGURE 19-8 Muscles of mastication. **A:** Masseter muscle. **B:** Temporalis muscle. (**A** and **B** from Fehrenbach MJ, Herring SW: Illustrated Anatomy of the Head and Neck, ed 3, WB Saunders, Philadelphia, 2007.)

muscles. Muscle pain can sometimes be associated with muscle tissue trigger points, which is known as *myofascial pain dysfunction
syndrome*. These trigger points can be localized by digital palpation, both intraorally and extraorally. Studies do not support the
role of TMD in directly causing headaches, neck pain, back pain, or
instability. However, cyclic episodes of TMD, and other incidents
of chronic body pain, are commonly encountered in the population
with TMD.

Joint sounds can occur because of disc derangement as the posterior part of the disc becomes caught between the condyle head and the
articular eminence. Joint sounds are not a reliable indicator of TMD,
because they can change over time in a patient. The clicking, grinding,
and popping sounds of the joint during movement, which are commonly present with TMD, are also found in persons without TMD.

Many controversies surround the treatment of TMD, and fewer
than half of patients with TMD seek treatment for their disorder. Most

C

FIGURE 19-8, cont'd **C:** Medical and lateral pterygoid muscles.

recent studies have determined that **malocclusion** and occlusal discrepancies are not involved in most cases of TMD, but lack of **overbite** may be an additive factor. Thus, occlusal adjustment, jaw repositioning jaw, and orthodontic treatment are not the treatments of choice for all patients with TMD, nor do these treatments seem to prevent TMD.

Most cases of TMD improve over time with inexpensive and reversible treatments, including patient-based or prescription pain control, relaxation therapy, stress management, habit control, moderate home-based muscular exercises, and **orofacial myology** (see **Chapter 20**). Many of the homecare steps to treat TMJ problems can prevent such problems in the first place, for instance, by avoiding eating hard foods and chewing gum, learning relaxation techniques to reduce overall stress and muscle tension, and maintaining good posture, especially when working at a computer. Pausing often to change position, and resting hands and arms, can relieve stressed muscles. It is always important to use safety measures to reduce the risk of fractures and dislocations.

A flat-plane, full-coverage oral appliance, for instance, a nonrepositioning stabilization splint, often is helpful to control bruxism and take stress off the TMJ, although some individuals may bite harder on it, thus worsening their condition. The anterior splint, with contact at the front teeth only, may then prove helpful if used short-term. Such

inexpensive and reversible treatments (i.e., ones not causing permanent jaw or dentition changes) show the same success as more expensive and irreversible treatments such as surgery. Thus, few patients with TMD require surgery or other extensive treatment. Surgery of the TMJ can now make use of arthroscopy with an endoscope and lasers. Replacement of the jaw joint(s) or disc(s) with TMJ implants is considered as a treatment of last resort.

An acute episode of TMD can occur when a patient opens too wide, causing maximal depression and protrusion of the mandible, as when yawning or receiving prolonged dental care. This causes subluxation, or partial dislocation of both joints. Subluxation occurs when the head of each condyle moves too far anteriorly past the articular eminence. Then, when the patient tries to close and elevate the mandible, the condylar heads cannot move posteriorly because both the bony relationships prevent this, and the muscles have become spastic.

Treatment of subluxation consists of relaxation of these muscles and careful movement of the mandible downward and back. The mandibular condylar heads can then assume the normal posterior position, in relation to the articular eminence, by the muscular action of the elevating muscles of mastication. Subsequently, these patients must refrain from extreme depression of the mandible, such as can occur with prolonged dental work.

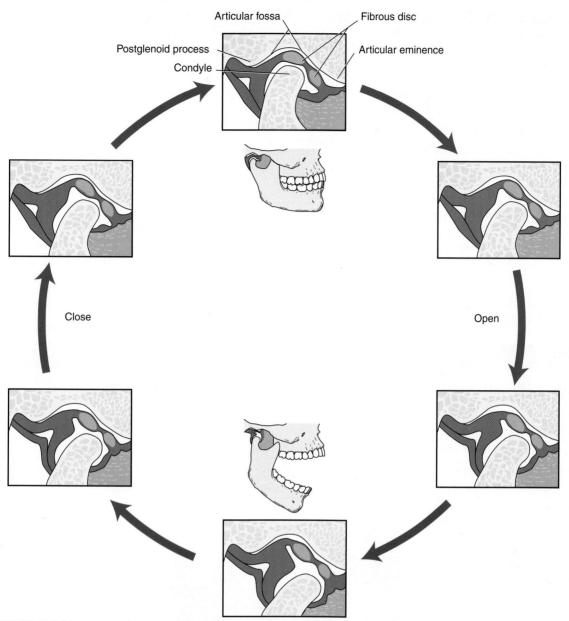

FIGURE 19-9 Movements of the mandible related to the temporomandibular joint to show opening and closing of the mouth.

TABLE 19-1	The Origin and Insertion of the Muscles of Mastication with Associated Movements of the Mandible		
MUSCLES	**ORIGIN**	**INSERTION**	**ASSOCIATED MOVEMENTS OF MANDIBLE**
Masseter	**Superficial head:** anterior two thirds of the lower border of the zygomatic arch	**Superficial head:** angle of mandible	Elevation of mandible (during jaw closing)
	Deep head: posterior one third and medial surface of zygomatic arch	**Deep head:** ramus of mandible	
Temporalis	Temporal fossa	Coronoid process of mandible	Elevation of mandible (during jaw closing) and retraction of mandible (lower jaw backward)
Medial pterygoid	Pterygoid fossa of the sphenoid bone	Angle of mandible	Elevation of mandible (during jaw closing)
Lateral pterygoid	**Superior head:** greater wing of sphenoid bone	**Both heads:** pterygoid fovea of the mandibular condyle	**Inferior heads:** slight depression of mandible (during jaw opening)
	Inferior head: lateral pterygoid plate from the sphenoid bone		**One muscle:** lateral deviation of mandible (to shift the lower jaw to the opposite side)
			Both muscles: protrusion of mandible (lower jaw forward)

(From Fehrenbach MJ, Herring SW: *Illustrated Anatomy of the Head and Neck,* ed 3, WB Saunders, Philadelphia, 2007.)

TABLE 19-2	Movements of the Mandible and Temporomandibular Joint
MANDIBULAR MOVEMENTS	**TEMPOROMANDIBULAR JOINT MOVEMENTS**
Protrusion of mandible, moving lower jaw forward	Gliding in both upper synovial cavities
Retraction of mandible, moving lower jaw backward	Gliding in both upper synovial cavities
Elevation and retraction of mandible, closing the jaws	Gliding in both upper synovial cavities and rotation in both lower synovial cavities
Depression and protrusion of the mandible, opening the jaws	Gliding in both upper synovial cavities and rotation in both lower synovial cavities
Lateral deviation of mandible, to shift lower jaw to the opposite side	Gliding in one upper synovial cavity and rotation in the opposite upper synovial cavity

(From Fehrenbach MJ, Herring SW: *Illustrated Anatomy of the Head and Neck,* ed 3, WB Saunders, Philadelphia, 2007.)

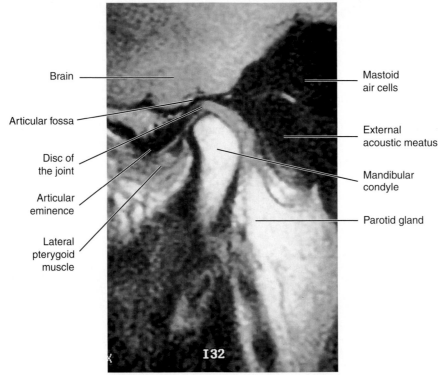

FIGURE 19-10 Coronal magnetic resonance imaging of the temporomandibular joint of an asymptomatic individual. *(From Quinn PD:* Color Atlas of Temporomandibular Joint Surgery, *Mosby, St Louis, 1998.)*

CHAPTER 20

Occlusion

●●● CHAPTER OUTLINE

Occlusion
Normal occlusion
Centric occlusion
   Arch form
   Dental curvatures and angulations
   Centric stops and relation
   Lateral and protrusive occlusion
   Mandibular rest position

Primary occlusion
Malocclusion
   Classification of malocclusion
   Skeletal considerations
   Parafunctional habits and myofunctional
     considerations

●●● LEARNING OBJECTIVES

- Define and pronounce the key terms in this chapter.
- Describe centric occlusion and its relationship to functional movements and patterns of the mandible.
- Outline Angle's classification of malocclusion and how it relates to patient care.
- Discuss orofacial myofunctional patterns, parafunctional habits, myofunctional and skeletal considerations, occlusal trauma, and their relationship to occlusion.

- Integrate the knowledge of occlusion and orofacial myofunctional considerations into the dental treatment of a patient in order to promote orofacial health.

●●● NEW KEY TERMS

Balancing interference
Bracing
Bruxism (bruk-sizm)
Canine rise (kay-nine)
Centric relation, stops
Clenching
Crossbite
Curve of Spee, Wilson
Distal step (dis-tl)
End-to-end bite
Flush terminal plane
Gnathic index (nath-ick)
Group function
Interlabial gap (in-ter-lay-be-al)

Interocclusal clearance (in-ter-ah-kloo-zhal)
Leeway space
Malocclusion (mal-ah-kloo-zhun): Angle's classification of, Class I, Class II (division I, division II), Class III
Mesial step (me-ze-il)
Mesognathic (me-so-nath-ik)
Occlusal trauma (ah-klooz-l)
Occlusion (ah-kloozh-n): centric, lateral, primary, protrusive
Open bite
Orofacial myofunctional disorders (my-oh-funk-shun-al), therapy
Orofacial myology (my-ol-oh-je)

Overbite
Overjet
Parafunctional habits (pare-ah-funk-shun-al)
Premature contacts
Prognathic (prog-nath-ik)
Range of motion (ROM)
Retrognathic (ret-row-nath-ik)
Resting posture
Side: balancing, working
Supporting cusps (kusp)
Terminal plane
Tongue thrusting
Underbite

OCCLUSION

Occlusion is the contact relationship between the **maxillary teeth** and **mandibular teeth** when the jaws are in a fully closed (occluded) position, as well as the relationship between the teeth in the same arch. Many patterns of tooth contact are possible; part of the reason for the variety is the substantial range of movement of the **mandibular condyle** within the **temporomandibular joint (TMJ)** (see Figure 19-9).

Occlusion develops in a child as the primary teeth erupt. During this time, oral motor behaviors develop and the masticatory skills are acquired. The deglutition skills to accommodate the mastication process begin to develop in utero, and are modified on a developmental continuum as the **primary dentition** erupts. Occlusion of the erupting **permanent dentition** is dependent on the primary teeth shedding, with the exception of the permanent molars, as these erupt distal to the primary dentition.

Interrelated factors are involved in the development of the occlusion, such as the associated musculature, neuromuscular patterns, TMJ functioning (see Chapter 19), tongue functioning and posturing, orofacial behaviors, and habit patterns. Thus, occlusion is only one aspect of an entire developing orofacial masticatory and deglutition system that includes many other factors and variables. The teeth, in proper alignment, are relatively self-cleansing by action of the cheek and lip musculature, with the neutralizing flow of saliva over the smooth tooth surfaces.

When the teeth in the dentition are not aligned properly, or there are orofacial myofunctional imbalances and/or parafunctional habit patterns present, they lose the ability to self cleanse. More importantly, when teeth of either **dentition** are not occluding properly, the teeth and **periodontium** may not be able to perform the functions for which they were designed. Unnatural occlusal stress is then placed on the dentition, which often results in occlusal disharmony. Occlusal disharmony may then lead to occlusal trauma. The dentition and the periodontium are able to withstand many of these daily stresses; however, these stresses are often excessive, such as with incorrect tongue, lip, and/or mandibular resting posture patterns and/or parafunctional habits (discussed later). Microscopic changes within the periodontium can occur with occlusal trauma (see Figures 14-33 and 14-34).

Dental professionals must remember that occlusal trauma does not directly cause bacterial-based periodontal disease, but may create an overriding adverse force factor in initiating or contributing to an already weakened and diseased periodontium. It also may be associated, on an acute basis, with the production of a cracked tooth from masticatory impact on a hard object, and fracture of the restoration margin may also occur. Occlusal trauma can usually be stopped if the etiological factors are eliminated, or if the involved teeth are protected from these stresses.

Unfortunately, the effects of occlusal trauma are often irreversible, if not intercepted early enough. These occlusal disharmonies, orofacial myofunctional patterns, and parafunctional habits should be controlled or eliminated during dental treatment and preventive maintenance therapy before initiating occlusal therapy (see later discussion). Signs or symptoms indicating abnormal patterns and habits must be addressed to eliminate the harmful occlusal disharmonies on a long-term basis. The effects on a patient's occlusion must also be kept in mind during all phases of dental treatment, especially during restorative treatment or when treating a **temporomandibular disorder (TMD)** (see Chapter 19).

NORMAL OCCLUSION

An ideal occlusion rarely exists, but the concept of a normal occlusion provides a basis for treatment. The optimum 138 occlusal contacts for the permanent dentition in the closure of 32 teeth are seldom, if ever,

achieved. When occlusion is considered, the position of the dentition in centric occlusion serves as the basis for reference (discussed next). Thus, centric occlusion serves as the standard for describing a normal occlusion. Ideally, a normal centric resting posture of the tongue, lips, and mandible is also present (discussed later). To prevent occlusal disharmony, all patients should have an occlusal evaluation before and after completion of their dental treatment plan, with reevaluation occurring on a regular basis (see the *Workbook for Illustrated Dental Embryology, Histology, and Anatomy* for guidelines and techniques).

CENTRIC OCCLUSION

Centric occlusion (CO), or habitual occlusion, is the voluntary position of the dentition that allows the maximum contact when the teeth occlude (Figure 20-1). It is the centered contact position of the occlusal surfaces of mandibular teeth on the occlusal surface of the maxillary

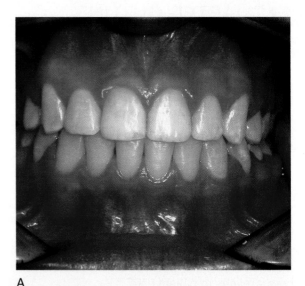

A

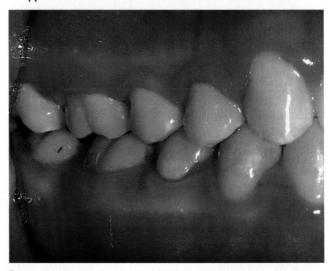

B

Figure 20-1 Permanent dentition in centric occlusion. **A:** Facial view. **B:** Buccal view. With a normal amount of overjet present, which is the horizontal overlap between the two arches. Also with a normal amount of overbite, which is the vertical overlap between the two arches. Note the three different segments to describe arch form: anterior, middle, and posterior. *(Courtesy of Dona M. Seely, DDS, MSD, Orthodontics, Seattle and Bellevue, WA.)*

teeth. CO is related to the functioning of the dentition. However, even when the teeth are in full closure, discrepancy between the relationships of the mandible, TMJs, and/or the maxilla may be significant (skeletal discrepancies are discussed later).

When the teeth of a normal occlusion are in the position of CO, each tooth of one arch is in occlusion with two others in the opposing arch, except for the mandibular central incisors and maxillary third molars. This structure serves to equalize the forces of impact in occlusion. Another benefit of this arrangement is that if a tooth is lost in one jaw, the alignment of the opposing jaw is not immediately disturbed or impaired. One antagonist remains until adequate restorative treatment can be performed.

If a tooth is lost for a longer period, the neighboring teeth usually tip in an effort to fill the edentulous space. The teeth become inclined, malaligned, and supereruption of the tooth opposing the space then occurs (see Figures 17-43 and 17-55). Thus, loss of one tooth disturbs the contact relationships in that area, as well as those teeth in the opposing arch, their antagonist(s), possibly causing changes in the occlusion of the entire dentition. Patients must understand when discussing tooth replacement that teeth are like building blocks: Pull one out of the construction, and they all fall down, possibly resulting in occlusal disharmonies.

In addition to tooth loss, abnormal pressure or force of movement from the tongue, such as in tongue thrusting or an incorrect resting posture of the tongue, may create occlusal disharmony. An open mouth resting posture of the lips or chronic mouth breathing result in inadequate closure of the lips needed to maintain an equilibrium between the lips and teeth as well as the surrounding orofacial structures. This most often leads to the teeth not being retained in a normal arch shape and thus malocclusion occurs (discussed later).

When the teeth normally occlude in CO, the maxillary arch horizontally overlaps the mandibular arch, a position called overjet (Figure 20-2). This normal amount of horizontal overlap, usually 1 to 3 mm, between the anterior segment of the two arches associated with the overjet allows extensions in the movement of the range of motion (ROM) of the mandible, and assists in keeping the soft tissue of the oral cavity out of the way during mastication. The ROM is a normal physiological and functional reciprocal ROM for opening or closure of the mandible.

Overjet is measured in millimeters with the tip of a periodontal probe, once a patient is in centric occlusion. The probe is placed at a right angle to the labial surface of a mandibular incisor at the base of the incisal edge of a maxillary incisor. The measurement is taken from the labial surface of the mandibular incisor to the lingual surface of the maxillary incisor. Note that the labiolingual width of the maxillary incisor is not included in the measurement.

In centric occlusion, the maxillary arch also vertically overlaps the mandibular arch, a position called overbite (see Figure 20-2). This normal amount of vertical overlap, normally 2 to 5 mm between the anterior segment of the two arches allows contact between the posterior teeth during mastication. It is usually expressed as a percentage at around 20% to 30%. Excessive amounts of either overjet or overbite are classified as a malocclusion (discussed later, see Figures 20-21, *A* and 20-22, *A*).

Overbite is measured in millimeters with the tip of a periodontal probe after a patient is placed in CO. The probe is placed on the incisal edge of the maxillary incisor at right angles to the mandibular incisor. As patients open their mouths or depress their jaws, the probe is then placed vertically against the mandibular incisor to measure the distance to the incisal edge of the mandibular incisor.

Studies show that overjet measurements were equally distributed among women and men, but overbite was noted more often in women. However, neither measurement was predictably associated with any particular craniofacial pattern. Both overjet and overbite tend to diminish with age, initially because of mandibular growth and later overbite due to incisal wear. When the reverse is the case, and the mandibular arch extends forward beyond the maxillary arch, the condition is referred to as an underbite (or retrognathia) (see Figure 20-26, *B*).

Within each dental arch, the teeth also create contact areas as they contact their same-arch neighbors on their proximal surfaces; the exception is the last tooth in each arch of each dentition, which lacks a distal contact (see Chapters 16 and 17). This contact between neighboring teeth serves two purposes: It protects the **interdental papillae** and stabilizes each tooth in the dental arch.

Open contacts allow areas of food impaction from opposing cusps, called plunging cusps, resulting in trauma to the interdental gingiva. Open contacts also do not allow mesiodistal stability between the teeth. Correct restorative treatment should not allow any open contacts, unless tooth position and tooth loss make this impossible. Although the practice is controversial, periodontal splints are often placed in the mouth lingually with tooth-colored resins and wires to simulate this stability needed for the teeth within the dental arch. All prosthetic treatment within the mouth, including the placement of bridges, implants, and removable dentures, is an attempt to simulate this stability.

Certain topics must be considered when studying CO: arch form and its development, dental curvatures and angulations, centric stops, centric relation, lateral and protrusive occlusion, mandibular rest position, and chewing patterns.

ARCH FORM

Each **dental arch** of the permanent dentition is divided into three segments when describing arch form: anterior, middle, and posterior (see Figure 20-1). The anterior segment includes the anterior teeth, the middle segment includes the premolars, and the posterior segment includes the molars. The concept of arch segments allows the arches to overlap slightly so that canines and first molars are cooperating in more than one segment. This arrangement serves to indicate that the canines and first molars function as anchor supports for both arches.

The anterior segment of each dental arch is curved and ends at the labial ridges of the canines. The middle segment is straight and extends from the distal part of the canines to the buccal cervical ridge of the mesiobuccal cusp of the first molar in each arch. The posterior segment creates a straight line, starting from the buccal cusps of the first molars and remaining in contact with the buccal surfaces of the second and third molars.

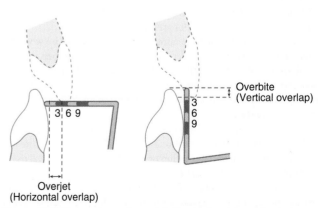

Figure 20-2 Comparison of overjet, the horizontal overlap between the two arches, and overbite, the vertical overlap between the two arches.

PHASES OF ARCH DEVELOPMENT

Each dental arch goes through phases of development as the permanent teeth erupt and the primary teeth are being shed (see Figure 6-22 for chronological timetable). During this time, the ramus and body of the jaw develops and undergoes lengthening and horizontal growth to achieve its mature form and accommodate the larger permanent teeth.

Phase one occurs when the permanent first molars erupt (see Figure 18-17). These teeth add dramatically to chewing efficiency and jaw development during a period of rapid growth of the child. They help support the jaws while the primary anterior teeth are being shed and the other permanent teeth are erupting. The **primate spaces** in the primary dentition are still present to allow future space for the permanent teeth (see Chapter 18).

Phase two occurs with eruption of the permanent anterior teeth near the midline of the oral cavity. First, the centrals, then the laterals generally erupt lingually to the primary anterior roots. However, shedding of the primary teeth and jaw growth finally place them labial to the position of the primary teeth they replaced (see Figures 6-26 and 18-17).

In addition, the permanent location of the anteriors is not established until the development of the arch form is complete. Thus, some degree of transient anterior crowding may occur between 8 to 9 years of age and persist until the emergence of the canines, when the space for the teeth is adequate again. However, incisor crowding that persists into a permanent dentition is considered a type of malocclusion (discussed later).

Phase three in the development of the form of the dental arches begins when the premolars erupt anterior to the permanent molars (see Figures 6-27 and 6-28). Developmentally, this is quite significant because the premolars are so much smaller than the primary molars they replace. This difference in size, mesiodistally between the two types of teeth, is called the leeway space (Figure 20-3). The contour of the bone covering the narrower roots of the premolars, in addition to the state of flux of the bone formation in this area, furnishes adjustment for dental arch measurements, making the middle segment of the arches important architecturally. Thus, this space allows the future forward movement of the permanent molars, which is discussed later with regard to the occlusion of the primary teeth.

However, if there is early loss of the primary second molars and **impaction** of the second premolar, leeway space can become compromised. Also, if permanent second molars erupt before the premolars, the arch perimeter is significantly shortened and occlusal disharmony is likely to occur, as is malocclusion (discussed later), because the second premolar is also unable to erupt. A fixed or removable space maintainer may be used to save this leeway space from the shed primary molars for the permanent premolars (Figure 20-4).

Phase four begins when the canines wedge themselves between the lateral incisors and the first premolars. Contact relations between the teeth are established, and the arch is complete from the permanent first molar forward. Simultaneously, the second molars are due to emerge distally to the first molars and support them during the wedging activity of the canines.

Phase five is the final phase of the development of the final dental arch form and consists of eruption of the third molars. Often the jaw length is not sufficient for eruption of these last teeth and dental treatment plans changes need to be considered (see Chapter 17).

Thus, the usual sequence for eruption of both the primary and permanent dentition is favorable to the development of the arches (Figures 20-5 and 20-6). Keeping this sequence in mind for each dentition is part of the treatment to prevent disruption in patients with

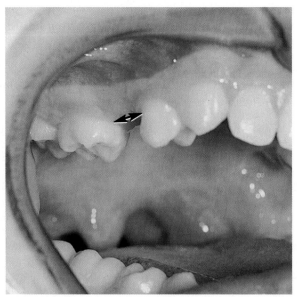

Figure 20-3 Leeway space in the maxillary arch (*double-headed arrow*) during the mixed dentition period and phase three of the dental arch development. This space is due to the difference in size, mesiodistally, between primary molars and permanent premolars.

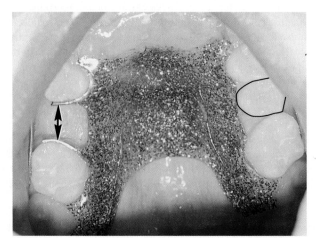

Figure 20-4 Removable maxillary space maintainer (*sparkle variety*) to hold the leeway space from the shed primary molar (*double-headed arrow*), so as to allow future eruption of the permanent second premolar. The permanent second molars have already erupted and may narrow the existing space in the premolar segment. Note that the permanent second premolar on the contralateral side is already fully erupted (*outlined*), so leeway space does not need to be maintained any longer.

primary and mixed dentition. Disruption of this sequence, with overlong retention or too-early loss of primary teeth, may allow complications to occur with the eruption of the permanent dentition. Proper treatment of these cases of disruption in the eruption sequence, and early orthodontic interceptive therapy, increases the chances for a normal occlusion. Panoramic radiographs of the mixed dentition are important in order to monitor tooth eruption sequence and arch development (see Figure 6-27, *A*).

It is important to note that **attrition** of the proximal surfaces also reduces the mesial-distal dimensions of the teeth and significantly reduces arch length over a lifetime, which causes crowding or spacing problems after age 40.

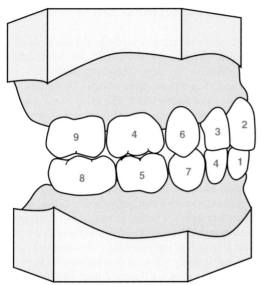

Figure 20-5 Favorable sequence of eruption per dental arch of the primary dentition.

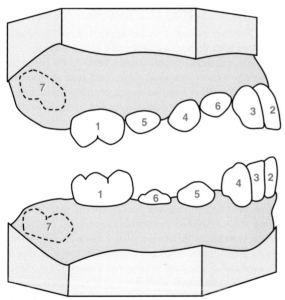

Figure 20-6 Favorable sequence of eruption per dental arch of the permanent dentition.

DENTAL CURVATURES AND ANGULATIONS

A common mistake is to assume that the forces of occlusion act on squared and flat teeth in straight lines or planes and that the axes of the teeth are at right angles to their masticatory surfaces. Many dental curvatures and angulations are present in normal occlusion and must be considered.

If imaginary planes are placed on the masticatory surfaces of each dental arch, the arches do not conform to these flat planes; the maxillary arch is convex occlusally, and the mandibular arch is concave (Figure 20-7, *A*). Thus, when the maxillary and mandibular teeth come into centric occlusion, they align along anteroposterior and lateral curves. This anteroposterior curvature is called the curve of Spee, which is produced by the curved alignment of all the teeth and is especially evident when viewing the posterior teeth from the buccal view.

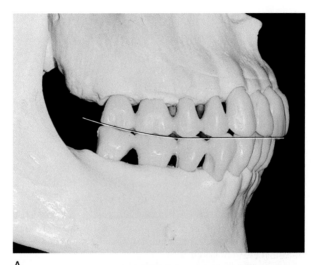

A

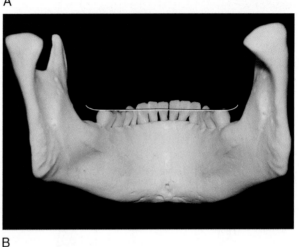

B

Figure 20-7 Curves of the teeth noted within the permanent dental arches. **A:** Curve of Spee with the maxillary arch convex and the mandibular arch concave. **B:** Curve of Wilson with a concave curve that occurs when a frontal section is taken through each set of molars.

Another curve of the dentition is the curve of Wilson (see Figure 20-7, *B*). This lateral curve results when a frontal section is visually compared to each set of maxillary and mandibular molars—the firsts, seconds, and then thirds. These imaginary dental curvatures are interesting, but it is important to note that modern dentistry does not use these curves often, in practice, because they have only a remote association with functional relationships. Both of these curves tend to be lost with age as a result of **attrition** (Figure 20-8). The composite of these curves created by the contact of the maxillary and mandibular teeth forms a line called the *occlusal plane.*

Individual teeth also exhibit some forms of curvature. Curves are found in the basic form of each tooth. Every third of a tooth represents a curved surface, except where a tooth is worn or fractured. These curvatures of the teeth should be noted when studying the dentitions, and especially when drawing them hoping to achieve lifelike drawings of each tooth. These curves also must be noted when restoring the teeth for proper function and esthetics.

When a tooth is bisected by its **root axis line (RAL),** the angulations of each tooth's root (or roots) within the alveolar bone are noted (Figure 20-9, discussed per tooth type in Chapters 16 and 17). This angled arrangement of the teeth allows proper spacing between the roots for blood and nerve supply, and for securing anchorage of the roots in the jaws.

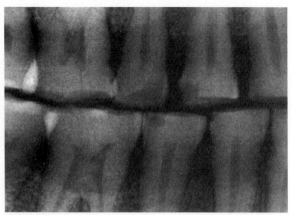

Figure 20-8 Attrition, or wear, of the masticatory surfaces of the teeth is noted on a radiograph. The result is a loss of the curvatures of the teeth within the dental arches.

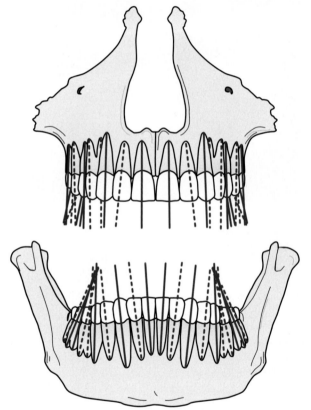

Figure 20-9 Each tooth of both arches of the permanent dentition is bisected by its root axis line, showing the angulations of the root within the alveolar bone of the arch.

Each tooth is placed at the angle that best withstands the lines of forces brought against it while functioning in normal occlusion. The angle at which it is placed depends on the function that the tooth must perform. If the tooth is placed at a disadvantage because of misalignment in the dental arch or continued incorrect pressures against it from the tongue, lips, or cheeks, its functional efficiency is limited, and the permanence of its position is endangered. The anteriors seem to be placed at a disadvantage because they are more vertically situated in the alveolar bone, but their function is only the momentary biting and cutting of food, not the full force of

chewing that occurs in the posterior teeth, which usually have more angulation.

The **masticatory surfaces** of teeth do not have any flat planes, unless some are created by wear, orofacial myofunctional disorders, or traumatic accident. Therefore, during occlusion, the curved surface of one tooth always comes into contact with the curved surfaces of another tooth. The escapement space for food during mastication is provided by the form of the individual tooth's **cusps, ridges, sulci, developmental grooves,** and **embrasures,** when the teeth come together in occlusion (see Figure 15-11). These escapement spaces are necessary for efficient occlusion during mastication.

The location and form of the escapement spaces can be changed when the occlusal relation is changed, as with attrition, inappropriate functional patterning of the mandible, tongue thrusting, or even with restorative treatment. These changes can be related to loss of function of the teeth, tongue, lip, and mandibular function and the masticatory system. Additionally, knowing the angulation of the roots within the alveolar bone is essential for the proper adaptation during the taking of radiographs and performing instrumentation. This measurement is also considered when evaluating a patient's smile.

CENTRIC STOPS

When the teeth are in centric occlusion, they should have maximal interdigitation with the locking of the two arch positions. The three areas of centric contacts, or centric stops, between the two arches are height of cusp contour, marginal ridges, and central fossae (Figure 20-10). Those cusps that function during centric occlusion are called the **supporting cusps** and include the lingual cusps of the maxillary posterior teeth and the buccal cusps of the mandibular posterior teeth. The incisal edges of the mandibular anterior teeth are usually included as supporting cusps.

These centric stops and supporting cusps are checked using articulating paper when restorative or prosthetic treatment is performed (Figure 20-11). An occlusal adjustment involving the removal of restorative, prosthetic, or natural tooth material may be necessary, depending on the results of the occlusal evaluation.

A dental manikin with unworn plastic teeth can show the ideal location of these centric stops and supporting cusps, if articulating paper is used and mastication is simulated. However, the relationship of centric stops to the masticatory surfaces is not rigidly set and may in reality vary considerably among individuals. Centric stops are often in the central fossa and are related to the inner surface of the marginal ridges rather than the embrasure surfaces of the ridges, as indicated in an ideal mapping of centric stops.

These contact relationships change with wear of the dentition. With advancing **attrition,** the supporting cusps are seated closer and closer to the bottoms of the opposing fossae. This process continues until the development of numerous flat surface contacts, which are termed *occlusal wear facets.* This process can result in the loss of a definite locking of the two jaws in centric occlusion, in addition to creating an unstable occlusal environment.

The position of the centric stops helps determine the height of the lower one third of the **vertical dimension of the face** when the teeth are in centric occlusion (see Figure 14-22). This dimension cannot be exactly measured in patients with teeth, and thus its loss requires clinical judgment and is based on the **Golden Proportion** as it relates to the face. This dimension is involved in the proper functioning of the teeth and jaws and the esthetic appearance of a patient. Loss of this part of the vertical dimension is based on **alveolar bone** loss and attrition (see Figure 14-22).

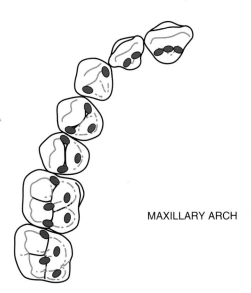

MAXILLARY ARCH

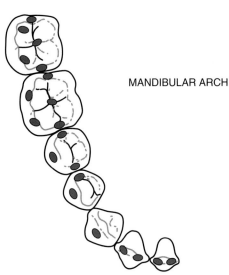

MANDIBULAR ARCH

Figure 20-10 Ideal centric stops showing articulation between the two arches are highlighted. Note that the stops include the height of cusps, incisal ridges, marginal ridges, or cingulums, as well as any central fossae of the teeth.

CENTRIC RELATION

Centric relation (CR) is the end point of closure of the mandible; the mandible is in the most retruded position to which it can be carried by the musculature and ligaments (see **Chapter 19**). Even though a patient is rarely in CR, except sometimes when swallowing, centric relation is a base measurement from which to evaluate a patient's occlusion because it can be easily repeated.

To attain CR, the mandible must undergo complete retraction (Figure 20-12). CR must be determined by the clinician without a patient's muscle participation. To do this, the clinician must gently establish the hinge movement of the mandible on the patient by gently arcing the mandible with the fingers in a closing and opening manner several times, before attempting placement of the loosened jaw into CR. Researchers are currently exploring various ways of clinically relaxing patients' jaws to determine this position of the mandible more precisely in addition to myofascial release and orofacial myofunctional therapy (discussed later).

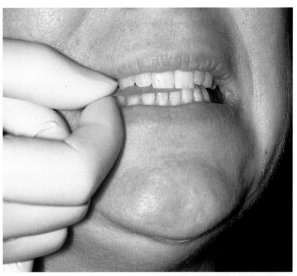

Figure 20-11 Articulating paper is used to check the centric stops during an occlusal evaluation or after restorative treatment.

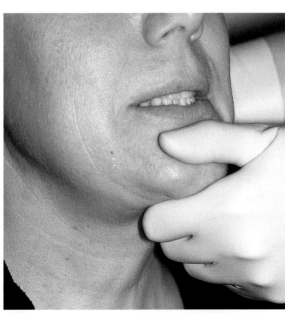

Figure 20-12 Attaining centric relation by establishing the hinge movement of the mandible by gently arching the mandible with the fingers in a closing and opening manner, several times. This is performed before attempting placement of the loosened jaw into centric relation—the end point of mandible closure in which the mandible is in the most retruded position.

Ideally, when the mandible is in CR, the dentition should be in CO (thus centric relation equals centric occlusion, or CR = CO). The centric resting position also remains in a neutral pattern with an adequate freeway space maintained. Therefore, no major shift of the dentition from centric relation occlusion to centric occlusion should occur. However, the average distance of shift or slide from a patient's occlusion in CR to CO is approximately 1 mm or less.

The position of CO can be attained by having a patient who is in centric relation squeeze his or her teeth together after achieving CR. The amount and pathway of shift in the dentition can then be recorded during the occlusal evaluation. One can easily simulate this procedure with their own dentition by putting the head back (centric relation) and then closing their teeth when they bring their head forward (centric occlusion).

However, if disorders such as those related to function (for instance, orofacial myofunctional disorders, discussed later) are present, striving to achieve CR in this manner may exacerbate the disorder. Clinicians should seat the patient in an upright position, inform the patient where the correct tongue placement is on the palate and having him or her bite the molars together (centric occlusion), followed by relaxing the mandible and allowing the maxillary and mandibular teeth to gently come apart until the masseter muscle is relaxed (centric relation that is also the same as centric rest).

A slide or shift in the position of the dentition from centric relation to centric occlusion (centric relation does not equal centric occlusion, or CR ≠ CO) should be noted. It is most often caused by premature contacts, where one or two teeth initially contact before the other teeth, or an orofacial myofunctional disorder (discussed later), as well as an incorrect habit pattern of the tongue and/or mandible, or deviation in the ROM patterning of the TMJ. The premature tooth contact, orofacial myofunctional disorder, and ROM deviation may contribute to occlusal disharmony. Additional slide between the teeth in centric relation to centric occlusion is also associated with tooth malalignment, improper intercuspation of the teeth, improper restorative treatment, and inherited arch lengths and relationships.

LATERAL AND PROTRUSIVE OCCLUSION

Masticatory movement entails not only the mandible going through elevation and depression but also deviations or excursions from side to side and forward duirng lateral and protrusion occlusion (see Figure 19-9). Therefore, other movements besides centric occlusion and its relationship to the teeth must be evaluated.

Evaluation of lateral occlusion is made by undergoing *lateral deviation* or excursion by moving the mandible either to the right or to the left until the canines on that side are in a cusp-to-cusp relationship (Figure 20-13).

Before the canines contact on each side, no other individual teeth should be contacting during lateral occlusion. The side to which the mandible has been moved is called the working side. Two working sides are noted in an occlusal evaluation: right lateral and left lateral. The side of the arch contralateral to the working side during lateral occlusion is called the balancing side.

In normal occlusion, the canine should be the only tooth in function during lateral occlusion; this is called canine rise (or cuspid rise). Thus, the mandible is moved to the working side when checking lateral occlusion, until the contralateral canines are edge to edge. If other teeth are involved in function during lateral occlusion, they must be noted; for example, the first molars if in function may present problems for the dentition.

If the canine rise does not exist on the working side because of cusp wear caused by parafunctional habits or tooth malalignment, it is acceptable that most of the entire posterior quadrant functions during lateral occlusion. This is called group function, because all contralateral posterior teeth are sharing the occlusal stress during function.

No teeth should make contact on the contralateral balancing side during lateral occlusion. If teeth are in contact on the balancing side, this is called a balancing interference. Balancing interference can be involved in occlusal disharmonies. For further confirmation of any balancing interferences during lateral deviation, floss can be placed over the occlusal surfaces on the appropriate side (Figure 20-14).

With the mandible in protrusive occlusion, all eight of the most anterior teeth (centrals and laterals) of both arches are normally in contact as the mandible undergoes protrusion (Figure 20-15). If only one or two assume the stress of protrusion, occlusal disharmony may occur.

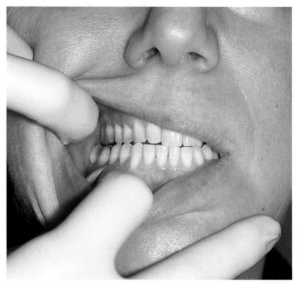

Figure 20-13 Undergoing lateral deviation, or excursion, to check the lateral occlusion on the working side (side to which the mandible has been moved) and balancing side (other side of the arch from working side). Note that the mandible is being moved until the contralateral arch canines are edge to edge during canine rise.

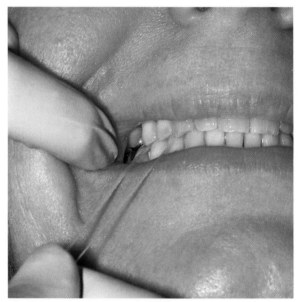

Figure 20-14 Using floss to confirm balancing interferences where teeth contact on the balancing side during lateral occlusion.

MANDIBULAR REST POSITION

The physiological rest position of the mandible is achieved when the mandible is being held in a relaxed state and is not being used in mastication, speech, or respiratory movements (Figure 20-16). With this rest position, an average space of 2 to 3 mm is noted between the masticatory surfaces of the maxillary and mandibular teeth. This space between the arches, when the mandible is at rest, is the interocclusal clearance, or, as more commonly called, *freeway space*.

This position of the mandible at rest is considered fairly stable, although it can be influenced by posture, fatigue, and tension. Thus, failure to assume this position when the jaws are not at work may mean that the patient is temporarily tense or has parafunctional habits such as clenching, grinding (bruxism), or bracing which may be involved in occlusal problems (discussed later).

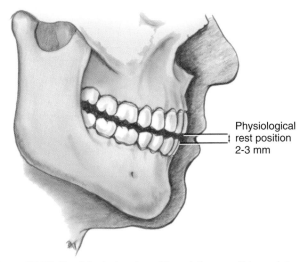

Figure 20-15 Undergoing protrusion to evaluate protrusive occlusion.

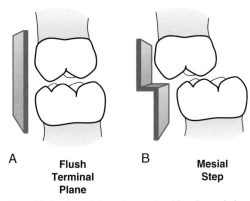

Figure 20-17 Evaluation of the primary dentition (buccal view of right side). **A:** Flush terminal plane, in which the primary maxillary and mandibular second molars are in an end-to-end relationship. This allows a normal molar relationship to occur in the permanent dentition. **B:** Mesial step in which the mandibular second molar is mesial to the maxillary molar. This will most likely allow a normal molar relationship to occur in the permanent dentition.

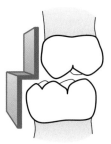

Distal Step

Figure 20-18 Primary dentition (buccal view of right side) in which distal step relationship exists with the primary mandibular second molar distal to the maxillary second molar. This is not a beneficial molar relationship because it will not usually result in a normal molar relationship in the permanent dentition when molar eruption occurs and the primary teeth are shed.

A **distal step** relationship, in which the primary mandibular second molar is distal to the maxillary second molar, is not an ideal molar relationship in the primary dentition and thus is not a type of terminal plane relationship (Figure 20-18). With the presence of a mesial step, an ideal permanent molar relationship most likely occurs after the eruption of the permanent dentition. An ideal molar relationship in the permanent dentition may still occur with a flush terminal plane, but rarely with the presence of a distal step relationship.

Within a primary dentition, **primate spaces** may occur between the primary teeth; a space is noted between the maxillary lateral incisor and the canine, and between the mandibular first molar and canine (see Figure 18-1). If primate spacing exists in the primary mandibular arch, after the eruption of the permanent first molar, the permanent first molar puts pressure on the primary second and first molars, causing forward movement of the primary mandibular canine and first molar (discussed earlier with regard to arch development). Thus, this primate space actually allows for this movement, which then facilitates the development of an ideal permanent molar relationship, along with the presence of a mesial step relationship.

When the child patient enters the *mixed dentition period*, analysis of space is performed so as to allow for early interceptive orthodontic therapy (see Figures 15-4 and 18-17). This analysis can range from

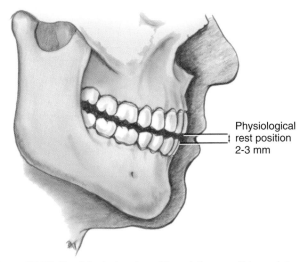

Physiological rest position 2-3 mm

Figure 20-16 Physiological rest position of the mandible, or interocclusal clearance of about 2 to 3 mm.

Overall, **resting posture** is the normal physiological position of the tongue, lips, and mandible when not functioning for chewing, swallowing, or speech. Correct physiological rest is when the tongue is resting on the palate, the teeth are not in occlusion, and the lips are gently closed without any signs of facial grimacing.

PRIMARY OCCLUSION

Similar to the permanent dentition, the primary dentition also has an ideal form (Figure 20-17). The canine relationship between the arches in primary teeth is the same as that of the permanent dentition. The ideal molar relationship in the primary dentition, when in centric occlusion, is referred to as the **terminal plane**. This can involve either a **flush terminal plane,** in which the primary maxillary and mandibular second molars are in an end-to-end relationship, or a **mesial step,** in which the primary mandibular second molar is mesial to the maxillary molar.

TABLE 20-1	**Angle's Classification of Malocclusion***		
CLASS	**MODEL**	**ARCH RELATIONSHIPS**	**DESCRIPTIONS**
Class I	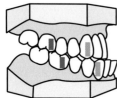	Molar: MB cusp of the maxillary first occluding with the MB groove of the mandibular first molar Canines: maxillary occluding with the distal half of the mandibular canine and the mesial half of the mandibular first premolar	Dental malalignment(s) present (see text), such as crowding or spacing; mesognathic profile
Class II	Division I Division II	Molar: MB cusp of the maxillary first occluding (by more than the width of a premolar) mesial to the MB groove of the mandibular first molar Canines: distal surface of the mandibular canine distal to the mesial surface of the maxillary canine by at least the width of a premolar	Division I: maxillary anteriors protruding facially from the mandibular anteriors, with deep over-bite; retrognathic profile Division II: maxillary central incisors either upright or retruded, and lateral incisors either tipped labially or overlapping the central incisors with deep overbite; mesognathic profile
Class III		Molar: MB cusp of the maxillary first occluding (by more than the width of a premolar) distal to the MB groove of the mandibular first molar Canines: distal surface of the mandibular mesial to the mesial surface of the maxillary by at least the width of a premolar	Mandibular incisors in complete crossbite; prognathic profile

*Note that this system deals with the classification of the permanent dentition.
MB, Mesiobuccal.

a general examination to a specific arch length analysis by radiographs, size of erupted permanent mandibular incisors, and prediction scheme by orthodontists. This analysis is performed during this period because there is no appreciable growth of the jaws anterior to the permanent first molars after age 7 or 8 without intervention.

MALOCCLUSION

Malocclusion is related to lack of an overall ideal form in the dentition while in centric occlusion. Rarely, malocclusion is directly associated with severe occlusal trauma. Malocclusion may affect patients by having a negative impact on their appearance and increasing their difficulty with homecare procedures. Poor homecare favors dental biofilm retention and increases the possibility that periodontal disease will affect the dentition with a malocclusion. Many malocclusions stem from hereditary factors.

An orthodontist working with other specialists, such as an orofacial myologist or a dental hygienist or speech therapist specifically trained in orofacial myology, can correct many malocclusions related to the teeth, and possibly to the rest of the masticatory system (see Figure 14-14). Thus, when correcting a malocclusion to achieve a more ideal form for the dentition, the occlusal functioning of the dentition also must be considered. Early intervention in the primary and mixed dentitions can prevent many malocclusions from occurring.

Approximately 80% of children and teenagers show some degree of malocclusion. The most common problems are crowding, a type of malocclusion that affects 40% of children and 80% of teenagers. The second most common type of malocclusion is excessive overjet of the maxillary incisors, which affects approximately 15% of children and teenagers.

Other factors are also involved in the consideration of smile design, such as gender, symmetry of color or shape, and position of teeth about the midline. A negative space (dark area) is also a consideration within an ideal smile and highlights the rest of the smile. The back of the mouth is considered a desired negative space because no light enters when standing. An example of an undesirable negative space is anterior or lateral crowded teeth creating shadows, a diastema, or even a loss of a prominent tooth that stands out from the whiteness of the rest of the teeth.

For a long time, clinicians have used Angle's classification of malocclusion, because it has not been adequately replaced by another system (Table 20-1). Although Angle's system has many inadequacies, it does serve to initially and simply address malocclusion. However, many malocclusions do not fit neatly into Angle's system, but this classification system of malocclusion does give clinicians a starting point in describing a particular case.

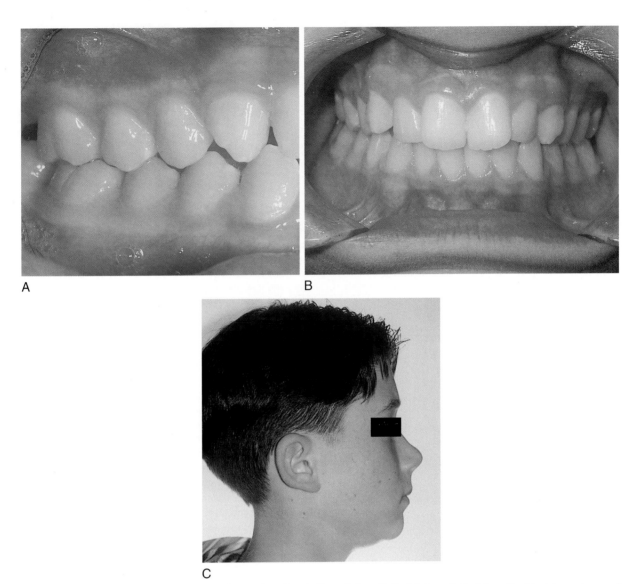

Figure 20-19 Class I malocclusion in a permanent dentition. **A:** Buccal view. **B:** Facial view. **C:** Facial profile. Mesiobuccal cusp of the maxillary first molar occludes with the mesiobuccal groove of the mandibular first molar, and the maxillary canine occludes with the distal half of the mandibular canine and the mesial half of the mandibular first premolar. Malocclusion in this case is due to dental malalignments, such as anterior crowding with a normal, or mesognathic, profile (see completed orthodontic therapy case in Figure 20-1). *(Courtesy of Dona M. Seely, DDS, MSD, Orthodontics, Bellevue and Seattle, WA.)*

CLASSIFICATION OF MALOCCLUSION

Angle's classification of malocclusion does *not* describe normal or even ideal occlusion, only malocclusion of the molars and canines. The basis of Angle's classification system was the simple hypothesis that the permanent maxillary first molar was the key to occlusion. Later, the relationship of the opposing canines was also evaluated. Therefore, Angle's system does not describe lateral or protrusive discrepancies, only those that are mesiodistally placed as related to the molars or canines.

Angle's system also assumes that a patient is occluding in a position of centric occlusion; thus it does not address the potential functional discrepancies between centric relation and centric occlusion. Thus, additional information is needed to more fully evaluate a patient's occlusion than just a basic classification system. It was also assumed that patients in malocclusion had all their permanent teeth. Thus, this classification system does not describe primary or mixed dentition malocclusions, although there are specific ways to classify the relationships of canines and molars in a primary dentition (discussed later).

In Angle's classification, most cases of malocclusion are grouped into three main classes, according to the position of the permanent maxillary first molar to the mandibular first molar. Thus, this classification system is based on the relationship of the teeth and *not* the skeletal considerations that are due to the disproportionate size or position of the jaws (discussed later). These three main classes are designated by Roman numerals (*I–III*), and they assume that both sides of the dentition are affected equally, unless specifically noted. Thus, separate classifications can be made, depending on which side is affected. Placement into Angle's system is only a classification, and *not* a complete diagnosis of a complex occlusal situation.

CLASS I MALOCCLUSION

All cases in a **Class I malocclusion** (neutroclusion) are characterized by an ideal mesiodistal relationship of the jaws and dental arches (Figure 20-19). In these cases of the permanent dentition, the mesiobuccal cusp of the maxillary first molar occludes with the mesiobuccal

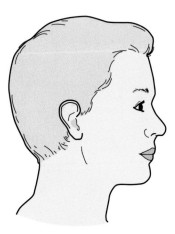

Mesognathic

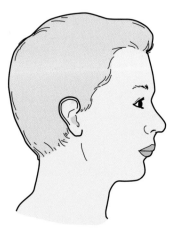

Retrognathic

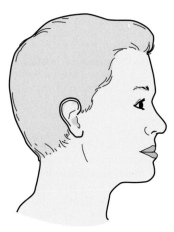

Prognathic

Figure 20-20 Three facial profiles: mesognathic, retrognathic, and prognathic, which can be measured by the **gnathic index** (or alveolar index), that is, the ratio of the distance from the middle of the nasion to the basion. This gives the degree of prominence of the maxilla as opposed to the mandible jaw. Note that an index below 98 is retrognathic, from 98 to 103 is mesognathic, and above 103 is prognathic.

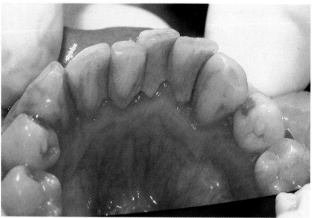

Figure 20-21 Mesial drift is a normal, natural movement phenomenon in which all the teeth move slightly toward the midline of the oral cavity over time. It can cause crowding, late in life, of a once-perfect dentition, and may lead to poor homecare in the area of crowding, as the presence of calculus demonstrates.

groove of the mandibular first molar. In relation to the opposing canines, the maxillary canine occludes with the distal half of the mandibular canine and the mesial half of the mandibular first premolar.

Class I malocclusion is due to dental malalignments, such as crowding ("crooked teeth") or spacing within normal jaws (see Figure 20-19). These patients have a normal facial profile, described by many clinicians with the older term mesognathic. The facial profile in centric occlusion has slightly protruded jaws, giving the facial outline a relatively flat appearance or straight profile (Figure 20-20); see discussion of later cases for the differing facial profiles.

Problems with crowding, in which the teeth are out of line within the dental arch, occur because of a disproportion between the size of the teeth and arch size. Spacing problems occur within an arch where the teeth are small relative to the size of the arch or where teeth are missing. Included in this class of malocclusion is crowding that occurs because of **mesial drift** as the dentition ages (Figure 20-21; see Chapter 14). Mesial drift, or physiological drift, is a normal, natural movement phenomenon in which all the teeth move slightly toward the midline of the oral cavity over time. This can cause crowding of a once-perfect dentition late in life. It occurs rather slowly, depending mostly on the degree of wear of the contact points between adjacent teeth and on the number of missing teeth. Overall, drift distances usually total no more than 1 cm over a lifetime. However, even this small amount may eventually lead to poor homecare and esthetics in the area of crowding.

Class I cases frequently have some protrusive or retrusive discrepancies in the anterior teeth, but other classes can also have these discrepancies (Figure 20-22). Within this grouping, overbites may be slight, moderate, or severe. Certain Class I cases have an open bite, in which the anterior teeth do not occlude (see Figure 16-8, *B*; for other class involvement, see Figure 20-26, *B*). In addition, Class I cases may have an end-to-end bite, or edge-to-edge bite, in which the teeth occlude without the maxillary teeth overlapping the mandibular teeth. With this type of occlusion, the anterior teeth of both jaws meet along their incisal edges when the teeth are in centric occlusion. An end-to-end bite can occur both anteriorly and posteriorly, unilaterally or bilaterally.

Class I cases can also include a crossbite, which occurs when a mandibular tooth or teeth are placed facially to the maxillary teeth (for other class involvement, see Figure 20-26, *A* and *B*). A crossbite can occur either anteriorly or posteriorly, unilaterally or bilaterally.

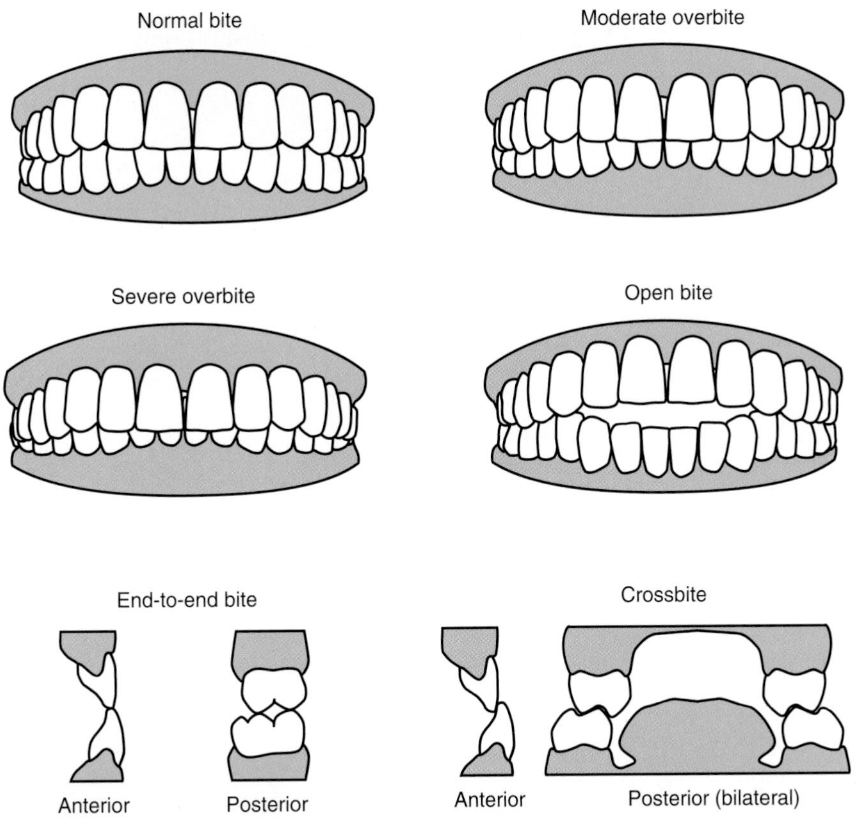

Normal bite

Moderate overbite

Severe overbite

Open bite

End-to-end bite

Crossbite

Anterior   Posterior

Anterior   Posterior (bilateral)

Figure 20-22 Slight, moderate, and severe overbites; open bite, end-to-end bites, and crossbites.

Individual teeth may be slightly deviated labially or lingually relative to the adjoining teeth in the same arch; they may be in labioversion or linguoversion.

CLASS II MALOCCLUSION

All cases in Class II malocclusion (distoclusion) in the permanent dentition are characterized by the mesiobuccal cusp of the maxillary first molar occluding (by more than the width of a premolar) mesial to the mesiobuccal groove of the mandibular first molar (Figure 20-23). The distal surface of the mandibular canine is distal to the mesial surface of the maxillary canine by at least the width of a premolar. A tendency to this type of malocclusion (less than the width of a premolar) can be noted. The major group of Class II malocclusion has two subgroups, division I and division II, based on the position of the anteriors, shape of the palate, and resulting facial profile.

In Class II malocclusion, division I in the permanent dentition, the maxillary anteriors protrude facially from the mandibular anteriors (Figure 20-24). The mandibular incisors usually overerupt, causing a severe overbite (deep overbite). The palate is often narrow and V-shaped. The facial profile shows an underbite, protruding upper lip, or recessive mandible and chin, or convex profile. The older term for describing the facial profile in Class II, division I is retrognathic (see Figure 20-20).

In Class II malocclusion, division II in a permanent dentition, the molars are in the same position, but rather than having protrusive maxillary anteriors, the maxillary central incisors are either upright or retruded (Figure 20-25). The maxillary lateral incisors are either tipped labially or overlap the central incisors. Overbite is severe (deep overbite), yet the palate is either normal or wide compared with

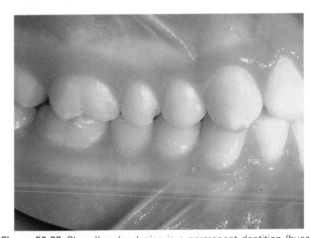

Figure 20-23 Class II malocclusion in a permanent dentition (buccal view). Mesiobuccal cusp of the maxillary first molar is occluding (by more than the width of a premolar) mesial to the mesiobuccal groove of the mandibular first molar, and the distal surface of the mandibular canine is distal to the mesial surface of the maxillary canine by at least the width of a premolar. *(Courtesy of Dona M. Seely, DDS, MSD, Orthodontics, Bellevue and Seattle, WA.)*

division I. The facial profile for Class II, division II is usually a normal or mesognathic profile, often with a rather prominent chin (see Figure 20-20).

CLASS III MALOCCLUSION

In all cases of a Class III malocclusion (mesioclusion) in a permanent dentition, the mesiobuccal cusp of the maxillary first molar occludes (by more than the width of a premolar) distal to the mesiobuccal

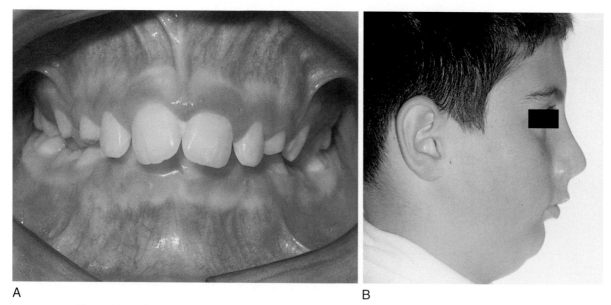

A

B

Figure 20-24 Class II malocclusion, division I in a permanent dentition. **A:** Facial view. **B:** Facial profile. Maxillary anteriors also protrude facially from the mandibular anteriors, causing a deep overbite, and the facial profile is convex, or retrognathic. *(Courtesy of Dona M. Seely, DDS, MSD, Orthodontics, Bellevue and Seattle, WA.)*

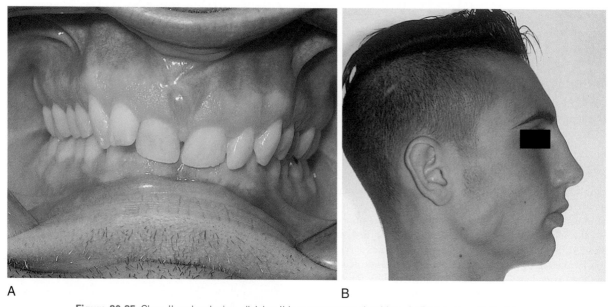

A

B

Figure 20-25 Class II malocclusion, division II in a permanent dentition. **A:** Facial view. **B:** Facial profile. Central incisors are in a retruded position, and the lateral incisors are tipped labially, with a deep overbite, but the facial profile is normal, or mesognathic. *(Courtesy of Dona M. Seely, DDS, MSD, Orthodontics, Bellevue and Seattle, WA.)*

groove of the mandibular first molar (Figure 20-26). The distal surface of the mandibular canine is mesial to the mesial surface of the maxillary canine by at least the width of a premolar.

In comparison with Class II, division I cases, in which the maxillary incisors are flared mesially, the mandibular incisors are usually in complete crossbite. In most cases, the mandibular incisors are also inclined lingually despite the crossbite. The facial profile usually shows a rather prominent mandible and possibly a normal or even retrusive maxilla, thus a concave profile. The older term that describes the facial profile with a Class III malocclusion is prognathic (see Figure 20-20). A tendency to this type of malocclusion (less than the width of a premolar) can be noted.

SUBDIVISIONS OF MALOCCLUSION

Angle's system recognized that a case of malocclusion did occasionally have differing classifications on each side of the dentition. These asymmetrical cases are labeled *subdivisions* and usually demonstrate the main characteristics of the main class and division.

Thus, Angle's classification of malocclusion allows for a Class II malocclusion, division I subdivision in which the patient has both a Class II and Class I malocclusion, showing a division I anterior pattern. Another situation that may present is a Class II malocclusion, division II subdivision, in which a patient has both a Class II and Class I, showing a division II anterior pattern. Finally, yet another situation that may

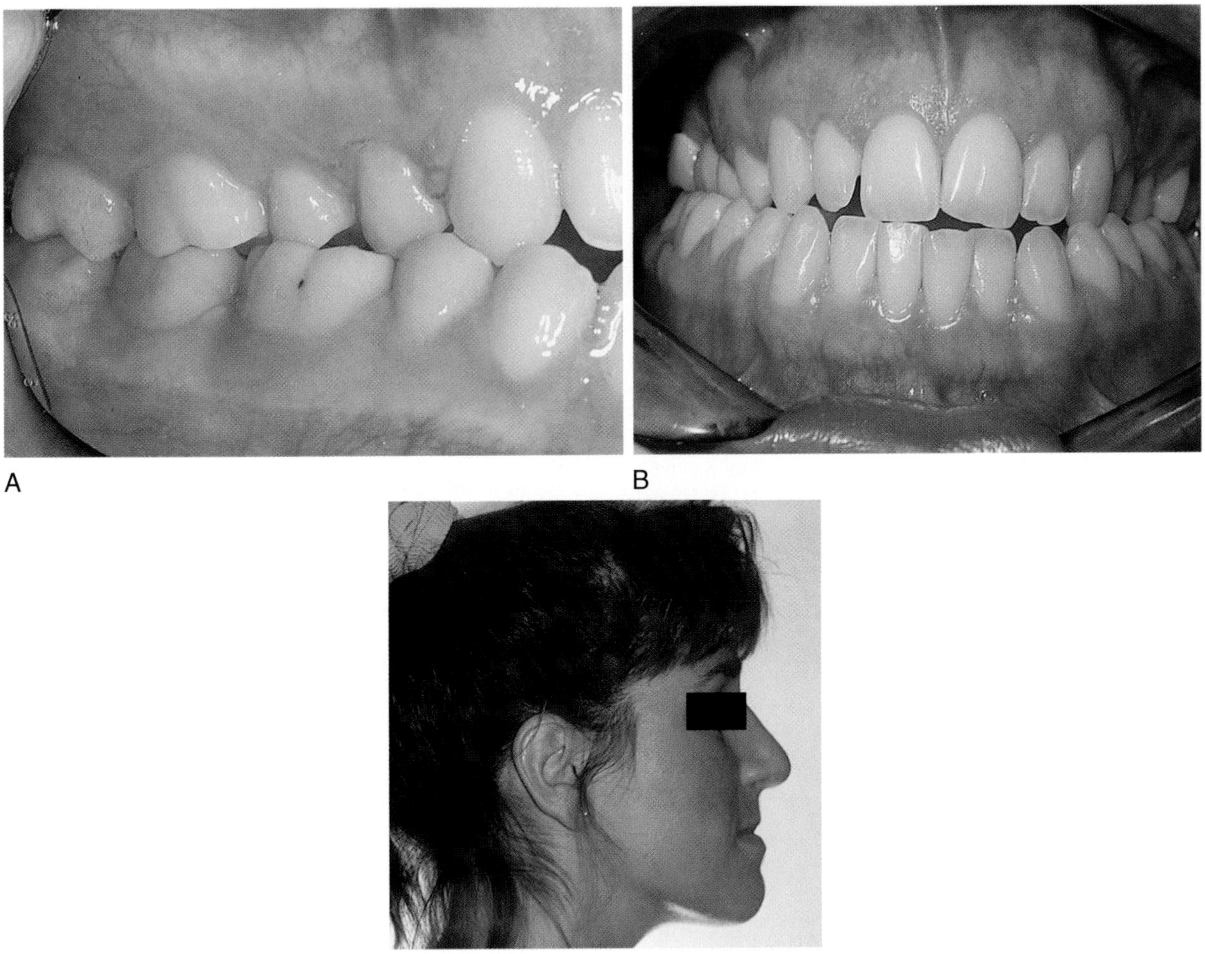

A

B

C

Figure 20-26 Class III malocclusion in a permanent dentition. **A:** Buccal view. **B:** Facial view. **C:** Facial profile. Mesiobuccal cusp of the maxillary first molar is occluding (by more than the width of a premolar) distal to the buccal groove of the mandibular first molar, and the distal surface of the mandibular canine is mesial to the mesial surface of the maxillary canine by at least the width of a premolar. Mandibular incisors are also in crossbite, as are other teeth, and the facial profile is concave, or prognathic. *(Courtesy of Dona M. Seely, DDS, MSD, Orthodontics, Bellevue and Seattle, WA.)*

present is a Class III malocclusion subdivision, in which a patient has both a Class III and Class I malocclusion on each side of the dentition.

SKELETAL CONSIDERATIONS

Many malocclusions are linked not only to the teeth, such as in Angle's classification of malocclusion, but also to discrepancies between the maxilla and mandible, which then affect the occlusion of the teeth. These skeletal abnormalities of the jaws can be corrected by an oral surgeon, working with an orthodontist; orthodontic therapy with tooth movement alone is not effective. In many cases, timely orthodontic intervention in young children, using certain orthodontic appliances, can direct bone growth of the jaws by arch expansion and by increasing arch length and level. These interventions may prevent the need for surgical intervention. In adults and those patients whose bone growth is complete, however, orthognathic surgery may be the only remedy for jaw discrepancies, because orthodontic appliances do not in themselves produce ideal results.

Generally, orthodontic patients requiring orthognathic surgical intervention undergo an initial period of orthodontic treatment before surgery so that the teeth occlude properly after surgery. Any orthodontic appliances used to align the teeth before surgery are left in place during the surgical procedure to stabilize the teeth and

jaws. After surgery, a period of follow-up orthodontic treatment helps achieve the final alignment of the teeth.

Most commonly corrected problems include a protruding or retruding chin, unsightly display of gingiva superior to the maxillary anterior teeth, an inability to achieve resting lip closure, and an overall elongation of the face. TMDs may also be minimized with surgery in severe cases (see Chapter 19).

Three basic spatial planes are involved in the classification of skeletal malocclusions: horizontal, vertical, and transverse. Horizontal malocclusions are further classified as either Class II or Class III malocclusions, similar to Angle's classification system. Vertical malocclusions include open bites and severe overbites. Transverse malocclusions include crossbites. Most patients undergoing orthognathic surgery have a combination of these types of skeletal malocclusions.

PARAFUNCTIONAL HABITS AND MYOFUNCTIONAL CONSIDERATIONS

Parafunctional habits are those movements of the mandible that are *not* within the normal ROM associated with mastication, speech, or respiratory movements. Thus, these habits occur more commonly

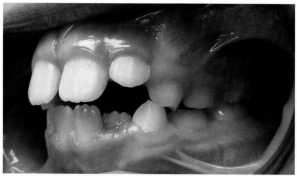

Figure 20-27 Primary canines in an end-to-end bite within a mixed dentition showing wear facets on the cusps. This is due to incorrect tongue posturing and parafunctional jaw patterns that can be addressed with orofacial myofunctional therapy by an orofacial myologist, especially before full disruption of the permanent dentition. *(Courtesy of Kimberly K. Benkert, RDH, BSDH, MPH, COM; Midwest Orofacial Myology, a Division of MYO USA, Inc., Glen Ellyn, IL.)*

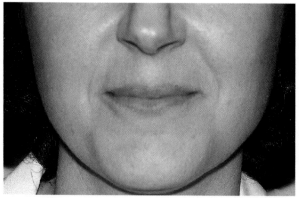

Figure 20-28 Overdevelopment of the masseter muscles with bilateral enlargement. Patient has a related history of the parafunctional habit of bruxism (grinding). *(From Fehrenbach MJ, Herring SW. Illustrated Anatomy of the Head and Neck, ed 3. WB Saunders, Philadelphia, 2007.)*

and in longer duration than motions associated with normal functioning.

Parafunctional habits include clenching the teeth in centric occlusion or a pattern deviation for long periods, without breaking into a mandibular rest position or interocclusal clearance. Grinding the teeth, or bruxism, is also a parafunctional habit. Grinding the teeth involves forceful meshing of the teeth, often causing audible noises. Attrition of the masticatory surfaces of differing levels is evident in cases of grinding, causing *wear facets*, especially in the canines' cusp tips (Figure 20-27 and see Figure 20-8, **Chapters 16 and 17**).

In contrast to the resting position discussed earlier, bracing is the sustained contraction, or tightening, of the musculature. With bracing, there is sustained contraction of muscles and suctioning of the buccal mucosa against the dentition without work purpose, and possibly rigid and sustained pressure of the tongue against the palate, mandible, and/or dentition while at rest or during function.

Parafunctional habits can be related to **gingival recession** and **abfraction** including a sheering or flaking of the enamel surface (see **Chapter 10** and Figure 12-1, *B*). Also, in many cases of parafunctional habits, a larger area of the **buccal mucosa** than just the **linea alba** can become **hyperkeratinized** (see Figure 9-6).

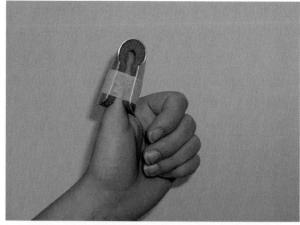

Figure 20-29 An intervention in prolonged nonnutritive sucking includes a digit cover (splint) during the night in order to fully interrupt and stop the sucking pattern of the digit as part of a behavior modification program. *(Courtesy of Kimberly K. Benkert, RDH, BSDH, MPH, COM; Midwest Orofacial Myology, a Division of MYO USA, Inc., Glen Ellyn, IL.)*

These parafunctional habits are often subconscious and occur when a person is sleeping or concentrating deeply, such as when driving, reading, watching television, or using the computer. Normally, around 20 to 30 pounds per square inch are exerted on molars during mastication, but grinders, especially at night without restraint, can exert as much as 200 pounds per square inch on their teeth. A person with these habits may have overdeveloped **masseter muscles** and consider it normal to feel facial and masticatory tension (Figure 20-28). Stress may be a factor in the etiology of these habits, although it is not always present. Parafunctional habits may be linked to the individual ways a person processes neurological impulses; about 10% to 15% of adults grind their teeth moderately to severely.

Patients who grind their teeth can wear a professionally made flatplane, nonrepositioning oral splint, or *nightguard* during waking hours or when sleeping. This oral splint consists of a removable hard plastic, acrylic or silicone appliance that covers the dental arch (or arches). This device can protect the teeth from further damage, such as attrition or recession from abfraction, and can reduce the occlusal stress of the habit throughout the dentition. In contrast, individuals who brace or clench need an oral splint or *nightguard* made of a softer material in order to provide a cushion to the teeth. An oromotor chewing appliance also can be worn during the daytime or nighttime to cushion and protect the buccal, lingual, and occlusal surfaces of the teeth.

The parafunctional habit of nonnutritive sucking of the thumb or fingers in children or young adults can cause an excessive anterior overjet, lips irreversibly stretched by protruding teeth, a deep narrow palate, and a callus on the thumb or fingers. Again, this activity, similar to other parafunctional habits, is largely unconscious.

The main suggested intervention in prolonged nonnutritive sucking includes a behavior modification program using auto-suggestion affirmations, gentle conscious reminders, a digit cover during the night in order to fully interrupt and stop the sucking pattern of the digit (Figure 20-29). This evidence-based Rapid Elimination Program (REP) is extremely effective in gently increasing the child's awareness of the habit by gently discussing and handling the problem. A REP may be initiated by the time the child is 4 years of age, however, it is also documented to work on ages as early as 2.5 to 3 years old.

Similar problems are associated with the prolonged overuse of pacifiers in young children. A pacifier should be taken away by age 12 to 14 months before disruption of the occlusion occurs. A REP is extremely effective when used with individuals having extended use of the pacifier or any other non-nutritive sucking, chronic nail biting, hair chewing, or other noxious oral related habit. Contrary to popular belief, research shows that no emotional trauma results from stopping prolonged nonnutritive sucking in children.

Severe dentofacial functional and structural changes can occur due to parafunctional habits of digit sucking, lip biting, chronic nail biting, and other prolonged noxious parafunctional and oral behavioral habits. Elimination of those parafunctional and noxious oral habits at an earlier age reduces the risk of negative changes to the dentition and assists in enhancing the normal growth and developmental patterns. Muscle balance, appropriate orofacial muscle pressures, and correct tongue function assist with guided growth and development of the dentition, lower third of the face, and overall orofacial environment. Oromotor patterns of the tongue, lips, resting posture, along with the mandibular patterns related to chewing, swallowing, and functional speech patterning can be normalized as digit sucking and/or parafunctional patterns are eliminated.

Another consideration when discussing parafunctional habits and occlusion is orofacial myology, which is the study and therapeutic treatment of the orofacial musculature and function to improve muscle balance, function, and tonicity. It focuses on establishment of correct functional activities of the tongue, lips, and mandible to enable normal growth, and so that development may take place in a stable, homeostatic environment. It may include treatment of parafunctional habits for the elimination of noxious oral habits, TMD related to bruxism, clenching, bracing, ROM activities, or postural habits.

Individuals practicing in this specialty area are licensed in dental hygiene, dentistry, and speech pathology. The certified orofacial myologist has been trained to identify, diagnose, and treat an orofacial myofunctional disorder (OMD) (Figure 20-30). Orofacial myologists work in a collaborative and team approach with dental professionals, especially orthodontists, periodontists, oral surgeons, and other health professionals such as speech pathologists, physical therapists, and occupational therapists.

OMDs include any disturbances in the normal, physiological functioning of the musculature of the orofacial environment, including muscles of the tongue, face, head, neck, and TMJ region, as well as functional activities of the tongue, lips, and mandible. In addition, OMD includes parafunctional habits that apply inappropriate pressures to the orofacial musculature or dentition such as tongue thrusting, clenching, bracing, bruxism, digit sucking, chronic nail biting, lip biting or chewing.

The most common OMD cited by many orofacial myologists relative to occlusion is tongue thrusting, which is the functional deviations occurring with habitual incorrect placement and use of the tongue, lips, and mandible during physiological rest, chewing, swallowing, and/or functional speech patterning. During the act of swallowing, rest posture, and functional speech patterning, the tongue influences and contributes to the orofacial environment and formation of the dental arches. The retained infantile habit of tongue thrusting in between the dental pads or the maladaptive pattern of resting it against or between the teeth to form an oral seal creates abnormal pressures/forces.

Incorrect functional patterns of resting position, chewing, swallowing, or speech movements have the ability to create occlusal and developmental facial change. As a result, the term tongue thrusting is used when describing an open mouth resting posture, oral breathing patterns related to lip incompetence, anterior or posterior open bite with tongue protrusion, other malocclusions where the tongue is an interference, deformation of the jaw functional patterns, abnormal functioning of the tongue, lips, ROM patterns of the mandible as they relate to chewing, swallowing, and speech functional patterning.

Another OMD cited by many orofacial myologists is an incorrect resting position of the lips, which can affect the position of the anterior teeth and facial esthetics. Also, an **interlabial gap** is recorded, which is the distance between the inferior border of the upper lip and the superior border of the lower lip in a physiologic resting position.

The competency of the lips to maintain a lip seal at rest can affect the position of the maxillary incisors, canines and even the premolars. Competent lips, buccinator, masseter, and mentalis action allow balanced muscle function with appropriate labial and buccal pressure against the teeth to maintain normal anterior and arch formation, curvature and inclination. Incompetent lips or failure to provide a lip seal does not control the labial pressures (Figure 20-31). When the tongue is also positioned incorrectly in an anterior or lateral/posture with additional force applied against the arch form and lack of pressure against the palate the curvature may change and the inclination increase allowing the maxillary incisors to lie in front of the lower lip, exaggerating already buccally inclined teeth or teeth that have not been able to fully erupt into position. When the tongue rests in between the teeth, an open bite development is often seen.

The tongue posture may be in the anterior, lateral or posterior positions. In the posterior when the tongue overlaps the dentition, the teeth often remain unerupted altering the normal arch curvature development or preventing complete eruption of the posterior teeth. The mandible may be more retruded during development in these situations or when a parafunctional habit, such as digit sucking, is present due to the excessive pressures of the thumb or hand resting against the mandible or the increased muscle activation of the mentalis muscle to help support an incompetent or everted lower lip pattern (see Figure 20-32). Tongue thrusting may also be associated with each of these problems, further adding to the presence of orofacial muscle imbalances. In comparison, overactive and imbalanced tight lips can cause the maxillary incisors to become lingually inclined.

Speech functional movement problems may be associated with OMDs. Many times these are only considered to be important if a lisping pattern is present, and often professionals assume traditional articulation speech therapy is the only answer. When disruptive oromotor and myofunctional patterns are present, it is these functional movements or patterning of the tongue, lip and jaw motions that create the most significant impairment to correct speech production. It is also important with functional speech pattern evaluation to also assess the balanced and sustainable rest posture of the tongue, lips, and mandible.

Of major importance seems to be the resting posture of the lips and tongue. Habitual open mouth rest posture does not allow the tongue to provide the valuable pressure in the palate that helps to widen the maxillary arch along with stimulating circulation and oxygenation to the palatal tissues. The palatal tissues appear cyanotic when lack of normalized pressures from the tongue is present. The palatal tissue color becomes more normalized once the tongue posture and neuromuscular functional patterning of the tongue improves.

Another issue is the length of the lingual frenulum. If the lingual frenum is restricted, as with **ankyloglossia**, it limits the possibility of creating appropriate pressure against the maxillary arch for normal expansion (see Figure 5-12). It also increases the risk factors of having incorrect functional speech patterns and articulation problems. Breathing issues, as well as untreated asthma and allergies, must also be addressed in order to reduce oromotor and orofacial myofunctional

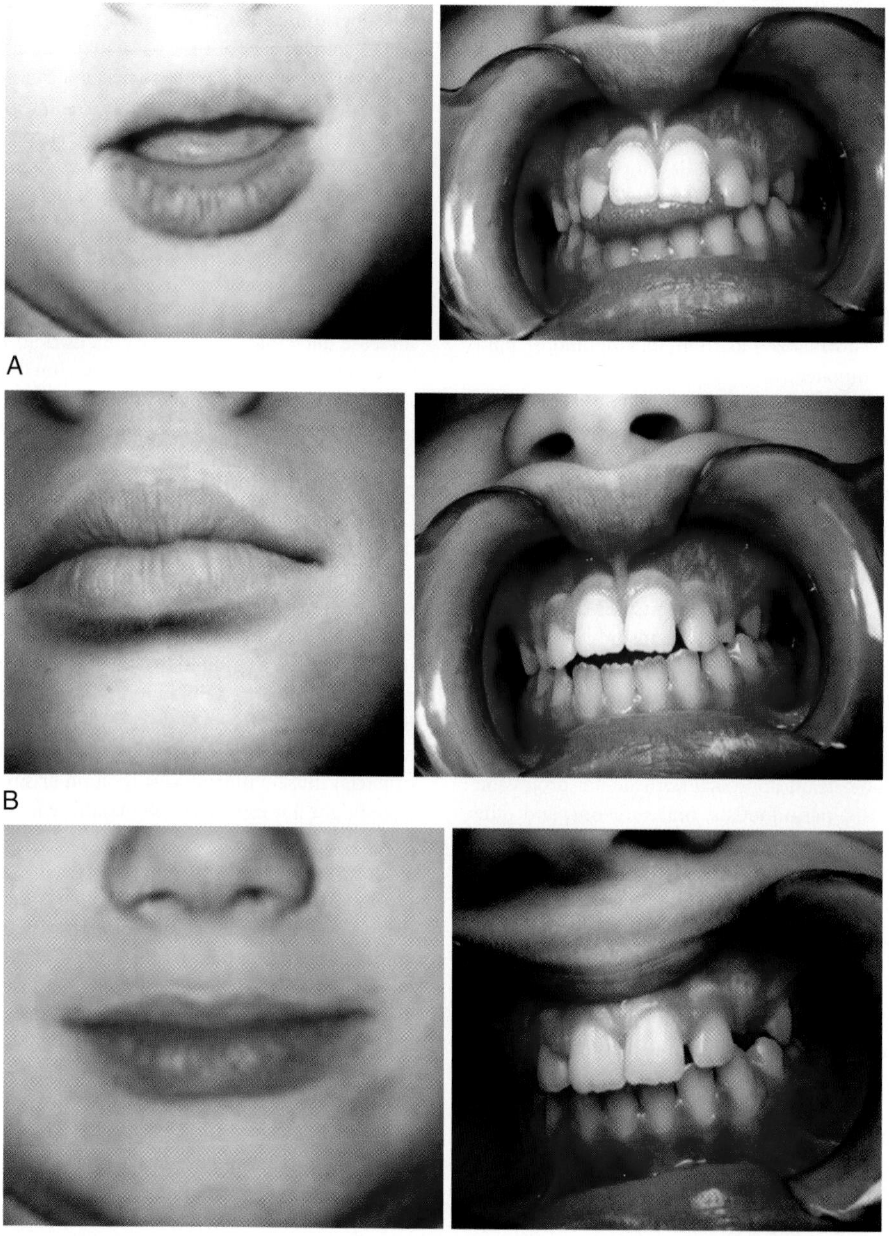

Figure 20-30 Before (**A**) and after six weeks of orofacial myofunctional therapy (**B**) and then after twelve weeks of therapy (**C**) *(Courtesy of Kimberly K. Benkert, RDH, BSDH, MPH, COM; Midwest Orofacial Myology, a Division of MYO USA, Inc., Glen Ellyn, IL.)*

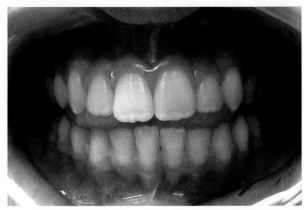

Figure 20-31 Incompetent lips or failure to provide a lip seal, which can affect the position of the maxillary incisors, canines and even the premolars. Note the dehydration of anterior teeth at incisal edges due to open mouth resting posture of the lips. *(Courtesy of Kimberly K. Benkert, RDH, BSDH, MPH, COM; Midwest Orofacial Myology, a Division of MYO USA, Inc., Glen Ellyn, IL.)*

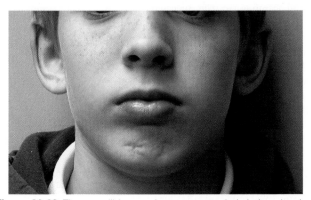

Figure 20-32 The mandible may be more retruded during development with the increased muscle activation of the mentalis muscle to help support an incompetent or everted lower lip pattern. *(Courtesy of Kimberly K. Benkert, RDH, BSDH, MPH, COM; Midwest Orofacial Myology, a Division of MYO USA, Inc., Glen Ellyn, IL.)*

risk factors since they present an increased challenge in achieving proper tongue, lips and mandibular resting posture; it is important to note that these health issues seem to be increasing in all ages of the population. A patent airway is always a major goal; airway structures, especially tonsils, adenoids, and nasal turbinates are included in the assessment and examination process.

After a differential diagnosis, the orofacial myologist prepares a patient-centered treatment plan taking into account collaboration with other oral and health care professionals and institutes orofacial myofunctional therapy (OMT). This consists of protocols, which include therapeutic neuromuscular training/reeducation incorporating oromotor exercises and activities, behavior modification and behavioral retraining, elimination of parafunctional habits/patterns, outcome evaluations and follow-up. These protocols may include neuromuscular retraining programs and elimination of digit sucking, muscle bracing, clenching, bruxism, and other noxious oral habits preventing the tongue, lips, and mandible from maintaining their physiologic rest and correct functional patterns discussed earlier. It includes establishing an appropriate interocclusal clearance and retraining the resting posture of the tongue, lips, and mandible. It means also creating correct bilateral chewing patterns, negative air pressure swallowing, functional eating patterns, and correct ROM of the mandible, as well as correct tongue, lip, and jaw movements for correct functional speech patterning.

An evidence-based and individualized, patient-centered treatment plan involves working in a collaborative manner with the other health professionals treating the patient (as discussed earlier). It includes making the patient aware of the OMD, retraining neuromuscular patterns, retraining the oromotor and muscular functions, toning appropriate musculature, and helping instruct the patient how to habituate the newly established patterns for long-term stability. Orofacial myologists believe early identification and treatment is the best advantage, but individuals at any age can benefit from therapy. Individuals with special needs and syndromes also may benefit significantly from including an OMT program into their health treatment plan.

Orofacial myolofunctional therapy has a traceable history through dental/dental hygiene and speech professions. It is an evolving area of specialization that has the potential of positively impacting the overall orofacial and oromotor function and even strongly influence the structures of the orofacial environment. An orofacial myofunctional and parafunctional habit pattern assessment should be incorporated into every examination process by dental hygienists, dentists, speech pathologists, and physicians to benefit from this area of specialized treatment.

Bibliography

Fehrenbach MJ, Herring SW: *Illustrated Anatomy of the Head and Neck,* ed 2, Phildelphia, 2007, WB Saunders.

Ibsen OAC, Phelan JA: *Oral Pathology for Dental Hygienists,* ed 5, Philadelphia, 2009, WB Saunders.

Mosby: *Mosby's Dental Dictionary,* ed 2, St Louis, 2007, Mosby.

Nanci A: *Ten Cate's Oral Histology,* ed 7, St Louis, 2008, Mosby.

Nelson S: *Wheeler's Dental Anatomy, Physiology and Occlusions,* ed 9, Philadelphia, 2009, WB Saunders.

Newman MG, Takei HH, Carranza FA: *Clinical Periodontology,* ed 7, Philadelphia, 2008, WB Saunders.

Okeson JP: *Management of Temporomandibular Disorders and Occlusion,* ed 6, St Louis, 2008, Elsevier.

Perry DA, Beemsterboer PL, Taggart EJ: *Clinical Periodontology for Dental Hygienists*, ed 3, Philadelphia, 2006, WB Saunders.

Stevens A, Lowe J: *Human Histology,* ed 3, St Louis, 2005, Mosby.

Young B, Heath JW: *Wheater's Functional Histology,* ed 5, 2006, Churchill Livingstone.

Arambawatta K, Peiris R, Nanayakkara D: Morphology of the cemento-enamel junction in premolar teeth. *J Oral Sci* 51(4):623–627.

Bosshardt DD, Lang NP: The junctional epithelium: from health to disease, *J Dent Res* 84(1):9–20, 2005.

Brocklehurst PR, Baker SR, Speight PM: Oral cancer screening: what have we learnt and what is there still to achieve? *Future Oncol* 6(2):299–304, 2010.

Cogulu D, Becerik S, Emingil G, et al: Oral rehabilitation of a patient with amelogenesis imperfecta, *Pediatr Dent* 31(7):523–527, 2009.

Coppe C, Zhang Y: Den Besten PK: Characterization of primary dental pulp cells in vitro, *Pediatr Dent* 31(7):467–471, 2009.

Dahlström L, Carlsson GE: Temporomandibular disorders and oral health-related quality of life. A systematic review, *Acta Odontol Scand* 68(2):80–85, 2010.

Dimitriu B, Vârlan C, Suciu I, et al: Current considerations concerning endodontically treated teeth: alteration of hard dental tissues and biomechanical properties following endodontic therapy, *J Med Life* 2(1):60–65, 2009.

Fleischmannova J, Matalova E, Sharpe PT, et al: Formation of the tooth-bone interface, *J Dent Res* 89(2):108–815, 2010.

Ghaname ES, Ritter AV, Heymann HO, et al: Correlation between laser fluorescence readings and volume of tooth preparation in incipient occlusal caries in vitro, *J Esthet Restor Dent* (1):31–39, 2010.

Gordan VV, Bader JD, Garvan CW, et al: Restorative treatment thresholds for occlusal primary caries among dentists in the dental practice-based research network, *J Am Dent Assoc* 141(2):171–184, 2010.

Huang GT: Pulp and dentin tissue engineering and regeneration: current progress, *Regen Med* 4(5):697–707, 2009.

Iorgulescu G: Saliva between normal and pathological. Important factors in determining systemic and oral health, *J Med Life* 2(3):303–307, 2009.

Martin-Biedma B, Gonzalez-Gonzalez T, Lopes M, et al: Colorimeter and scanning electron microscopy analysis of teeth submitted to internal bleaching, *J Endod* 36(2):334–337, 2010.

Martinez EF, da Silva LA, Furuse C, et al: Dentin matrix protein 1 (DMP1) expression in developing human teeth, *Braz Dent J* 20(5):365–369, 2009.

Mason RM: A retrospective and prospective view of orofacial myology, *Int J Orofacial Myology* 34:5–14, 2008.

Miller JR, Mancl L: Risk factors for the occurrence and prevention of temporomandibular joint and muscle disorders: lessons from 2 recent studies, *Am J Orthod Dentofacial Orthop* 134(4):537–542, 2008.

Patil MS, Patil SB, Acharya AB, et al: Palatine rugae and their significance in clinical dentistry: a review of the literature, *J Am Dent Assoc* 139(11):1471–1478, 2008.

Pessoa RS, Oliveira SR, Menezes HH, de Magalhaes D: Effects of platelet-rich plasma on healing of alveolar socket: split-mouth histological and histometric evaluation in *Cebus apella* monkeys, *Indian J Dent Res* 20(4):442–447, 2009.

Rath-Deschner B, Daratsianos N, Duhr S, et al: The significance of RUNX2 in postnatal development of the mandibular condyle, *J Orofac Orthop* 71(1):17–23, 2010.

Rinaldi JC, Arana-Chavez VE: Ultrastructure of the interface between periodontal tissues and titanium mini-implants, *Angle Orthod* 80(3):459–465, 2010.

Ricucci D, Lin LM, Spangberg LS: Wound healing of apical tissues after root canal therapy: a long-term clinical, radiographic, and histopathologic observation study, *Oral Surg Oral Med Oral Pathol Oral Radiol Endod* 108(4):609–621, 2009.

Shashikiran ND, Babaji P, Reddy W: Double facial and a lingual trace talon cusps: a case report, *J Indian Soc Pedod Prev Dent* 23:89–91, 2005.

Terrer E, Raskin A, Koubi S, et al: A new concept in restorative dentistry: LIFEDT-light-induced fluorescence evaluator for diagnosis and treatment: part 2-treatment of dentinal caries, *J Contemp Dent Pract* 11(1):E095–E102, 2010.

Vidal R, Greenwell H, Hill M, et al: Success rate of immediate implants placed and restored by novice operators, *Implant Dent* 19(1):81–90, 2010.

Villar CC, Cochran DL: Regeneration of periodontal tissues: guided tissue regeneration, *Dent Clin North Am* 54(1):73–92, 2010.

Wenzel A, Møystad A: Work flow with digital intraoral radiography: a systematic review, *Acta Odontol Scand* 68(2):106–108, 2010.

Glossary

A

Abfraction (ab-frak-**shen)** Hard tooth tissue loss from tensile and compressive forces during tooth flexure.

Abrasion (u-brey-**zhun)** Hard tooth tissue loss caused by friction from toothbrushing and/or toothpaste.

Accessory canals Extra openings located on lateral parts of roots.

Accessory root Extra root on tooth.

Acellular cementum First layers of cementum deposited without embedded cementocytes.

Acinus (plural, acini) (as-i-nus, **as-**i-ny) Group of secretory cells of salivary gland.

Active eruption Vertical tooth movement through oral tissue.

Adipose connective tissue (ad-i-pose) Specialized connective tissue composed of fat, little matrix, adipocytes.

Afferent vessels (af-er-int) Lymphatic vessels that allow flow of lymph into lymph node.

Ala (plural, alae) (ah-lah, **a-**lay) Winglike cartilaginous structure bounding nares laterally.

Alveolar bone (al-vee-o-lar) Part of maxilla or mandible that supports teeth.

Alveolar bone proper Bone lining alveolus.

Alveolar crest Most cervical rim of alveolar bone proper.

Alveolar crest group Alveodental ligament subgroup originating in alveolar crest to insert into cervical cementum.

Alveolar mucosa Oral mucosa immediately apical to mucogingival junction.

Alveolar process Dental arch or tooth-bearing part of each jaw that contains alveoli.

Alveolodental ligament (al-vee-o-lo-**den-**tl) Main principal fiber group with subgroups: alveolar crest, horizontal, oblique, apical, interradicular.

Alveolus (plural, alveoli) (al-vee-o-lus, al-**vee-**o-lie) Socket of tooth.

Ameloblasts (ah-mel-oh-blasts) Cells that differentiate from preameloblasts to form enamel during amelogenesis.

Amelogenesis (ah-mel-oh-**jen-**i-sis) Apposition of enamel matrix by ameloblasts.

Amelogenesis imperfecta (im-per-fek-**tah) Hereditary enamel dysplasia with absent or thin enamel.

Amniocentesis (am-nee-o-sen-**tee-**sis) Prenatal diagnostic procedure sampling amniotic fluid.

Amniotic cavity (am-nee-**ot-**ik) Fluid-filled cavity facing epiblast layer.

Anaphase (an-ah-faz) Third phase of mitosis with separation of two chromatids of each chromosome and migration.

Anatomical crown Part of crown covered by enamel.

Anatomical root Part of root covered by cementum.

Anchoring collagen fibers Fibers from connective tissue involved in basement membrane.

Angle of the mandible Thickened area on posterior-inferior border of mandibular ramus.

Angle's classification of malocclusion System used to initially classify malocclusion.

Ankyloglossia (ang-kel-o-**gloss-**ee-ah) Lingual frenum with abnormally short attachment.

Anodontia (an-ah-**don-**she-ah) Absence of single tooth or multiple teeth owing to lack of initiation.

Anterior teeth Incisors and canines at front of the oral cavity.

Anterior faucial pillar (faw-shawl) Anterior lateral folds of tissue in pharynx created by underlying muscle forming the fauces.

Apex of the nose Tip of nose.

Apical foramen (ay-pi-kl for-**ay-**men) Opening from pulp near apex of tooth.

Apical group Alveolodental ligament subgroup radiating apically from cementum to insert into alveolar bone proper.

Apposition (ap-oh-**zish-**in) Layered growth of a firm or hard tissue such as cartilage, bone, enamel, dentin, cementum.

Appositional growth (ap-oh-**zish-**in-al) Growth by addition of layers to outside of tissue mass.

Arrest lines Smooth, stained microscopic lines caused by apposition in cartilage, bone, cementum.

Articular eminence (ar-tik-**you-ler) Rounded protuberance on inferior aspect of zygomatic process for articulation of temporomandibular joint.

Articular fossa Depression on inferior aspect of temporal bone for articulation of temporomandibular joint.

Articulating surface of the condyle (ar-tik-**you-late-ing **kon-**dyl) Head of mandibular condyle within the temporomandibular joint.

Attached gingiva Gingiva that tightly adheres to alveolar bone around the roots of teeth.

Attrition (ah-trish-**un) Hard tooth tissue loss caused by tooth-to-tooth contact during mastication or parafunctional habits.

Avulsion (ah-vul-**shin) Complete tooth displacement from socket due to extensive trauma.

B

Balancing interference Teeth in contact on balancing side during lateral occlusion.

Balancing side Other side of the arch from the working side during lateral occlusion.

Basal bone (bay-sal) Part of jaws that forms the body of the maxilla or mandible.

Basal lamina (lam-i-nah) Superficial part of basement membrane; within dentogingival junction has both an external and internal basal lamina surrounding junctional epithelium.

Basal layer Single layer of cuboidal epithelial cells overlying basement membrane.

Basement membrane Extracellular material consisting of basal and reticular lamina produced by either epithelium or connective tissue.

Base of the tongue Most posterior part of tongue.

Basophil (bay-sah-fil) White blood cell containing granules of histamine.

B-cell Lymphocyte that matures in lymph nodes and works during humoral immune response.

Bell stage Fourth stage of odontogenesis with enamel organ assuming bell shape.

Bicuspid (bi-**kus-**pid) Older dental term for premolar.

Bifurcated (bi-fer-**kay-**ted) Tooth having two root branches.

Bilaminar embryonic disc (by-**lam-**i-nar) Circular plate of bilayered cells developed from blastocyst.

Bilateral symmetry (sim-me-try) Each half of embryo mirrors the other half.

Black hairy tongue Tongue lesion marked by dead cells and keratin buildup that becomes extrinsically stained.

Blastocyst (blas-tah-sist) Structure formed during prenatal development consisting of trophoblast cells and inner mass of cells that develop into embryo.

Blood Fluid connective tissue containing cells and plasma.

Body of the mandible (man-di-bl) Horizontal part of lower jaw inferior to teeth.

Body of the maxilla (mak-sil-ah) Horizontal part of upper jaw superior to teeth.

Body of the tongue Anterior part of the tongue.

Bone Rigid connective tissue.

Bone marrow (mar-oh) Innermost part of bone in medullary cavity.

Bracing Sustained contraction or tightening of the musculature.

Branchial apparatus (brang-ke-al ap-pah-**ra-**tis) Group that includes branchial arches, branchial grooves and membranes, pharyngeal pouches.

Branchial arches Six stacked bilateral swellings of tissue that appear inferior to stomodeum, including mandibular arch.

Branchial grooves Grooves between neighboring branchial arches on each side of embryo.

Bruxism (bruk-sizm) Parafunctional habit of tooth grinding.

Buccal (buk-al) Structures or facial surfaces of tooth close to inner cheek.

Buccal developmental depressions Depression on each side of the buccal ridge on posteriors.

Buccal fat pad Pad of underlying adipose connective tissue in vestibules.

Buccal mucosa Mucosa that lines inner cheek.

Buccal region Region of face composed of the soft tissue of cheek.

Buccal ridge Ridge extending vertically in the center of the crown's buccal surface of posteriors.

Bud stage Second stage of tooth development marked by growth of dental lamina into buds.

C

Calcium hydroxyapatite (hy-drox-see-**ap-**ah-tite) Main inorganic crystal with chemical formula of $Ca_{10}(PO_4)_6(OH)_2$ in enamel, alveolar bone, dentin, cementum.

Canaliculi (kan-ah-**lik-**u-lie) Tubular canals in both bone and cementum.

Cancellous bone (kan-**sel-**us) Spongy bone within compact bone with trabeculae instead of Haversian system.

Canine eminence (kay-nine **em-**i-nins) Vertically oriented and labially placed bony ridge of alveolar bone.

Canine rise Contralateral canine should be only tooth in function during lateral occlusion.

Canines Anteriors that are third teeth from midline in each quadrant.

Cap stage Third stage of tooth development with dental lamina growing into cap shape.

Capillary blood plexus (cap-ih-lary) Capillaries between papillary layer and deeper layers of lamina propria.

Capsule (kap-sule) Connective tissue that surrounds outer part of entire gland or lesion.

Cartilage (kar-ti-lij) Firm, nonmineralized connective tissue.

Caudal end (kaw-dal) Tail end of structure.

Cell Smallest unit of organization in the body.

Cell membrane Membrane that completely surrounds a cell.

Cellular cementum (see-**men-**tum) Outer layers of cementum which contain embedded cementocytes.

Cemental caries (see-**men-**tal) Shallow carious lesion of cementum.

Cemental spurs Symmetrical spheres of cementum attached to the root surface.

Cementicles (see-**men-**ti-kuls) Mineralized bodies of cementum either attached to root or free in periodontal ligament.

Cementoblasts (see-**men-**toe-blasts) Cells that form cementoid and are differentiated from the dental sac.

Cementocytes (see-**men-**toe-sites) Cementoblasts entrapped by the cementum they produce.

Cementoenamel junction (CEJ) Tooth anatomy where crown enamel and the root cementum are close.

Cementogenesis (see-men-toe-**jen-**i-sis) Apposition of cementum in the root area.

Cementoid (see-**men-**toyd) Cementum matrix laid down by cementoblasts.

Cementum (see-**men-**tum) Outermost layer of the root of a tooth.

Central cells of the dental papilla Primordium of the pulp.

Central fossa Fossa located at convergence of cusp ridges in a central point on occlusal surface of posteriors.

Central groove Most prominent developmental groove on posteriors, traveling mesiodistally to separate occlusal table buccolingually.

Central incisor Incisor closest to the midline.

Centric occlusion (CO) Voluntary position of dentition that allows maximal contact when teeth occlude.

Centric relation (CR) End point of closure of mandible in which the mandible is in most retruded position.

Centrioles (sen-tree-ols) Pair of cylindrical structures in centrosome.

Centromere (sen-tro-mere) Clear constricted area where two chromatids of chromosome are joined.

Centrosome (sen-tro-some) Organelle associated with centrioles.

Cephalic end (se-**fal-**ik) Head end of structure.

Cervical cysts (ser-vi-kal) Developmental cysts formed when branchial grooves are not obliterated.

Cervical loop Most cervical part of enamel organ responsible for root development.

Cervical ridge Ridge running mesiodistally in cervical one third of buccal crown surface on primary dentition and permanent molars.

Cheek Buccal region that forms side of face between nose, mouth, ear.

Chondroblasts (kon-dro-blasts) Cells that produce cartilage tissue.

Chondrocytes (kon-dro-sites) Mature chondroblasts.

Chromatids (kro-mah-tids) Two filamentous daughter chromosomes joined at a centromere during cell division.

Chromatin (kro-mah-tin) Chief nucleoprotein in the nondividing nucleoplasm.

Chromosomes (kro-mah-somes) Separate concentrations of chromatin in a dividing nucleus of a cell.

Cingulum (sin-gu-lum) Raised and rounded area on the cervical third of lingual surface on anteriors.

Circumpulpal dentin (serk-um-pul-pal) Layer of dentin around the outer pulpal wall.

Circumvallate lingual papillae (serk-um-val-ate) Larger mushroom-shaped lingual papillae that line up along the anterior side of the sulcus terminalis on the tongue.

Class I malocclusion Malocclusion characterized by ideal mesiodistal relationship of jaws and dental arches with minor dental malalignments.

Class II malocclusion Malocclusion with mesiobuccal cusp of the maxillary first molar occluding by more than the width of a premolar mesial to the mesiobuccal groove of the mandibular first molar.

Class III malocclusion Malocclusion with mesiobuccal cusp of maxillary first molar occluding by more than width of a premolar distal to mesiobuccal groove of mandibular first molar.

Class II malocclusion, division I Class II malocclusion with permanent maxillary anteriors protruding facially.

Class II malocclusion, division II Class II malocclusion with maxillary central incisors either upright or retruded.

Cleavage (kleve-ij) Process during prenatal development when mitosis converts a zygote to a blastocyst.

Cleft lip (kleft) Developmental disturbance of upper lip from failure of fusion of maxillary processes with medial nasal process.

Cleft palate Developmental disturbance from failure of fusion of palatal shelves with primary palate or with each other.

Cleft uvula Mildest form of cleft palate.

Clenching Parafunctional habit with teeth held in centric occlusion for long periods without interocclusal clearance.

Clinical crown Part of anatomical crown visible in the oral cavity and not covered by gingival tissue.

Clinical root Part of anatomical root visible in the oral cavity and not covered by gingival tissue.

Cloacal membrane (klo-ay-kal) Membrane at caudal end of embryo that is the location of future anus.

Col (kohl) Interdental gingiva apical to contact area assumes nonvisible concave form between facial and lingual gingival surfaces.

Collagen fibers (kol-ah-jen) Main protein fiber.

Colloid (kol-oid) Material in follicles of thyroid reserved for production of thyroxine.

Compact bone (kom-pak) Bone deep to periosteum with Haversian system of bone with lamellae.

Concrescence (kahn-kres-ens) Union of root structure of two or more teeth through cementum only.

Congenital malformations (kon-jen-i-til mal-for-**may**-shins) Birth defects or developmental problems evident at birth.

Connective tissue Basic tissue mainly composed of cells and matrix.

Connective tissue papillae (pah-pil-ay) Interdigitation of loose connective tissue with epithelium.

Connective tissue proper Two adjacent layers consisting of loose and dense connective tissue.

Contact area Tooth anatomy where adjacent tooth crowns in same arch touch on each proximal surface.

Contour lines of Owen Adjoining imbrication lines in dentin that demonstrate disturbance in body metabolism.

Copula (kop-u-lah) Posterior swelling formed from third and fourth branchial arches which overgrows second arches to form tongue base.

Coronal pulp Pulp located in tooth crown.

Coronoid notch (kor-ah-noid) Main part of anterior border of mandibular ramus.

Coronoid process Bony projection at anterior border of mandibular ramus.

Cortical bone (kor-ti-kal) Plates of compact bone on facial and lingual surfaces of alveolar bone.

Crossbite Malocclusion in which mandibular tooth or teeth are placed facially to maxillary teeth.

Crown Part of tooth composed of dentin and pulp covered by enamel.

Curve of Spee Anteroposterior curvature produced by planes placed on masticatory surfaces of each dental arch.

Curve of Wilson Concave curve produced when frontal section is taken through maxillary and mandibular molars.

Cusp (kusp) One or more major elevations on masticatory surface of canines and posteriors.

Cuspid (kus-pid) Older dental term for canine.

Cusp of Carabelli Small cusp on permanent maxillary first molar.

Cusp of Carabelli groove Groove associated with a cusp of Carabelli.

Cusp ridges Ridges that descend from each cusp tip on posteriors.

Cusp slopes Two ridges on incisal edge of canines divided by cusp tip.

Cusp tip Tip of cusp on incisal surface of canines and occlusal table of posteriors.

Cytodifferentiation (sy-to-dif-er-en-she-ay-shin) Development of different cell types.

Cytoplasm (sy-to-plazm) Fluid part contained within cell membrane.

Cytoskeleton (sy-to-skel-it-on) Three-dimensional system of support within cell.

D

D-A-Q-T System System to designate teeth: *D* for dentition, *A* for arch, *Q* for quadrant, *T* for tooth type.

Dens in dente (denz in **den**-tay) Developmental disturbance caused by invagination of enamel organ into dental papilla.

Dense connective tissue Deepest layers of dermis or lamina propria.

Dental anatomy Area of dental sciences dealing with tooth morphology.

Dental arch Alveolar process or tooth-bearing part of each jaw in either maxillary or mandibular arch.

Dental lamina (lam-i-nah) Growth from oral epithelium giving rise to tooth buds.

Dental papilla (pah-pil-ah) Inner mass of ectomesenchyme of tooth germ that produces dentin and pulp.

Dental sac Tooth germ part consisting of ectomesenchyme surrounding outside of enamel organ.

Dentigerous cyst (den-ti-jer-os) Odontogenic cyst that forms from reduced enamel epithelium.

Dentin (den-tin) Hard inner layer of tooth crown overlying pulp.

Dentin dysplasia (den-tin dis-**play**-ze-ah) Faulty development of dentin.

Dentinal fluid (den-tin-al) Fluid within dentinal tubule in dentin.

Dentinal hypersensitivity (hi-per-sen-si-tiv-it-ee) Exposed dentin sensitive to various stimuli.

Dentinal caries (den-tin-al) Carious lesion gone beyond dentinoenamel junction from enamel invasion.

Dentinal tubules Long tubes in dentin.

Dentinocemental junction (DCJ) Junction between dentin and cementum formed during root development.

Dentinoenamel junction (DEJ) Junction between dentin and enamel formed by mineralization of disintegrating basement membrane.

Dentinogenesis (den-tin-oh-**jen**-i-sis) Apposition of predentin by odontoblasts.

Dentition (den-**tish**-in) Natural teeth in jaws of either primary and permanent or mixed grouping of teeth.

Dentition periods Three periods that occur throughout lifetime: primary, mixed, permanent.

Dentogingival junction (den-to-jin-**ji**-val) Junction between tooth surface and gingival tissue.

Dentogingival junctional tissue Tissue that includes sulcular epithelium and junctional epithelium.

Depression of the mandible (de-**presh**-in) Lowering of lower jaw.

Dermis (der-mis) Connective tissue proper in the skin.

Desmosome (**dez**-mo-some) Intercellular junction between cells.

Developmental depression Depression usually evident in specific tooth area.

Developmental groove Primary groove that marks junction among developmental lobes on lingual surface of anteriors or occlusal table of posteriors.

Developmental pits Pits on lingual surface of anteriors or on occlusal table and buccal and lingual surface of posteriors.

Diastema (di-ah-**ste**-mah) Open contact that can exist between permanent maxillary central incisors.

Differentiation (dif-er-en-she-**ay**-shin) Change in embryonic cells to become quite distinct structurally and functionally.

Dilaceration (di-las-er-**ay**-shun) Crown or root(s) showing angular distortion.

Disc of the joint Disc of temporomandibular joint located between temporal bone and mandibular condyle.

Distal (**dis**-tl) Surface of tooth farthest away from midline.

Distal contact Contact area on distal tooth surface.

Distal marginal ridge Marginal ridge on distal part of lingual surface of anteriors or distal part of occlusal table on posteriors.

Distal step No terminal plane relationship exists because primary mandibular second molar is distal to maxillary second molar.

Distolingual marginal groove Developmental groove that crosses distal marginal ridge on lingual surface and extends onto root of anteriors.

Dorsal surface of the tongue Top surface of tongue.

Down syndrome Developmental defect involving trisomy of chromosome no. 21.

Duct Passageway that allows glandular secretion to be directly emptied.

E

Early childhood caries (ECC) Extensive acute caries of primary teeth.

Ectoderm (**ek**-toe-derm) Layer in trilaminar embryonic disc derived from epiblast layer and lining stomodeum.

Ectodermal dysplasia (dis-**play**-ze-ah) Syndrome involving abnormal development of one or more ectodermal structures including anodontia.

Ectomesenchyme (**ek**-toe-mes-eng-kime) Mesenchyme from ectoderm influenced by neural crest cells.

Ectopic pregnancy (ek-**top**-ik) Implantation occurring outside the uterus.

Edentulous (e-**den**-tu-lus) Dentition with either partial or complete loss of teeth.

Efferent vessel (**ef**-er-ent) Lymphatic vessel in which lymph flows out of lymph node.

Elastic cartilage (**kar**-ti-lij) Cartilage found in ear and epiglottis.

Elastic connective tissue (e-**las**-tik) Specialized connective tissue with mostly elastic fibers.

Elastic fibers (e-**las**-tik) Protein fiber in connective tissue composed of microfilaments.

Elevation of the mandible (el-eh-**vay**-shun) Raising of lower jaw.

Embrasures (em-**bray**-zhers) Spaces formed from curvatures where two teeth in same arch contact.

Embryo (**em**-bre-oh) Structure derived from implanted blastocyst.

Embryoblast layer (**em**-bre-oh-blast) Small inner mass of embryonic cells in blastocyst.

Embryology (em-bre-**ol**-ah-jee) Study of prenatal development.

Embryonic cell layers (em-bre-**on**-ik) Germ layers derived from increased number of embryonic cells.

Embryonic folding Embryonic folding of embryo placing tissue in proper position.

Embryonic period Prenatal developmental time period for embryo from second to eighth week.

Enamel (ih-**nam**-l) Hard outer layer of tooth crown.

Enamel caries Carious lesion invaded through enamel either by pits and grooves or through smooth surface.

Enamel dysplasia (dis-**play**-ze-ah) Faulty development of enamel.

Enamel knot Region noted in molars' enamel organ orchestrating crown form.

Enamel lamellae Partially mineralized vertical sheets of enamel matrix.

Enamel matrix Matrix of enamel formed during amelogenesis by the ameloblasts.

Enamel organ Cap or bell-shaped part of tooth germ that produces enamel.

Enamel pearl Small spherical enamel projections on tooth surface.

Enamel rod Crystaline structural unit of enamel.

Enamel spindles Microscopic feature present in mature enamel as short dentinal tubules near dentinoenamel junction.

Enamel tufts Microscopic feature in mature enamel of small dark brushes near dentinoenamel junction.

Endochondral ossification (en-do-**kon**-dril os-i-fi-**kay**-shun) Formation of osteoid within cartilage model.

Endocrine gland (**en**-dah-krin) Ductless gland that secretes directly into the blood.

Endocytosis (en-do-sigh-**toe**-sis) Uptake of materials from extracellular environment into cell.

Endoderm (**en**-doe-derm) Layer in trilaminar embryonic disc derived from hypoblast layer.

Endoplasmic reticulum (ER) (en-do-**plas**-mik rey-**tik**-u-lum) Membrane-bound organelle with channels that is either rough or smooth.

Endosteum (en-**dos**-te-um) Lining of medullary cavity of bone.

Endothelium (en-do-**theel**-ee-um) Unstratified squamous epithelium lining vessels and serous cavities.

End-to-end bite Teeth that occlude without maxillary teeth overlapping mandibular teeth.

Eosinophil (e-ah-**sin**-ah-fil) White blood cell involved in parasitic diseases since primary function is phagocytosis of immune complexes.

Epiblast layer (**ep**-i-blast) Superior layer in bilaminar disc.

Epidermis (ep-i-**der**-mis) Superficial layers of skin.

Epiglottic swelling (ep-ee-**glot**-ik) Posterior swelling that develops from fourth branchial arches marking development of future epiglottis.

Epithelial attachment (EA) Device that attaches junctional epithelium to tooth surface.

Epithelial rests of Malassez (ep-ee-**thee**-lee-al mal-ah-**say**) Epithelial cell groups in periodontal ligament after disintegration of Hertwig's epithelial root sheath.

Epithelium (ep-ee-**thee**-lee-um) Basic tissue that covers and lines external and internal body surfaces.

Erectile tissue (e-**rek**-tile) Thin-walled vessels in nasal cavity capable of considerable engorgement.

Erosion (e-**ro**-zhun) Hard tooth tissue loss through chemical means not involving bacteria.

Excretory duct (ex-**kreh**-tor-ee) Duct of salivary gland through which saliva exits into the oral cavity.

Exocrine gland (ek-sah-krin) Gland having duct associated with it.

Exocytosis (ek-so-sigh-**toe**-sis) Active transport of material from vesicle out into extracellular environment.

Exostoses (ek-sos-**toe**-sese) Small localized bone growths noted usually on facial surface of alveolar process of maxilla.

F

Facial (**fay**-shal) Structures or tooth surfaces closest to facial surface.

Fauces (**faw**-seez) Opening posteriorly from the oral cavity proper into pharynx.

Fertilization (fur-til-uh-**zay**-shun) Process by which sperm penetrates ovum during preimplantation period.

Fetal alcohol syndrome Syndrome in infant during embryonic period resulting from ethanol ingested by pregnant woman.

Fetal period (**fete**-il) Prenatal development period for fetus from third to ninth month.

Fetus (**fete**-is) Structure of fetal period of prenatal development derived from enlarged embryo.

Fibroblast (**fi**-bro-blast) Cell that synthesizes protein fibers and intercellular substance.

Fibrocartilage (fi-bro-**kar**-ti-lij) Cartilage of parallel, thick, compact collagenous bundles.

Fifth branchial arch (**brang**-ke-al) Rudimentary embryonic branchial arch that is absent or included with fourth branchial arch.

Filiform lingual papillae (**fil**-i-form) Slender threadlike lingual papillae giving dorsal surface of tongue its velvety texture.

First branchial arch (**brang**-ke-al) Mandibular arch in embryo.

First molar Molar closest to midline and at sixth position.

First premolar Premolar closer to midline and at fourth position.

Floor of the mouth Area of oral cavity proper underneath ventral surface of tongue and bordered by mandibular arch.

Flush terminal plane Terminal plane relationship where primary maxillary and mandibular second molars are in end-to-end relationship.

Fluting Elongated developmental depression on the surface root branches.

Foliate lingual papillae (**fo**-le-ate) Vertical ridges of lingual papillae on lateral tongue surface.

Follicles (**fol**-i-kls) Masses embedded in meshwork of reticular fibers within lobules of thyroid.

Foramen cecum (for-**ay**-men **se**-kum) Small pitlike depression located where sulcus terminalis points backward toward pharynx.

Fordyce's spots (for-**die**-seez) Small yellowish elevations of sebaceous glands on oral mucosa.

Foregut (**fore**-gut) Anterior part of future digestive tract or primitive pharynx that forms oropharynx.

Fossa (plural, fossae) (**fos**-ah, **fos**-ay) Shallow, wide depressions on lingual surface of anteriors or occlusal table of posteriors.

Fourth branchial arch (**brang**-ke-al) Branchial arch in embryo that participates in formation of laryngeal cartilages.

Free gingival crest Most superficial part of marginal gingiva.

Free gingival groove Groove that separates attached gingiva from marginal gingiva.

Frontal region (**frunt**-il) Region of face that includes forehead and area above the eyes.

Frontonasal process (frun-to-**na**-zil) Prominence in upper facial area at cephalic end of embryo.

Fungiform lingual papillae (**fun**-ji-form) Smaller mushroom-shaped lingual papillae on dorsal tongue surface.

Furcation (fer-**kay**-shin) Area between two or more root branches before division from root trunk.

Furcation crotches Spaces between roots at the furcation.

Fusion (fu-zhin) Joining of embryonic tissue of two separate surfaces or elimination of a furrow between two adjacent swellings or developmental disturbance in which adjacent tooth germs unite to form large tooth.

G

Gemination (jem-i-**nay**-shin) Developmental disturbance with single tooth germ trying to divide forming large single-rooted tooth.

Generalized resorption Resorption of hard tissue or entire skeleton of bone in varying amounts resulting from endocrine activity.

Geographic tongue Lesion that appears as red and then paler pink to white patches on tongue body.

Germinal center (**jurm**-i-nil) Center region of lymphatic nodule of a lymph node where lymphocytes mature.

Gingiva (jin-**ji**-vah) Gum tissue composed of mucosa surrounding maxillary and mandibular teeth in alveoli and covering alveolar processes.

Gingival fiber group (jin-**ji**-val) Fiber groups within gingiva that have no bony attachments.

Gingival crevicular fluid (GCF) ((jin-**ji**-val kre-**vik**-koo-ler) Fluid in gingival sulcus.

Gingival hyperplasia (hi-per-**play**-ze-ah) Overgrowth of mainly interproximal gingiva.

Gingival recession (re-**sesh**-un) Inferiorly placed margin of free gingival crest.

Gingival sulcus (**sul**-kus) Space facing sulcular gingiva.

Gingival tissue Tissue that covers alveolar process including attached gingiva and marginal gingiva.

Gland Structure that produces secretion necessary for normal body functioning.

Globular dentin Dentin with both primary and secondary mineralization.

Gnathic index (**nath**-ick) Measurement that gives degree of maxillary arch prominence.

Goblet cells Cells in respiratory mucosa that produce mucus for moisture.

Goiter (**goy**-ter) Enlarged thyroid.

Golden Proportions Principle that provides guide for esthetically pleasing proportion.

Golgi complex (**gol**-jee) Organelle of cell involved in protein segregation, packaging, transport.

Granular layer Layer superficial to prickle layer in some forms of keratinized epithelium.

Granulation tissue (gran-yoo-**lay**-shin) Immature connective tissue formed during initial repair.

Group function Entire posterior quadrant functions during lateral occlusion.

H

Hard palate Anterior part of palate.

Haversian canal (hah-**ver**-zi-an) Vascular tissue space in osteon.

Haversian system Organized arrangement of lamellae and canals in compact bone.

Height of contour Crest of curvature which is the greatest elevation of the tooth crown either incisocervically or occlusocervically.

Hemidesmosome (hem-eye-**des**-mah-some) Forms intercellular junction involving attachment of cell to nearby noncellular surface.

Hertwig's epithelial root sheath (HERS) (hirt-**wigz**) Part of cervical loop that functions to shape the root(s) and induce root dentin formation.

Hilus (**hi**-lus) Depression on one side of lymph node.

Hindgut (**hind**-gut) Posterior part of future digestive tract.

Histodifferentiation (his-toe-dif-er-en-she-**ay**-shin) Development of different tissue types.

Histology (his-**tol**-oh-je) Study of microscopic structure and function of tissue.

Horizontal group Alveodental ligament subgroup originating in alveolar bone proper to insert horizontally into cementum.

Howship's lacuna (**how**-ships) Large shallow pit in bone created by osteoclast.

Hutchinson's incisors (**hutch**-in-suns in-**sigh**-zers) Developmental disturbance in permanent incisors with screwdriver-shaped crowns caused by congenital syphilis.

Hyaline cartilage (hi-ah-line **kar**-ti-lij) Cartilage that contains no nerves or blood vessels serving as growth center in temporomandibular joint.

Hyoid arch (**hi**-oid) Second branchial arch that lies inferiorly to mandibular arch in embryo.

Hyoid bone Bone suspended in anterior midline of neck that has many muscle attachments.

Hypercementosis (hi-per-see-men-**toe**-sis) Excessive production of cellular cementum.

Hyperkeratinized (hi-per-**ker**-ah-tin-izd) Excessive production of keratin.

Hypoblast layer (**hi**-po-blast) Inferior layer in bilaminar disc.

Hyposalivation (hi-po-sal-i-**vay**-shen) Decreased production of saliva.

I

Imbrication lines (im-bri-**kay**-shun) Slight ridges that extend mesiodistally in cervical third associated with lines of Retzius in enamel.

Imbrication lines of von Ebner (von **eeb**-ner) Incremental lines in mature dentin.

Immature bone First bone to be produced by either ossification method.

Immunogen (**im**-un-ah-jen) Antigen treated as foreign capable of triggering immune response.

Immunoglobulin (Ig) (im-u-no-**glob**-u-lin) Blood protein or *antibody* produced by plasma cells during immune response.

Impacted (im-**pak**-ted) Unerupted or partially erupted tooth positioned against another tooth, bone, or soft tissue preventing eruption.

Implantation (im-plan-**ta**-shin) Embedding of blastocyst in endometrium.

Incisal angles (in-**sigh**-zl) Two angles on permanent incisors formed from incisal ridge or edge and each proximal surface.

Incisal edge Incisal ridge on permanent incisors that flattens after eruption.

Incisal ridge Linear elevation on incisal or masticatory surface of permanent incisors when newly erupted.

Incisal surface Masticatory surface for anteriors.

Incisive papilla (in-**sy**-ziv pah-**pil**-ah) Small bulge of tissue at anterior hard palate.

Incisors (in-**sigh**-zers) Anteriors first and second from midline: centrals and laterals.

Inclined cuspal planes (**kusp**-al) Sloping planes located between cusp ridges on posteriors.

Inclusions (in-**kloo**-zhins) Metabolically inert substances or transient structures within cell.

Induction (in-**duk**-shin) Action of one group of cells on another leading to developmental pathway in responding tissue.

Infraorbital region (in-frah-**or**-bit-al) Facial region located both inferior to orbital region and lateral to nasal region.

Initiation stage First stage of tooth development.

Inner enamel epithelium (IEE) Innermost cells of enamel organ which form ameloblasts.

Intercalated duct (in-**tur**-kah-lay-ted) Duct associated with acinus or terminal part of salivary gland.

Intercellular junctions Mechanical attachments between cells or between cells and nearby noncellular surfaces.

Intercellular substance Transparent substance that fills in spaces between tissue cells.

Interdental ligament Principal fiber subgroup that inserts interdentally into cervical cementum of neighboring teeth.

Interdental papilla (in-ter-**den**-tal pah-**pil**-ay) (plural, **papillae** [(pah-**pil**-ay)]) Extension of attached gingiva between adjacent teeth.

Interdental septum Alveolar bone between two neighboring teeth.

Interglobular dentin Dentin with only primary mineralization.

Interlabial gap (in-ter-**lay**-be-al) Distance between inferior border of upper lip and superior border of lower lip when at physiologic resting position.

Intermaxillary segment (in-ter-**mak**-si-lare-ee) Growth from paired medial nasal processes on inside of stomodeum.

Intermediate filaments (**fil**-ah-ments) Components of cytoskeleton.

Intermediate layer Layer of epithelium superficial to basal layer in nonkeratinized epithelium.

International Standards Organization Designation System for Teeth (ISO System) International system for tooth designation using two-digit code.

Interocclusal clearance (in-ter-ah-**kloo**-zhal) Space between dental arches when mandible is at rest.

Interphase (**in**-ter-faz) Period when cell is between divisions but is growing and functioning.

Interprismatic region (in-ter-**priz**-mat-ik) Outer region surrounding each enamel rod.

Interproximal space (in-ter-**prok**-si-mal) Area between adjacent tooth surfaces.

Interradicular group (in-ter-rah-**dik**-u-lar) Alveolodental ligament subgroup on multirooted teeth inserted on cementum of one root to cementum of other root(s).

Interradicular septum Alveolar bone between the roots of same tooth.

Interstitial growth (in-ter-**stish**-il) Growth from deep within tissue or organ.

Intertubular dentin (in-ter-**tube**-u-lar) Dentin between dentinal tubules.

Intramembranous ossification (in-trah-**mem**-bran-us os-i-fi-**kay**-shun) Formation of osteoid within dense connective tissue.

J

Joint capsule Two-layered connective tissue that completely encloses temporomandibular joint.

Junctional epithelium (JE) (jungk-shun-al) Deeper extension of sulcular epithelium.

K

Karyotype (kare-e-oh-tipe) Photographic analysis of chromosomes.

Keratin (ker-ah-tin) Intermediate protein filament found in calloused epithelium consisting of opaque waterproof substance.

Keratin layer Most superficial layer in keratinized epithelium.

Keratohyaline granules (ker-ah-toe-**hi-**ah-lin) Prominent granules in cytoplasm of epithelial cells that form keratin chemical precursor.

L

Labial (lay-be-al) Structures or facial surfaces of the teeth close to lips.

Labial commissures (kom-i-shoors) Corners of the mouth where upper and lower lips meet.

Labial frenum (plural, **frena**) (**free-**num, **free-**nah) Fold(s) of tissue located at midline between labial mucosa and alveolar mucosa on dental arch(es).

Labial mucosa Mucosal lining of inner parts of the lips.

Labial ridge Central ridge on labial surface of canines from greater development of middle labial developmental lobe.

Lacuna (plural, **lacunae**) (lah-**ku-**nah, lah-**ku-**nay) Small space that surrounds chondrocyte or osteocyte within cartilage matrix or bone.

Lamellae (lah-**mel-**ay) Closely apposed sheets of bone tissue in compact bone.

Lamina dura (lam-i-nah **dur-**ah) Radiopaque line representing alveolar bone proper.

Lamina propria (pro-pree-ah) Connective tissue–proper region of oral mucosa.

Laryngopharynx (lah-**ring-**gah-**fare-**inks) Most inferior part of pharynx close to laryngeal opening.

Larynx (lare-inks) Voice box in midline of neck.

Lateral deviation of the mandible (de-vee-**ay-**shun) Shifting lower jaw to one side.

Lateral incisor Incisor second from midline.

Lateral lingual swellings Parts of developing tongue that form on each side of tuberculum impar.

Lateral nasal processes Tissue on outer part of nasal pits that forms nasal alae.

Lateral occlusion Movement that occurs when mandible moves to the side until canines are in cusp-to-cusp relationship.

Lateral surface of the tongue Side of tongue.

Leeway space Space created when primary molars are shed to make room for smaller mesiodistal permanent premolars.

Lens placodes (plak-odz) Placodes forming eyes and related tissue.

Line angle Line formed by junction of two crown surfaces.

Linea alba (lin-ee-ah **al-**bah) White ridge of keratinized epithelium on buccal mucosa at the level where teeth occlude.

Lines of Retzius (ret-zee-us) Incremental lines in mature enamel.

Lingual (ling-gwal) Structures or tooth surfaces closest to tongue.

Lingual fossa Fossa on lingual surface of anteriors.

Lingual frenum (free-num) Midline fold of tissue between ventral surface of tongue and floor of the mouth.

Lingual groove Groove on lingual surface of anteriors.

Lingual papillae (pah-**pil-**ay) Small elevated structures of specialized mucosa on the tongue.

Lingual pit Developmental pit on lingual surface of anteriors or lingual surface of maxillary posteriors.

Lingual ridge Vertically oriented and centrally placed ridge that extends from cusp tip to cingulum on lingual surface of canines.

Lingual tonsil (ton-sil) Irregular mass of tonsillar tissue located posteriorly on dorsal surface of the tongue.

Linguogingival groove Vertically placed groove on lingual surface of anteriors that originates in lingual pit extending cervically and slightly distally onto cingulum.

Linguoincisal edge Raised edge on incisal border of lingual fossa of maxillary central incisor.

Lining mucosa Mucosa associated with nonkeratinized stratified squamous epithelium.

Lobes Large inner parts of glands or regions of tooth during development.

Lobules (lob-ules) Smaller inner parts of glands.

Localized resorption Resorption of bone or other hard tissue that occurs in specific area.

Loose connective tissue Superficial layer of dermis of the skin or lamina propria of the oral mucosa.

Lumen (loo-men) Central opening where saliva is deposited into duct after production by secretory cells.

Lymph (limf) Tissue fluid that drains from surrounding region into lymphatic vessels.

Lymph nodes Bean-shaped filtering bodies grouped in clusters along connecting lymphatic vessels.

Lymphadenopathy (lim-fad-uh-**nop-**ah-thee) Enlarged and palpable lymph nodes.

Lymphatic ducts (lim-**fat-**ik) Ducts that smaller lymphatic vessels containing lymph converge into and that then empty into the venous system.

Lymphatic nodules (nah-jools) Masses of lymphocytes in lymph node.

Lymphatic vessels System of endothelium-lined channels that carry lymph.

Lymphatics Network of lymphatic vessels that collect and transport lymph linking lymph nodes.

Lymphocyte (lim-fo-site) Second most common white blood cell in the blood involved in immune response.

Lysosomes (li-sah-somes) Organelles of cell functioning in both intracellular and extracellular digestion.

M

Macrodontia (mak-roe-**don-**she-ah) Abnormally large teeth.

Macrophage (mak-rah-faje) Most common white blood cell in connective tissue proper or *monocyte* before migration from blood.

Major salivary glands Large paired glands that have named associated ducts.

Malocclusion (mal-ah-**kloo-**zhun) Failure to have overall ideal form to the dentition while in centric occlusion.

Mamelons (mam-ah-lons) Rounded enamel extensions on incisal ridge of anteriors.

Mandible (man-di-bl) Lower jaw.

Mandibular arch (man-dib-you-lar) Lower dental arch with mandibular teeth or first branchial arch in embryo.

Mandibular condyle (kon-dyl) Bony projection off posterior and superior border of mandibular ramus.

Mandibular notch Depression between coronoid process and condyle.

Mandibular processes Processes of first branchial arch that fuse at midline to form mandibular arch.

Mandibular symphysis (sim-fi-sis) Midline area of mandible formed by fusing two mandibular processes.

Mandibular teeth Teeth in mandibular arch of lower jaw or mandible.

Mandibular torus (plural, **tori**) (**tore-**us, **tore-**eye) Bone growth noted on lingual aspect of mandibular arch.

Mantle dentin Outermost layer of dentin found in crown region adjacent to dentinoenamel junction.

Marginal gingiva Gingiva at gingival margin of each tooth.

Marginal grooves Developmental grooves that cross either marginal ridge.

Marginal ridges Rounded raised borders on mesial and distal parts of lingual surface of anteriors or occlusal table of posteriors.

Mast cell White blood cell similar to basophil due to involvement in allergic responses.

Mastication (mass-ti-kay-shin) Chewing process.

Masticatory mucosa (mass-ti-ka-tor-ee) Mucosa associated with keratinized stratified squamous epithelium.

Masticatory surface Chewing surface on crown.

Matrix (may-triks) Substance in connective tissue composed of intercellular substance and fibers or extracellular substance that is partially mineralized and serves as a framework for later mineralization.

Maturation (ma-cher-**ray-**shin) Attainment of adult size as well as adult form and function.

Maxilla (mak-**sil-**ah) Upper jaw.

Maxillary arch (mak-si-lar-ee) Upper dental arch with maxillary teeth.

Maxillary process Prominence from mandibular arch that grows superiorly and anteriorly on each side of stomodeum.

Maxillary teeth Teeth in maxillary arch or maxilla or upper jaw.

Maxillary tuberosity (too-beh-ros-i-tee) Tissue-covered bony elevation just distal to last tooth of maxillary arch.

Meckel's cartilage (mek-els **kar-**ti-lij) Cartilage that forms within each side of mandibular arch and that disappears as bony mandible forms.

Medial nasal processes Middle part of the tissue growing around nasal placodes located between nasal pit.

Median lingual sulcus Midline depression on dorsal surface of the tongue.

Median palatine raphe (pal-ah-tine **ra-**fe) Midline ridge of tissue on hard palate that overlies bony fusion marked by median palatine suture.

Meiosis (my-**oh-**sis) Process of reproductive cell production that ensures correct number of chromosomes.

Melanin pigmentation (mel-**a-**nin) Localized macules of pigmentation caused by presence of melanin.

Mental region (ment-il) Region of the face with chin as major feature.

Mesenchyme (mes-eng-kime) Embryonic connective tissue.

Mesial (me-ze-il) Surface of tooth closest to midline.

Mesial contact Contact area on mesial surface of tooth.

Mesial drift Natural movement of teeth over time toward midline of the oral cavity.

Mesial marginal ridge Marginal ridge on mesial part of lingual surface of anteriors or mesial part of occlusal table of posteriors.

Mesial step Terminal plane relationship with primary mandibular second molar is mesial to maxillary molar.

Mesiodens (me-ze-oh-denz) Supernumerary tooth between two permanent maxillary central incisors.

Mesoderm (mes-oh-derm) Embryonic layer located between ectoderm and endoderm.

Mesognathic (me-so-**nath-**ik) Facial profile in centric occlusion with slightly protruded jaws, giving facial outline a relatively flat appearance or straight profile.

Metaphase (met-ah-faz) Second phase of mitosis in which chromosomes are aligned into equatorial position.

Microdontia (mi-kro-**don-**she-ah) Abnormally small teeth.

Microfilaments (my-kroh-**fil-**ah-ments) Components of cytoskeleton that are delicate and threadlike.

Microtubules (my-kroh-**too-**bules) Components of the cytoskeleton that are slender tubular microscopic structures.

Midgut (mid-gut) Middle part of future digestive tract.

Minor salivary glands Small salivary glands with short unnamed ducts.

Mitochondria (mite-ah-**kon-**dree-ah) Organelles associated with manufacture of energy for cell.

Mitosis (my-**toe-**sis) Cell division that occurs in phases and results in two daughter cells.

Molars (mo-**lerz**) Most posterior teeth with firsts, seconds, thirds.

Monocyte (mon-ah-site) White blood cell that becomes *macrophage* after migration from the blood into the tissue.

Morphodifferentiation (mor-foe-dif-er-en-she-**ay-**shin) Development of the differing form that will create a specific structure.

Morphogenesis (mor-fo-**jen-**is-is) Process of development of specific tissue morphology.

Morphology (mor-**fol-**ah-je) Form of structure.

Mucobuccal fold (mu-ko-**buk-**al) Area within vestibule where labial mucosa or buccal mucosa meets alveolar mucosa.

Mucocele (mu-kah-sele) Lesion due to retention of saliva in minor salivary gland.

Mucogingival junction (mu-ko-**jin-**ji-val) Line of demarcation between attached gingiva and alveolar mucosa.

Mucoperiosteum (mu-ko-per-ee-**os-**te-im) Loose connective tissue acting as periosteum to underlying bone.

Mucosa (mu-**ko-**sah) Mucous membrane lining.

Mucoserous acinus (mu-ko-**sere-**us) Group of mucous cells surrounding lumen with serous demilune producing mixed secretory product.

Mucous acinus (mu-kis) Group of mucous cells producing mucous secretory product.

Mucous cells Secretory cells that produce mucous secretory product.

Mulberry molars (mull-bare-ee) Developmental disturbance resulting from congenital syphilis forming enamel nodules on molars' occlusal surface.

Multirooted Teeth with two or more root branches.

Muscles of mastication (mass-ti-**kay-**shin) Muscles involved in mastication: masseter, temporalis, medial and lateral pterygoid.

Myoepithelial cells (my-oh-ep-ee-**thee-**lee-al) Contractile epithelial cells on acini that facilitate the flow of saliva out of each lumen into connecting ducts.

N

Naris (plural, **nares**) (**nay-**ris, **nay-**rees) Nostril of nose.

Nasal ala (plural, **alae**) (**nay-**zil **a-**lah, **a-**lay) Winglike cartilaginous structures of the nose that bound nares laterally.

Nasal cavity (**kav-**it-ee) Inner space of nose.

Nasal conchae (**kong-**kay) Projecting structures that extend inward from each lateral wall of the nasal cavity.

Nasal pits Depressions in center of each nasal placode that evolve into the nasal cavities.

Nasal placodes (plak-odz) Placodes that develop into olfactory organ for the sensation of smell located in mature nose.

Nasal region Region of the face occupied by external nose.

Nasal septum (sep-tum) Midline part of the nose that separates the nares.

Nasmyth's membrane (nas-miths) Residue on newly erupted teeth that may become extrinsically stained.

Nasopharynx (nay-zo-**fare**-inks) Division of pharynx superior to level of soft palate.

Neonatal line (ne-oh-**nate**-l) Accentuated incremental line of Retzius in enamel or contour line of Owen in dentin from birth process.

Nerve Bundle of neural processes outside central nervous system.

Neural crest cells (noor-al) Specialized group of cells developed from neuroectoderm that migrate from the crests of the neural folds and disperse to specific sites within the mesenchyme.

Neural folds Raised ridges in the neural plate that surround deepening neural groove.

Neural groove Groove from further growth and thickening of neural plate.

Neural plate Centralized band of cells that extends length of embryo.

Neural tube Tube formed when neural folds meet and fuse superior to neural groove.

Neuroectoderm (noor-oh-**ek**-toe-derm) Specialized group of cells that differentiates from ectoderm.

Neuron (noor-on) Functional cellular component of nervous system.

Nicotinic stomatitis (nik-ah-**tin**-ik sto-mah-**ti**-tis) Whitish lesion on hard palate caused by heat from smoking or hot liquid consumption.

NK-cell Large lymphocyte or natural killer cell involved in first line of defense.

Nonkeratinized stratified squamous epithelium (non-**ker**-ah-tin-izd) Epithelium in superficial layers of lining mucosa.

Nonsuccedaneous (non-suk-seh-**dane**-ee-us) Permanent teeth without primary predecessors, namely the molars.

Nuclear envelope (noo-kle-er) Double membrane completely surrounding nucleus.

Nuclear pores Avenues of communication between inner nucleoplasm and outer cytoplasm.

Nucleolus (noo-**kle**-ah-lis) Rounded nuclear organelle centrally placed in nucleoplasm.

Nucleoplasm (noo-kle-ah-plazm) Semifluid part within nucleus.

Nucleus (plural, **nuclei**) (**noo**-kle-eye) Largest, densest, most conspicuous organelle in cell.

O

Oblique group (o-**bleek**) Alveolodental ligament subgroup originating in alveolar bone proper to extend apically and obliquely to insert into cementum.

Oblique ridge Transverse ridge that crosses occlusal table obliquely from mesiolingual to distobuccal on most maxillary molars.

Occlusal developmental pits (ah-**klooz**-l) Pits in fossae on occlusal table of posteriors.

Occlusal surface Masticatory surface of posteriors.

Occlusal table Part of occlusal surface of posteriors bordered by marginal ridges.

Occlusal trauma Trauma to periodontium from occlusal disharmony.

Occlusion (ah-**kloozh**-n) Anatomical alignment of teeth and relationship to masticatory system.

Odontoblastic process (oh-don-toe-**blast**-ik) Attached cellular extension of odontoblast within dentinal tubule.

Odontoblasts (oh-**don**-toe-blasts) Cells that produce dentin and differentiate from outer cells of the dental papilla.

Odontoclasts (oh-**don**-toe-klasts) Cells that resorb dentin, cementum, enamel.

Olafactory mucosa (**ol**-fak-tor-e) Mucosa in the roof of each part of the nasal cavity that carries sense of smell receptors.

Open bite Malocclusion without anteriors occluding.

Oral cavity proper Inside of mouth.

Oral epithelium (ep-ee-**theel**-ee-um) Embryonic lining of oral cavity derived from ectoderm.

Oral mucosa (mu-**ko**-sah) Mucosa or mucous membrane lining oral cavity.

Oral region Region of face that contains the lips and oral cavity.

Orbit (or-bit) Bony socket that contains eyeball.

Orbital region (or-bit-al) Facial region that includes bony orbit and eyeball.

Organ Somewhat independent body part formed from tissue.that performs specific function or functions

Organelles (or-gah-**nels**) Specialized structures within cell that are permanent and metabolically active.

Orofacial myology (**my**-ol-oh-je) Study and therapeutic treatment of orofacial musculature and function to improve muscle balance, function, tonicity.

Orofacial myofunctional disorders (OMD) (my-oh-**funk**-shun-al) Disturbances in normal, physiologic functioning of musculature of orofacial environment.

Orofacial myofunctional therapy (OMT) Therapeutic neuromuscular reeducation program incorporating oromotor expertises, behavior modification, behavioral retraining to eliminate orofacial myofunctional disorders.

Oronasal membrane (or-oh-**nay**-zil) Embryonic membrane that disintegrates to bring the nasal and oral cavities into communication.

Oropharyngeal membrane (or-oh-fah-**rin**-je-al) Membrane at cephalic end of embryo.

Oropharynx (or-o-**fare**-inks) Oral division of pharynx.

Orthokeratinized stratified squamous epithelium (or-tho-**ker**-ah-tin-izd) Epithelium that demonstrates keratinization of epithelial cells.

Ossification (os-i-fi-**kay**-shun) Bone formation.

Osteoblasts (**os**-te-oh-blasts) Bone-forming cells.

Osteoclast (**os**-te-oh-klast) Cell that functions in resorption of bone.

Osteocytes (**os**-tee-oh-sites) Mature osteoblasts entrapped in bone matrix.

Osteoid (**os**-te-oid) Initially formed bone matrix.

Osteons (**os**-te-onz) Concentric layers of lamellae in compact bone.

Otic placodes (o-tik **plak**-odz) Placodes in embryo forming future internal ear.

Outer cells of the dental papilla (pah-**pil**-ah) Cells of dental papilla tissue that differentiate into odontoblasts.

Outer enamel epithelium (OEE) Outer cells of enamel organ that serve as protective barrier.

Overbite Maxillary arch vertically overlaps mandibular arch.

Overjet Maxillary arch horizontally overlaps mandibular arch.

Ovum (oh-vum) Female reproductive cell or egg which can be fertilized.

P

Palatal (pal-ah-tal) Lingual structures or tooth surfaces closest to palate.

Palatal shelves Two processes derived from maxillary processes during prenatal development.

Palatal torus (tore-us) Normal variation of bone growth noted on midline of hard palate.

Palate (pal-it) Roof of mouth.

Palatine rugae (ru-ge) Firm, irregular ridges of tissue directly posterior to incisive papilla.

Palatine tonsils (pal-ah-tine **ton**-sils) Tonsillar tissue located between faucial pillars.

Palmer Notation Method System of tooth designation commonly used in orthodontics with oral cavity is divided into quadrants and each tooth is designated by a numeral 1 to 8.

Papillary layer (pap-i-lar-ee) Layer of loose connective tissue of dermis or lamina propria.

Parafunctional habits (pare-ah-**funk**-shun-al) Mandible movements not within normal motions associated with mastication, speech, or respiratory movements.

Parakeratinized stratified squamous epithelium (pare-ah-**ker**-ah-tin-izd) Keratinized epithelium associated with masticatory mucosa of attached gingiva.

Paranasal sinuses (pare-ah-**na**-zil **sy**-nus-es) Paired air-filled cavities in bone.

Parathyroid glands (par-ah-**thy**-roid) Endocrine glands along posterior aspects of thyroid.

Parotid duct (pah-**rot**-id) Duct associated with parotid.

Parotid papilla (pah-**pil**-ah) Small elevation of tissue on inner part of the buccal mucosa that protects parotid duct.

Parotid salivary gland Major salivary gland located irregularly from zygomatic arch to posterior border of the mandible.

Passive eruption Eruption that takes place when gingiva recedes with no actual tooth movement.

Peg lateral Lateral incisor crown that is smaller from partial microdontia.

Peg third molar Small molar crown with one cusp from partial microdontia.

Perichondrium (per-ee-**kon**-dre-im) Outermost connective tissue layer surrounding most cartilage.

Perikymata (per-ee-**ki**-mot-ah) Grooves evident on teeth associated with the lines of Retzius in enamel.

Periodontal ligament (PDL) (pare-ee-o-**don**-tal) Ligament surrounding the teeth that supports and attaches them to alveoli bony surface.

Periodontal ligament space Radiolucent area representing periodontal ligament on radiographs.

Periodontium (per-e-o-**don**-she-um) Supporting hard and soft dental tissue between and including parts of tooth and alveolar bone.

Periosteum (per-ee-**os**-te-im) Dense connective tissue layer on outer part of bone.

Peripheral cells of the dental papilla Outer cells of the dental papilla that become odontoblasts.

Peritubular dentin (pare-i-**tube**-u-lar) Dentin that creates wall of dentinal tubule.

Permanent dentition or teeth (den-**tish**-in) Second and final dentition.

Phagocytosis (fag-oh-sigh-**toe**-sis) Engulfing and then digesting of solid waste or foreign material by cell.

Pharyngeal pouches (fah-**rin**-je-il) Four pairs of evaginations lining the pharynx between branchial arches.

Pharyngeal tonsils Located on superior and posterior walls of nasopharynx.

Pharynx (fare-inks) Muscular tube of neck or throat.

Philtrum (fil-trum) Vertical groove on midline of upper lip.

Pit and groove patterns Patterns formed from pits and grooves on lingual surface of anteriors or occlusal surface of permanent posteriors.

Placenta (pla-**sen**-tah) Temporary prenatal organ that provide support to developing embryo.

Placodes (plak-odz) Areas of ectoderm found at location of developing special sense organs on the embryo.

Plasma (plaz-mah) Fluid substance in the blood vessels that carries blood cells and metabolites.

Plasma cells White blood cells derived when B-cell lymphocytes form immunoglobulins or *antibodies*.

Platelets (plate-lits) Blood cell fragments functioning in clotting mechanism.

Plica fimbriata (plural, **plicae fimbriatae**) (**pli**-kah fim-bree-**ay**-tah, **pli**-kay fim-bree-**ay**-tay) Fold with fringelike projections on ventral surface of the tongue.

Pocket epithelium (PE) Epithelium lining periodontal pocket.

Point angle Imaginary line formed by junction of three crown surfaces.

Polymorphonuclear leukocyte (PMN) (pol-ee-mor-fah-**noo**-klee-er **loo**-ko-site) Most common white blood cell involved in inflammatory response or *neutrophil*.

Posterior teeth Molars, and premolars if present, in the back of the mouth.

Posterior faucial pillar (faw-shawl) Posterior lateral folds of tissue in pharynx created by underlying muscle forming the fauces.

Postglenoid process (post-**glen**-oid) Sharp ridge posterior to articular fossa.

Preameloblasts (pre-ah-**mel**-oh-blasts) Cells from inner enamel epithelium of enamel organ that differentiate into ameloblasts.

Preimplantation period (pre-im-plan-**ta**-shin) Period of unattached conceptus taking place during first week of prenatal development.

Predentin Dentin matrix laid down by apposition by odontoblasts.

Premature contacts Situation in which one or two teeth initially contact before other teeth.

Premolars (pre-**mo**-lerz) Posteriors fourth and fifth teeth from midline in permanent dentition including firsts and seconds.

Prenatal development (pre-**nay**-tal) Processes that occur from start of pregnancy to birth.

Prickle layer Layer that is superficial to basal layer in keratinized epithelium.

Primary dentin Dentin formed before completion of apical foramen.

Primary dentition (den-**tish**-in) First dentition or *deciduous*.

Primary palate Anterior part of final palate derived from intermaxillary segment during prenatal development.

Primary teeth First teeth present or *deciduous*.

Primate spaces Developmental spaces between primary teeth.

Primitive pharynx Cranial part of foregut that forms oropharynx.

Primitive streak Furrowed, rod-shaped thickening in middle of embryonic disc.

Primordium (pry-**more**-de-um) Earliest indication of part or organ during prenatal development.

Principal fibers Collagen fibers organized into groups on the basis of orientation to tooth and related function.

Prognathic (prog-**nath**-ik) Facial profile with rather prominent mandible and possibly normal or even retrusive maxilla or concave profile.

Proliferation (pro-lif-er-**ay**-shin) Controlled cellular growth.

Prophase (**pro**-faz) First phase of mitosis with chromatin condensing into chromosomes.

Protrusion of the mandible (pro-**troo**-zhin) Moving lower jaw forward.

Protrusive occlusion Occlusion when mandible undergoes protrusion.

Proximal root concavities (**prok**-si-mal) Depressions on proximal root surfaces.

Proximal surfaces Mesial and distal surfaces between adjacent teeth.

Pseudostratified columnar epithelium (soo-doh-**strat**-i-fide) Simple epithelium that falsely appears as multiple cell layers.

Pterygomandibular fold (teh-ri-go-man-**dib**-yu-lar) Tissue fold that extends from junction of hard and soft palates down to mandible.

Pulp Soft innermost connective tissue in both crown and root.

Pulp cavity Part of tooth composed of pulp and covered by dentin.

Pulp chamber Part of the tooth containing mass of pulp.

Pulp horns Extensions of coronal pulp into cusps of posteriors.

Pulp stones Masses of mineralized dentin in pulp.

Pulpitis (pul-**pie**-tis) Inflammation of pulp.

Q

Quadrants (**kwod**-rints) Division of each dental arch into two parts with four quadrants in oral cavity.

R

Radicular pulp (rah-**dik**-u-lar) Pulp located in the root area of tooth.

Ramus (**plural, rami**) (**ray**-mus, **rame**-eye) Mandible plate(s) that extends upward and backward from the body on each side.

Ranula (**ran**-u-lah) Lesion from retention of saliva usually in submandibular salivary gland.

Red blood cell (RBC) Blood cell whose cytoplasm contains hemoglobin which binds and then transports the oxygen.

Reduced enamel epithelium (REE) (ep-ee-**thee**-lee-um) Layers of flattened cells overlying enamel surface from compressed enamel organ.

Regions of the face Facial surface areas: frontal, orbital, nasal, infraorbital, zygomatic, buccal, oral, mental.

Regions of the neck Areas that extend from the skull and mandible inferior to clavicles and sternum.

Reichert's cartilage (**rike**-erts **kar**-ti-lij) Cartilage in second branchial arch that eventually disappears.

Remodeling Process by which bone is replaced over time.

Repolarization (re-po-ler-i-**za**-shun) Process that occurs in cell with nucleus moving away from the center to a position farthest away from basement membrane.

Resorption (re-**sorp**-shun) Removal of hard tissue such as bone, enamel, dentin, or cementum.

Respiratory mucosa Mucosa that consists of pseudostratified ciliated columnar epithelium.

Range of motion (ROM) Normal physiologic and functional reciprocal range of motion/movement for mandibular opening or closure.

Resting posture Normal physiologic position of tongue, lips, and mandible when not in function of chewing, swallowing, or speech.

Rete ridge (**ree**-tee) Interdigitation of epithelium into connective tissue.

Reticular connective tissue (re-**tik**-u-ler) Delicate network of interwoven reticular fibers.

Reticular fibers Fibers in embryonic tissue.

Reticular lamina (**lam**-i-nah) Deeper part of basement membrane.

Retraction of the mandible (re-**trak**-shun) Moving lower jaw backward.

Retrognathic (re-tro-**nath**-ik) Facial profile with protruding upper lip with recessive mandible and chin and convex profile.

Retromolar pad (re-tro-**mo**-ler) Dense pad of tissue just distal to last tooth of mandibular arch.

Reversal lines Stained, scalloped microscopic lines caused by resorption in cartilage, bone, cementum.

Ribosomes (**ry**-bo-somes) Organelles of cell associated with protein production.

Ridges Linear elevations on masticatory surface of either anterior or posterior teeth.

Root Part of a tooth composed of dentin covered by cementum.

Root axis line (RAL) Imaginary line representing long axis line of tooth drawn to bisect cervical line.

Root concavities Indentations on the surface of the root(s).

Root fusion Developmental disturbance that creates deep developmental grooves with root fusion.

Root of the nose Nose located between the eyes.

Root trunk Root of multirooted teeth where the root originates from crown.

Rubella (roo-**bell**-ah) Viral infection that can serve as teratogen transmitted by way of placenta to embryo.

S

Saliva (sah-**li**-vah) Secretion from salivary glands that lubricates and cleanses the oral cavity and helps in digestion.

Salivary glands (**sal**-i-ver-ee) Glands that produce saliva.

Second branchial arch (**brang**-ke-al) Branchial arch inferior to mandibular arch in embryo or *hyoid arch*.

Second molar Molar distal to first molar and in seventh position from midline.

Second premolar Premolar in fifth position from midline.

Secondary bone Mature bone tissue that replaces immature bone.

Secondary dentin Dentin that is formed after completion of apical foramen.

Secondary palate Posterior part of final palate formed by fusion of two palatal shelves.

Secretory cells (sek-**kre**-tory) Epithelial cells that produce saliva.

Septum (**plural, septa**) (**sep**-tum, **sep**-tah) Connective tissue divides inner part of glands.

Serous acinus (**sere**-us) Group of serous cells producing serous secretory product.

Serous cells Secretory cells that produce serous secretory product.

Serous demilune (**dem**-ee-lune) Serous cells superficial to mucous secretory cells in mucoserous acinus.

Sextants (**sex**-tants) Dental arch division into three parts based on relationship to midline.

Sharpey's fibers (**shar**-peez) Collagen fibers from periodontal ligament partially inserted into both cementum and bone.

Simple epithelium (un-**strat**-i-fide) Epithelium that consists of a single layer of cells.

Simple squamous epithelium (**skway**-mus) Lining of blood and lymphatic vessels, heart, serous cavities, lung, kidney interfaces.

Sinusitis (sy-nu-**si**-tis) Inflamed mucosal tissue in paranasal sinus.

Sixth branchial arch (**brang**-ke-al) Branchial arch in embryo that fuses with fourth branchial arch to participate in formation of laryngeal cartilages.

Skeletal muscles Striated muscles under the voluntary control of central and peripheral nervous systems.

Soft palate Posterior part of palate.

Somites (**so**-mites) Paired cuboidal aggregates of cells differentiated from mesoderm.

Specialized mucosa Mucosa found on dorsal and lateral surface of tongue in the form of the lingual papillae.

Sperm Cell containing male contribution of chromosomal information that fertilizes female ovum.

Spina bifida (**spi**-nah **bif**-ah-dah) Neural tube defect affecting vertebral arches.

Squames (skwaymz) Flattened platelike epithelial cells.

Stellate reticulum (**stel**-ate reh-**tik**-u-lum) Star-shaped cell layer between outer and inner enamel epithelium of enamel organ.

Sternocleidomastoid muscle (stir-no-klii-do-**mass**-toid) Large strap muscle of neck.

Stippling Pin-point depressions present on surface of attached gingiva.

Stomodeum (sto-mo-**de**-um) Primitive mouth in embryo.

Stratified epithelium (**strat**-i-fide) Epithelium consisting of two or more layers.

Stratified squamous epithelium (**skway**-mus) Epithelium of skin and oral mucosa.

Stratum intermedium (**stra**-tum in-ter-**mede**-ee-um) Compressed layer between outer and inner enamel epithelium of enamel organ.

Striated duct (**stri**-ate-ed) Larger duct connecting lobules of salivary gland.

Sublingual caruncle (sub-**ling**-gwal **kar**-unk-kl) Small papilla at anterior end of each sublingual fold.

Sublingual duct Short duct associated with sublingual gland.

Sublingual fold Ridge of tissue on each side of the floor of the mouth.

Sublingual salivary gland Major salivary gland located in neck.

Subluxation (sub-luk-**say**-shun) Partial dislocation of both temporomandibular joints.

Submandibular duct (sub-man-**dib**-you-lar) Duct associated with submandibular gland.

Submandibular salivary gland Major salivary gland located in neck.

Submucosa (sub-mu-**ko**-sah) Tissue deep to oral mucosa composed of loose connective tissue.

Succedaneous (suk-seh-**dane**-ee-us) Permanent teeth with primary predecessors: anteriors, premolars.

Successional dental lamina (suk-**sesh**-shun-al) Extension of dental lamina into ectomesenchyme forming succedaneous permanent teeth.

Sulcular epithelium (**sul**-ku-lar ep-ee-**thee**-lee-um) Epithelium that stands away from the tooth creating gingival sulcus.

Sulcus terminalis (**sul**-kus ter-mi-nal-is) Groove located posteriorly on dorsal tongue surface.

Superficial layer Most superficial layer in nonkeratinized epithelium.

Supernumerary teeth (soo-per-**nu**-mer-air-ee) Developmental disturbance characterized by one or more extra teeth.

Supplemental groove Secondary groove on lingual surface of anteriors and occlusal table on posteriors.

Supporting alveolar bone Consists of both cortical bone and trabecular bone.

Supporting cusps (kusp) Cusps that function during centric occlusion: lingual cusps of maxillary posteriors, buccal cusps of mandibular posteriors, incisal edges of mandibular anteriors.

Synapse (**sin**-aps) Junction between two neurons or between neuron and effector organ where neural impulses transmit.

Synovial cavities (sy-**no**-vee-al) Upper and lower compartments divided by disc of temporomandibular joint.

Synovial fluid Fluid in the joint capsule that fills and lubricates temporomandibular joint.

Synovial membrane Inner layer of temporomandibular joint capsule producing synovial fluid.

Syphilis (**sif**-i-lis) Infective teratogen spirochete *Treponema pallidum* that can produce dental anomalies and other defects.

System Group of organs functioning together.

T

Taste buds Barrel-shaped organs of taste associated with lingual papillae.

Taste pore Opening in taste bud.

T-cell Lymphocyte that matures in thymus working during cell-mediated immune response.

Telophase (**tel**-oh-faz) Final phase of mitosis with division into two daughter cells and reappearance of nuclear membrane.

Temporomandibular disorder (TMD) (tem-poh-ro-man-**dib**-you-lar) Disorder associated with one or both temporomandibular joints.

Temporomandibular joint (TMJ) Joint where temporal bone of the skull articulates with mandible.

Teratogens (**ter**-ah-to-jens) Environmental agents or factors such as infections, drugs, radiation causing malformations.

Terminal plane Ideal molar relationship in primary dentition when in centric occlusion.

Tertiary dentin Dentin formed in response to localized injury to exposed dentin.

Tetracycline stain (tet-rah-**si**-kleen) Intrinsic tooth stain from ingestion of antibiotic tetracycline during tooth development.

Third branchial arch (**brang**-ke-al) Branchial arch in embryo responsible for formation of parts of hyoid bone.

Third molar Molar distal to second molar and in eighth position from midline.

Thirds Crown surface or root division into three parts: crown horizontally and vertically and root horizontally.

Thyroid cartilage (**thy**-roid **kar**-ti-lij) Midline prominence of larynx.

Thyroid gland Endocrine gland in neck.

Thyroglossal duct (**thy**-ro-**gloss**-al) Temporary tube that connects thyroid with tongue base during prenatal development.

Tissue Structure formed by grouping of cells with similar characteristics of shape and function.

Tissue fluid Interstitial body fluid.

Tomes' granular layer (tomes) Dentin beneath cementum and adjacent to dentinocemental junction that looks granular.

Tomes' process Secretory surface of each ameloblast.

Tongue thrusting Functional deviations with habitual incorrect placement and use of tongue.

Tonofilaments (**ton**-oh-fil-ah-ments) Intermediate filaments having major role in intercellular junctions.

Tonsillar tissue Nonencapsulated masses of lymphoid tissue.

Tooth fairy Mythological creature takes children's shed primary teeth from under the pillow and leaves a sum of cash during the night; helpers are always appreciated.

Tooth germ Primordium of tooth consisting of enamel organ, dental papilla, dental sac.

Trabeculae (trah-**bek**-u-lay) Joined matrix pieces forming lattice in cancellous bone or bands of connective tissue in lymph node that separate lymphatic nodules.

Trabecular bone (trah-**bek**-u-lar) Cancellous bone between alveolar bone proper and places of cortical bone.

Transverse ridge (trans-**vers**) Ridge formed by joining of two triangular ridges crossing occlusal table transversely or from labial to lingual outline.

Triangular fossa Fossa that has triangular shape where triangular grooves terminate.

Triangular grooves Grooves that separate a marginal ridge from the triangular ridge of cusp, and which at the termination of the ridges form triangular fossae.

Triangular ridges Cusp ridges that descend from the cusp tips toward the central part of occlusal table.

Trifurcated (try-fer-**kay**-ted) Tooth having three root branches.

Trilaminar embryonic disc (try-**lam**-i-ner) Embryonic disc with three layers: ectoderm, mesoderm, endoderm.

Trophoblast layer (**trof**-oh-blast) Layer of peripheral cells of blastocyst.

Tubercle of the upper lip (**too**-ber-kl) Midline thickening of upper lip.

Tubercles (**too**-ber-kls) Accessory cusps on cingulum of anteriors or occlusal tables of permanent molars.

Tuberculum impar (too-**ber**-ku-lum **im**-par) Initial part of developing tongue located in midline.

Turnover time Time that it takes for newly divided cells to be completely replaced throughout entire tissue.

U

Underbite When lower jaw extends forward beyond upper jaw.

Universal Tooth Designation System Numbering system for permanent teeth by using Arabic numerals #1 through #32 and for primary teeth by using capital letters *A* through *T*.

Uvula (**u**-vu-lah) Midline muscular structure hanging down from posterior margin of soft palate.

V

Vacuoles (**vak**-you-oles) Spaces or cavities within cytoplasm.

Ventral surface of the tongue Underside of tongue.

Vermilion border (ver-**mil**-yon) Transition zone outlining lips from surrounding skin.

Vermilion zone Darker appearance of the lips compared with surrounding skin.

Vertical dimension of the face Dividing face into three horizontal parts.

Vestibular fornix (ves-ti-bu-lar **fore**-niks) Deepest recess of each vestibule.

Vestibules (**ves**-ti-bules) Maxillary and mandibular spaces between the lips and cheeks anteriorly and laterally and the teeth and gingiva medially and posteriorly.

Volkmann's canals (**volk**-manz) Vascular canals in compact bone other than Haversian canals.

von Ebner's salivary glands (von **eeb**-ners) Serous minor salivary glands associated with circumvallate lingual papillae.

W

White blood cell (WBC) Blood cells from bone marrow's stem cells that mature there or in other lymphatic tissue.

Working side Side to which mandible has been moved during lateral occlusion.

X

Xerostomia (zer-oh-**sto**-me-ah) Dry mouth.

Y

Yolk sac Fluid-filled cavity that faces hypoblast layer.

Z

Zygomatic arch (zy-go-**mat**-ik) Bony support for cheek.

Zygomatic region Facial region that overlies zygomatic arch.

Zygote (**zy**-gote) Fertilized egg from union of ovum and sperm.

Anatomical Position

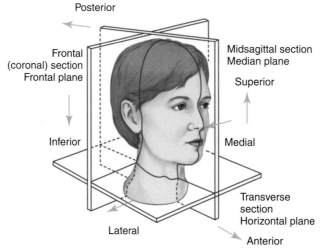

A-1 Head and neck in anatomical position showing the midsagittal, transverse, and frontal sections. *(Fehrenbach MJ, Herring SW. Illustrated Anatomy of the Head and Neck, ed 2. WB Saunders, Philadelphia, 2002.)*

Units of Measure

UNIT	ABBREVIATION	EQUIVALENT	MEASUREMENT APPLICATION
Centimeter	cm	0.4 inch	Naked eye: pathological lesions
Millimeter	mm	0.1 cm	Naked eye: extremely large human cells (muscle, liver), periodontal pockets
Micrometer	mm	0.001 mm	Light microscopy: most human cells; large organelles and bacteria, ameloblasts
Nanometer	nm	0.001 μm	Electron microscopy: smaller organelles, largest of macromolecules, dental tissue units

APPENDIX C

Tooth Measurements

(All adapted from Nelson S: *Wheeler's Dental Anatomy, Physiology, and Occlusion*, ed 9, Saunders, Philadelphia, 2009.)

TABLE 1	Measurements of the Permanent Incisors (in Millimeters)						
	CERVICOINCISAL LENGTH OF CROWN	LENGTH OF ROOT	MESIODISTAL DIAMETER OF CROWN	MESIODISTAL DIAMETER OF CROWN AT CERVIX	LABIOLINGUAL DIAMETER OF CROWN	LABIOLINGUAL DIAMETER OF CROWN AT CERVIX	CURVATURE OF CERVICAL LINE: MESIAL	CURVATURE OF CERVICAL LINE: DISTAL
Maxillary central incisor	10.5	13.0	8.5	7.0	7.0	6.0	3.5	2.5
Maxillary lateral incisor	9.0	13.0	6.5	5.0	6.0	5.0	3.0	2.0
Mandibular central incisor	9.0	12.5	5.0	3.5	6.0	5.3	3.0	2.0
Mandibular lateral incisor	9.5	14.0	5.5	4.0	6.5	5.8	3.0	2.0

TABLE 2	Measurements of the Permanent Canines (in Millimeters)						
	CERVICOINCISAL LENGTH OF CROWN	LENGTH OF ROOT	MESIODISTAL DIAMETER OF CROWN	MESIODISTAL DIAMETER OF CROWN AT CERVIX	LABIOLINGUAL DIAMETER OF CROWN	LABIOLINGUAL DIAMETER OF CROWN AT CERVIX	CURVATURE OF CERVICAL LINE: MESIAL	CURVATURE OF CERVICAL LINE: DISTAL
Maxillary canine	10.0	17.0	7.5	5.5	8.0	7.0	2.5	1.5
Mandibular canine	11.0	16.0	7.0	5.5	7.5	7.0	2.5	1.0

TABLE 3	Measurements of the Permanent Premolars (in Millimeters)							
	CERVICO-OCCLUSAL LENGTH OF CROWN	LENGTH OF ROOT	MESIODISTAL DIAMETER OF CROWN	MESIODISTAL DIAMETER OF CROWN AT CERVIX	BUCCOLINGUAL DIAMETER OF CROWN	BUCCOLINGUAL DIAMETER OF CERVIX	CURVATURE OF CERVICAL LINE: MESIAL	CURVATURE OF CERVICAL LINE: DISTAL
Maxillary first premolar	8.5	14.0	7.0	5.0	9.0	8.0	1.0	0.0
Maxillary second premolar	8.5	14.0	7.0	5.0	9.0	8.0	1.0	0.0
Mandibular first premolar	8.5	14.0	7.0	5.0	7.5	6.5	1.0	0.0
Mandibular second premolar	8.0	14.5	7.0	5.0	8.0	7.0	1.0	0.0

TABLE 4	Measurements of the Permanent Maxillary Molars (in Millimeters)							
	CERVICO-OCCLUSAL LENGTH OF CROWN	LENGTH OF ROOT	MESIODISTAL DIAMETER OF CROWN	MESIODISTAL DIAMETER OF CROWN AT CERVIX	BUCCOLINGUAL DIAMETER OF CROWN	BUCCOLINGUAL DIAMETER AT CERVIX	CURVATURE OF CERVICAL LINE: MESIAL	CURVATURE OF CERVICAL LINE: DISTAL
Maxillary first molar	7.5	Buccal = 12 Lingual = 13	10.0	8.0	11.0	10.0	1.0	0.0
Maxillary second molar	7.0	Buccal = 11 Lingual = 12	9.0	7.0	11.0	10.0	1.0	0.0
Maxillary third molar	6.5	11.0	8.5	6.5	10.0	9.5	1.0	0.0

TABLE 5	Measurements of the Permanent Mandibular Molars (in Millimeters)							
	CERVICO-OCCLUSAL LENGTH OF CROWN	LENGTH OF ROOT	MESIODISTAL DIAMETER OF CROWN	MESIODISTAL DIAMETER OF CROWN AT CERVIX	BUCCOLINGUAL DIAMETER OF CROWN	BUCCOLINGUAL DIAMETER AT CERVIX	CURVATURE OF CERVICAL LINE: MESIAL	CURVATURE OF CERVICAL LINE: DISTAL
Mandibular first molar	7.5	14.0	11.0	9.0	10.5	9.0	1.0	0.0
Mandibular second molar	7.0	13.0	10.5	8.0	10.0	9.0	1.0	0.0
Mandibular third molar	7.0	11.0	10.0	7.5	9.5	9.0	1.0	0.0

TABLE 6	Measurements of the Primary Teeth (in Millimeters)						
	LENGTH OVERALL	LENGTH OF CROWN	LENGTH OF ROOT	MESIODISTAL DIAMETER OF CROWN	MESIODISTAL DIAMETER AT CERVIX	FACIAL-LINGUAL DIAMETER OF CROWN	FACIAL-LINGUAL DIAMETER AT CERVIX
Maxillary Teeth							
Central incisor	16.0	6.0	10.0	6.5	4.5	5.0	4.0
Lateral incisor	15.8	5.6	11.4	5.1	3.7	4.8	3.7
Canine	19.0	6.5	13.5	7.0	5.1	7.0	5.5
First molar	15.2	5.1	10.0	7.3	5.2	8.5	6.9
Second molar	17.5	5.7	11.7	8.2	6.4	10.0	8.3
Mandibular Teeth							
Central incisor	14.0	5.0	9.0	4.2	3.0	4.0	3.5
Lateral incisor	15.0	5.2	10.0	4.1	3.0	4.0	3.5
Canine	17.0	6.0	11.5	5.0	3.7	4.8	4.0
First molar	15.8	6.0	9.8	7.7	6.5	7.0	5.3
Second molar	18.8	5.5	11.3	9.9	7.2	8.7	6.4

Tooth Development

TABLE 1	Development of Permanent Incisors			
	Maxillary Central Incisor	**Maxillary Lateral Incisor**	**Mandibular Central Incisor**	**Mandibular Lateral Incisor**
Number of lobes	4 lobes			
First evidence of calcification	3–4 months	1 year	3–4 months	3–4 months
Completion of enamel	4–5 years	4–5 years	4–5 years	4–5 years
Eruption date	7–8 years	8–9 years	6–7 years	7–8 years
Completion of root	10 years	11 years	9 years	10 years

TABLE 2	Development of Permanent Canines	
	Maxillary Canine	**Mandibular Canine**
Number of lobes	4 lobes	
First evidence of calcification	4–5 months	4–5 months
Completion of enamel	6–7 years	6–7 years
Eruption date	11–12 years	9–10 years
Completion of root	13–15 years	12–14 years

TABLE 3	Development of Permanent Premolars			
Specific Teeth	**Maxillary First Premolar**	**Maxillary Second Premolar**	**Mandibular First Premolar**	**Mandibular Second Premolar**
Number of lobes		4 lobes		4 or 5 lobes
First evidence of calcification	1½–1¾ years	2–2½ years	1¾–2 years	2¼–2½ years
Completion of enamel	5–6 years	6–7 years	5–6 years	6–7 years
Eruption date	10–11 years	10–12 years	10–12 years	11–12 years
Completion of root(s)	12–13 years	12–14 years	12–13 years	13–14 years

TABLE 4	Development of Permanent Maxillary Molars		
	Maxillary First Molar	**Maxillary Second Molar**	**Maxillary Third Molar**
Number of lobes	5 lobes	4 lobes	
First evidence of calcification	Birth	2½ years	7–9 years
Completion of enamel	3–4 years	7–8 years	12–16 years
Eruption date	6–7 years	12–13 years	17–21 years
Completion of root(s)	9–10 years	14–16 years	18–25 years

TABLE 5	Development of Permanent Mandibular Molars		
	Mandibular First Molar	**Mandibular Second Molar**	**Mandibular Third Molar**
Number of lobes	5 lobes	4 lobes	
First evidence of calcification	Birth	2½–3 years	8–10 years
Completion of enamel	2½–3 years	7–8 years	12–16 years
Eruption date	6–7 years	11–13 years	17–21 years
Completion of roots(s)	9–10 years	14–15 years	18–25 years

(All adapted from Nelson S: *Wheeler's Dental Anatomy, Physiology, and Occlusion,* ed 9, Saunders, Philadelphia, 2009.)

Index

Page references followed by *f* indicate figure, by *b* indicate box, and by *t* indicate table.